SECOND EDITION

ISSUES and TRENDS in NURSING

PRACTICE, POLICY, AND LEADERSHIP

GAYLE ROUX, PHD, NP-C, FAAN
Dean and Professor
College of Nursing and
Professional Disciplines
University of North Dakota
Grand Forks, North Dakota

JUDITH A. HALSTEAD, PHD, RN, ANEF, FAAN
Executive Director
NLN Commission for Nursing
Education Accreditation
Washington, DC
Professor Emerita
School of Nursing
Indiana University
Indianapolis, Indiana

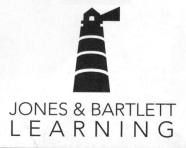

JONES & BARTLETT
LEARNING

World Headquarters
Jones & Bartlett Learning
5 Wall Street
Burlington, MA 01803
978-443-5000
info@jblearning.com
www.jblearning.com

Jones & Bartlett Learning books and products are available through most bookstores and online booksellers. To contact Jones & Bartlett Learning directly, call 800-832-0034, fax 978-443-8000, or visit our website, www.jblearning.com.

Substantial discounts on bulk quantities of Jones & Bartlett Learning publications are available to corporations, professional associations, and other qualified organizations. For details and specific discount information, contact the special sales department at Jones & Bartlett Learning via the above contact information or send an email to specialsales@jblearning.com.

10498-1

Production Credits
VP, Executive Publisher: David D. Cella
Executive Editor: Amanda Martin
Editorial Assistants: Emma Huggard, Christina Freitas
Production Editor: Vanessa Richards
Production Assistant: Molly Hogue
Senior Marketing Manager: Jennifer Scherzay
Product Fulfillment Manager: Wendy Kilborn

Composition: S4Carlisle Publishing Services
Cover Design: Scott Moden
Rights & Media Specialist: Wes DeShano
Media Development Editor: Troy Liston
Cover and chapter opener image: © Smart Design/Shutterstock
Printing and Binding: Edwards Brothers Malloy
Cover Printing: Edwards Brothers Malloy

Library of Congress Cataloging-in-Publication Data
Names: Roux, Gayle M., editor. | Halstead, Judith A., editor.
Title: Issues and trends in nursing: practice, policy, and leadership / edited by Gayle Roux, Judith A. Halstead.
Description: Second edition. | Burlington, MA: Jones & Bartlett Learning, [2018] | Preceded by Issues and trends in nursing: essential knowledge for today and tomorrow/edited by Gayle Roux, Judith A. Halstead. 2009. | Includes bibliographical references and index.
Identifiers: LCCN 2016038355 | ISBN 9781284104899
Subjects: | MESH: Nursing—trends | Nursing Care—trends | United States
Classification: LCC RT4 | NLM WY 16 AA1 | DDC 610.73—dc23
LC record available at https://lccn.loc.gov/2016038355

6048

Printed in the United States of America
21 20 19 18 17   10 9 8 7 6 5 4 3 2

Contents

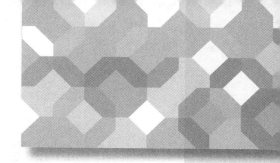

     Wendy Stoelting-Gettelfinger

     Introduction   63
     The Regulation of Nursing Practice   64
     Accessing Your State's Nurse Practice Act and
          Administrative Rules   66
     The History of State Boards and Their Regulatory Functions   67
     The Nurse Licensure Compact and Advance Practice Registered
          Nurse Compact   69
     Nursing Licensure   72
     Certification   74
     The Regulation of Advanced Practice Registered Nurses   76
     Standard of Care   77
     Summary   80
     Reflective Practice Questions   81
     References   81

4   **Understanding the NCLEX-RN**   85
     Judith A. Halstead

     Introduction   85
     Purpose of the NCLEX-RN   86
     Components of the NCLEX-RN Test Plan   90
     Framework of Client Needs   91
     Computer Adaptive Testing   94
     The Passing Standard   95
     Types of Questions on the NCLEX-RN Examination   96
     Preparing for the NCLEX-RN   99
     Taking the NCLEX-RN   103
     Summary   104
     Reflective Practice Questions   104
     References   105

5   **Professional Nursing Organizations**   107
     Judith A. Halstead

     Introduction   108
     The Nature of Professional Nursing Organizations   108
     The Mission and Impact of Professional Nursing
          Organizations   109
     Professional Nursing Organizations with Clinical,
          Political, and Regulatory Focus   111
     Professional Organization Membership and Involvement   115
     Summary   117

Unit II   The *Environment* and *Nursing* Practice

UNIT III   THE *PERSON* IN HEALTH CARE

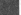

Preface

From its origins, nursing was described by Florence Nightingale as a distinct discipline concerned with the relationship between the patient, nurse, and environment. Nightingale defined nursing as having "charge of the personal health of somebody. . .and what nursing has to do. . .is to put the patient in the best condition for nature to act upon him" (1859/1992, p. 75). Nursing has advanced as a scientific discipline, with a wide scope of responsibility as a goal-directed and evidence-based practice within a complex healthcare system. The goal of health and "putting the patient in the best condition for nature to act" require the nurse to address a constantly expanding body of knowledge, technology, and sociocultural change. It is with this challenge in mind that the first edition of this textbook was originally created. This second edition continues to address the challenges facing nurses with updated and newly added chapters on contemporary nursing and healthcare topics. The graduating nurse must understand the complicated context of the issues that affect the nurse–patient relationship including political policy, professional organizations, safety and other performance outcomes, emergency preparedness, and global health issues, to name a few.

Although many different viewpoints of nursing theory have been debated, there is general agreement on the domains of nursing. Fawcett concluded there is a consensus about the central concepts of the discipline—person, environment, health, and nursing. These concepts constitute nursing's metaparadigm (Fawcett, 1989). Therefore, the concepts of nursing, environment, person, and health were selected to form the organizational units of this textbook. The chapter topics do indeed aggregate into these four concepts, lending validity to the umbrella of the metaparadigm to describe the essence of nursing.

Unit I addresses *The Nursing Profession,* beginning with a discussion of the historical origins of nursing with emphasis on the history and development of the nursing profession in the United States. Nursing education is also addressed with a description of the various educational nursing programs that exist within the profession and a focused discussion on contemporary issues impacting nursing education curricula. Other chapter topics in Unit I identify the essential information a graduating nurse needs to know to be socialized into the profession including preparing for the NCLEX-RN examination, understanding professional licensure and regulation, developing professionally through membership in professional nursing organizations, and transitioning into practice as a new registered nurse.

Unit II focuses on *The Environment and Nursing Practice*. To be safe and effective practitioners, nurses must fully understand and appreciate the complexity of the healthcare environment within which they practice. Having systematized knowledge about safety, research, and the regulatory mechanisms in health care is essential for nurses to produce safe, cost-effective, and evidence-based patient health outcomes. The chapters within Unit II address current trends and issues existing within the healthcare environment including the movement toward a culture of interprofessional practice; safety, quality, and performance outcomes in the workplace; disaster preparedness; and evidence-based practice. Acknowledging the importance of achieving a healthy work–life balance, the personal responsibility of the nurse in maintaining a balanced and healthy lifestyle across one's career is also addressed in a chapter to this edition of the text.

In Unit III, *The Person in Health Care*, the patient becomes the focus of discussion. Maintaining a caring relationship with the patient that facilitates health and healing requires the nurse to be socially conscious. Sociocultural changes in the United States, increasing numbers of clients without insurance, bioethical dilemmas, legal directives, the Affordable Care Act, and federal and state policy embody an infrastructure for the person seeking health care. The increasing cultural diversity of the United States' population and rising numbers of vulnerable patients requiring access to health care has multiple implications for nurses in their role as patient advocates. The legal and ethical issues related to nursing care are discussed with an emphasis on the nurse's advocacy role in ensuring attention to the legal and ethical rights of clients.

Unit IV addresses *Health and Nursing Issues*. Risk factors and health issues related to care of individuals in rural, urban, and global settings are important considerations for nurses. Informatics and health information technology are increasingly influential in delivering effective, high-quality health care, thus requiring nurses to be knowledgeable and competent in understanding how technology affects their daily practice. Nurses are also personally accountable for increasing their understanding of emerging disciplines, an example of which is genomics. All nurses need to incorporate nursing genomic competencies into their practice regardless of practice setting and this text edition has added a chapter addressing this topic that will only continue to grow in importance in coming years.

The four units provide a wealth of information that prepare the graduate to transition into nursing and confidently face the challenges of the future of the nursing profession. The essentials of information given in each chapter are intended to provide the undergraduate nursing student with the necessary details to think critically about issues and trends in nursing, engage in relationships with patients within an informed context of the issues and their environment, and create therapeutic plans to improve health outcomes. The editors and authors are sensitive to the fact that this text is one of a multitude of resources that is needed to achieve excellence in nursing.

The editors, authors, and Jones & Bartlett Learning staff have shared their expertise as a commitment to nursing education. We hope the contributions of this textbook are a valuable component of your knowledge development, making a significant difference in how you think about and practice nursing.

Gayle Roux, PhD, NP-C, FAAN
Judith A. Halstead, PhD, RN, ANEF, FAAN

References

Fawcett, J. (1989). *Analysis and evaluation of conceptual models of nursing* (2nd ed.). Philadelphia, PA: Davis.

Nightingale, F. (1859/1992). *Notes on nursing*. Philadelphia, PA: J.B. Lippincott.

Contributors

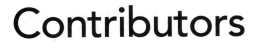

Darla Adams, CRNA, PhD
Clinical Associate Professor and
   Associate Dean
College of Nursing & Professional
   Disciplines
University of North Dakota
Grand Forks, North Dakota

Paula Clutter, PhD, RN, CNL, CNE,
   CENP, CMSRN
Associate Professor
College of Nursing
Texas Woman's University
Houston, Texas

Barbara deRose, PhD, NP-C
Clinical Assistant Professor
School of Nursing
Indiana University
Indianapolis, Indiana

Catherine Dingley, PhD, RN, FNP
Associate Professor
School of Nursing
University of Nevada, Las Vegas
Las Vegas, Nevada

Patricia Ebright, PhD, RN, FAAN
Associate Professor Emerita
School of Nursing
Indiana University
Indianapolis, Indiana

Karen J. Egenes, EdD, RN
Associate Professor
Marcella Niehoff School of Nursing
Loyola University Chicago
Chicago, Illinois

Rebecca A. Feather, PhD, RN,
   NE-BC, FNAP
Faculty, Course Mentor, Nursing
College of Health Professions
Western Governors University
Indianapolis, Indiana

Joan L. Frey, EdD, MSN, BS
Professor
Interim Academic President and Dean
Galen College of Nursing
Louisville, Kentucky

Eileen K. Fry-Bowers, PhD, JD,
   RN, CPNP
Associate Professor
Hahn School of Nursing and Health Science
Betty and Bob Beyster Institute for Nursing
   Research, Advanced Practice, and
   Simulation
University of San Diego
San Diego, California

Cathy R. Fulton, DNP, RN, ANP-BC,
   FNP-BC
Clinical Assistant Professor
School of Nursing
Indiana University
Indianapolis, Indiana

Judith A. Halstead, PhD, RN, ANEF,
   FAAN
Executive Director
NLN Commission for Nursing Education
   Accreditation
Washington, DC
Professor Emerita
School of Nursing
Indiana University
Indianapolis, Indiana

Brian W. Higgerson, DNSc, RN, FNP-BC, CNE
Clinical Associate Professor
College of Nursing & Professional Disciplines
University of North Dakota
Grand Forks, North Dakota

Josette Jones, PhD, RN
Associate Professor, Health Informatics and Nursing
Director, Health Informatics
School of Informatics and Computing
School of Nursing
Indiana University
Indianapolis, Indiana

Peggy Mancuso, PhD, RN, CNM, CNE
Professor and Associate Dean for Research and
    Clinical Scholarship
College of Nursing
Texas Woman's University
Denton, Texas

Christine K. Murphy, MA
Director of Public Policy and Advocacy
National League for Nursing
Washington, DC

G. Elaine Patterson, EdD, RNC, NP-C, CNE
Professor of Nursing
Nursing Programs
Ramapo College of New Jersey
Mahwah, New Jersey

Deanna L. Reising, PhD, RN, ACNS-BC, FNAP, ANEF
Associate Professor
School of Nursing
Indiana University
Bloomington, Indiana
Magnet Program Co-Director/System Magnet
    Coordinator
Bloomington Hospital
Indiana University Health
Bloomington/Indianapolis, Indiana

Monique Ridosh, PhD, RN
Assistant Professor
Marcella Niehoff School of Nursing
Loyola University Chicago
Maywood, Illinois

Mary E. Riner, PhD, RN, CNE, FAAN
Professor
Associate Dean for Global Affairs
School of Nursing
Indiana University
Indianapolis, Indiana

Gayle Roux, PhD, NP-C, FAAN
Dean and Professor
College of Nursing and Professional Disciplines
University of North Dakota
Grand Forks, North Dakota

Martha Scheckel, PhD, RN
Professor and Chair
College of Nursing and Health Sciences
Department of Nursing
Winona State University
Winona and Rochester, Minnesota

Susan Sheriff, PhD, RN, CNE
Professor
College of Nursing
Texas Woman's University
Denton, Texas

Phyllis Ann Solari-Twadell, PhD, RN, MPA, FAAN
Associate Professor
Marcella Niehoff School of Nursing
Loyola University Chicago
Chicago, Illinois

Janice Springer, DNP, MA, RN
Public Health Nursing Consultant
Disability Integration Advisor
Disaster Health Services Volunteer
American Red Cross
Washington, DC

Jo-Ann Stankus, PhD, RN
Assistant Professor
College of Nursing
Texas Woman's University
Denton, Texas

Wendy Stoelting-Gettelfinger, PhD, JD, FNP, APN, NP-C
Associate Professor
FNP Program Coordinator
School of Nursing
University of Indianapolis
Indianapolis, Indiana

Donna Zucker, PhD, RN, FAAN
Professor
Associate Dean for Academic Affairs and Graduate
  Program Director
College of Nursing
University of Massachusetts, Amherst
Amherst, Massachusetts

Unit I

The *Nursing* Profession

History of Nursing

Karen J. Egenes

LEARNING OUTCOMES

After reading this chapter you will be able to:

- Discuss the importance for nursing to understand its own history.
- Identify the contributions of selected leaders in the development of U.S. nursing.
- Trace the origins of major professional nursing organizations.
- Describe the impact of war on the development of nursing.
- Discuss the influences of faith traditions on the history of nursing.
- Analyze the relationship of history with the current healthcare delivery system.

Introduction

History can be defined as a study of events from the past leading up to the present time. However, the study of history focuses on not just the chronology of events but also the impact and influence those events continue to have throughout time. Over the passage of time, events unfold and trends emerge. These historical trends, in turn, influence or shape the destiny of an individual or a group. The development and evolution of the nursing profession is intricately connected to historical influences throughout the ages, beginning in antiquity. The study of the history of nursing helps us to better understand the societal forces and issues that continue to confront the profession. Understanding the history of nursing also allows nurses to gain an appreciation of the role the profession has played in the healthcare system of the United States (Donahue, 1991). The purpose of this chapter is to provide an overview of the history of nursing with an emphasis on nursing in the United States, describe the influence of societal trends on the development of nursing as a profession, and identify the contributions of selected leaders in U.S. nursing.

Nursing in Antiquity

In primitive societies, the decision to be a caregiver was often made for a person long before he or she had the ability to make such a choice. For example, among the members of the Zuni tribe, if an infant was born with a part of the placenta covering the face, it was taken as a sign that he or she had been marked as one who was destined to be a caregiver (Henly & Moss, 2007). In many societies, the provision of nursing care was a role that was assigned to female members. Because women traditionally provided nurturance to their own infants, it was assumed these same caring approaches could be extended to sick and injured community members as well. Yet in other societies, care of the sick was a role assigned to medicine men, shamans, or other male tribe members.

Because no formal education in the care of the sick was available, the earliest nurses learned their art through oral traditions passed from generation to generation, from observations of others caring for the sick, and many times, through a process of trial and error. Those who acquired a reputation for expert care of the sick with a succession of positive outcomes were often sought after to provide care to friends and relatives. In this way, they established themselves in a practice of nursing care.

Available evidence indicates that nurses first formed themselves into organized groups during the early Christian era. The nursing ideals of charity, service to others, and self-sacrifice were in harmony with the teachings of the early Christian church. The role of **deaconess** gave women a meaningful way of participating in the work of the church. Deaconesses were often Roman matrons or widows with some educational background who were selected by the church's bishops to visit and care for the sick in their homes. Fabiola was a deaconess who is credited with the establishment and operation of the first Christian hospital in Rome. The deaconess Phoebe is often cited as the first "visiting nurse" because of the expert home nursing care she provided (Nutting & Dock, 1907).

> **KEY TERM**
>
> **Deaconess:** Woman with some educational background who was selected by the church to provide care to the sick.

Throughout antiquity, the preferable, and often safest, nursing care was provided in one's own home, where one was cared for by family members, clansmen, or friends. Care in a hospital was sought only by those who had no family members nearby, such as persons whose work took them away from their homes or persons who had been ostracized or who were destitute. Early hospitals were begun by members of religious communities—nuns and monks who devoted their lives to the care of the sick. One example is the convent hospital at Beaune in France, where the sick were cared for in beds that lined the walls surrounding the main altar of the convent's church. Another example was the Hôtel-Dieu in Paris, a hospital operated by the Augustinian sisters, which was founded by the bishop of Paris in 651 AD. Since its founding, the hospital has had an unbroken record of care "for all who suffer." The detailed records that survive from this hospital provide many interesting insights into the state of medical and nursing care during the Middle Ages. More than one patient was placed in each bed, with the feet of one patient opposite the face of another. Because patients received no diagnosis upon admission, a patient with a leg fracture might be placed in the same bed with a patient with smallpox and another with tuberculosis (Robinson, 1946).

Nursing in Early Modern Europe

In England, in the wake of the Protestant Reformation, monasteries and convents were closed and their lands were seized. Care of the sick fell to "common" women, often those of the lower classes who were too old or too ill to find any other type of work. Hospital records of the day report that nurses were often sanctioned for fighting, use of foul language, petty theft, and extortion of money from patients (Pavey, 1953). The sick who lacked families to tend to their needs were warehoused in almshouses and municipal hospitals, overseen by attendants who lacked any knowledge of nursing care. Charles Dickens, a Victorian-era author who championed social reform, described the poor conditions of nursing care through his characters Sairey Gamp and Betsy Prig in his novel *Martin Chuzzlewit*. Dickens's nurses were often drunk while on duty, engaged in intimate relationships with their patients, and took delight in their patients' deaths (Dolan, 1968).

During the first half of the 19th century, a variety of British social reformers advocated for the formation of groups of religious women to staff the existing hospitals. To answer this need, Elizabeth Fry, a Quaker who had earlier fought for prison reform in England, founded the Protestant Sisters of Charity in 1840. Members of this sisterhood received only a rudimentary education in nursing; their only practical nursing experiences consisted of observing patients at two London hospitals.

The nurses of St. John's House, an English Protestant sisterhood founded in 1848, lived together as a community under the direction of a clergyman and a lady superintendent. Pupils paid 15 pounds sterling for a training program that was 2 years in length but were then required to work for St. John's House for 5 years in return for room and board and a small salary. Although they received instruction in nursing in the Middlesex, Westminster, and King's College hospitals in London, they nursed for only a few hours each day, spending the remainder of their time engaged in religious instruction and prayer (Pavey, 1953).

On the European continent, Theodor Fliedner, a German Lutheran pastor, in an attempt to create a role for women in the church, established a Deaconess Home and Hospital at Kaiserswerth, a city in Germany on the Rhine River. Pastor Fliedner had traveled to England, where he was impressed with the work of Elizabeth Fry. Together with his wife, Frederike, Pastor Fliedner founded a deaconess training program. Although the deaconesses' primary instruction was in nursing, they also received education in religious instruction and in the provision of social services. According to the plan of Pastor Fliedner, deaconesses took no vows but instead promised to continue to carry out their work as long as they felt called to this role. In return, the deaconesses were cared for by their motherhouse, which provided them with a permanent home. Although they were sent on assignments, they remained under the protection of their home organization (Gallison, 1954).

Florence Nightingale and the Origin of Professional Nursing

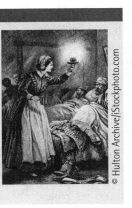

KEY TERM

Florence Nightingale: The founder of professional nursing in England.

© Hulton Archive/iStockphoto.com

Into this setting entered **Florence Nightingale**, the woman who would not only reform nursing as it existed at that time but also lay the foundation for nursing as a profession. Florence Nightingale was born into a wealthy British family. For their honeymoon, her parents embarked on an extensive tour of Europe. Their first child, Parthenope (the Greek name for Naples), was born while they visited Naples, and their second child, Florence, was born in the Italian city of that name. When the family returned to England, Mr. Nightingale took charge of the education of his daughters. Florence was educated in Greek and Latin, mathematics, natural science, ancient and modern literature, German, French, and Italian (Nutting & Dock, 1907).

It was assumed that Florence would follow the traditional path dictated for women of the upper class during the Victorian era, which included marriage and the rearing of a family. Although Florence was courted by various wealthy suitors, she rebuffed their approaches, stating she instead believed she had been called to dedicate her life to the service of humanity. Nightingale's parents at first were appalled by her desire to care for the sick, because such work was considered improper for a woman of her class. As steadfast members of the Church of England, they were even more shocked at her suggestion that she might seek admission to a convent of Irish Catholic nursing sisters. With time they consented to her attendance for a 2-week period at Pastor Fliedner's Deaconess Home and Hospital in Germany. In July 1851, she was able to return to Kaiserswerth for 3 months, during which time she worked with the deaconesses, learned basic information about patient care, and observed the Fliedners' methods of instruction in nursing.

When Nightingale returned to England, she was appointed superintendent of the Upper Harley Street Hospital, a small hospital for sick and elderly women of the upper class who had experienced financial difficulties. During her time in this position, she also made a journey to Paris to observe the hospital work of the Catholic Sisters of Charity and volunteered as a nurse at the Middlesex Hospital during a cholera epidemic there.

In 1854, the Crimean War broke out, in which Russia waged war against the combined armies of England, France, and Turkey. Nightingale was appalled to learn that the mortality rate for British troops was 41 percent. More disturbing was the fact that whereas the French had nursing nuns to care for their troops, the British army lacked any kind of nurses. In fact, most British soldiers were dying from disease rather than from injuries incurred on the battlefield. From her travels, observations of nursing care provided in hospitals abroad, and practical experiences in nursing, she had a far greater knowledge of the elements of skilled nursing care than the majority of medical workers of her time (Pavey, 1953).

Using her political influence, Nightingale sought permission for her and a band of ladies drawn from the upper class to travel to the Crimea and to care for the sick and wounded. Because Nightingale believed that dirt, rather than microscopic pathogens, was the cause of disease, she embarked on a campaign to thoroughly scrub the soldiers' barracks and hospital wards and to let in sunshine and fresh air. Within months, the number of deaths decreased dramatically. Nightingale, who had learned the principles of statistics from her father's tutelage, carefully documented the results of her care and used these as the basis for further interventions (Woodham-Smith, 1951). Through her work, she laid the foundation for modern evidence-based practice.

When Nightingale returned to England, she was hailed as a heroine. The British people, in recognition for her work, established a trust fund to be used at her discretion. Through this Nightingale Fund, she established the Nightingale School of Nursing at **St. Thomas' Hospital** in London for the education of professional nurses. The school differed from earlier forms of nursing education because student nurses received classes in theory coupled with clinical experiences on hospital wards. In addition, a set curriculum guided the students' experiences, so that during their program, they received training in various aspects of nursing care for patients in many of the hospital's specialty areas. Because the Nightingale School had the Nightingale Fund as its financial base, students' experiences were planned by Nightingale and her instructors (Baly, 1997; Seymer, 1960). Emphasis was placed on the proper education of the nurse, rather than on the needs of the hospital.

> **KEY TERM**
>
> **St. Thomas' Hospital:** A hospital in London where Florence Nightingale established the Nightingale School of Nursing.

Origins of Professional Nursing in the United States

Within a decade of Nightingale's return from the Crimea, the United States experienced the outbreak of civil war. When the war began, there was no provision for military nurses in either the Union or the Confederacy. At the time, there were no nursing schools, no "trained" nurses, and no nursing credentials. The title "nurse" was also rather vague and could refer to an officer's wife who accompanied her husband to the battlefield, a woman who came to care for a wounded son or husband and remained to care for others, a member of a Catholic religious community in a hospital that cared for military personnel, or a volunteer. It is estimated that more than 3,000 women served as nurses during the Civil War, caring for sick or wounded soldiers on the battlefields, in field hospitals, in hospitals removed from battle sites, or even in their own homes. These female volunteer nurses went to the war with only the most basic knowledge of nursing care derived from their personal experiences caring for loved ones. They learned about the care of battle-related injuries and illnesses through their own wartime experiences (Livermore, 1888). **Table 1-1** identifies some of the nurses who provided care to soldiers during the Civil War, such as Clara Barton.

Clara Barton.
Courtesy of Library of Congress Prints &
Photographs Online Catalog,
LC-USZ62-75827.

Influences of the U.S. Civil War

The Civil War nurses listed in Table 1-1 laid the foundation for professional nursing in the United States. The work they performed changed the public's perception of work by women outside of their homes. Many Civil War nurses had left their husbands and/or families to serve in situations that had not previously been considered a proper "place" for ladies. The work of the Civil War nurses also changed public opinion about women's work in health care. Women, who had volunteered as nurses during the Civil War, had come to realize the value of formal education in the care of the sick. Some of them became instrumental in the establishment of the first nurse training schools (schools of nursing) in the United States. In 1868, just 3 years after the end of the war, Samuel Gross, MD, president of the American Medical Association, strongly endorsed the formation of training schools for nurses (Larson, 1997).

The Effects of Social Change in the United States

Following the Civil War, cities in the United States experienced a rapid growth. Fueled by the rise of industries, many persons from rural areas flocked to cities to

TABLE 1-1 CIVIL WAR NURSES

Nurse	Role
Dorothea Dix (1802–1887)	Dix was a superintendent of Union Army nurses during the war. She was a teacher and reformer of mental hospitals who, at the outbreak of the war, was charged with recruitment of nurses and supervision of nursing activities.
Kate Cummings (1836–1909)	Cummings was a nurse for the Confederate Army. During the war, she kept a diary that she later published. Her book presents a realistic record of Confederate hospitals and nursing.
Jane Woolsey (1830–1900)	Woolsey was a volunteer nurse for the Union Army. She became a superintendent of a Union hospital in Virginia. She later published her memoirs, which describe medical practices, the work of nurses, and the lives of wounded soldiers. Following the war, she helped to found the nurse training school at Presbyterian Hospital in New York City.
Clara Barton (1821–1912)	Barton was a volunteer nurse who served in battlefield hospitals and prisoner of war camps. Following the war, she founded and became the first president of the American Red Cross.
Walt Whitman (1819–1892)	Whitman was a poet who worked as a volunteer nurse in a Union military hospital in Washington, DC. He later memorialized in his poetry the work of wartime nurses in the care of wounded and dying soldiers.
Harriet Tubman (1820–1913)	Tubman was born into slavery and escaped to Philadelphia. During the war she nursed soldiers using herbs and other home remedies.
Mary Livermore (1820–1905)	Livermore was a teacher and abolitionist who served as a volunteer nurse. As director of the Northwestern branch of the U.S. Sanitary Commission, she directed the solicitation and distribution of food and medical supplies to military hospitals.
Louisa May Alcott (1832–1888)	Alcott was an author and volunteer nurse for the Union Army. Her book *Hospital Sketches*, which was based on letters she had written home from an army hospital, aroused public awareness of the work of nurses in the grim environments of military hospitals.
Mary Ann "Mother" Bickerdyke (1817–1901)	Bickerdyke was a nurse for the Union Army. Before the war she had studied botanic medicine. She is renowned for her work in founding, cleaning, and sanitizing Union military hospitals in the face of opposition from Union officers. She also collected food and medical supplies for Union military hospitals.

find work in factories. Hordes of immigrants from Eastern and Southern Europe came to the cities to meet the factories' insatiable appetite for manpower. In fact, the population of many U.S. cities nearly doubled during each decade from 1880 until 1920. Crowded living conditions in the burgeoning cities often fostered the spread of disease. Because these new arrivals to cities often lacked family members with sufficient resources to care for them in time of illness and need, their only option was to seek care in municipal almshouses.

In many large cities in the United States, the sick wards of the almshouses evolved into public hospitals. Conditions in these municipal institutions in the United States were equal to the horrible environments in England that were described by Dickens.

A group of reform-minded citizens who visited public charitable facilities in New York City during the 1870s reported that much of the nursing care was provided by drunkards and former convicts. It was reported that prostitutes sentenced in the city's courts were given the choice of going to prison or going into hospital service. No nurses were on duty at night; instead, the patients were supervised by night watchmen (Pavey, 1953).

Establishment of the First Nurse Training Schools

The success of the Nightingale School of Nursing became known around the world. Social activists in many countries wrote to Nightingale with requests for her to send one of her graduates to found a nurse training school and hospital in their city. It was not long before social reformers and some physicians in the United States espoused the idea that provision of safe nursing care was important and could best be delivered by persons who had received a formal education in nursing. Small groups of public-minded women grew increasingly concerned about the welfare of the patients housed in the massive hospitals and almshouses and worked to establish nurse training schools to sanitize the institutions and to give patients care far better than that rendered by the untrained and politically chosen attendants then employed (Schryver, 1930).

The first permanent school of nursing in the United States is reputed to be the **nurse training school of Women's Hospital of Philadelphia**, which was established in 1872. The staff members of the hospital were predominantly female physicians, who sought to open the field of nursing to a better quality type of woman. Following the Nightingale model, the school had a set curriculum, paid instructors, equipment for the practice of nursing skills, provision for student experiences in other Philadelphia hospitals, and a nurses' library.

> **KEY TERM**
>
> **Nurse training school of Women's Hospital of Philadelphia:** Established in 1872, reputed to be the first permanent school of nursing in the United States.

In the same year, a training school for nurses was founded at the New England Hospital for Women and Children, another hospital with a staff composed of female physicians. Located in Boston, the school was founded and administered by two physicians, Dr. Susan Dimrock, who had been educated in Switzerland and was familiar with the educational methods of Kaiserswerth, and Dr. Marie Zakrzewska, who taught bedside nursing. **Linda Richards**, who is purported to be the first educated nurse in the United States, was a graduate of this program. Another notable graduate was **Mary Mahoney**, the first African American graduate nurse (Dolan, 1968). **Table 1-2** describes some of the early leaders in nursing from this era.

Unfortunately, physicians' support for the formal education of nurses was absent in the establishment of other early nurse training schools. Indeed, for many years a number of eminent physicians were opposed to any education for nurses other than the most basic training (Goodnow, 1953). Despite this, in 1873, three notable nurse training schools were established: the Bellevue Hospital Training School in New York City, the Connecticut Training School in New Haven Hospital, and the Boston Training School in Massachusetts General Hospital. It is significant that these schools were founded through the efforts of committees of laywomen, rather than physicians.

Conditions in Nurse Training Schools

In 1883, 10 years after the first training schools were founded, the number of training schools across the country had grown to 35. The majority of these schools were located on the east and west coasts, with isolated schools located in large cities across the nation's heartland. However, unlike the Nightingale School, training schools in the United States were economically dependent upon the hospitals in which they were located. Because of this, the needs of the hospital took precedence over the students' educational needs.

Hospital boards and physicians soon realized the economic advantages of the use of student labor, under the aegis of "clinical training," in the delivery of care to hospitalized patients. Because students tended to be compliant and obedient, the care they provided was cheap, efficient, and more cost effective than if graduate nurses had been hired by hospitals. The student nurses in effect traded their labor for the opportunity to be educated in a profession. Students worked 12-hour shifts with little or no clinical supervision. Some were required to sleep on hospital wards in beds that adjoined those of their patients. Classes were irregularly scheduled and were often cancelled when students were needed to staff the wards. Some hospitals earned additional funds by sending students to care for patients in private homes, a setting in which students were typically overworked and lacked both supervision and access to instruction (Kalisch & Kalisch, 1995).

By 1900, the number of schools had increased to 432. Many of these schools had been founded in state mental hospitals, tuberculosis sanatoria, and other "specialty"

TABLE 1-2 EARLY LEADERS IN NURSING

Early Leader	Contribution to Nursing
Linda Richards (1841–1930)	Richards was awarded the title "America's first trained nurse." She was the first graduate of the yearlong nurse training program at the New England Hospital for Women and Children. She established the first nurse training program in Japan, and then returned to the United States to found nurse training programs in Michigan, Massachusetts, and Pennsylvania.
Isabel Hampton Robb (1860–1910)	Robb was the superintendent of nurses at the Illinois Training School and the Johns Hopkins School for Nurses. She became the first president of the Society of Superintendents of Training Schools for Nurses (forerunner of the National League for Nursing) and the Associated Alumnae Association (forerunner of the American Nurses Association).
Sophia Palmer (1853–1920)	Palmer was a founder of the New York State Nurses Association and campaigner for nurse licensure in New York. She became the first editor of the *American Journal of Nursing*. She authored a history of nursing, as well as other nursing textbooks and journal articles.
Lavinia Dock (1858–1956)	Dock was a lecturer, author, and activist. Her campaign for women's suffrage and participation in antiwar protests sometimes led to her arrest. She authored many nursing textbooks and, because of her leadership in the International Council of Nurses, served as editor for the *American Journal of Nursing*'s Foreign Department.
Mary Adelaide Nutting (1858–1948)	Nutting was the appointed head of the Department of Nursing and Health at Teachers College of Columbia University. She became the world's first professor of nursing.
Isabel Maitland Stewart (1878–1947)	Stewart was a professor of nursing at Teachers College of Columbia University. She worked tirelessly for the establishment of a standardized nursing curriculum. She insisted on the need for nursing research to give the profession a solid scientific base.
Lillian Wald (1867–1940)	From her work providing home nursing care and teaching home nursing to immigrant women on New York City's Lower East Side, Wald went on to found the Henry Street Settlement and the first Visiting Nurse Association.
Mary Breckinridge (1881–1965)	Breckinridge was a nurse–midwife. She founded the Frontier Nursing Service to provide maternity services to women in the Appalachian Mountains of eastern Kentucky. Nurses visited families on horseback. This service significantly lowered the maternal mortality rate of the region served.

hospitals that provided very limited experiences. Still other schools were founded in hospitals with fewer than 25 beds, which because of their size, provided less than adequate clinical experiences (Baer, 1990).

Following the completion of their training, only a select handful of graduates were offered hospital positions as supervisors and clinical faculty. The majority of graduates found employment in the homes of clients who could afford their services. The need for these private duty nurses was great because the majority of infants were delivered in the home, and some surgical procedures were performed there. In addition, many medical conditions, such as typhoid fever and pneumonia, were treated in the home setting. Often a private duty nurse slept in the same room as her patient and was also responsible for laundry chores and meal preparation. Despite these harsh work conditions, nursing offered women a socially acceptable means of self-support and economic independence.

Advances in Science and Medicine

The 19th century was marked by vigorous intellectual activity and the expansion of knowledge in the sciences. These advances profoundly influenced both medicine and the burgeoning profession of nursing. By the beginning of the 20th century, the symptoms and natural life histories of many diseases had been identified. Because of advances in the development of microscopes, in some cases, the causative organisms of disease had been identified as well. Newly developed instruments aided in the assessment of bodily function. Through the development of antiseptic agents and anesthesia, complicated surgical procedures were possible. Increasingly the practice of medicine was based on scientific knowledge and aimed to both control and cure disease.

The expansion of scientific knowledge and the increased use of complex technological procedures were linked to the growth of schools of nursing. The work of curing patients was best carried out in hospitals where physicians and surgeons had access to modern technology. With the expansion of medical care, educated nurses were needed to aid in the care and treatment of patients with increasingly more complex conditions and needs.

The Origins of Public Health Nursing

At the end of the 19th century, the field of public health nursing was instituted, which provided a new area in which nurse graduates could find employment. District nursing originated in England during the 1860s. Through funding from wealthy philanthropists, nurses provided care to "sick poor" persons in their homes, and also provided food and medical supplies. In 1886, the idea spread to the United States, and two district nurse associations were established in Boston and Philadelphia.

In 1893, **Lillian Wald** originated settlement house nursing, an offshoot of district nursing, among the immigrant populations on the Lower East Side of New York.

Following her graduation from the New York Hospital Training School, Wald taught a home nursing class in a neighborhood populated by recent immigrants. One day a young child came to her, asking for her aid in the care of his mother who had given birth only 2 days before. He escorted her to a dreary apartment where she found the young mother lying on a bed in a pool of blood. Wald was so moved by this scene that she made the commitment to care for the destitute immigrant population of her city. With funding provided by women of the upper class, she and a classmate, Mary Brewster, moved into a small apartment in the neighborhood, offering nursing care to recent immigrants who sought their help. They were soon joined by other nurses and by social workers. Within 2 years, they helped to found the Henry Street Settlement House to provide both home nursing care and a variety of social services to New York's immigrant population (Wald, 1934).

In an attempt to demonstrate the positive outcomes that could be realized by a public health nurse in a school setting, in October 1902 Wald sent one of her Henry Street nurses, Lina Ravanche Rogers, to work for a month in the New York public schools. At that time, any child could be barred from school if the teacher believed there was reason for the exclusion. However, no attempt was made to determine whether there was a medical cause for the exclusion, nor was any attempt made to secure treatment for the child if this were necessary. The school nurse experiment was so successful in reducing the number of absences among schoolchildren that by December 1902, Lina Rogers was appointed to the Board of Health and 12 additional nurses were employed to aid her provision of school health services.

Wald was the first person to use the term *public health nursing* to describe the work of nurses in patients' homes as well as in other community settings. This field of nursing gained such prominence that in 1912 the National Organization for Public Health Nursing (NOPHN) was founded to set standards and to plan for the expansion of community-based nursing services (Randall, 1937).

The Origins of Nursing Associations

The World's Fair and Colombian Exposition was held in Chicago from May until October 1893 to celebrate the 400th anniversary of Columbus' arrival in the New World. Various conventions and conferences were held at the exposition, including the International Congress of Charities, Correction and Philanthropy. A section of this conference was chaired by Isabel Hampton. Prominent nurses presented papers on topics related to nursing. Of concern to the nurses gathered was the fact that at that time, only one-tenth of the persons who practiced nursing in the United States were graduates of hospital nurse training schools. The other 90 percent, who received equal pay for their care of the sick, had little or no formal education in nursing. Nurse licensure was considered vital to the protection of the public by providing a distinction between educated nurses and uneducated nurses. Nurse leaders voiced their concerns about the need for licensure, called for nurses to unite to advance their new profession, and proposed strategies to unite nurses.

In 1896, the **Nurses' Associated Alumnae of the United States and Canada,** which later became the American Nurses Association (ANA), was founded with the intent of achieving licensure for nurses. This escalating concern for nurse licensure led to the formation of state nurses' associations that were committed to the attainment of nurse registration through the passage of a nurse practice act in each state of the union. Other goals of the association included the establishment of a code of ethics, promotion of the image of nursing, and provision of attention to the financial and professional interests of nursing (ANA & National League of Nursing Education, 1940).

> **KEY TERM**
>
> **Nurses' Associated Alumnae of the United States and Canada:** Originally founded in 1896 with the intent of achieving licensure for nurses; became the American Nurses Association.

Another concern voiced was the lack of educational standards in nursing. The programs offered in nurse training schools varied in length from a few months to 3 years, and curricula and entrance requirements varied greatly. This issue was of particular concern to the 18 superintendents of nurse training schools who attended the Congress. As a result of their conversations, they joined together in 1893 to form the **American Society of Superintendents of Training Schools of Nursing**, a national nursing organization focused on elevating the standards of nursing education. This association later became the National League for Nursing Education, and still later, the National League for Nursing (NLN).

> **KEY TERM**
>
> **American Society of Superintendents of Training Schools of Nursing:** A national nursing organization founded in 1893 to elevate the standards of nursing education; later became the National League for Nursing Education, and ultimately, the National League for Nursing.

Licensure for Nurses

In 1901, New York, New Jersey, Illinois, and Virginia were the first states that organized state nurses' associations with the goal of enacting a nurse practice act for their states. In 1903, North Carolina passed the first nurse licensure act in the United States. By 1921, 48 states, as well as the District of Columbia and the territory of Hawaii, had enacted laws that regulated the practice of professional nursing. These early versions of nurse practice acts provided for licensure as a "registered nurse" (Birnbach, 1999).

Although the passage of these acts marked a tremendous milestone in the professionalization of nursing, a serious weakness of the early nurse practice acts was that they were permissive laws, rather than mandatory. They were "permissive" in that only nurses who were licensed were permitted to use the title "registered nurse." Thus, untrained persons were not prohibited from practice as nurses as long as they did not use the title "registered nurse."

This deficiency caused hardships for registered nurses during the Great Depression of the 1930s. Because the states lacked mandatory nurse licensure, any person was legally able to work as a "nurse" for pay. Thus licensed graduate nurses competed with uneducated "nurses" for the few available positions. The ANA argued that if only licensed nurses were allowed to practice, there would be enough work for each of them. Mandatory licensure laws, which made it unlawful for any person to practice nursing without a valid nursing license, were not passed by states until the late 1940s.

Effects of the Great Depression on Nursing

The stock market crash of 1929 plunged the United States into the throes of the Great Depression. Although every group of workers was devastated by the collapse of the nation's economy, nurses were particularly affected. Most nurses were independent practitioners, self-employed in private duty work in patients' homes. However, the patients who once employed private duty nurses were now unable to pay for this service.

Nurses who attempted to move from private duty work in patients' homes to hospital settings encountered problems in this venture. The depression years saw reductions in the number of hospital beds occupied. Patients who were forced to seek medical care were often without financial resources. Most hospitalized patients were in hospitals with training schools that used their students for bedside care. Hospitals without training schools were usually staffed with uneducated attendants. It is estimated that of the hospitals with training schools, 73 percent had no graduate nurse employees, and of these, only 15 percent had four or more graduate nurse employees. Graduate nurses who engaged in bedside patient care were looked down on as nurses not able to succeed in private duty work. After much debate, some hospital administrators decided to accept the services of unemployed registered nurses in exchange for a room, meals, and laundry but offered the nurses no salary (Kalisch & Kalisch, 1995).

The National Recovery Act, passed by the U.S. Congress in 1933 in an effort to find employment for those without work, did not apply to unemployed nurses. The law stated that the agreement "shall not apply to. . . professional persons employed in their profession" (Roosevelt, 1933). In response to the implications of the National Recovery Act for the nursing profession, the Board of Directors of the ANA issued the following position statements:

1. Any plan for economic recovery must consider the thousands of unemployed graduate registered nurses.

2. In all cases, the most effective type of nursing service should be made available to patients.

3. Wherever possible, the nurse should be employed on the basis of an 8-hour day or 48-hour week.

4. The salaries of nurses should be kept above sustenance levels.

5. Nurses caring for acutely ill patients should not be expected to work more than 8 hours out of 24.

By 1933, the 8-hour day for hospital nurses was gaining ground. This schedule for nurses gained support because it helped to alleviate the problem of unemployment of nurses. When nurses were on duty for 8 hours instead of 12 hours, three nurses, rather than two, could work during each 24-hour period.

A milestone was reached in 1933 when the federal government announced that a program offered through the Civil Works Service would provide funds for bedside nursing care in the homes of recipients of unemployment relief. The care would be paid for with Federal Emergency Relief Administration funds at a set rate per visit, not to exceed the established rate charged by accredited visiting nurse associations in the local district. The program also included the use of graduate nurses for instruction to home workers, health education programs, instruction in hygiene, preventative measures, care of infants and children, first aid, and nutrition. This program served to interest many nurses in the specialty area of public health nursing ("The NRA and Nursing," 1933).

Nursing and Times of War

Times of war have increased both the nation's need for nurses and the public's recognition of nurses' work in saving lives. Educated nurses first served as army nurses in 1898, in the Spanish–American War. At the outbreak of the war, nurse training schools had been educating nurses for nearly 20 years. Congress authorized the Surgeon General to hire as many nurses as would be needed. At first, the educated nurses had difficulty winning acceptance from medical officers, but because they had been approved by the Surgeon General, their presence was tolerated. However, as the war progressed, their skills in caring for ill and wounded soldiers won recognition, and army doctors came to depend on them. More than 1,500 nurses entered the army during the war. **Table 1-3** presents information about some of the early military nurses in our country's history.

In 1901, an act of Congress established a permanent Army Nurse Corps, followed in 1908 by the establishment of the Navy Nurse Corps. However, military nursing did not achieve prominence until 1917, when the United States entered World War I. At the beginning of the war there were fewer than 500 nurses in the Army Nurse Corps. However, by the war's end, aided by reserve nurses from the

TABLE 1-3 MILITARY NURSES

Nurse	Role
Clara Maas (1876–1901)	Following service in the Spanish–American War, Maas participated in a study to determine the cause of yellow fever. She allowed herself to be bitten by a mosquito known to have bitten infected patients, contracted the disease, and died a few days later.
Jane Delano (1862–1919)	Delano is credited with the creation of American Red Cross Nursing. She recruited nurses for army service in World War I through the American Red Cross. While touring Red Cross hospitals in France following the Armistice, she contracted an ear infection and died a few days later.
Annie Goodrich (1866–1954)	Goodrich was a professor at Teachers College of Columbia University. During World War I, she organized and served as dean of the Army School of Nursing. Following the war, she served as the first dean of the Yale University School of Nursing.
Julia Stimson (1881–1948)	During World War I, Stimson served as chief nurse of the American Expeditionary Forces. Following the war, she served as dean of the Army School of Nursing and was appointed the first superintendent of the Army Nurse Corps. During World War II she recruited nurses for military service.
Florence Blanchfield (1882–1971)	Blanchfield was superintendent for the Army Nurse Corps during World War II. She was one of a few women to reach the rank of colonel. Following the war, she worked for passage of the bill that granted army and navy nurses the pay, benefits, and privileges prescribed for commissioned officers.
Lucile Petry (1902–1999)	Petry served as head of the Cadet Nurse Corps during World War II. This program provided a free nursing education to women who agreed to provide military service until the end of the war.

American Red Cross National Nursing Service, the number had increased to over 21,000 army nurses and 1,386 navy nurses. During the war, over 10,000 U.S. nurses served overseas.

In 1914, when war first broke out in Europe, Jane Delano was appointed Director of Nursing Services for the American Red Cross Department of Nursing. Because the American Red Cross was regarded as the unofficial reserve for the military in times of national emergency, it became Delano's responsibility to recruit nurses for the Army Nurse Corps, Navy Nurse Corps, and U.S. Public Health Service, as well as to equip nurses for duty overseas. Traditionally, only graduates of nurse training school were eligible for military service. However, as the war progressed and the supply of nurses became depleted, society women, filled with a spirit of patriotism but unwilling to commit to a formal educational program in nursing, increasingly pressured the government for the right to serve as volunteer nurses. Although various schemes were developed to conserve the supply of nurses through the uses of volunteer nurses' aides, nurse leaders remained resolute that only educated nurses could serve as military nurses.

In an effort to recruit college-educated women into military nursing, in 1918 Vassar College offered its campus as a training camp to provide a 12-week preclinical program in basic science and basic nursing skills as part of a nursing program for college women. Upon successful completion of the Vassar Training Camp program, the college women were assigned to select nurse training schools as regular students for the completion of their education in nursing. During that summer, 432 women from 115 colleges and representing 41 states participated in the Vassar program. Their enthusiasm spread interest in nursing across U.S. college campuses. Many graduates of the Vassar Training Camp became leaders in nursing education during the following decades.

In a related effort, the Army School of Nursing was founded in 1918, with Annie Goodrich, a former faculty member from Teachers College of Columbia University, as its dean. Following the model used by the best civilian hospitals of the time, Goodrich's goal in founding the school was to provide patients in military hospitals with quality care provided by student nurses supervised by educated faculty. The school's curriculum was 3 years in length, with 9 months credit awarded to college graduates. Most clinical experiences were provided in army hospitals, with affiliations in civilian hospitals for pediatrics and other experiences. There were 500 students in the class of 1921, the first class to graduate from the Army School of Nursing. Although the school had been planned to be a permanent institution, it was closed in 1933 because of financial constraints imposed by the Great Depression (see **Contemporary Practice Highlight 1-1**). However, the Army School of Nursing was well organized and offered a high standard of nursing education that served as a model for nurse training schools in the civilian sector (Jensen, 1950).

In 1940, as a second world war threatened, the ANA and other nursing organizations established the Nursing Council of National Defense to recruit more student nurses as well as to assess the number of graduate nurses who might be available for military service. The council worked closely with the American Red Cross in attempts to recruit registered nurses for military service. When a national inventory of nursing personnel conducted by the National Nursing Council revealed an acute shortage of nurses, the council joined with U.S. Representative Frances Payne Bolton of Ohio in the sponsorship of the first bill passed by Congress that provided government funding for the education of nurses for national defense. This bill was followed closely by the **Bolton Act of 1942**, which created the U.S. Cadet Nurse

KEY TERM

Bolton Act of 1942: Legislation that created the U.S. Cadet Nurse Corps, a program subsidized by the federal government and designed to quickly prepare nurses to meet the needs of the armed forces, civilian and government hospitals, and war industries.

CONTEMPORARY PRACTICE HIGHLIGHT 1-1

OPIATES

Opium trade and opiate addiction threads throughout history. Nurses recognized opiate addiction as a public health issue with increasing prominence in the United States after World War I. Social determinants of international countries supplying the drug trade included inexpensive land to grow opium, cheap labor forces, and a steady flow of revenue for unstable governments and cartels. Consider how opiate addiction is managed as a public health issue today. Deaths from opiates have increased 200% in the United States since 2000 (Rudd, Aleshire, Zibbell, & Gladden, 2016). What can we learn from examining the historical background of opiate addiction and comparing the current public health issues facing the United States today? What strategies and legislation can affect international drug trade? How can nursing practice and education play a role in preventing overprescribing pain medications and early recognition and treatment of substance disorders?

Corps, a program to prepare nurses as quickly as possible to meet the needs of the armed forces, civilian and government hospitals, and war industries. The entire nursing education of students enrolled in this program, including tuition, housing, uniforms, books, and monthly stipends, was subsidized by the federal government. Students were required to promise to work in either civilian or military nursing roles that were deemed essential to the national defense for the duration of the war. The Bolton Act further stipulated that the length of study for members of the Cadet Nurse Corps be reduced from 36 months to 30 or fewer months. By the beginning of 1944, students in the Cadet Nurse Corps began reporting to military hospitals for the clinical experiences that composed their senior year. The Bolton Act had a widespread influence on nursing education, mandating standards for nursing education programs and the removal of school policies that discriminated against students' gender, marital status, ethnicity, or race.

During the war, over 77,000 nurses, more than two-fifths of the active nurses at the time, served in the armed forces. Despite these valiant efforts, the number of nurses in military service remained inadequate. In his address to Congress in January 1945, President Roosevelt requested a national draft of nurses. Although the leading nursing organizations were supportive of a national service act for all men and women, they opposed a law aimed specifically at nurses. Discussion about the bill ended with the Allies' victory in Europe.

During times of war, the profession of nursing has attained a positive image and has enjoyed the highest level of respect from members of the lay public (Kalisch & Kalisch, 1981). During World War II, the great need for nurses caused the U.S. government to provide the resources that were needed to both increase the supply of nurses and improve the quality of nursing education. Nurse leaders seized on this opportunity to advance not only military nursing but also the profession in general.

Collective Bargaining in Nursing

Following World War II, the United States experienced one of its most drastic shortages of nurses. Many nurses who returned from the war sought the role of wife and mother. Until the 1960s, nurses who worked in hospitals were expected to resign from their positions when they married. In addition, returning military nurses who had experienced such profoundly autonomous roles during the war were now reluctant to return to the subservient role of staff nurse in a hospital.

During the years that immediately followed the end of the war, despite the acute nursing shortage, nurses were paid far less than elementary school teachers, the professional group to whom nurses were most often compared. In fact, a study conducted in 1946 by the California Nurses Association found that the majority of staff nurses were paid only slightly more than hotel maids and seamstresses.

During the 1940s, Shirley Titus, executive director of the California Nurses Association, lobbied for economic empowerment for nurses. At the ANA convention of 1946 she successfully argued for nurses' rights to economic security through collective bargaining, insurance plans, benefit packages, and access to consultation from state nurses' associations. In 1949, the ANA approved state nurses' associations as collective bargaining agencies for nurses. However, a 1947 revision of the Taft-Hartley Labor Act exempted not-for-profit institutions such as hospitals from the requirement to enter into labor negotiations with their employees to address workplace grievances. Because the ANA had adopted a "no-strike" policy, and hospitals were not required to enter into labor negotiations with nurse employees, nurses often had no means to improve their work conditions other than by threats of mass resignation. Although hospitals were not required to enter into collective bargaining agreements with nurses, many times nurses working collectively were able to pressure their employers into voluntary labor agreements.

In 1966, the ANA rescinded its no-strike clause, opening the way for nurses' strikes for improvements in work conditions and salaries. Although relatively few strikes by nurses have occurred, when they have, nurses have ensured that care for those in need continued to be provided. Both nurses and members of the general public are often opposed to the idea of nurses entering into labor negotiations with employers, which they view as "unprofessional." However, collective bargaining has provided nurses with both increased economic security and a greater voice in decisions that affect patient care (Stafford et al., 2000).

Advances in Nursing Education

The apprentice system that initially was used in nursing education was often criticized by academicians and external review agencies because of its lack of intellectual rigor and its exploitation of student labor. In 1919, a Committee for the Study of Nursing Education, supported by the Rockefeller Foundation, was established to examine the state of both public health nursing and nursing education. The committee's published report, the **Goldmark Report** (1923), recommended that nursing education should have educational standards, and that schools of nursing should have a primary focus on education, rather than on care of patients. The report further recommended that nursing education be moved to universities, and that nurse educators receive the advanced education that was required for their roles. Although some changes in nursing education were implemented after the publication of the Goldmark Report, the changes were neither far reaching nor permanent. Hospital administrators resisted change in nursing education that would eliminate the "free" labor provided by nursing students.

> **KEY TERM**
>
> **Goldmark Report:** Published in 1923, this report recommended that nursing education develop educational standards, schools of nursing adopt a primary focus on education and be moved to universities, and nurse educators receive advanced education.

In 1926, the Committee on the Grading of Nursing Schools was organized to analyze the work of nurses and to study the educational preparation of student nurses. The committee's published report, *Nurses, Patients, and Pocketbooks*, became known as the Burgess Report (1928). The committee recommended that admission criteria be adopted for applicants to schools of nursing, and that hospital nursing schools focus on education of students rather than provision of patient care. The report further decried a hospital's use of funds collected for care of the sick to finance its nurse training school. Unfortunately, the recommendations of the Burgess Report were also largely ignored.

A third evaluation of nursing education, *The Future of Nursing*, authored by Esther Brown (1948), was funded by the Carnegie Foundation. Like the two previous reviews, Brown recommended that schools of nursing strive for autonomy from hospital administration, improve the quality of their programs, recruit faculty with baccalaureate or graduate degrees, and use discretion in the selection of sites to be used for students' clinical experiences. To relieve the acute shortage of nurses that followed World War II, Brown strongly advocated the employment of married nurses and the recruitment of men into nursing. Brown further recommended that nursing practice be based on principles from the physical and social sciences.

The years that followed World War II saw a significant increase in the number of students who sought college degrees. This trend was coupled with dramatic changes in health care as technological advances increasingly led to specialized practice in medicine and nursing (Kalisch & Kalisch, 1995). However, during the 1950s and 1960s, the number of baccalaureate programs in nursing grew at a very slow rate.

The vast majority of schools of nursing continued to be hospital-based diploma programs. Many of the diploma nursing programs had improved in quality as a result of the Brown Report. Improvements were also linked to measures instituted by the NLN, such as the publication of a standardized curriculum and the establishment of a process of voluntary accreditation. However, the diploma programs continued to be dependent on hospitals for financial support and continued to give higher priority to the service needs of the hospitals rather than to their students' educational needs.

In response to the acute nursing shortage that followed World War II, an associate degree in nursing (ADN) was initiated. The ADN program was conceived by **Mildred Montag** as the topic of her doctoral dissertation. It was initiated on an experimental basis in 1951 to provide a large number of nurses in a relatively short time period. It was intended that the ADN nurse would practice solely at the bedside and would have a significantly narrower scope of practice than the traditional registered nurse. The ADN programs were tested for 5 years (1952–1957) and successfully produced nurses who were proficient in technical skills and could successfully function as registered nurses despite the fact that their program was only 2 years in length (Haase, 1990). The number of ADN programs increased as the number of community colleges increased. The ADN programs provided a pathway to the nursing profession for men, married women, mature students, and other groups who had traditionally been excluded from admission to nursing programs. By the end of the 1970s, the number of graduates from ADN programs exceeded the number of graduates from baccalaureate programs and diploma programs. As the number of ADN programs increased, the number of diploma programs rapidly declined.

> **KEY TERM**
>
> **Mildred Montag:** Developed the concept for associate degree in nursing programs.

In 1965, the ANA published the document *Educational Preparation for Nurse Practitioners and Assistants to Nurses*, which became known as the ANA position paper. This document reaffirmed the stand that nursing education should occur in institutions of higher education, rather than in hospitals. In addition, the position paper stated that the minimum preparation for beginning professional nurses should be a baccalaureate degree, the minimum preparation for beginning technical nurses should be an associate degree, and the educational preparation of nursing assistants should be a short, intensive preservice program in an institution that offered vocational education (ANA, 1965). Although the ANA position paper arose from the association's concern that societal changes and advances in technology required significant changes in nursing education, publication of this document led to an enduring rift in the profession and has discouraged movement toward the baccalaureate degree as the requirement for entry level into practice for professional nursing.

During the first half of the 20th century, the number of baccalaureate and graduate programs in nursing increased slowly. The slow rate of growth of collegiate programs can be partly attributed to the nursing profession's uncertainty about the curriculum these programs should follow and the ways in which they should differ from diploma programs. At the beginning of the 1960s, only 14 percent of all basic students in nursing were enrolled in baccalaureate programs. In addition, there were only 14 higher degree programs in nursing to prepare the faculty needed to staff schools of nursing. A study commissioned in 1963 by the Surgeon General of the U.S. Public Health Service revealed that faculty in all schools of nursing, including baccalaureate programs, lacked the minimal educational preparation required for teaching. The published report of the study, *Toward Quality in Nursing, Needs and Goals*, recommended increased federal funding for nursing programs, and led to the passage of the Nurse Training Act of 1964 (Kalisch & Kalisch, 1995). This federal assistance was particularly important in the development of graduate programs in nursing. Prior to this time, nurses were often required to seek graduate degrees in education or in related disciplines. The 1970s saw a rapid increase in graduate programs focused on clinical specialties and laid the basis for an expansion in advanced practice roles in nursing.

Advances in Nursing Practice

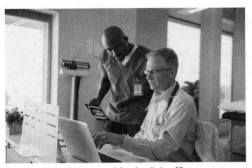

Nurse and physician consulting in clinic office.
© Hero Images/Getty

The growth of master's degree programs in nursing opened many new advanced practice roles for nurses, including the roles of clinical specialist, nurse practitioner, researcher, and nurse administrator. Clinical nurse specialists have expertise in a defined clinical area. They are educated to provide expert care to patients who have complex health problems that require specialized care, to serve as role models for staff nurses, to provide consultation to nurses from other clinical areas, and to identify and research clinical problems associated with patient care. By the 1970s, clinical specialist roles had been developed in a variety of nursing practice areas including psychiatric/mental health nursing, cardiac nursing, oncology nursing, and community health nursing.

During the 1960s, concern for extending access to primary care services to traditionally underserved populations led to the evolution of the nurse practitioner role. It was long believed that the role of the nurse could be expanded and that nurses with specialized education could perform many of the primary care functions traditionally performed by physicians, but at a substantially lower cost. The title *nurse practitioner* was first used in a demonstration project at the University of Colorado, which was designed to prepare nurses to deliver well child care in ambulatory care settings. By the 1970s nurse practitioner preparation increasingly occurred in graduate programs in nursing. Provision of primary care by nurse practitioners became widely accepted by the general public.

The expansion of nurses' roles necessitated changes in the extant state nurse practice laws. At times, the extended roles for nurses, especially prescriptive authority for nurses, were met with criticism and opposition by medical associations. Nurses in advanced practice roles honed their skills in political activism as they fought for the changes in legislation that were required for roles for which they had been educated.

Advances were also made in nursing research. Over time, nurse leaders had struggled to establish nursing as a discipline that was separate and unique from medicine. However, this could be accomplished only when nursing developed its own unique theory base and body of knowledge. In addition, technological advances in medicine called for concurrent advances in clinical nursing practice, which could best be developed and validated through research. The journal *Nursing Research*, which was first published during the 1950s, provided a great impetus to nursing scholarship. The National Institutes of Health, Division of Nursing Research, was initiated in 1956. This body provided extramural grants for nursing research projects, and primarily funded proposals focused on applied research aimed to improve nursing practice. Nursing research further spawned the development of nursing theory by nurse scholars such as Martha Rogers, Hildegarde Peplau, Imogene King, Myra Levine, and Dorothy Orem. Prior to the work by these nurse theorists, frameworks for nursing research had often been "borrowed" from other disciplines. The new emphasis on the development and refinement of nursing theories allowed nursing to be established as a distinct discipline.

As early as the mid-1930s hospital and public health nursing administration were identified as areas of graduate study for nurses. It was acknowledged that nursing administration required a specialized set of knowledge and skills. Therefore, in the 1950s the W. K. Kellogg Foundation funded 13 universities in order to establish graduate nursing programs that prepared nurses for hospital nursing administration. This emphasis continued into the 1970s as nursing administration was increasingly recognized as a practice area and certification for the specialty of nursing administration was established. However, the increasing emphasis on clinical specialization in nursing during the 1970s and early 1980s eventually resulted in decreased numbers of nurses enrolling in educational programs that were focused on nursing administration (Simms, 1989). Today nursing administration is recognized as an advanced practice role requiring graduate education to adequately prepare nurses to lead in complex healthcare practice and educational settings.

Nursing History and Health Policy

During the past 2 decades scholars of the history of nursing have made great strides in conveying to colleagues the importance of history to the present and to the future of the nursing profession. Increasingly, the history of the profession has moved from mere accounts of significant events in the lives of nursing leaders. The newer focus aims to identify links that connect past events to present concerns, with an eye toward the formulation of plans for the future.

Analysis of historical trends has made us increasingly aware that the debate surrounding many of our current healthcare policies has origins rooted in the past. One example is the challenges modern healthcare professionals face in their attempts to ensure the delivery of safe and affordable high-quality health care to traditionally underserved populations. Although this issue is not new, a review of the history of health care reveals a variety of perceptions of this issue accompanied by diverse opinions about the best interventions to address the issue. Examination of these various perceptions helps us to understand the forces that have contributed to the shaping of healthcare policy. Consideration of these forces provides a framework for formulation of plans for the future.

Noted nurse historian Joan Lynaugh has often stated, "What happens in the present is not an accident. It has a past" (Fairman & D'Antonio, 2013, p. 347). Examination of this "past" provides insights into the events that led to policy decisions. Fairman and D'Antonio (2013) offer the example that the rise of the earliest nurse training schools can be linked to the rise in technological innovations in medicine and physicians' concurrent need for educated colleagues to help protect patients as they underwent these advanced procedures.

Examination of the history of nursing will help those engaged in shaping health policy to comprehend the continuity of nursing's values over time. For example, the profession's ongoing concern for quality in patient care and the maintenance of safe environments for the delivery of care have influenced many of the policy issues the profession has embraced over the decades. Indeed, the profession's early involvement in collective bargaining can be linked to nurses' advocacy for safe environments in which they could maintain the standards of practice advanced by the ANA. Nurses' ability to influence the development of policies that are congruent with our professional ideals will depend on our skill in articulation of our values, standards, and concerns for patients' welfare that have endured over time.

Summary

From the beginning of humanity, persons have been designated, called, or educated to perform the functions we now refer to as nursing care. The history of nursing has been distinctly linked to a tradition of caring. Nurses have felt a true responsibility to reach out to those in need and to advocate on their behalf. **Contemporary Practice Highlight 1-2** further illustrates this call to caring.

The history of nursing reveals a pattern of recurrent issues that the profession has been required to confront over time. Some of these issues have included maintenance of standards for the profession, autonomy for nurses, and maintenance of control of professional nursing practice. Over time, the profession has also addressed phenomena such as nursing shortages, new categories of healthcare providers, and ethical dilemmas. Each decade has brought new insight into ways the profession can better meet these challenges.

Nurses of the future must continue to monitor changes in technology, advances in scientific knowledge, and changes in society and in the healthcare delivery system. Perhaps through study of the challenges of the past we will have the insights to best meet our future.

CONTEMPORARY PRACTICE HIGHLIGHT 1-2

CARING IN NURSING

Susan Reverby, a noted historian, argues that "caring" is the central dilemma of U.S. nursing. She asserts that the history of nursing is intimately entwined with the history of U.S. womanhood. She believes that throughout history, nurses have viewed caring as the basis of their practice. Indeed, nurses believe it their "order," or mandate, to care if they are to fulfill the proper role of a professional nurse. However, nurses have difficulty fulfilling this mandate in a society that varies in the value held for caring.

In her historical research article, she traces the history of the "mandate" to care from Florence Nightingale, through the origins of U.S. nurse training schools, to the present day. In her analysis, she suggests that nursing continues to be plagued by the dilemma of "altruism versus autonomy" and offers implications of this dilemma for modern professional nursing practice. Too often nurses have equated the "order" to care and empower others with the need for self-immolation. She suggested that nurses need "to create a new political understanding for the basis of caring and to find ways to gain the power to implement it" (p. 10) and in the process gain an understanding of how to practice altruism *with* autonomy.

Reflect on ways you can establish you nursing practice of altruism *with* autonomy.

Data from Reverby, S. (1987). A caring dilemma: Womanhood and nursing in historical perspective. Nursing Research, 36(1), 5–11.

Reflective Practice Questions

1. Reflect on one of the infectious disease issues that the profession of nursing has confronted in the past such as tuberculosis. What solutions were proposed or implemented? What can we learn from these successful (or unsuccessful) efforts? How does the management of clients with tuberculosis differ today?

2. What contributions has military nursing made to the entire profession? What current nursing practices are the legacy of military nursing?

3. Although advanced practice nursing roles were formally introduced to the profession during the latter half of the 20th century, it has been argued that nurses began to function in expanded roles long before that time. Give examples of expanded roles assumed by nurses (community health nurses, military nurses) early in the 20th century. What do you envision for the profession of nursing 20 years from now? What current trends in nursing practice do you believe will be the basis for future practice?

References

American Nurses Association. (1965). American Nurses Association's first position paper on education for nursing. *American Journal of Nursing, 65*(12), 106–111.

American Nurses Association, & National League of Nursing Education. (1940). *Nurse practice acts and board rules: A digest.* New York, NY: Authors.

Baer, E. (1990). *Editor's notes for nursing in America: A history of social reform.* New York, NY: National League for Nursing.

Baly, M. (1997). *Florence Nightingale and the nursing legacy* (2nd ed.). London, England: Whurr.

Birnbach, N. (1999). Registration. In T. Schorr & M. Kennedy (Eds.), *100 years in American nursing: Celebrating a century of caring* (pp. 17–22). Hagertown, MD: Lippincott Williams and Wilkins.

Brown, E. L. (1948). *Nursing for the future.* New York, NY: Russell Sage Foundation.

Burgess, M. A. (1928). *Nurses, patients, and pocketbooks.* New York, NY: Committee on the Grading of Nursing Schools.

Dolan, J. A. (1968). *History of nursing* (12th ed.). Philadelphia, PA: W.B. Saunders.

Donahue, P. (1991). Why nursing history? *Journal of Professional Nursing, 7,* 77.

Fairman, J., & D'Antonio, P. (2013). History counts: How history can shape our understanding of health policy., *Nursing Outlook, 61,* 346–352.

Gallison, M. (1954). *The ministry of women: One hundred years of women's work at Kaiserswerth, 1836–1936.* London, England: Butterworth.

Goldmark, J. (1923). *Nursing and nursing education in the United States.* New York, NY: Macmillan.

Goodnow, M. (1953). *Nursing history* (9th ed.). Philadelphia, PA: W.B. Saunders.

Haase, P. (1990). *The origins and rise of associate degree education.* Durham, NC: Duke University Press.

Henly, S. J., & Moss, M. (2007). American Indian health issues. In S. Boslaugh (Ed.), *Encyclopedia of epidemiology* (Vol. 1, pp. 25–30). Thousand Oaks, CA: Sage.

Jensen, D. (1950). *History and trends of professional nursing* (2nd ed.). St. Louis, MO: Mosby.

Kalisch, P., & Kalisch, B. (1981). When nurses were national heroines: Images of nursing in American film, 1942–1943. *Nursing Forum, 20*(1), 14–61.

Kalisch, P., & Kalisch, B. (1995). *The advance of American nursing* (3rd ed.). Philadelphia, PA: Lippincott.

Larson, R. D. (1997). *White roses: Stories of Civil War nurses*. Gettysburg, PA: Thomas.

Livermore, M. (1888). *My story of the war: A woman's narrative of four years' experience as a nurse in the Union Army*. Hartford, CT: A.D. Worthington.

The NRA and Nursing. (1933). *Illinois State Nurses' Association Bulletin, 30*, 6.

Nutting, M. A., & Dock, L. (1907). *A history of nursing: The evolution of nursing systems from the earliest times to the foundation of the first English and American training schools for nurses*. New York, NY: G. P. Putnam's Sons.

Pavey, A. E. (1953). *The story of the growth of nursing as an art, a vocation, and a profession* (4th ed.). Philadelphia, PA: J.B. Lippincott.

Randall, M. G. (1937). *Personnel policies in public health nursing*. New York, NY: Macmillan.

Reverby, S. (1987). A caring dilemma: Womanhood and nursing in historical perspective. *Nursing Research, 36*(1), 5–11.

Robinson, V. (1946). *White caps: The story of nursing*. Philadelphia: J.B. Lippincott.

Roosevelt, F. D. (1933). The President's reemployment agreement. In G. Peters, & J. T. Woolley (Eds.), *The American Presidency Project*. Retrieved from http://www.presidency.ucsb.edu/ws/?pid=14492

Rudd, R. A., Aleshire, N., Zibbell, J. E., & Gladden R. M. (2016). Increases in drug and opioid overdose deaths—United States, 2000–2014. *Morbidity & Mortality Weekly Report, 64*(50), 1378–1382.

Schryver, G. F. (1930). *A history of the Illinois Training School for Nurses, 1880–1929*. Chicago, IL: Board of Directors of the Illinois Training School for Nurses.

Seymer, L. (1960). *Florence Nightingale's nurses: The Nightingale Training School, 1860–1960*. London, England: Pitman Medical.

Simms, L. (1989). The evolution of education for nursing administration. In B. Henry, C. Arndt, M. Di Vincenti, & A. Marriner-Tomey (Eds.), *Dimensions of nursing administration: Theory, research, education, practice* (pp. 459–467). Cambridge, MA: Blackwell Scientific Publications.

Stafford, M., Taylor, J., Zimmerman, A., Henrick, A., Perry, K., & Lambke, M. (2000). Letters to the editor: "A new vision for collective bargaining." *Nursing Outlook, 48*(2), 92.

Wald, L. (1934). *Windows on Henry Street*. Boston, MA: Little, Brown.

Woodham-Smith, C. (1951). *Florence Nightingale*. New York, NY: McGraw-Hill.

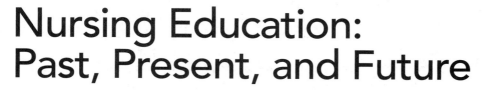

Nursing Education: Past, Present, and Future

Martha Scheckel

LEARNING OUTCOMES

After reading this chapter you will be able to:

- Develop an understanding of the historical evolutions, contributions, and differences of various nursing education programs.
- Critique contemporary options for nursing education in the context of social, political, and economic trends and issues.
- Explain the process of accreditation in nursing education.
- Analyze curriculum and instruction in relation to learning nursing practice.
- Develop a personal philosophy of nursing education that reflects trends and issues in nursing education and practice.

Introduction

This chapter provides a descriptive account of nursing education including how its past has shaped its present and how current times are influencing its future. Understanding the historical development of nursing education promotes an awareness of the diversity that exists within nursing education

31

and an understanding of the various academic pathways that have developed within nursing education and the complexities surrounding educational preparation for nursing practice.

This chapter begins with a discussion of the types of nursing education prevalent since the turn of the 20th century (see **Table 2-1**) and the issues associated with each program. The discussion covers practical/vocational nursing and progresses through the academic spectrum describing undergraduate programs for preparing registered nurses (RNs; associate and baccalaureate) and master's and doctoral graduate programs for providing advanced nursing education. The second half of the chapter focuses on curriculum and instruction in nursing education, including exemplars that describe what students learn and how they learn it in today's nursing schools. One might wonder why it is important for nursing students to understand curriculum and instruction. In the past, what and how students learned was the specialty of faculty. However, recent evidence suggests that learner-centered curriculum and instruction can improve student learning outcomes (Weimer, 2013), and the focus is on creating learning environments in which students play an increasingly active role in their own learning. Therefore, a goal of the latter part of this chapter is to promote dialogue between teachers and students to encourage

TABLE 2-1 THE HISTORICAL EVOLUTION OF NURSING EDUCATION PROGRAMS

Early 1900s	1920s–1930s	1940s–1950s	1960s–Present	Programs No Longer in Existence
Practical nursing	Practical nursing	Practical nursing	Practical nursing	
Nightingale Schools	Diploma schools	Diploma schools	Diploma schools	
Baccalaureate nursing programs	BSN	BSN	BSN	
Associate degree nursing programs		ADN	ADN	
Postgraduate nursing education	EdDs	Master's degrees	Master's degrees, PhD, DNS/DNSc, ND, DNP	ND

Abbreviations: ADN, associate degree in nursing; BSN, bachelor of science in nursing; DNP, doctor of nursing practice; DNS/DNSc, doctor of nursing science; EdD, doctor of education; ND, nursing doctor; PhD, doctor of philosophy.

mutual trust, respect, and understanding of the content and processes involved in preparing nursing students for contemporary nursing practice.

Students and teachers are encouraged to use this chapter as a platform for discussion, which can be further enriched by exploring the reference list provided at the end of the chapter. In this way, this chapter provides an excellent gateway to engage readers in the study of nursing education and to pursue ways of integrating its content with other sources of knowledge.

Understanding Nursing Education Programs

To gain an understanding of the various types of nursing education programs and the context within which they were developed, the discussion for each program provides a comprehensive overview that includes a historical account of the program's development, the unique and significant issues and challenges associated with the program, and information on contemporary trends related to the program. A description of academic progression (mobility) programs and a discussion of the educational accreditation process and its important role in ensuring high-quality nursing education programs are also included.

Practical/Vocational Nursing Education

Unlike the historically untrained or poorly trained practical nurse, who had unlimited and unsupervised freedom to practice, the present practical nurse is now often a hybrid. Today's practical/vocational nursing student (SPN/SVN) is being taught basic skills during the nursing program. After licensing, the LPN/LVN [practical nurse] is permitted to perform complex nursing, as assigned by the registered nurse (RN) and allowed by their state's nurse practice act. (Hill & Howlett, 2013, p. 71)

Responding to a Need: A Historical Overview of Practical/Vocational Nursing Education

Practical/vocational nursing began with the industrial revolution of the late 1800s. To meet workforce demands during this time, many people moved from rural areas to urban areas. Women needing employment often provided domestic services, including those associated with caring for the sick (Kurzen, 2012). To support the skills of this new healthcare provider, in 1892 the Young Women's Christian Association (YWCA) located in Brooklyn, New York, offered the first formal practical nursing course. Over time, landmark reports about the state of nursing education contributed to the development of practical/vocational nursing programs. For example, in 1923 Josephine Goldmark compiled a report titled *Nursing and Nursing Education in the United States* (see **Table 2-2**). In it she recommended higher education standards for practical nurses, laws regulating their practice, and improved environments for their training. In 1948 Lucille Brown compiled another report, *Nursing for the Future*, which hastened the growth of

TABLE 2-2 DOCUMENTS INFLUENCING TRENDS AND ISSUES IN NURSING EDUCATION

Name of Document	Year Published	Contribution to Nursing Education
Goldmark Report	1923	Studied the field of nursing education and recommended minimal education standards
Burgess Report	1928	Studied nursing practice and education and addressed the need for major changes in the profession and for the development of a more comprehensive educational philosophy
Brown Report	1948	Recommended vocational education for practical nurses and recommended that education for RNs be in an institution of higher learning
Ginzberg Report	1949	Suggested it would be more economical for hospitals to eliminate diploma nursing programs and begin a 2-year course of study for student nurses in colleges
Nursing Schools at the Mid-Century (West & Hawkins)	1950	Identified that many schools of nursing were not meeting standards, which provided evidence for reforming diploma nursing education
Community College Education for Nursing (Montag)	1959	Established the validity of the ADN (2-year nursing) program as adequate preparation for nursing practice
Toward Quality in Nursing (U.S. Public Health Service)	1963	Cautioned against preparing all nurses at the baccalaureate level
American Nurses' Association Position Statement (ANA)	1965	Stated that those licensed to practice nursing should be educationally prepared in institutions of higher education
National Commission for the Study of Nursing and Nursing Education	1970	Cautioned against preparing all nurses at the baccalaureate level
Pew Health Professions Report (O'Neil et al.)	1988	Identified competencies nurses would need to prepare for nursing practice in the 21st century
Institute of Medicine's *Future of Nursing* report	2011	Recommended strategies by which nurses could be maximally prepared to provide patient care in a reformed healthcare system

practical nursing programs by emphasizing vocational schools as good environments for practical nursing programs.

Working as a Practical/Vocational Nurse: Scope and Function

Since the first half of the 20th century, the scope and function of practical/vocational nurses have become increasingly sophisticated. Licensed to practice either as licensed practical nurses (LPNs) or as licensed vocational nurses (LVNs), they work under the supervision of RNs. Nurse practice acts for the practical/vocational nurse vary from state to state, but generally, the practical/vocational nurse is responsible for stable patients and patients with common health conditions. They also are responsible for collecting and reporting abnormal data, offering suggestions for developing and changing nursing care, providing bedside care, teaching health maintenance, and participating with the healthcare team in evaluating nursing care (Kurzen, 2012).

Understanding Practical/Vocational Nursing Education Today

The scope and function of practical/vocational nurses reflect the need for appropriate knowledge and skills, which are provided under the supervision of an RN or primary care provider (Kurzen, 2012). Practical/vocational nursing education programs are often offered in community colleges. Most programs are 12 to 18 months in length, and graduates of these programs complete a national practical/vocational nursing exam (National Council Licensure Examination for Practical Nurses [NCLEX-PN/VN]; see Chapter 4) prior to being employed. For some individuals, this short course of study is a stepping-stone to pursuing further nursing education to become an RN. It also allows them to work as a practical/vocational nurse while obtaining more nursing education. For others, practical/vocational nursing becomes a long-term career option. In either case, employment possibilities for practical/vocational nurses vary and are more plentiful in some states than in others. Long-term care facilities, clinics, hospitals, and home health care are the largest employers of practical/vocational nurses, with home health care leading the way in employment options.

According to the Bureau of Labor Statistics (2014), the need for practical/vocational nurses is expected to increase 25 percent from 2012 to 2022. The bureau reports that the increased need for practical/vocational nurses is primarily due to rising elderly populations who will need practical/vocational nurses to care for them in residential care facilities and home care.

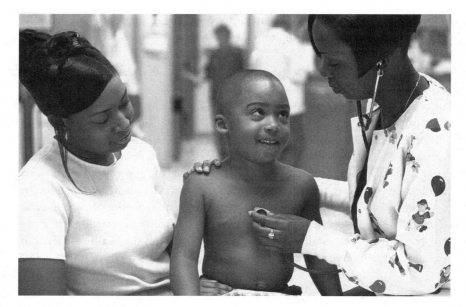

Nurse assessing patient's heart rate.
© Creatas/Alamy Images

Diploma Nursing Education

Your own first steps toward a nurse's skill—and toward the coveted nurse's cap," Miss Reamer said, "Will be classes. But not for long." They [student nurses] would learn the hospital routine gradually on the wards, then more and more, until each student would be responsible for her own patients. (Wells, 1943, p. 29)

Training vs. Educating: The History of Diploma Nursing Education

The quotation is from *Cherry Ames*, a popular fictional series of books about nurses that enamored many, encouraged the pursuit of nursing careers, and indeed reflected diploma nursing programs of that time in nursing education's history. Diploma nursing (originally known as "hospital nursing") began during the latter part of the 19th century with a growth in hospitals. Training of hospital nurses at this time was based on an **apprenticeship model** where nursing students provided service (direct patient care) in exchange for a few educational lectures, room and board, and a monthly allowance (King, 1987). The apprenticeship model flourished because it offered women an opportunity for a vocation, it improved care of the sick, and decreased the cost of nursing service in hospitals while student nurses provided patient care services for a minimal allowance (Bullough & Bullough, 1978).

Despite the benefits of the apprenticeship model, it underwent criticism from nursing education leaders. Goldmark (1923) in

> **KEY TERM**
>
> **Apprenticeship model:** A model of nursing education that was prevalent during the first half of the 20th century, where student nurses learned nursing practice by providing service to hospitals.

particular emphasized that the training needs of students and the service needs of hospitals were incongruent. She wrote that when "the needs of the sick must predominate; the needs of education must yield" (p. 195). Training in the care of children, for example, was relinquished if students were needed to care for patients on the surgical ward. Similarly, May Ayres Burgess published a report in 1928 titled *Nurses, Patients, and Pocketbooks* (later known as the Burgess Report), which contended that within the apprenticeship model, students' patient assignments were based on the hospital's needs rather than on the educational needs of the students.

To balance the academic needs of nursing students with their need for clinical experiences, Dr. Richard Olding Beard advocated for university education for nursing students, and in 1909 he founded a nursing program at the University of Minnesota. This program is often heralded as the first baccalaureate nursing program. However, it closely resembled diploma education because, even though nursing students met university standards for admission and coursework, they were required to work 56 hours a week on the hospital ward (Bullough & Bullough, 1984).

Shifting to a New Era in Diploma Nursing Education

Following Dr. Beard's efforts, the **National League for Nursing Education (NLNE)** made numerous attempts to redesign diploma nursing education programs. In 1917, 1919, 1927, and 1937 the NLNE published *Standard Curriculum for Schools of Nursing,* encouraging diploma programs to decrease students' time working on the ward and to increase their education by offering 3 years of coursework in the sciences and clinical experiences caring for diverse populations (e.g., medical–surgical, pediatric, and obstetric patients).

> **KEY TERM**
>
> **National League for Nursing Education (NLNE):** A professional nursing organization that fostered excellence in nursing education by supporting nursing education research, engaging in policymaking and advocacy efforts related to nursing education, and promoting faculty development. It was the precursor to the National League for Nursing.

During the middle of the 20th century, diploma nursing programs continued to thrive. However, changes in health care such as rapid advances in medical technology and the expansion of knowledge in disease treatment required nurses to have sound theoretical preparation (Melosh, 1982). These changes signified a decline in hospital-based diploma programs and the beginning of a new era in nursing education where education would occur predominantly in colleges and universities.

Understanding Diploma Nursing Education Today

As of 2012 there were approximately 60 diploma programs in the United States (National League for Nursing [NLN], 2013). Hospitals that continue to support diploma programs maintain this educational option because these programs supply the nurses needed in their hospitals, provide a geographically accessible program for some students, and offer a nursing degree in a short length of time. To meet further educational needs of students enrolled in diploma programs, many of these programs collaborate with colleges and universities to offer students options to obtain associate and baccalaureate degrees.

Associate Degree Nursing Education

Every story in the mosaic of history has a beginning, a cast of characters, a set of social circumstances, and its own momentum. The development of a new, two year program for educating professional nurses during the years just after World War II is no exception. (Haase, 1990, p. 1)

Creating New Models of Nursing Education: The History of Associate Degree Nursing Education

The development of associate degree nursing (ADN) education began in response to the post–World War II nursing shortage and gained momentum following the Ginzberg Report (1949), which suggested that, in comparison to a 4-year nursing program, it would be more efficient and economical for colleges to offer a 2-year course of study in nursing. Ginzberg did not believe that all nurses needed baccalaureate education to provide patient care. Through associate degree programs, nurses could be prepared to provide safe and competent patient care in less time than required in baccalaureate education, which would provide a feasible solution to the nursing shortage.

It was at this time that Mildred Montag (1951) described how 2-year ADN programs, housed in community colleges, could prepare RNs as semiprofessionals. This group of RNs would meet the demand for nurses by acquiring enough nursing skill and judgment to provide nursing care but not the expert skill and judgment of baccalaureate-prepared nurses. Further study by Montag (1959) suggested that nurses prepared with an associate degree were performing similarly to staff nurses prepared with baccalaureate degrees. Moreover, those within the nursing profession believed that, with the exception of preparation in leadership and public health, nurses with an associate degree provided outstanding bedside nursing care (Smith, 1960). Others contended the associate degree program's focus on learning rather than on service to hospitals provided educationally sound preparation for nursing practice (Lewis, 1964). For the first time in the history of nursing education, the associate degree in nursing offered those with little access to baccalaureate nursing programs the opportunity to become RNs (Hassenplug, 1965).

KEY TERM

American Nurses Association (ANA): A professional organization for nurses that develops various standards of nursing practice and promotes change through policy development.

Controversies in Associate Degree Nursing Education

Historically there have been many advantages identified with ADN education, and these advantages remain present in today's ADN programs. Nevertheless, in 1965 at the height of the success of ADN programs, the **American Nurses Association (ANA)** published a position paper stating that those licensed to practice nursing should be prepared in institutions of higher education (universities) and that the minimum preparation for the professional nurse should be a baccalaureate degree. This potentially meant that associate degree–prepared nurses could not practice as RNs unless they had licensure requirements that were different from baccalaureate-prepared nurses.

Despite these challenging circumstances, studies conducted since the ANA's position paper through the 1990s showed that, especially in hospital settings, there were unclear differentiations between nurses prepared in ADN programs and those prepared in baccalaureate degree programs (Bullough, Bullough, & Soukup, 1983; Bullough & Sparks, 1975; Haase, 1990). In fact, many studies showed RNs performed essentially the same in practice regardless of academic preparation. Studies occurring in the 2000s, however, began to present a different picture. Research suggests that baccalaureate-prepared nurses are equipped to fulfill complex contemporary nursing roles through a broad range of competencies (e.g., leadership and systems thinking skills, evidence-based practice and research skills), contribute to improved patient outcomes and lower patient mortality rates, and are preferred by hospitals, particularly teaching, children's, and "magnet" hospitals (Institute of Medicine [IOM], 2011). This is not to say that ADN programs will cease to exist. However, these studies do indicate that academic progression (mobility) programs in which associate degree–prepared nurses obtain baccalaureate and higher degrees in nursing, will take on even greater significance than they have in the past.

Understanding Associate Degree Nursing Education Today

According to the U.S. Department of Health and Human Services Health Resources and Services Administration (2010), 45.4 percent of those wishing to become nurses enter ADN or associate degree in science (ASN) programs. As a result, these programs remain one of the most feasible options for becoming an RN. Faculty of ADN/ASN programs take responsibility for preparing graduates for RN roles within structured settings such as medical-surgical nursing, maternity, and pediatrics in hospitals (Hendricks, 2016). However, it is important to note that only 20.8 percent of ADNs return to school for baccalaureate and higher degrees (U.S. Department of Health and Human Services Health Resources and Services Administration, 2010). Because the associate degree in nursing is considered an entry-level degree into practice as an RN, it is important to support efforts toward creating seamless academic progression programs that facilitate ADNs' attainment of a baccalaureate or higher degree in nursing (Organization for Associate Degree Nursing & American Nurses Association, 2015).

Baccalaureate Nursing Education

Very many private schools [hospital schools] of nursing still exist, but like the private schools of medicine that remain, there is a handwriting upon the walls of their future. . . .

It says that their days are numbered, that 'the old order changeth, giving place to the new,' that the day of the university education of the nurse has come. (Beard, 1920, p. 955)

Advocating for University Education: The History of Baccalaureate Nursing Education

Dr. Richard Olding Beard (just quoted), a great supporter of baccalaureate nursing education, followed the thinking of Florence Nightingale and the **Nightingale Schools**. Nightingale believed that nursing education should occur outside of hospitals and the medical model (Stewart, 1943). This model of nursing education would avoid apprenticeships where nursing students received less education in the principles of nursing care because they were providing long hours of service to hospitals. Nightingale advocated for nursing students to learn sound theory in anatomy and physiology, surgery, chemistry, nutrition, sanitation, and professionalism; to train under the guidance of ward sisters who were nurses with experience and dedication to the profession; and to be part of a system that was financially independent from hospitals (Stewart, 1943).

> **KEY TERM**
>
> **Nightingale Schools:** Schools of nursing developed by Florence Nightingale that promoted student nurses learning the theory and practice of nursing outside of hospital control.

The Nightingale philosophy initially succeeded in the United States when Bellevue School of Nursing in New York adopted it in 1873. However, opposition to it, which included arguments that nurses do not need to be overeducated, that hospitals needed nurses for service, and that independent funding for nursing schools was unrealistic, maintained diploma nursing education. Despite the overwhelming support for diploma schools, several nursing education leaders during the early 1900s continued to advocate for baccalaureate nursing education. For example, in 1901, Ethel Gordon Bedford Fenwick, founder of the International Council of Nurses, asserted it was time for nurses to be educated in universities where they could become skilled practitioners able to address local, national, and international health issues (Fenwick, 1901). In 1909 the University of Minnesota established the first baccalaureate nursing program in the United States beginning the slow movement toward baccalaureate education for nurses in place of diploma education.

Struggling to Develop Baccalaureate Nursing Education

Many schools followed the University of Minnesota's example of offering students courses that supplemented diploma education. The most progressive of these programs was started at Teachers College, Columbia University, in 1917. Here students received 2 years of science at the university, 2 years of nursing at Presbyterian Hospital in New York, and 1 year of specialization in either public health or education (Bullough & Bullough, 1978). By the 1930s the number of students completing this "collegiate curricula" doubled, but these emerging baccalaureate programs remained chaotic and often resembled today's graduate education with an emphasis on specialization in public health, teaching, administration, and clinical specialties (Stewart, 1943, p. 276).

In the 1940s the development of baccalaureate nursing education continued, but the struggle to develop curricula for it and define nursing roles from within it remained problematic. The Brown Report was especially helpful in making bold statements about baccalaureate nursing education. Brown (1948) wrote that nursing education belonged in institutions of higher education and that curricula in higher education for nursing education be integrated to include both liberal and technical training to support professional nursing practice. Brown also stated that the degree granted should be the bachelor of science in nursing and that these nurses be prepared for complex clinical situations requiring high levels of education and skill.

By the 1960s baccalaureate education was becoming increasingly differentiated from diploma or associate degree education. In particular, preparation in liberal education, intellectual skills, and content in leadership, management, community health, and teaching contributed to this differentiation (Kelly & Joel, 2002). The struggle for baccalaureate education seemed to be resolving, and the ANA position paper (1965) calling for the baccalaureate to be the entry-level degree for nursing strengthened the argument for baccalaureate education. Nonetheless, other groups, including the Surgeon General's Consultant Group's document *Toward Quality in Nursing* (U.S. Public Health Service, 1963) and the National Commission for the Study of Nursing and Nursing Education (1970) were cautious in firmly stating that all licensed nurses needed baccalaureate preparation. These groups advocated for additional research to understand the skills and responsibilities required for high quality patient care. But this specific research (described in the next section) would not occur until nearly 40 years later.

Understanding Baccalaureate Nursing Education Today

Since the 1960s, baccalaureate nursing education programs have doubled. Today there are approximately 696 baccalaureate programs (National League for Nursing, 2013). Enrollments in these programs steadily increased for 13 consecutive years, until 2012 when there was only a 2.6 percent increase in program enrollments, which was the lowest increase since 2007 (American Association of Colleges of Nursing, 2014a). Until the 2000s, little research existed that responded to calls put forth in the 1960s to understand the relationship between educational preparation and high-quality patient care. A series of contemporary studies has shown that hospitals with more baccalaureate-prepared nurses have better patient outcomes, including lower patient mortality rates (Blegen, Goode, Park, Vaughn, & Spetz, 2013; Kutney-Lee, Sloane, & Aiken, 2013; Yakusheva, Lindrooth, & Weiss, 2014).

As evidence mounts showing the relationship between higher education for nurses and improved patient outcomes, the momentum for the baccalaureate degree as the degree needed for entry-level practice as an RN has increased.

Contemporary Practice Highlight 2-1 details the IOM's (2011) recommendation regarding increasing the number of baccalaureate-prepared nurses, and subsequent employer preferences for hiring nurses with a baccalaureate degree. What matters here is that support for baccalaureate nursing education does not mean opposing practical, associate, or diploma nursing education. Rather, it means encouraging nurses without baccalaureate degrees to pursue this degree, becoming active in making baccalaureate education accessible and affordable, and working as a team regardless of the academic preparation of a nurse.

Graduate Education: Master's and Doctoral Degrees

When one turns to the other . . . he [sic] finds a distinct possibility that a fresh and conspicuously enlarged contribution may soon come from many more nurses who find places of great social and professional usefulness in consultation, planning, research, writing, and the promotion of health services. (Brown, 1948, p. 98)

Advancing Nursing Education: The History of Master's Preparation in Nursing Education

The quote by Esther Lucille Brown was a prelude to the formation of nursing education programs that granted master's degrees in nursing. At the time of her statement in 1948 few nurses had master's degrees (known at that time as "specialties");

CONTEMPORARY PRACTICE HIGHLIGHT 2–1

BACCALAUREATE EDUCATION POLICY INITIATIVES

In 2011 the Institute of Medicine (IOM) published a report titled *The Future of Nursing: Leading Change, Advancing Health*. The purpose of the report was to identify and recommend ways nurses could be maximally prepared to provide patient-centered, safe, high-quality, and equitable nursing care in reformed healthcare systems. One of the recommendations was to increase the number of nurses with a baccalaureate degree to 80 percent by 2020. The report suggests that nurses with a baccalaureate degree have the educational preparation to provide nursing care in a manner that meets the demands of contemporary healthcare systems. The report further emphasizes that an all-baccalaureate prepared nursing workforce will provide "a uniform foundation" (p. 170) for nursing roles within a reformed healthcare system. Since the publication of the IOM report and ongoing studies linking baccalaureate nursing education with improved patient outcomes, 79.6 percent of healthcare employers are demonstrating a preference for hiring nurses with baccalaureate nursing degrees, and 45.1 percent of healthcare employers are requiring that newly hired nurses have a baccalaureate degree (American Association of College of Nursing, 2014b).

instead, many with preparation beyond basic nursing education had postgraduate education. Postgraduate education was training nurses received through internships in specific clinical areas or theoretical preparation in public health and nursing education (Bullough et al., 1983). It also included additional training for nursing supervision and administration (Brown, 1948). Prior to the 1950s, if nurses wanted to obtain a master's degree rather than postgraduate education, they had to seek an advanced degree in another field such as sociology or psychology (Bullough & Bullough, 1984).

During the 1950s the first master's degree in nursing was established when Rutgers University in New Jersey offered a master's degree in psychiatric nursing. As master's in nursing programs grew, support for them also increased. In 1969 and 1978 the ANA advocated for advanced preparation of nurses in theory to improve practice. They also advocated for specialty nursing roles to offer high-level competence in particular areas of nursing practice. By the 1970s societal trends encouraged an even greater demand for master's in nursing programs (Murphy, 1981). For instance, healthcare environments needed nurses with advanced preparation in areas such as research, teaching, administration, and clinical areas of nursing practice. The Council of Baccalaureate and Higher Degree Programs (1985) of the NLN provided further support for master's preparation by stating that the nation needed nurses prepared with master's degrees in nursing to meet society's nursing needs.

Despite support for master's education for nurses, Starck (1987) argued that by the 1980s there were far too many (totaling 257 titles) master's degree nursing programs, which served only to confuse the public. Starck recommended the curriculum of master's programs be reformed so that all master's-prepared nurses would receive core preparation in "leadership, management, teaching, intellectual curiosity, creative inquiry, collaborative and consultative skills, and professionalism" (p. 20). This preparation would prepare nurses to work in settings where autonomy and fiscal management skills were needed. Starck projected increases in healthcare costs would lead to the need for master's-prepared nurses to manage community-based nursing centers and to oversee companies providing services to hospitals.

Understanding Master's Preparation in Nursing Education Today

Starck (1987) was correct in projecting the need for master's-prepared nurses to function within a greater scope (e.g., there are now community-based clinics managed by nurse practitioners). Today there are over 330 master's nursing programs in existence in the United States, including but not limited to, clinical nurse specialist, nurse educator, nurse practitioner, midwifery, and nurse anesthetist (Dracup, 2015). In recent years, the rise of the Doctor of Nursing Practice (DNP) degree is creating questions about the continued need for the master's degree in nursing, causing a decline in the number of clinically oriented master's programs (Gerard, Kazer, Babington, & Quell, 2014). In 2004 the American Association of Colleges of Nursing's *Position Statement on the Practice Doctorate in Nursing* identified a need for nurses to use high levels of clinical, fiscal, organizational, and leadership expertise to ensure high-quality healthcare outcomes. These high levels of expertise require that nurses be prepared at the doctoral level. Subsequently, with the exception of the clinical nursing leader (CNL), the need for master's-prepared nurses may decrease in the future.

The CNL is a master's degree in nursing that focuses on generalist preparation, rather than specialist preparation (American Association of Colleges of Nursing [AACN], 2007). The reason for developing such a role comes from evidence suggesting a need for nurses with master's education and an understanding of the broader healthcare system to develop methods for improving patient outcomes, coordinate evidence-based practice, and promote client self-care and client decision making. The development of the CNL has been controversial. There are those who contend that the CNL only adds confusion to the multiple existing graduate education pathways, that its development undermines the roles of other nursing specialists (e.g., nurse practitioners and clinical nurse specialists), and that it minimizes the leadership role of every professional nurse (Gardenier, 2012). However, recent evidence suggests that, when healthcare systems implemented the CNL role, there were improvements in patient care outcomes (Bender, 2014). Bender (2014) also points out that studies suggest CNLs do continue to experience

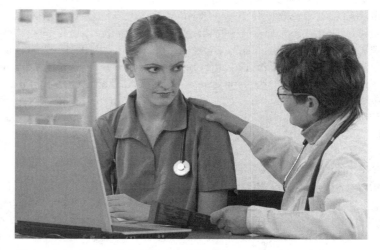

Nursing student with clinical nursing instructor.
© NotarYES/Shutterstock

challenges in defining their role. These challenges highlight the need for continued dialogue about the role of the CNL, the continued need for research about its efficacy, and the overall impact of this role in nursing practice specifically and in healthcare systems generally. It is clear that there remains a need in the United States for nurses prepared at the master's-degree level. The complexity of the healthcare system, the critical shortage of nurse educators, and the need for advanced practice nurses to deliver cost-effective, evidence-based patient care are just three of the driving forces that require nurses be prepared beyond the baccalaureate level to provide leadership in nursing administration, education, and practice.

Developing the Discipline of Nursing: The History of Doctoral Education in Nursing

Doctoral education for nurses has existed since the 1920s. Doctoral programs originally prepared nurses for administrative and teaching roles. The first program was offered in 1924 at Teachers College, Columbia University, where nurses received an educational doctorate (EdD). Nurses received EdDs because the nursing profession had not developed its own doctoral programs, these doctorates were accessible through programs that offered part-time study, and the programs discriminated less against women as compared to programs in other fields (Bullough & Bullough, 1984). It was not until the latter part of the 20th century that doctoral programs in nursing developed. They developed out of recognition that the nursing profession needed its own research and theoretical base. As a result, doctoral programs in nursing dramatically increased, and offered nurses the opportunity to conduct research and develop theory within their own discipline.

The PhD (doctorate of philosophy) in nursing is the terminal degree for ensuring nurses are competent to conduct research, which develops nursing knowledge and theory (Bednash, Breslin, Kirschling, & Rosseter, 2014). Despite the long established merit of the PhD, in the 1960s Boston University initiated another doctoral degree, the DNSc, or the clinical doctorate. The intent of the DNSc was to prepare nurses for doctoral-level work in clinical practice, rather than research and theory (Ponte & Nicholas, 2015). Regardless of its original intent as a clinical doctorate, studies over time have indicated that the DNSc (also known as the DNS or DSN), is in many respects equivalent to the PhD (Ponte & Nicholas, 2015).

Another alternative option to the PhD was developed in the 1970s when Margaret Newman of New York University advocated for the ND (doctor of nursing) program. Similar to the DNSc, with the noted exception that the ND also prepared individuals for basic licensure as an RN, she believed an ND would prepare nurses just as medical schools prepare physicians—for application of advanced knowledge in clinical practice. The first ND program began in 1979 at Case Western Reserve

University in Cleveland, Ohio. An educational option that was never extensively embraced by the profession, all ND programs subsequently closed as the PhD in nursing programs expanded, and the ND degree is no longer in existence.

Understanding Doctoral Preparation in Nursing Education Today

There are presently 133 PhD (research-focused) doctoral programs in the United States, up from 103 programs in 2006 (Kirschling, 2014). The steady increase in research-focused doctoral programs reflect a strong interest in doctoral programs that ensure the generation of nursing knowledge.

The DNP (doctor of nursing practice), proposed by the **American Association of Colleges of Nursing** in 2004 (AACN, 2004), is the newest nursing doctorate. It is the terminal degree for advanced practice nursing roles, which include, but are not limited to, nurse administrator, certified registered nurse anesthetist, nurse midwife, and nurse practitioner. The DNP is comparable to practice doctorates in fields such as pharmacy and physical therapy. The DNP provides advanced preparation in scientific foundations of nursing practice, leadership, evidence-based practice, healthcare technologies, healthcare policy, interprofessional collaboration, clinical prevention and population-based health care, and advanced nursing practice in specialty areas (AACN, 2006). This preparation provides the basis for building a cadre of nurses who can assess and design healthcare systems that are responsive to rapidly changing and complex healthcare environments (AACN, 2015a).

> **KEY TERM**
>
> **American Association of Colleges of Nursing (AACN):** A professional organization in nursing that serves baccalaureate nursing and higher degree nursing education programs by influencing the quality of nursing education and practice through research, advocacy efforts, policymaking, development of high-quality educational standards and indicators, and faculty development.

Today there are 246 DNP programs (AACN, 2015a), including both RN-to-DNP and MSN-to-DNP programs. As increasing numbers of nurses prepared with the DNP enter the workforce, it is important to understand how DNP-prepared advanced practice nurses are contributing to the nursing profession and healthcare delivery, particularly how they are affecting changes in practice (Redman, Pressler, Furspan, & Potempa, 2015; see **Contemporary Practice Highlight 2-2**). It will also be essential to help the public and other healthcare providers understand the role of the nurse prepared with the DNP degree.

Nurses who are considering the pursuit of doctoral education will need to carefully consider which doctoral degree is the best fit for their professional career goals—the PhD, DNS, or DNSc degree with a research focus or a practice focused doctorate such as the DNP. The PhD, DNS, and DNSc degrees prepare nurses to conduct research and add to nursing science, whereas a DNP degree prepares nurses to improve patient outcomes and translate research for use in practice (AACN, 2014c).

CONTEMPORARY PRACTICE HIGHLIGHT 2-2

ADOPTING THE BSN-TO-DNP AS ENTRY INTO ADVANCED PRACTICE REGISTERED NURSE ROLES

In 2013, the AACN asked the RAND Corporation, a nonprofit institution aimed at improving policy and decision making through research, to explore nursing program offerings that prepare advanced practice registered nurses (APRNs). The AACN wanted RAND to identify barriers and facilitators to nursing programs fully adopting the DNP. In other words, they were interested in knowing why some schools continue APRN master's programs whereas others have eliminated the master's degree for APRN preparation and offer only the DNP for attaining an APRN. The RAND Corporation's report provided six recommendations, which included a need for the AACN to (a) conduct studies documenting the impact of the DNP on patient care; (b) provide outreach and data to healthcare facilities for the purpose of understanding DNP skills sets; (c) document strategies schools are using to overcome barriers to offering the BSN-to-DNP; (d) showcase academic-practice collaborations providing clinical practicum experiences for DNP students; (e) provide clarity and guidance for capstone projects; and (f) assist schools to overcome challenges to offering BSN-to-DNP programs. The RAND Corporation suggested that full adoption of the BSN-to-DNP will be slow unless policies require the DNP as entry into APRN roles and students and employers better understand the benefits of the DNP role.

Data from American Association of Colleges of Nursing. (2015b). *The DNP by 2015: A study of the institutional, political, and professional issues that facilitate or impede establishing a post-baccalaureate doctor of nursing practice program.* Retrieved from http://www.aacn.nche.edu /dnp/DNP-Study.pdf

Academic Progression in Nursing Education

There is more depth to my practice now. I see nursing theory behind everything I do. (Delaney & Piscopo, 2007, p. 170)

Deepening one's knowledge base and understanding of nursing as well as advancing one's nursing career often occur through programs that support academic progression in nursing education. **Academic progression programs** (also known as educational mobility or career ladder programs) enable individuals to enter the nursing profession from different educational points or pursue professional career development through a seamless articulation between programs, without losing credits from previous degree work. This additional academic preparation often involves articulating or making a transition from one nursing degree to another, more advanced nursing degree.

For example, there are LPN/VN, RN-to-BSN, RN-to-MSN, and BSN-to-PhD (or DNP) academic progression options. The RN-to-BSN or RN-to-MSN degree programs enable RNs who hold a diploma in nursing or an

> **KEY TERM**
>
> **Academic progression programs:** Nursing programs that facilitate the seamless articulation or transition from one degree in nursing to another degree (e.g., LPN to RN, ASN to BSN, ASN to MSN, BSN to PhD).

ADN (ASN) degree to return to school to pursue either a BSN or an MSN degree and receive credit for their previous coursework and possibly their work experience. There are also programs for those individuals who hold previous nonnursing baccalaureate degrees that enable them to complete a BSN in an accelerated time frame, usually within 12 to 18 months. These are commonly referred to as second-degree, fast track, or accelerated nursing programs. Accelerated programs for those individuals with previous nonnursing baccalaureate degrees who wish to receive a generic master's degree in nursing (leading to licensure as an RN), also exist.

The commonality in all of the academic progression options is that they enable the learner to achieve the advanced degree in a timely manner by recognizing and giving credit for previous academic accomplishments. Obtaining credit for previous academic accomplishments is often referred to as prior learning assessment (PLA). PLA is "the process of granting college credit, certification, or advanced standing toward further education or training" (Klein-Collins & Wertheim, 2013, p. 51). For example, PLA can include permitting the learner to prepare a portfolio documenting prior academic or work experiences that are evaluated for potential academic credit.

Advancing one's nursing practice can also occur through continuing education programs that result in specialized credentials, certifications, or continuing education credits. For example, nurses can obtain additional education to become certified in diabetes education, critical care, or wound and ostomy care. They can also obtain continuing education by attending conferences or completing online courses or independent studies on particular topics relevant to their area of practice.

Supporting Academic Progression Programs

Academic progression programs have a long history in nursing education and, in recent years, many of these programs have increased in enrollment due to progress in distance education technologies, making advanced education more accessible. These programs have also flourished with support from various professional organizations in nursing, health care, and education to promote baccalaureate and higher degrees in nursing. For example, in 2012 the American Association of Community Colleges, AACN, Association of Community College Trustees, NLN, and National Organization for Associate Degree Nursing issued a "Joint Statement on Academic Progression for Nursing Students and Graduates" (AACN, 2012). The statement promoted seamless progression to higher degrees in nursing and access to advanced nursing degrees for every nursing student and nurse. The Future of Nursing: Campaign for Action is a national initiative that supports the statement (see http://www.campaignforaction.org) and promotes the development of innovative and seamless academic progression educational models through its Academic Progression in Nursing (APIN) program (Gerardi, 2014).

Reflecting on the Advantages and Disadvantages of Academic Progression Programs

Academic progression programs offer students flexible and dynamic options for advancing nursing careers. They are also often affordable and accessible and can expedite the attainment of advanced degrees. For instance, students who wish to start their nursing career as an associate degree–prepared RN can attend a community college. Once they decide to pursue a baccalaureate degree, they can continue working as an RN and complete an online baccalaureate completion program or a program at a nearby college or university. Or they may decide to pursue a master's degree in nursing and opt to enroll in an RN-to-MSN program.

Disadvantages of academic progression options can include, but are not limited to, increased time commitments to complete coursework, problems with transferring credits from school to school and gaining credit for prior learning, and risks associated with returning to school when one is faced with competing career and family demands. Students who are considering academic progression programs are encouraged to investigate programs prior to enrollment to ensure they have a comprehensive understanding of admission policies and curricular requirements.

Accreditation in Nursing Education

Accreditation is a process by which an institution's (e.g., school of nursing's) programs, policies, and practices are reviewed by an external accrediting body to determine whether professional standards are being met. Accreditation is also considered to be a means of fostering continuous quality improvement in programs because faculty participate in the process to review and reflect upon all aspects of their program, with the goal of maintaining and improving quality.

In the United States there are three national nursing accrediting bodies. Schools of nursing can be accredited by the **Accreditation Commission for Education in Nursing (ACEN)**, the American Association of Colleges of Nursing **Commission on Collegiate Nursing Education (CCNE)**, or the **National League for Nursing Commission for Nursing Education Accreditation (NLN CNEA)**. ACEN and NLN CNEA accredit all programs of nursing, whereas the CCNE limits their accreditation activities to BSN, MSN, and DNP programs. **Contemporary Practice Highlight 2-3** presents the NLN CNEA as the newest nursing accreditation body and its accreditation standards.

KEY TERM

Accreditation: A process by which an institution's (e.g., school of nursing's) programs, policies, and practices are reviewed by an external accrediting body to determine whether professional standards are being met.

KEY TERM

Accreditation Commission for Education in Nursing (ACEN): This commission is an accrediting body and Title IV gatekeeper for federal funds for all types of nursing education programs.

KEY TERM

Commission on Collegiate Nursing Education (CCNE): Affiliated with the American Association of Colleges of Nursing, this commission is an accrediting body for baccalaureate and higher degree nursing education programs.

KEY TERM

National League for Nursing Commission for Nursing Education Accreditation (NLN CNEA): Affiliated with the National League for Nursing, this commission is an accrediting body for PN/VN, Diploma, ASN/ADN, BSN, MSN, and DNP nursing programs.

NATIONAL LEAGUE FOR NURSING COMMISSION FOR NURSING EDUCATION ACCREDITATION

The National League for Nursing Commission for Nursing Education Accreditation (NLN CNEA) is the newest nursing accrediting body established in 2013. The mission of NLN CNEA is to promote excellence and integrity in nursing education through accrediting all types of nursing education programs. This accrediting body values a culture of caring, diversity, integrity, and excellence. Its standards for accreditation include Standard I–Culture of Excellence: Program Outcomes; Standard II–Culture of Integrity and Accountability: Mission, Governance, and Resources; Standard III–Culture of Excellence and Caring: Faculty; Standard IV–Culture of Excellence and Caring: Students; Standard V–Culture of Learning and Diversity: Curriculum and Evaluation Processes. These standards are intended to respect the diversity of nursing programs, promote a culture of ongoing quality improvement, and prepare a competent and caring nursing workforce.

Data from National League for Nursing Commission for Nursing Education Accreditation. (2016). Accreditation standards for nursing education programs. Retrieved from http://www.nln.org/docs/default-source /accreditation-services/cnea-standards-final-february -201613f2bf5c78366c709642ff00005f0421.pdf?sfvrsn=4

Participation in the accreditation process of any of the nursing accrediting bodies is usually a voluntary activity that schools undertake for the professional and public acknowledgment of the quality of their programs. In recent times, some states have passed legislation to make nursing program accreditation mandatory. Although accreditation has historically been a voluntary activity, it is an extremely meaningful one to the school and its students, because in some cases, students can be denied access to scholarships/grants or admission to undergraduate or graduate programs if they are not enrolled in or graduates of a professionally accredited school. When choosing a nursing program, prospective students should always investigate whether or not the program is accredited by a nursing accrediting body. In addition to nursing's professional accrediting bodies, all schools of nursing are required to be approved for operation by the appropriate state board of nursing. Rules and regulations governing the operation of nursing programs can be found in state board of nursing nurse practice acts. State boards of nursing have the statutory authority to close down the operation of nursing schools if school performance does not meet the standards set forth by the respective state board.

The quality of nursing programs is measured through nationally established standards or criteria. Standards can include such things as how the school is fulfilling its mission and philosophy, how its curriculum is preparing students for nursing practice, and how academically and experientially qualified the faculty are to fulfill their teaching role.

Nursing accrediting bodies accredit nursing programs for a set period of time, usually 5 to 10 years, depending upon the agency and the review findings. Throughout the accreditation period, schools continue to use professional standards as benchmarks to evaluate their program, making necessary changes to ensure they maintain quality.

Curriculum and Instruction in Nursing Education

Central to nursing education are curriculum and instruction. **Curriculum** is the overall structure of nursing education programs that reflects schools' mission and philosophy, course of study, and learning experiences faculty and students engage in to achieve learning outcomes. **Instruction** consists of the teaching and learning strategies faculty and students engage in to achieve the elements of a curriculum. Throughout the history of nursing education various trends and issues have influenced curriculum and instruction. For example, advances in germ theory added to what students learned about aseptic technique, progress in pharmacology changed what students learned about drug therapies, and research in educational theory changed how teachers taught as well as understanding how students learn.

KEY TERM

Curriculum: The overall structure of nursing education programs that reflects a school of nursing's mission and philosophy, program outcomes, course of study, learning experiences, and program evaluation methods.

KEY TERM

Instruction: Teaching and learning strategies faculty and students engage in to achieve the elements of a curriculum.

What follows are examples of current trends and issues influencing curriculum and instruction in nursing programs. The purpose of the overview is to provide an understanding of why students are learning what they are learning in their curriculum (i.e., important topics) and why teachers use particular methods of teaching and learning (i.e., important methods).

Learning Nursing: Important Topics in Nursing Education

Patient Safety

Teaching concepts related to patient safety remains a priority in nursing education. In recent years, due to widely publicized medical errors, patient safety has taken on even greater importance. This, in turn, sharpened the focus of patient safety in nursing education, as reflected by the Quality and Safety Education for Nurses (QSEN) project (Case Western Reserve University [CWRU], 2014). QSEN's goal is to prepare nursing students with the knowledge, attitudes, and skills to ensure quality and safety in healthcare (CWRU, 2014). Since its beginning in 2005, QSEN has influenced how nursing students are prepared to understand the practices and principles of reducing medical errors (refer to the QSEN website at www.qsen.org). Chapter 8 provides a further discussion of patient safety and creating a culture of safety in healthcare systems.

Cultural Competence

Cultural competence is the extent to which a nurse understands and has the skills required to effectively address the healthcare needs of individuals who hold cultural beliefs and values that are different from his or her own. As society becomes increasingly diverse and global in nature, there is an increased emphasis on teaching concepts related to cultural competence in nursing curricula. For example, according to the U.S. Census Bureau (2015), by 2020 it is anticipated that over 50 percent of children in the United States will be from a minority race or ethnic group, and that by 2060, only 36 percent of children will be single-race non-Hispanic white. The bureau predicts that this trend will result in the population of the United States becoming a majority-minority by 2044. Therefore, nurses will work with healthcare providers and provide care to patients who have cultural backgrounds with which they are not familiar. Nursing programs are integrating coursework and clinical experiences related to cultural diversity and global health care into the curriculum. These experiences can include, but are not limited to, clinical experiences in other countries and learning with nursing students who live in other countries (Edmonds, 2012). Chapter 14 provides a comprehensive discussion of cultural issues that affect nursing practice.

Gerontology

According to the Centers for Disease Control and Prevention (2013), by 2030 the number of people over the age of 65 will have doubled to 71 million, which will comprise 20 percent of the American population. In a response to this trend,

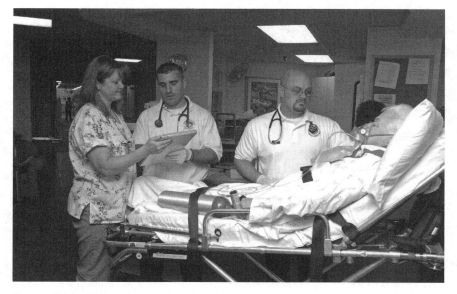

Nurses caring for an elderly patient in the emergency room.
© Jones and Bartlett Learning. Courtesy of MIEMSS.

professional nursing organizations such as AACN and NLN have developed a number of competencies, teaching resources, and curriculum guides to assist nursing faculty in preparing undergraduate and graduate nursing students to care for the elderly population. The importance of having a critical mass of nurses prepared to care for the growing population of elderly in the United States cannot be overstated. It is important for gerontology concepts and experiences to be integrated throughout nursing curricula to provide students with the skills required to care for both the well and ill elderly. The elderly as a vulnerable population is addressed in Chapter 13.

Evidence-Based Practice

Evidence-based practice is an approach to nursing care where nurses draw on the best research evidence available to make clinical decisions. In nursing, evidence-based practice includes nurses' use of research studies and theory from within nursing and outside of nursing (e.g., medicine, psychology, sociology) to make clinical decisions. Today's nursing students can expect to learn evidence-based practice through various activities where teachers provide instruction in best practices for gathering, analyzing, synthesizing, and using evidence. See Chapter 10 for a further discussion of evidence-based practice.

Technology and Informatics

Regardless of the practice setting in which students learn nursing care, it will include using various technologies and knowledge of informatics to assist with patient care. These technologies can include, but are not limited to, medical devices patients will use to provide self-care, as well as information retrieval, clinical information management, and documentation technologies. For example, students may have clinical experiences where they will use digital devices (e.g., tablet computers, phones) to assist them in providing patient care in the clinical setting. Students' use of these digital devices has important implications for improving their clinical decision-making skills, time management, and the provision of patient education (Brown & McCrorie, 2015). Students are also being exposed to the use of a variety of clinical management systems. For instance, there are electronic health records, telemedicine systems, and patient surveillance systems, many of which have implications for ensuring patient quality and safety. Chapter 20 further addresses health information technology and informatics and their implications for nursing practice.

Interprofessional Education

A major movement in healthcare education is that of interprofessional education. It is defined as occasions when professionals learn with, from, and about each other to improve collaboration and quality of care (World Health Organization, 2010). The need for such education originates from concerns about patient care quality and safety and the overall importance of innovative ways to ensure good patient care outcomes. Research on interprofessional education indicates that it can improve clinical outcomes, patient-centered communication, and collaborative team behavior (Reeves, Perrier, Goldman, Freeth, & Zwarenstein, 2013). Nursing students benefit from actively participating in emerging models of interprofessional education. Chapter 7 further explores the topic of interprofessional research and practice.

Learning Nursing: Important Methods in Nursing Education

New Pedagogies

Pedagogy is a term that refers to the processes of teaching and learning. Much attention is being given to the roles of teachers and students in the learning process. Teachers are urged to critically assess the pedagogies they are using in the classroom and clinical settings and to use active learning pedagogies to better prepare students for nursing practice. This movement, along with educational research providing evidence for best teaching practices, has led teachers to diminish their reliance on passive learning strategies (e.g., lectures) and increase their use of strategies that actively engage learners. For instance, problem-based learning, flipped classrooms, team-based learning, and service learning are examples of active learning strategies, all of which enhance learning nursing practice. Nursing students today can expect to be much more engaged and actively involved in the teaching and learning process as compared to nursing students of the past.

Thinking Practices

Critical thinking is the ability of nursing students to make sound clinical decisions and judgments and use clinical reasoning to provide high-quality and safe patient care. Traditionally, the nursing process has been used as a method for students to learning thinking in nursing practice. The nursing process does assist students in thinking through the assessment of a patient's health status, determining nursing diagnoses, planning care, selecting nursing interventions to support that care, and evaluating patients' responses to care. However, current research in nursing education suggests that students also need to engage in thinking practices that promote reflective thinking, where they build practical knowledge (knowledge from experience); embodied thinking, where they learn the importance of intuition; and pluralistic thinking, where they consider a clinical situation using many perspectives (Ironside, 2015). Today's nursing student can expect learning experiences where teachers use the nursing process but also use other strategies to develop students' clinical reasoning skills.

Distance Education

With the advent of new learning technologies there has been tremendous growth in the use of distance education. In learning experiences delivered through a distance education format, students and faculty interact with each other in physically separate environments (Friesth, 2016). Nursing students today can expect that many nursing programs, both undergraduate and graduate, will be offered in distance education formats. It is important for students to consider the role distance education may play in pursuit of their educational goals and if enrolling in a distance education program is the best choice for them.

Simulation

Simulation allows student nurses to practice their clinical decision making in an environment that is as close as possible to a real-life clinical situation. Examples of simulated learning experiences include the use of task trainers (e.g., arms for intravenous catheter insertion), standardized patients (live actors), computer-based programs, gaming, virtual reality, and mannequins (Ulrich & Mancini, 2014), as well as high-fidelity human patient simulators (HPSs). Teachers use these forms of simulation to foster students' understanding of patients' values and needs, clinical reasoning and decision-making skills, and "hands-on" psychomotor skills. One significant advantage to the use of simulated learning experiences is that they allow students to experience clinical scenarios that they may not get to experience in real clinical settings. Undergraduate nursing students as well as graduate nursing students can expect simulation to be an increasingly common teaching strategy in their nursing education.

The Future of Nursing Education

In 2011 the IOM published a report titled *The Future of Nursing: Leading Change, Advancing Health*. The purpose of the report was to document recommendations for transforming the nursing profession in a manner that maximizes nurses' abilities to meet the healthcare needs of society within a reformed health care system. The report's key messages (as stated on pages 4–9 of the report) include the following: (a) nurses should practice to the full extent of their education and training; (b) nurses should achieve higher levels of education and training through an improved education system that promotes seamless academic progression; (c) nurses should be full partners, with physicians and other health professionals, in redesigning health care in the United States; and (d) effective workforce planning and policymaking require better data collection and an improved information infrastructure. Eight recommendations follow the key messages. These recommendations reflect many of the issues and trends discussed in this chapter. For example, IOM recommendation five suggests that the proportion of nurses with a baccalaureate degree should increase to 80 percent by 2020. The information presented in this chapter about seamless academic progression demonstrates how nursing programs are implementing this recommendation.

Another way nursing programs are enacting the IOM's recommendations is described in **Contemporary Practice Highlight 2-4**. This highlight addresses the

---

CONTEMPORARY PRACTICE HIGHLIGHT 2–4

PREPARATION FOR THE PROFESSIONS PROGRAM

In 2004 and 2005 the Carnegie Foundation for the Advancement of Teaching, an organization committed to the improvement of teaching and learning, began a study to examine teaching and learning in schools of nursing. The Preparation for the Professions Program is a study where investigators compared nursing with other professions such as clergy, engineering, law, and medicine to determine commonalities and differences among these professions (Benner, Sutphen, Leonard, & Day, 2010). The study findings showed that nursing programs facilitate professional identity and ethical comportment among nursing students. The study also demonstrated that using clinical practice assignments that integrate classroom theory is a powerful mechanism for learning nursing practice. However, the study findings also showed that nurse educators need to improve how they teach students nursing science, social and natural sciences, the humanities, and technology. The findings of this study are reshaping curriculum and instruction in nursing programs across the country.

Carnegie Foundation for the Advancement of Teaching's Preparation for the Professions Program, a multiyear, multidisciplinary study that investigated learning and effective teaching for nursing and other professions. The results of this study has undoubtedly influenced trends in nursing education, which interface with all four of the IOM's key messages.

Summary

This chapter provided insight into how nursing education will match the healthcare needs of society with the educational preparation of nurses. In particular, practical/vocational nursing will continue to have a place in nursing practice, especially in home health care. Diploma and ADN programs will remain, but evidence linking baccalaureate education with improved patient outcomes is resulting in seamless academic progression programs that will increase the numbers of nurses prepared with baccalaureate degrees. Master's degree programs in nursing will continue, including clinical nurse leader (CNL) programs to prepare nurses who will provide oversight and coordination of nursing care at the individual, community, and systems levels. Doctoral education will continue with both the PhD in nursing to prepare nurses in research to generate new knowledge and the DNP as the primary advanced nursing practice degree to prepare nurses with a high level of competency in direct and indirect service roles for patients with complex healthcare needs.

Nursing education is dynamic. Throughout the history of nursing education the nursing programs offered have been a direct reflection of social, political, and economic trends and issues. Nursing leaders and nurses have responded to changing needs by offering a variety of nursing programs. A consistent theme throughout all of the changes in nursing education has been the presence of nursing leaders who diligently investigate the state of nursing education and advocate for reforms to improve the delivery of health care through high-quality nursing education. The accreditation standards that arose from leadership in nursing education and the flexibility of nursing educators and nursing students in changing curriculum and instruction are evidence of the patient-centered care the nursing profession strives to provide. Nursing students are beneficiaries of a long history in nursing education that has been characterized by a sustained emphasis on advocacy for ensuring they are prepared for nursing practice.

Reflective Practice Questions

1. As you reflect on this chapter, what are the advantages and disadvantages of the various degree options available in contemporary nursing education?
2. Nursing educators have often made changes in nursing education based on society's needs. How important is it to examine who decides what the needs of society are and who decides what changes are made in nursing education in response to these needs?
3. As knowledge in health care continues to proliferate, reflect on how you are learning to practice nursing. Is it possible to know "all there is to know" about nursing practice? Which is more important: learning to think like a nurse or memorizing information needed in nursing for practice?
4. A critique of nursing education is that its methods of curriculum and instruction have not changed—that is, teachers are still teaching using models of nursing education from the past. After reflecting on this chapter do you agree or disagree with this statement and why?

References

American Association of Colleges of Nursing. (2004). *Position statement on the practice doctorate in nursing.* Retrieved from http://www.aacn.nche.edu/publications/position/DNPpositionstatement.pdf

American Association of Colleges of Nursing. (2006). *The essentials of doctoral education for advanced practice.* Washington, DC: Author.

American Association of Colleges of Nursing. (2007). *White paper on the education and role of the clinical nurse leader.* Washington, DC: Author. Retrieved from http://www.aacn.nche.edu/publications/white-papers/ClinicalNurseLeader.pdf

American Association of Colleges of Nursing. (2012). Joint statement on academic progression for nursing students and graduates. Retrieved from http://www.aacn.nche.edu/aacn-publications/position/joint-statement-academic-progression

American Association of Colleges of Nursing. (2014a). *Press release. Enrollment growth slows at U.S. nursing schools despite calls for a more highly educated nursing workforce.* Retrieved from http://www.aacn.nche.edu/news/articles/2014/slow-enrollment

American Association of Colleges of Nursing. (2014b). Employment of new nurse graduates and employer preferences for baccalaureate-prepared nurses. Retrieved from http://www.aacn.nche.edu/leading_initiatives_news/news/2014/employment14

American Association of Colleges of Nursing. (2014c). Key differences between DNP and PhD/DNS programs. Retrieved from http://www.aacn.nche.edu/dnp/ContrastGrid.pdf

American Association of Colleges of Nursing. (2015a). Fact sheet: The doctor of nursing practice. Retrieved from http://www.aacn.nche.edu/media-relations/fact-sheets/DNPFactSheet.pdf

American Association of Colleges of Nursing. (2015b). *The DNP by 2015: A study of the institutional, political, and professional issues that facilitate or impede establishing a post-baccalaureate doctor of nursing practice program.* Retrieved from http://www.aacn.nche.edu/dnp/DNP-Study.pdf

American Nurses Association. (1965). American Nurses Association first position on education for nurses. *American Journal of Nursing, 65*(120), 106–111.

American Nurses Association. (1969). *Statement on graduate education in nursing.* Kansas City, MO: Author.

American Nurses Association. (1978). *Statement on graduate education in nursing.* Kansas City, MO: Author.

Beard, R. O. (1920). The social, economic and educational status of the nurse. *The American Journal of Nursing, 12*(20), 955–962.

Bednash, G., Breslin, E. T., Kirschling, J. M., & Rosseter, R. J. (2014). PhD or DNP: Planning for doctoral nursing education. *Nursing Science Quarterly, 27*(4), 296–301. doi: 10.1177/0894318414546415

Bender, M. (2014). The current evidence base for the clinical nurse leader: A narrative review of the literature. *Journal of Professional Nursing, 30*(2), 110–123. doi: 10.1016/j.profnurs.2013.08.006

Benner, P., Sutphen, M., Leonard, V., & Day, L. (2010). *Educating nurses: A call for radical transformation.* San Francisco, CA: Jossey-Bass.

Blegen, M. A., Goode, C. J., Park, S. H., Vaughn, T., & Spetz, J. (2013). Baccalaureate education in nursing and patient outcomes. *Journal of Nursing Administration, 43*(2), 89–94. doi: 10.1097/NNA.0b013e31827f2028

Brown, E. L. (1948). *Nursing for the future: A report prepared for the National Nursing Council.* New York, NY: Russell Sage Foundation.

Brown, J., & McCrorie, P. (2015). The iPad: Tablet technology to support nursing and midwifery student learning: An evaluation in practice. *Computer, Informatics, Nursing, 33*(3), 93–98. doi: 10.1097/CIN.0000000000000131

Bullough, B., Bullough, V., & Soukup, M. C. (1983). *Nursing issues and nursing strategies for the eighties.* New York, NY: Springer.

Bullough, B., & Sparks, C. (1975). Baccalaureate vs. associate degree nurses: The care–cure dichotomy. *Nursing Outlook, 23 (11),* 688–992.

Bullough, V. L., & Bullough, B. (1978). *The care of the sick: The emergence of modern nursing.* New York: Prodist.

Bullough, V. L., & Bullough, B. (1984). *History, trends, and politics of nursing*. Norwalk, CT: Appleton-Century-Crofts.

Bureau of Labor Statistics. (2014). *Occupational outlook handbook: Licensed practical and licensed vocational nurses*. Retrieved from http://www.bls.gov/ooh/healthcare/licensed-practical-and-licensed-vocational-nurses.htm

Burgess, M. A. (1928). *Nurses, patients and pocketbooks: Report of a study of the economics of nursing conducted by the Committee on the Grading of Nursing Schools*. New York: Committee on the Grading of Nursing Schools.

Case Western Reserve University. (2014). Project overview: The evolution of the quality and safety education for nurses (QSEN) initiative. Retrieved from http://qsen.org/about-qsen/project-overview

Centers for Disease Control and Prevention. (2013). *The state of aging and health in America 2013*. Retrieved from http://www.cdc.gov/aging/pdf/state-aging-health-in-america-2013.pdf

Council of Baccalaureate and Higher Degree Programs. (1985). *Master's education in nursing. Route to opportunities in contemporary nursing: 1984–1985*. New York, NY: National League for Nursing.

Delaney, C., & Piscopo, B. (2007). There really is a difference: Nurses' experiences with transitioning from RNs to BSNs. *Journal of Professional Nursing, 23*(3), 167–173.

Dracup, K. (2015). Master's nursing programs. Retrieved from http://www.aacn.nche.edu/education-resources/msn-article

Edmonds, M. L. (2012). An integrative literature review of study abroad programs for nursing students. *Nursing Education Perspectives, 33*(1), 30–34. http://dx.doi.org/10.5480/1536-5026-33.1.30

Fenwick, E. B. (1901). A plea for the higher education of trained nurses. *American Journal of Nursing, 2*(1), 4–8.

Friesth, B. (2016). Teaching and learning at a distance. In D. Billings & J. Halstead (Eds.), *Teaching in nursing: A guide for faculty* (5th ed., pp. 342–356). St. Louis, MO: Elsevier.

Gardenier, D. (2012). Does nursing need the clinical nurse leader? *Journal for Nurse Practitioners, 8*(1), 30–31. http://dx.doi.org/10.1016/j.nurpra.2011.11.007

Gerard, S. O., Kazer, M. W., Babington, L., & Quell, T. T. (2014). Past, present, and future trends of master's education in nursing. *Journal of Professional Nursing, 30*(4), 326–332. doi:10.1016/j.profnurs.2014.01.005

Gerardi, T. (2014). AONE and the academic progression in nursing initiative. *Journal of Nursing Administration, 44*(3), 127–128. doi: 10.1097/NNA.0000000000000038

Ginzberg, E. (1949). *A pattern for hospital care: Final report of the New York State hospital study*. New York, NY: Columbia University Press.

Goldmark, J. (1923). *Nursing and nursing education in the United States: The Committee for Study of Nursing Education*. New York, NY: Macmillan.

Haase, P. T. (1990). *The origins and rise of associate degree nursing education*. Durham, NC: Duke University Press.

Hassenplug, L. W. (1965). Preparation of the nurse practitioner. *Journal of Nursing Education, 1*, 29–33.

Hendricks, S. M. (2016). Curriculum models for undergraduate programs. In D. Billings & J. Halstead (Eds.), *Teaching in nursing: A guide for faculty* (5th ed., pp. 130–143). St. Louis, MO: Elsevier.

Hill, S. S., & Howlett, H. S. (2013). *Success in practical/vocational nursing: From student to leader* (7th ed.). St. Louis, MO: Elsevier Saunders.

Institute of Medicine. (2011). *The future of nursing: Leading change, advancing health*. Retrieved from http://www.thefutureofnursing.org/IOM-Report

Ironside, P. M. (2015). Narrative pedagogy: Transforming nursing education through 15 years of research in nursing education. *Nursing Education Perspective, 38*(2), 83–88: http://dx.doi.org/10.5480/13-1102

Kelly, L. Y., & Joel, L. A. (2002). *The nursing experience: Trends, challenges, and transitions* (4th ed.). New York, NY: McGraw-Hill.

King, M. G. (1987). *Conflicting interests: Professionalization and apprenticeship in nursing education. A case study of the Peter Bent Brigham Hospital* (Unpublished doctoral dissertation). Boston University, Boston, MA.

Kirschling, J. M. (2014). Reflections on the future of doctoral programs in nursing. Retrieved from http://www.aacn.nche.edu/dnp/JK-2014-DNP.pdf

Klein-Collins, R., & Wertheim, J. B. (2013). Growing importance of prior learning assessment in the degree completion toolkit. In R. G. White & F. R. DiSilvestro (Eds.), *New directions for adult and continuing education: No. 140. Continuing education in colleges and universities: Challenges and opportunities* (pp. 51–60). San Francisco, CA: Jossey-Bass. doi: 10.1002/ace.20073

Kurzen, C. R. (2012). *Contemporary practical/vocational nursing* (7th ed.). Philadelphia, PA: Wolters Kluwer-Lippincott Williams & Wilkins.

Kutney-Lee, A., Sloane, D. M., & Aiken, L. H. (2013). An increase in the number of nurses with baccalaureate degrees is linked to lower rates of postsurgery mortality. *Health Affairs, 32*(3), 579–586. doi: 10.1377/hlthaff.2012.0504

Lewis, E. P. (1964). The associate degree program. *American Journal of Nursing, 64*(5), 78–81.

Melosh, B. (1982). *"The physician's hand." Work culture and conflict in American nursing.* Philadelphia, PA: Temple University Press.

Montag, M. (1951). *The education of nursing technicians.* New York, NY: G. P. Putnam's Sons.

Montag, M. (1959). *Community college education for nurses.* New York, NY: McGraw-Hill.

Murphy, M. I. (1981). *Master's programs in nursing in the eighties: Trends and issues.* Washington, DC: American Association of Colleges of Nursing.

National Commission for the Study of Nursing and Nursing Education. (1970). Summary report and recommendations. *American Journal of Nursing, 70*(2), 279–294.

National League for Nursing. (2013). *Annual survey of schools of nursing, fall 2012.* Retrieved from http://www.nln.org/docs/default-source/newsroom/nursing-education-statistics/AS1112_F01.pdf-pdf.pdf

National League for Nursing Commission for Nursing Education Accreditation. (2016). *Accreditation standards for nursing education programs.* Retrieved from http://www.nln.org/docs/default-source/accreditation-services/cnea-standards-final-february-201613f2bf5c78366c709642ff00005f0421.pdf?sfvrsn=4

National League for Nursing Education. (1917). *Standard curriculum for schools of nursing.* Baltimore, MD: Waverly Press.

National League for Nursing Education. (1919). *Standard curriculum for schools of nursing.* New York, NY: Author.

National League for Nursing Education. (1927). *Standard curriculum for schools of nursing.* New York, NY: Author.

National League for Nursing Education. (1937). A *curriculum for schools of nursing.* New York, NY: Author.

O'Neil, E. H., & the Pew Health Professions Commission. (1998). *Recreating health professional practice for a new century: The fourth report of the Pew Health Professions Commission.* San Francisco, CA: Pew Health Professions Commission.

Organization for Associate Degree Nursing and American Nurses Association. (2015). *Organization for Associate Degree Nursing and American Nurses Association joint position statement on academic progression to meet the needs of the registered nurse, the health care consumer, and the U.S. health care system.* Retrieved from https://www.oadn.org/images/pdf/Position%20Statements/160113_OADN_ANA_PositionStatement_Academic_Progression_150602.pdf

Ponte, P. R. & Nicholas, P. K. (2015). Addressing the confusion related to DNS, DNSc, and DSN degrees, with lessons for the nursing profession. *Journal of Nursing Scholarship, 47*(4), 347–353. doi: 10.1111/jnu.12148

Redman, R. W., Pressler, S. J., Furspan, P., & Potempa, K. (2015). Nurses in the United States with a practice doctorate: Implications for leading in the current context of health care. *Nursing Outlook, 63,* 124–129. 10.1016/j.outlook.2014.08.003

Reeves, S., Perrier, L., Goldman, J., Freeth, D., & Zwarenstein, M. (2013). Interprofessional education: Effects on professional practice and healthcare outcomes (update). *Cochrane Database of Systematic Reviews, 3.* Retrieved from http://onlinelibrary.wiley.com/doi/10.1002/14651858.CD002213.pub3/full

Smith, D. W. (1960). Different programs; different objectives. *Nursing Outlook, 8*(12), 688–689.

Starck, P. L. (1987). The master's-prepared nurse in the marketplace: What do master's-prepared nurses do? What should they do? In S. E. Hart (Ed.), *Issues in graduate nursing education* (pp. 3–23). New York, NY: National League for Nursing.

Stewart, I. M. (1943). *The education of nurses: Historical foundations and modern trends.* New York, NY: Macmillan.

Ulrich, B., & Mancini, B. (2014). *Mastering simulation: A handbook for success.* Indianapolis, IN: Sigma Theta Tau International Honor Society of Nursing.

U.S. Census Bureau. (2015). *New census bureau report analyzes U.S. population projections.* Retrieved from http://www.census.gov/newsroom/press-releases/2015/cb15-tps16.html

U.S. Department of Health and Human Services Health Resources and Services Administration. (2010). *The registered nurse population: Findings from the 2008 national sample survey of registered nurses.* Retrieved from http://bhpr.hrsa.gov/healthworkforce/supplydemand/nursing/rnsamplesurvey/rnsurveyfinal.pdf

U.S. Public Health Service. (1963). *Toward quality in nursing.* Report of the Surgeon General's Consultant Group on Nursing (Pub No. 992). Washington, DC: U.S. Government Printing Office.

Weimer, M. (2013). *Learner-centered teaching: Five key changes to practice* (2nd ed.). San Francisco, CA: Jossey-Bass.

Wells, H. (1943). *Cherry Ames student nurse.* New York, NY: Grosset & Dunlap.

West, M. D., & Hawkins, C. (1950). *Nursing schools at the mid-century.* New York, NY: National Committee for the Improvement of Nursing Services.

World Health Organization. (2010). *Framework for action on interprofessional education & collaborative practice.* Geneva, Switzerland: Author. Retrieved from http://apps.who.int/iris/bitstream/10665/70185/1/WHO_HRH_HPN_10.3_eng.pdf

Yakusheva, O., Lindrooth, R., & Weiss, M. (2014). Economic evaluation of the 80% baccalaureate nurse workforce recommendation: A patient-level analysis. *Medical Care, 52*(10), 864–869. doi: 10.1097/MLR.0000000000000189

Nursing Licensure and Certification

Wendy Stoelting-Gettelfinger

LEARNING OUTCOMES

After reading this chapter you will be able to:

- Define nursing licensure.
- Define nursing certification.
- Explain the differences between nursing licensure and certification.
- Discuss the history of nursing licensure.
- Describe the purpose of state boards of nursing.
- Identify three functions of state boards of nursing.
- Identify who has the authority to define scope of nursing practice.
- Discuss the regulation of nursing practice.
- Locate current nurse practice act for current state of residence.
- Describe six essential elements of a nurse practice act.
- Discuss three benefits of the mutual recognition model.

Introduction

Healthcare professions that require specialized knowledge and skills such as nursing are regulated to ensure public safety and prevent inherent harm. As healthcare consumers, the trust that we place in our healthcare providers is based on the concept of competency; we often take it for granted that the nurse, dentist, or physician from whom we seek services is knowledgeable and qualified to provide those services. Regulation of healthcare providers exists to protect the public. Healthcare outcomes are directly affected by nursing practice, how it is defined, and ultimately how it is regulated. Nursing regulation is designed to protect public safety; therefore, effective regulation is essential to promote better patient safety and improved health outcomes. Nursing practice is governed by state and territorial nurse practice acts and regulatory procedures. This chapter discusses the regulation of nursing practice, licensure, and certification and how they function to protect consumers of nursing services.

The Regulation of Nursing Practice

The American Nurses Association (ANA) defines nursing as "the protection, promotion, and optimization of health and abilities, prevention of illness and injury, alleviation of suffering through the diagnosis and treatment of human response, and advocacy in health care for individuals, families, communities, and populations" (ANA, 2016a). Nursing, like most other health professions that require specialized knowledge and independent critical thinking, is regulated because individuals can be harmed by the actions of an incompetent or unqualified practitioner. The public relies upon this regulatory oversight of healthcare providers because they themselves may not be able to identify whether specific healthcare providers are competent or incompetent. In order to regulate the practice of nursing, governmental oversight is provided on a state level by a regulatory authority known as a state board of nursing.

A state board of nursing (BON) is a state-specific licensing or regulatory body that sets standards for safe nursing care, decides the scope of practice for nurses within that state's jurisdiction, and issues a **license** to a qualified nurse within the state that the board regulates (Graduate-NursingEDU.org, 2016). The structure for a BON is unique to each state along with its authority and decision-making powers (NCSBN, 2011a, 2016l). In 2007, the National Council of State Boards of Nursing (NCSBN), which has member representatives from all state and territories, adopted guiding principles for nursing regulation. These guiding principles include protection of the public, competence of all practitioners regulated by a BON, due process and ethical decision making, shared accountability, strategic collaboration, evidence-based regulation, response to marketplace, and globalization of nursing. These guiding principles provide the foundation for nursing regulation (NCSBN, 2016d).

Nursing practice is carefully defined within the profession's scope of practice through the **nurse practice acts (NPAs)** of

> **KEY TERM**
>
> **License:** Permission to engage in an activity; a professional license allows the holder to engage in a specific activity for compensation.

> **KEY TERM**
>
> **Nurse practice acts (NPAs):** State or territorial statutes that define the legal limits for the practice of nursing within that state or territory and explicitly identify the requirements for licensure.

individual states and territories. Each state or territory has enacted an NPA, which is a piece of state regulatory legislation that is enforced by its state or territorial BON to promote competent and safe nursing care (NCSBN, 2010). States and territories, through their police powers, enact laws to regulate nursing to protect persons from incompetent nursing care (NCBSN, 2016k). NPAs establish BONs that are authorized to define the scope of nursing practice, develop administrative rules to further define state law, create regulatory entities, empower delegated entities with regulatory authority, and ensure accountability for nurses. Although each state and territory's NPA differs, all NPAs include six critical elements. These include authority and composition of a BON, educational program standards, scope of nursing practice with accompanying standards, types of licenses and titles, licensure requirements, and grounds for disciplinary action (NCSBN, 2016k). In summary, the NPA is the most authoritative and controlling piece of governing law that regulates nursing practice within a state's jurisdiction.

According to Schmitt and Shimberg (1996), regulation is intended to guarantee that the public is protected from unscrupulous, incompetent and unethical practitioners; offer some assurance to the public that the person being regulated is competent to provide certain services in a safe and effective manner; and offer a means by which persons who fail to comply with the profession's standards can be disciplined, including the withdrawal of their licenses. NCSBN holds that state/territory nurse practice acts provide the legal basis for the regulation of nursing activities and that the responsibility for interpreting the legal scope of nursing practice rests solely with the individual BONs (NCSBN, 2016k).

Nurse practice acts vary among states; however, many of them are based on the model act that was originally published by the ANA in 1988. The NCSBN also maintains a model nurse practice act and model rules titled *NCSBN Model Nursing Practice Act and Model Nursing Administrative Rules* (NCSBN, 2016h). The model act and administrative rules provide recommended or model language that individual states or territories may use in the development of their state/territory specific nurse practice acts. The NCSBN Model Act and Rules contain exemplary legislation that can be used by any state or territorial BON. The current model act and rules were developed by NCSBN committees, approved by the Delegate Assembly in 2012, and then updated in 2014 (NCSBN, 2016h).

The *NCSBN Model Act* and *Model Rules* provide a resource that state legislators and members of individual state/territory BONs can use as a comparative guide to help write language for the existing nurse practice act of their respective state (NCSBN, 2016i). This comparison can identify language that may be missing in a state/territory's existing nurse practice act or provide language that can be used for new regulation. Because each state/territory has its own unique version of an NPA, models provide examples and guidance for the use of standardized or uniform language that helps to facilitate a shared knowledge or understanding of what constitutes the practice of nursing (NCSBN, 2016i). The challenge for many individual practicing nurses can be how to locate their own state or jurisdiction's current NPA.

Accessing Your State's Nurse Practice Act and Administrative Rules

Many states and jurisdictions now post the most current version of their nurse practice act on the Internet. The NCSBN, whose mission is to promote regulatory excellence, maintains a database on its website (http://www.ncsbn.org/contact-bon .htm) that contains electronic contact information for state BONs for all 50 states, the District of Columbia, and four U.S. territories (Guam, the Northern Mariana Islands, Puerto Rico, and the Virgin Islands).

Many of the state nursing board websites include links to the current state nurse practice act. For those states that do not include links, there is contact information. Your state or territory's state nursing board or designated regulatory agency also can help answer many of your questions concerning the practice of nursing within your jurisdiction. If you are not certain whether a website is official or up to date, call your state or territory's state BON, and they can direct you to the most current version of their jurisdiction's nurse practice act. Because nurse practice acts can be written in a legal format that may be difficult to interpret, you may also want to consult the accompanying administrative rules for the NPA. Administrative rules help to further define the NPA, providing additional details. Administrative rules are very helpful in answering specific questions that you might have about your NPA.

As a licensed registered nurse (RN), it is imperative that you also become familiar with your employer's practice policies and guidelines. For example, some employers will use more stringent guidelines concerning delegation than are dictated by the jurisdiction's NPA. The concept of delegation is specifically addressed in each state's NPA, a document that is always being updated and is subject to change. "All nurses have a duty to understand their NPA and to keep up with ongoing changes as this dynamic document evolves as the scope of practice expands" (Russell, 2012, p. 36).

Most states recognize the concept of **delegation.** Therefore, it is important for RNs to be familiar with the concept of delegation as many states' NPAs define parameters that authorize RNs to delegate certain tasks under specific conditions. "All decisions related to delegation and assignment are based on the fundamental principles of protection of the health, safety and welfare of the public" (NCSBN, 2007, para. 6). The Joint Statement on Delegation developed by the ANA and the National Council of State Boards of Nursing lists the five rights

KEY TERM

Delegation: The process by which a registered nurse directs another person to perform nursing skills and activities that the person would not normally carry out while still retaining accountability for those activities (National Council of State Boards of Nursing, 2016g).

of delegation that are applicable to each state's NPA. An RN must apply professional judgment when following the five rights of delegation within his or her state or terrority's NPA to ensure the following: the right task, under the right circumstances, to the right person, with the right directions and communication, and under the right supervision and evaluation (NCSBN, 2007, para. 7).

As the practice of nursing continues to evolve and expand, the concept of delegation also changes. It is critically important for RNs to be able to effectively work with others, delegate, manage, and appropriately supervise within the legal parameters of a governing jurisdiction's NPA. The nursing shortage and need for nursing services mandates that nurses understand and use delegation to meet the needs of healthcare consumers (NCSBN, 2016c).

The topic of delegation should be covered during your employment orientation. If the topic of delegation and your employer's policies are not discussed in your orientation, you should request copies of these policies for your review and use so that you can correctly apply this critical nursing skill.

The History of State Boards and Their Regulatory Functions

Prior to the Industrial Revolution, it was easier for persons to evaluate the quality of services that they received because communities were small and persons were well known by everyone in the community. Family members provided healthcare services and if outside services were required, the reputation of healthcare providers was well known within the community (Russell, 2012). The first state to pass a nursing regulation law protecting the title of "nurse" was North Carolina which did so in 1903. At that time it became the responsibility of the North Carolina Board of Nursing to develop the nursing licensure examination and issue nursing licenses (UNC-TV, 2012).

In the early 1900s, states initiated the development of government-established BONs to protect the public's health by overseeing and ensuring the safe practice of nursing (NCSBN, 2016d). At the turn of the century, New York, New Jersey, and Virginia developed some of the first nurse practice acts (Roberts, 1954). In addition to establishing standards for safe nursing care, BONs are responsible for accrediting or approving nursing education programs. Program approval is an essential component of state licensure because it ensures that state and territorial standards are being met. This process is different from national nursing accreditation that assesses and ensures that the quality of nursing programs is maintained on a national level.

In addition to protecting the public from harm, one of the most critical functions for BONs is the issuance of licenses to practice nursing. However, once a nursing license is issued, a nursing board's job is not complete. State and territorial

---

BOX 3-1 FUNCTIONS OF THE STATE BOARDS OF NURSING

Issue licenses and manage renewal process
Establish nursing practice standards
Regulate advanced practice nursing
Approve operation of nursing education programs
Investigate complaints against licensed practitioners

Hold disciplinary hearings, suspending or revoking
    licensure if necessary
Promulgate all rules related to the regulation of
    nursing practice

---

nursing boards continue to monitor each nurse's adherence to governing laws. If a nurse engages in an unsafe or unlawful practice of nursing, a BON can revoke a license (NCSBN, 2016d). **Box 3-1** provides a further description of the functions of BONs.

Individuals who serve on a BON are typically appointed to their position, in many states by the governor. Professional organizations nominate members in other states. The process can further differ between states and territories. For example, in North Carolina, state board members are elected. The legislature is also responsible for appointing board members in other states (Brent, 2012). Members of a BON generally report to the governor of a state or territory, both the governor and state or territorial agency, a state or territorial agency or another state or territorial official or organization. State or territorial law often determines the membership or composition of a state BON, which is usually a mix of different types of nurses with various educational backgrounds as well as healthcare consumers. Generally, BONs consist of licensed practical nurses (LPNs), RNs, advanced practice registered nurses (APRNs), and healthcare consumers. The members of a BON convene to oversee nursing activities, including nursing education within a state, and also to take regulatory actions including discipline on nurse licenses when the nurse practice act is violated (NCSBN, 2016m). In some states and territories, BONs also regulate certified nursing assistants (CNAs) and other healthcare professionals. Individual state nurse practice acts dictate the scope of regulatory authority and powers for individual state and territory BONs. Each state and territory is represented by the NCSBN, a not-for-profit organization that serves as the vehicle for BONs to act together to provide regulatory excellence for public safety, health, and welfare. The membership for the NCSBN is composed of members from the BONs in the 50 states, the District of Columbia, and four U.S. territories—Guam, the Virgin Islands, American Samoa, and the Northern Mariana Islands. Four states currently maintain two separate BONs for RNs and LPNs—California, Georgia, Louisiana, and West Virginia (NCSBN, 2016a).

The Nurse Licensure Compact and Advance Practice Registered Nurse Compact

The **Nurse Licensure Compact (NLC)** and Advance Practice Registered Nurse Compact are model pieces of legislation designed to advance "public protection and access to care through the mutual recognition of one state-based license that is enforced locally and recognized nationally" (NCSBN, 2016f). Compacts allow nurses to practice and communicate with patients across state lines. The enhanced model legislation addresses physical and electronic communication and practice.

> **KEY TERM**
>
> **Nurse Licensure Compact (NLC):** A form of interstate compact specific to nurse licensure that provides an agreement between two or more states for the purpose of recognizing nurse licensure between and among a group of participating states. States must enter into one in order to achieve mutual recognition (NCSBN, 2011b).

In 2000, the NCSBN launched the NLC initiative to advance the mobility of nurses' practice. Maryland was the first state to implement an NLC in 1999. Since that time, 25 states have enacted NLC legislation. In May 2015, new versions of the NLC and APRN Compact were adopted by the NCSBN. The enhanced model language will be adopted by future states enacting compacts. Compacts allow a nurse or advance practice nurse to be licensed in his or her state of primary residency and to practice in other compact states that agree to mutually recognize that nurse's single multistate license from the primary resident state. Essentially, the compacts authorize licensed nurses who reside in a compact-participating state to practice in another compact-participating state without obtaining additional practice licenses. Participating states acknowledge another state's licensure through an NLC or APRN Compact. Currently, multistate licensure privilege means that a nurse has the privilege of practicing in any participating compact state that is not his/her state of residency. As long as a nurse remains in good standing, renews his/her multistate licensure and continues to reside in a primary state of residence that is a compact state, there is no time limit for working in other compact states (NCSBN, 2016f).

Compacts allow nurses to practice in other states both physically and electronically through multistate licensure privilege. However, it is important to note that nurses residing in states that participate in an NLC or APRN compact who want to practice across state lines in other participating states are subject to the laws and regulations of each state they practice within. Although nursing licensure is tied to the nurse's state of primary residence, accountability for nursing practice is tied to the laws and regulations of the state where a patient is located at the time nursing care and services are rendered. This type of accountability is not unique to nursing licenses; it also applies to other licenses such as a driver's license. For example, a person driving in Indiana must obey the speeding laws of Indiana even if his or her driver's license was issued in Ohio. Similarly, nurses must abide by the nursing practice laws in the states where they are practicing (NCSBN, 2016f). For example, a nurse whose primary residence is in the state of Kentucky, but who is providing case management services through telehealth, Internet, or telephone connections to a patient who resides in South Carolina, would be governed by the South Carolina nurse practice act for care provided to that patient. Nursing practice is no longer limited to the provision of physical patient care but also includes nursing care such as counseling, education, and prior authorization of services through the use of technology. The expansion of digital and electronic services makes this concept even more significant for nurses.

To be eligible to hold multistate licensure through the NLC, a nurse must declare primary residence in a state that has joined the compact (NCSBN, 2016j, p. 1). A nurse's primary state of residence (PSOR) or home state is defined by the mutual recognition model as "the state of a person's declared fixed permanent and principal home or domicile for legal purposes" (New Hampshire Board of Nursing, 2016, para. 5). Sources used to verify a nurse's PSOR include federal income tax returns, driver's license, voter registration cards, etc. (NCSBN, 2016n). The state of primary residence is used to determine jurisdiction for nursing licensure. Nurses changing permanent residence from one NLC state to another NLC party state must relinquish their licensure in their previous home state and apply in their new home state. Nurses should apply for licensure in advance if they anticipate a change in their PSOR. Nurses generally have 90 days to obtain a license in their new PSOR. Nurses should not wait until their current license expires before applying for a license in their new home state (Ridenour, 2011). However, if a nurse moves from a non-NLC state to an NLC state and declares the NLC state as their PSOR, they must apply for a new license but can still keep their noncompact license. Although this may seem confusing, nurses are not allowed to have more than one multistate compact license at a time (Ridenour, 2011).

Licensure is not based on the state of practice because with the implementation of telenursing and other forms of nursing such as case management through managed care, it is sometimes difficult to determine the state of practice for the specific purpose of licensure. In addition, nurses who are not currently in the workforce or who are working temporarily could be subject to difficulties with state licensure. Tracing complaints and investigations is also facilitated by linking licensure to the state of primary residence rather than employment. For states not participating in the mutual recognition model, nurses must apply for separate licensure within the state where they are going to practice either physically or electronically, regardless of residence. Even though there is a national licensure examination, individual state licensure in noncompact participating states is required. There is no limit placed on the number of licenses that a nurse may hold from non-noncompact states (Ridenour, 2011).

There are many positive outcomes associated with the **mutual recognition model** and only very few potential negatives. The mutual recognition model and NLC clarify the practice of telehealth and interstate nursing practice. In addition, the NLC provides greater mobility for nurses and improves access to care. This is critical in times of disaster when nurses need to mobilize to areas of need. The NLC also promotes information sharing among participating NLC states that recognize the mutual recognition model to promote quality of care and discipline if necessary (NCSBN, 2016l). One potential negative is the need for increased vigilance on the part of nurses who practice across state lines to understand the particular standards of care, scope of practice, and state laws that apply within the state where care is rendered. Without separate application for licensure, it may be less apparent to nurses that they must fully understand each state's nurse practice act and governing laws where they render care.

> **KEY TERM**
>
> **Mutual recognition model:** A model that allows a nurse to have one license in his or her state of residency with the ability to practice (electronically or physically) across state lines in other states that participate in this model if there are no restrictions on his or her license and that person acknowledges that he or she is subject to each state's practice laws and rule (NCSBN, 2011b).

History of the Nurse Licensure Compact

The NCSBN Delegate Assembly began the creation of the NLC in 1996. At that time, NCSBN delegates voted to begin the process of studying and inspecting various mutual recognition models and report their findings. By 1997, the NCSBN Delegate Assembly unanimously agreed to endorse a mutual recognition model. In 1998, the NCSBN Board of Directors endorsed the goal to remove regulatory barriers to increase access to safe nursing care (Evans, 2015; NCSBN, 1996). The RNs and licensed practical nurses and vocational nurses (LPN/VN) compact was initiated on January 1, 2000. The first states to pass the RN and LPN/VN NLC into law were Maryland, Texas, Utah, and Wisconsin.

Also in 2000, the Nurse Licensure Compact Administrators (NLCA) was organized to protect the public's health and safety. The mission of the NLCA is to promote compliance with laws governing the practice of nursing in each party state through the mutual recognition of party state licenses (NLCA, 2014). In 2002, the NCSBN adopted the APRN Compact to complement the NLC for advanced practice nurses. However, due to lack of uniformity in advanced practice nursing, the compact faced implementation challenges and was only partially implemented in Iowa, Utah, and Texas. In 2008, the Consensus Model for APRN Regulation was adopted to promote uniformity in advance practice. Two years later, the APRN Consensus Model language was integrated into the APRN Compact. In May 2015, the NCSBN Delegate Assembly met and adopted enhanced compact language to align the NLC and APRN Compact and promote implementation (Evans, 2015).

Nursing Licensure

Nursing **licensure** is a form of credentialing or regulatory method that is used when the activities being regulated are complex and require specialized knowledge coupled with the ability to make independent decisions. At the very heart of licensure are public safety and the need to ensure minimal competency in a set of nursing skills that a licensed nurse must possess in order to competently provide consistent quality nursing care for a defined level of nursing practice. Nursing licensure is defined by the NCSBN as "the process by which BONs grant permission for an individual to engage in nursing practice after determining that the applicant has attained the competency necessary to perform a unique scope of practice" (NCSBN, 2016e, p. 1). The requirements for licensure define what is necessary for individuals to be able to practice the profession of nursing safely and ensure that each person meets those minimal requirements.

> **KEY TERM**
>
> **Licensure:** The process by which a state or governmental agency grants permission to an individual to engage in a given profession for compensation.

The licensure process addresses both qualification and disciplinary activities. First, licensure encompasses predetermination of the qualifications that are required to perform a defined scope of practice (e.g., LPN vs. RN) safely and an objective evaluation process to determine that the qualifications for the defined scope of practice are met. Generally speaking, the objective evaluation is accomplished through an examination (NCLEX-RN; NCLEX-PN) that must be passed before the individual can practice (NCSBN, 2016d, p. 1). In addition, licensure provides title protection for the roles and functions that RNs perform, and it gives authority to take disciplinary action against a licensee if he or she violates the nurse practice act and governing laws, thus ensuring that the public health, safety, and welfare are protected (NCSBN, 2011b).

In the United States, nursing licensure is a regulatory function of each state. Currently, each state's or territory's BON or a designated entity grants licensure to RNs within that jurisdiction. Each state has the ability through enforcement powers to designate an entity with licensing authority to ensure that each individual who claims to be a nurse can function at a minimal level of competency. Many states' nurse practice acts also contain language that provides protection for the title of "registered nurse" to persons who hold a valid license and prevents other persons from using the title or credentials. One example of this type of title protection can be found in Arizona's Nurse Practice Act (see **Box 3-2**).

The History of Nursing Licensure

Nursing licensure originally came about to protect the public from unsafe nursing practice. During the 1900s nurse practice acts consisted mainly of lists of the names of trained nurses. The state of North Carolina was the first state to enact

> **BOX 3-2   ARIZONA'S NURSE PRACTICE ACT**
>
> **Nurse Practice Act: Section 32-1636:** Only a person who holds a valid and current license to practice registered nursing in this state or in a party state pursuant to section 32-1668 may use the title "nurse," "registered nurse," "graduate nurse," or "professional nurse" and the abbreviation "R.N." No other person shall assume or claim any such titles or use such abbreviation or any other words, letters, signs or figures to indicate that the person using it is a registered, graduate or professional nurse.
>
> Reproduced from Arizona State Legislature. (1997). Arizona Nurse Practice Act. Chapter 140 - 431R - S Ver of SB1099. Section 32-1636. Retrieved from http://www.azleg.state.az.us/legtext/43leg/1r/laws/0140.htm

a nurse practice act, in 1903. By 1923, all states had enacted nurse practice acts. From the 1930s through the 1950s, nurse licensure laws were enacted to help define the practice of nursing and to prevent unlicensed individuals from practicing nursing. In 1955, the ANA issued a model definition of nursing that affirmed that not all nursing duties required physician supervision and that some duties were independent nursing functions. However, the definition did forbid nurses from diagnosing conditions or prescribing medications. Over time, the practice of nursing has expanded, with regulatory focus on professional accountability (Damgaard, Hohman, & Karpiuk, 2000).

Historically, when an RN wanted to work in a state other than his or her home state, he/she had to apply for licensure in that other state. In the past, there was no national licensure examination. That meant there was no consistency between states' nurse licensure exams. The NCSBN was instrumental in developing the national licensure exam for RNs, which changed in 1982 to the National Council Licensure Examination for Registered Nurses (NCLEX-RN). Thanks to the elimination of state-specific licensure exams, nurses can be more mobile and more easily pursue career opportunities in multiple states.

Requirements for Nursing Licensure

To ensure public protection, each state or territory in the United States through its state BON or designated licensure body requires a candidate for nursing licensure to pass the National Council Licensure Examination for Registered Nurses (NCLEX-RN) or the NCLEX for Practical Nurses (NCLEX-PN) and meet other requirements before granting a nursing license. The passing level for the exam is set to ensure that at a minimum, a sufficient skill set is demonstrated to protect the public. The NCLEX examination measures the competencies needed to perform safely and effectively as a newly licensed, entry-level nurse (NCSBN, 2016e). In 2011, the NCSBN Delegate Assembly adopted the Uniform Licensure Requirements (ULRs) to serve as standards for licensure for RNs and LPNs in all states and territories. The ULR provides for additional public protection by requiring disclosure of substance use disorders and prior actions taken or initiated against a professional or occupational license, registration, or certification. States have been encouraged to adopt the ULRs to promote consistency across all U.S. jurisdictions (McDougal et al., 2011). The requirements for nursing licensure for applicants who wish to become licensed RNs include successful graduation from high school or completion of a GED, successful graduation from an approved nursing school, application to the appropriate state agency for licensure, payment of required fees, and criminal background check in some states (NCSBN, 2016e). In addition, applicants must not have a criminal history such as a felony conviction that prohibits them from taking the NCLEX-RN. If an applicant successfully meets all these requirements, then a state nursing board or licensure body may grant the applicant a nursing license. Simply passing the NCLEX-RN is no guarantee that an applicant will automatically be granted a nursing license. Only after all state requirements have been satisfied will a candidate be considered for licensure. Although these requirements may seem extensive, the responsibility associated with nursing licensure and safely caring for patients demands such consideration. See Chapter 4 for more information on the NCLEX-RN.

> **KEY TERM**
>
> **Certification:** "A process by which a nongovernmental agency or association certifies that an individual licensed to practice a profession has met certain predetermined standards specified by that profession for specialty practice" (American Nurses Association, 1979, p. 67).

Certification

Certification is a form of credentialing that demonstrates attainment of increased knowledge but does not address a legal scope of practice like licensure does. Individual certification is the most common type of certification and is awarded when a nurse demonstrates a level of competency above the licensure level for a specific area of nursing practice. The American Association of Critical Care Nurses (AACN) defines certification as "a process by which a nongovernmental agency validates, based upon predetermined standards, an individual nurse's qualifications for practice in a defined functional or clinical area of nursing" (AACN, 2016, p. 1).

Numerous state BONs use professional certification as a requirement toward granting authority for APRNs. Organizations, like individuals, also can be certified. However, the certification process for organizations is very different from individual or personal certification. Organizations such as hospitals or healthcare institutions can be certified by external/reviewing entities. Organizational certification is referred to as *accreditation* (American Nurses Credentialing Center, 2016b, p. 1). The Joint Commission is one example of an external entity that accredits hospitals. Hospitals go through an accreditation process to ensure that they are achieving a defined set of performance measures. In essence, hospital accreditation provides a "gold seal of approval" for hospitals achieving those standards. This approval rating allows consumers to make choices based upon standardized measures that reflect the quality of care provided at that hospital (The Joint Commission, 2016a, para. 1).

Another type of organizational recognition that has particular meaning for nurses is "magnet status." Magnet status is an award given by the American Nurses Credentialing Center, an affiliate of the ANA, to hospitals that satisfy specific criteria based on the strength and quality of nursing in that facility (ANCC, 2016c). A magnet hospital is an organization or facility that exhibits nursing excellence through patient outcomes, communication, and delivery of care. Other entities provide voluntary accrediting services for community-based facilities. An example of such a voluntary accrediting agency is the Commission on Accreditation of Rehabilitation Facilities International (CARF International).

Potential for confusion exists because regulatory agencies and professional associations may use the term *certification* differently with individuals and organizations (The Joint Commission, 2016b). As technology advances and the number of nursing specialty areas continue to grow, nurses are pursuing certification to increase their knowledge and skill beyond what they learned in their basic nursing programs. For example, the American Nurses Credentialing Center offers certifications in over 40 areas of nursing practice.

However, certification is a concept that is frequently misunderstood by employers, the public, and even other nurses. Examining the current certification process for APRNs provides a unique opportunity for understanding nursing certification in general, because it mirrors the previous development of nursing licensure. APRN certification is in an earlier phase of evolution than is RN licensure. Therefore, APRNs today find that both the uniformity of standards and recognition of their advanced practice expertise lag behind those of their RN status (Evans, 2015). For example, APRNs' ability to prescribe medications, professional titles, and the ability to bill third-party payers continue to vary from state to state. Therefore, APRNs continue to face many of the challenges and barriers to practicing in different states that RNs faced prior to adoption of the NLC. As states adopt the APRN Compact, barriers to advance practice across jurisdictions will potentially decrease (Evans, 2015). However, nursing studies have demonstrated that nurses experience positive benefits if they obtain certification. Specialty certification provides positive benefits for patients, families, nurses, and employers (Kaplow, 2011). Certification is becoming the new standard measure for excellence in nursing care in this quickly changing healthcare system. Certification distinguishes mastery of skills and knowledge that go beyond the scope of nursing licensure. The American Association of Critical Care Nurses Malcolm Baldrige National Quality Award, Beacon Award of Excellence, and Magnet Recognition Program recognize certification as a critical component of nursing excellence in specialized practice. Healthcare consumers and nurses are becoming increasingly aware of the benefits of certification to help ensure safe and high-quality nursing care services (Fleishman, Meyer, & Watson, 2011).

Requirements for Certification

The requirements for certification are diverse and depend upon the organization granting certification. Requirements usually address the candidate's RN licensure status, educational preparation, and number of clinical practice hours in the chosen specialty. Historically, large numbers of professional and specialty groups have offered certification exams. Therefore, the requirements are extremely varied. For example, the AACN has different certification requirements than the American Association of Operating Room Nurses (AAORN). To determine the exact requirements for certification, nurses should check with the specialty organization through which they wish to become certified.

Differences Between Licensure and Certification

Certification, on its face, appears to be very similar to licensure. However, licensure and certification are two different terms that carry different meanings both professionally and legally. Certification is the granting of credentials that indicate a person has achieved a level of specialization higher than the minimal level of competency indicated by licensure (AACN, 2016). Licensure is technically a form of legal certification. Although some very specific forms of certification carry a legal status, most certifications only imply a specialized skill or knowledge set associated with specific professional status. Nursing licensure, on the other hand, implies a legal status because it establishes lawful authorization for a scope of nursing practice (NCSBN, 2011b).

The Regulation of Advanced Practice Registered Nurses

The regulation of APRNs differs significantly from state to state among BONs. In addition, it is important to note that in some states advanced practice nurses, such as certified registered nurse anesthetists (CNRAs), may be managed by the state's medical board. Currently, the NCSBN recommends the use of APRN certification examinations as a basis for determining APRN credentialing. However, the scope of practice and prescriptive privileges that APRNs have depend on each state's NPA. Until states adopt the APRN Compact, APRNs must seek and receive recognition from each state in which they practice. Currently, Texas, Utah, and Iowa are the only three APRN Compact states with partial implementation (Evans, 2015).

The NLC applies only to nursing licensure and currently does not apply to APRN certifications (NCSBN, 2016h). Generally, an APRN would need to contact the state in which he or she anticipates practicing as an APRN and meet the requirements for licensure and certification as an APRN with prescribing privileges (as permitted) in that state. The APRN who resides in a state that is part of the mutual recognition model and declares that state as their primary residence may go to another compact state and practice as an RN because he or she has a compact RN license but may *not* practice as an APRN *until* he or she receives advanced practice licensure and meets the certification requirements for that state.

It is important to know that regulatory state requirements can affect certification within a particular state. APRNs can track state legislative changes through the NCSCN website at https://www.ncsbn.org/aprn.htm and the ANA Advance Practice Nurses Consensus Model Toolkit at http://www.nursingworld.org/consensusmodel (ANCC, 2016a).

In 2008, the Consensus Model for APRN Regulation: Licensure, Accreditation, Certification and Education (LACE Model) was developed as a collaborative effort by more than 40 nursing organizations to make APRN practice and regulation more uniform and consistent. The APRN Regulatory Model (LACE) defines four advance nurse practice roles: certified nurse midwife (CNM), certified registered nurse anesthetist (CRNA), clinical nurse specialist (CNS), and certified nurse practitioner (CNP). Under the APRN Regulatory Model, certification and licensure must be congruent in terms of role and population focus.

With the progression of implementation of the APRN Consensus Model, certifying organizations such as ANCC are changing certification programs to more accurately reflect the roles and populations required by the Model (ANCC, 2016a). For example, the Adult Nurse Practitioner Primary Care Nurse Practitioner certification is being retired in December 2016 and is being replaced by the Adult Gerontology Primary Care Nurse Practitioner certification (ANCC, 2016d). As the APRN Regulatory Model and Enhanced Compact and new state legislative changes are implemented, it will be critically important for APRNs to understand the issues affecting their licensure, certification, and practice.

Standard of Care

A **standard of care** is a legal concept that all nurses should become familiar with and understand. This concept is used to depict a standard or measure of behavior that describes how a nurse is expected to act or professionally conduct him- or herself according to an accepted reasonable practice of nursing care. Standards of care and practice can be published within a state's administrative code, and are generally defined within each state's or territory's jurisdiction. For example, in the state of Indiana, RNs and LPNs have a defined responsibility to apply the nursing process and to act in a specific manner as a member of the registered nursing profession (Indiana Administrative Code, 2013).

RNs are mandated to function within the legal boundaries of nursing based on their knowledge of the statutes and rules governing nursing (Indiana Administrative Code, 2013). Therefore, it is imperative for nurses to be aware of and fully understand the rules and statutes that govern nursing practice in their state or territory. Nursing behaviors, including acts, knowledge, and practices that fail to meet defined minimal standards of acceptable current practice that could endanger the health, safety, and welfare of the public, represent unprofessional nursing conduct in Indiana (Indiana Administrative Code, 2013).

Nurses should conduct themselves with the degree of care, skill, and knowledge that reasonably competent nurses would exhibit in comparable situations. It is important to note that the standard of care represents a minimum level of practice that a nurse must stay within to avoid being found negligent or guilty of malpractice. Nurses must exercise good judgment using their nursing education to the best of their ability under the circumstances. In addition, a standard of care can be used to compare the performance of a nurse with another in the same specialty.

Standards of Care for Particular Areas of Nursing Practice

In malpractice actions, the adequacy of a nurse's performance is based on a professional standard that is then compared with the performance of other nurses in the same specialty area. This type of comparison allows nurses to be compared more accurately with the performance of their peers. For example, neonatal intensive care nurses determine the standard of care for other neonatal intensive care nurses. The conduct of a surgical nurse would not be compared with the conduct of a public health nurse. Standards of care apply to specific areas of nursing practice (ANA, 2016b).

Malpractice actions are premised on allegations of failure to comply with a professional standard of care or performance. If a nurse's actions fall below the accepted professional standard of care, he or she may be found guilty of malpractice. It is extremely important for nurses to be familiar with and understand the professional standard of care that applies to their practice area. There are various layers of accountability for nursing practice ranging from broad national/general practice guidelines to narrow specialty- and state-specific guidelines. Nurses can go to their professional organization's website to determine appropriate standards of care for particular practice settings also called standards of practice. For example, nurses can visit the ANA website to access information concerning appropriate standards of care and practice.

It is important to note that the Standards of Professional Nursing Practice are duties that are common to all RNs regardless of their role, specialty, or population that nurses are expected to perform with competence. These standards are used as evidence of standard or care with the understanding that standards are context dependent and vary upon clinical circumstances. For example, the application of standards could be different during a natural disaster such as a hurricane than a regular day (ANA, 2010). The ANA published the third edition of *Nursing: Scope and Standards of Practice* in 2015 (ANA, 2015).

The ANA states that "the public has a right to expect RNs to demonstrate professional competence throughout their careers" (ANA, 2010, p. 32). The ANA's *Scope and Standards of Nursing Practice* provides and outlines the expectations of the professional role for RNs including scope of practice and standards of professional practice and related competencies. The *Scope and Standards* also provide new information that can be incorporated into state nurse practice acts, which provide another layer of accountability. Rules and regulations promulgated by states that are specific to that state's nurse practice act, may further restrict the RN's practice. Additional restrictions upon nursing practice can be enforced by institutions or agencies of employment through policies and procedures (ANA, 2010). **Contemporary Practice Highlight 3-1** offers additional discussion of patient safety and standards of care.

CONTEMPORARY PRACTICE HIGHLIGHT 3-1

EMPHASIS ON PATIENT SAFETY

Since the Institute of Medicine (IOM) released its report *To Err Is Human: Building a Safer Healthcare System* (IOM, 2000), which revealed only 55 percent of patients received recommended care, reporting that approximately 98,000 died each year due to medical errors, there has been a renewed interest in patient safety and standards of care. In 2010, the U.S. Department of Health and Human Services, Office of Inspector General (2010). reported that below standard hospital care resulted in approximately 180,000 Medicare deaths. In 2013, the *Journal of Patient Safety* reported that deaths from preventable harm may be as high as 210,000–400,000 (James, 2013). This would make medical errors the third leading cause of death in the United States. Medication errors, in particular, provide an example of high-risk situations that can result in a breach of standards of care and patient safety while exposing nurses to potential liability. Fully engaging patients and their advocates during hospital stays, listening to patients to identify harms, and transparency in accountability will be necessary to decrease patient harm (James, 2013).

Official Resources for Determining Standards of Practice and Care

A variety of resources for nursing practice standards exist. Nurses may wish to use different resources depending on the states in which they decide to practice. In addition, standards are interpreted and applied differently depending on the state of jurisdiction. In malpractice actions, courts rely on some or all of these resources to help determine the applicable standard of care in each individual case. Some of these resources include:

- State statutes and administrative codes
- Nurse practice acts (a listing of resources concerning nurse practice acts can be found at http://www.ncsbn.org)
- American Nurses Association (a listing of specialty care nursing standards and scopes of practice can be found at http://www.nursingworld.org/Main MenuCategories/ThePracticeofProfessionalNursing/NursingStandards)
- The Joint Commission (www.jointcommission.org)
- State and federal case law and published opinions by judges
- Hospital policies
- Specialty nurse organizations, for example:
  - American Association of Critical Care Nurses (http://www.aacn.org)
  - Association of Public Health Nurses (http://phnurse.org)
  - American Association of Nurse Practitioners (https://www.aanp.org)

Summary

It is critically important for RNs to understand how and why nursing practice is regulated. By understanding the basic concepts of nursing regulation, licensure, certification, and standards of care, RNs are empowered with the necessary skills to provide safe nursing care. State nurse practice acts vary from state to state and territories, and nurses must be aware of their governing nurse practice act when delivering and/or delegating care. As nursing continues to advance, and with the emergence of the field of telehealth, it is becoming increasingly important for nurses to understand that the care they deliver across state lines is affected by varying state laws and the regulatory process.

Reflective Practice Questions

1. Have you ever read the NCSBN *Model Nursing Practice Act* and *Model Nursing Administrative Rules*? You can find a copy of both on the NCSBN website at http://www.ncsbn.org. Note the differences between the *Practice Act* and *Administrative Rules*. How are they different? Is one easier to read than the other? Do the *Administrative Rules* provide more detail? Do you think that your state or territory follows the NCSBN *Model Nursing Practice Act* and *Model Nursing Administrative Rules*? Explain why or why not.
2. Do you think it is important for various types of nurses to serve on state boards of nursing? What qualities do you think a state board of nursing member should exemplify? Why?
3. What state do you want to obtain nursing licensure from after graduating from nursing school? Can you list your state's nursing licensure requirements? Is it a Nurse Licensure Compact participating state? Do you plan to practice outside your state of residency? What entity should you contact to find out the exact requirements for nursing licensure?
4. How does certification affect an individual's nursing practice? What are some of the benefits associated with certification?

References

American Association of Critical Care Nurses. (2016). What is certification [Fact sheet] Retrieved from http://www.aacn.org/wd/certifications/content/consumer-whatiscert.pcms?menu=certification)

American Nurses Association. (1979). *The study of credentialing in nursing: A new approach.* Kansas City, MO: Author. Retrieved from http://www.nursecredentialing.org/CredentialingDefinitions

American Nurses Association. (2010). *Nursing: Scope and standards of practice* (2nd ed.). Silver Spring, MD: Author. Retrieved from www.nursesbooks.org/ebooks/download/NursingScopeStandards.pdf

American Nurses Association. (2015). *Nursing: Scope and standards of practice* (3rd ed.) Silver Spring, MD: Author.

American Nurses Association. (2016a). FAQ. Retrieved from http://www.nursingworld.org/FunctionalMenuCategories/FAQs

American Nurses Association. (2016b). Professional standards. Retrieved from http://www.nursingworld.org/MainMenuCategories/ThePracticeofProfessionalNursing/NursingStandards

American Nurses Credentialing Center. (2016a). Consensus model for APRN regulation: Frequently asked questions [Fact sheet]. Retrieved from http://www.nursecredentialing.org/Certification/APRNCorner/APRN-FAQ

American Nurses Credentialing Center. (2016b). *FAQs: About accreditation* [Fact sheet]. Retrieved from http://www.nursecredentialing.org/AboutAccreditationFAQ#accred

American Nurses Credentialing Center. (2016c). Magnet recognition program overview [Fact sheet]. Retrieved from http://www.nursecredentialing.org/Magnet/ProgramOverview

American Nurses Credentialing Center. (2016d). Nurse practitioner certifications. Retrieved from http://www.nursecredentialing.org/certification.aspx

Arizona State Legislature. (1997). Arizona Nurse Practice Act. Chapter 140 - 431R - S Ver of SB1099. Section 32-1636. Retrieved from http://www.azleg.state.az.us/legtext/43leg/1r/laws/0140.htm

Brent, N. J. (2012). Protect yourself: Know your nurse practice act [Online CE]. Retrieved from http://ce.nurse.com/course/ce548/protect-yourself--know-your-nurse-practice-act/

Damgaard, G., Hohman, M., & Karpiuk, K. (2000). *History of nursing regulation.* Colleagues in Caring Project. Retrieved from http://doh.sd.gov/boards/nursing/Documents/WhitePaperHistory2000.pdf

Department of Health and Human Services, Office of the Inspector General. (2010). *Adverse events in hospitals: National incidence among Medicare beneficiaries.* Washington, DC. Retrieved from https://oig.hhs.gov/oei/reports/oei-06-09-00090.pdf

Evans, S. (2015). The nurse licensure compact: A historical perspective. *Journal of Nursing Regulation, 6*(3), 11–16.

Fleischman, R. K., Meyer, L., & Watson, C. (2011). Best practices in creating a culture of certification. *AACN Advanced Critical Care, 22,* 33–49. doi: 10.1097/NCI.0b013e3182062c4e

GraduateNursingEDU.org. (2016). Retrieved from http://www.graduatenursingedu.org/state-board-of-nursing/

Indiana Administrative Code. (2013). Article 2. Standards for the competent practice of registered and licensed practical nursing. Retrieved from http://www.in.gov/legislative/iac/T08480/A00020.PDF

Institute of Medicine. (2000). *To err is human: Building a safer health system.* Washington, DC: National Academy Press.

James, J. T. (2013). A new, evidence-based estimate of patient harms associated with hospital care. *Journal of Patient Safety, 9*(3), 122–128.

Kaplow, R. (2011). The value of certification. *AACN Advanced Critical Care, 22,* 25–32. doi: 10.1097/NCI.0b013e3182057738.

McDougal, B., Bitz, K., Derouen, S., Nagel, J., Thomas, K., Newman, B., . . . Filippone, J. L. (2011). The 2011 uniform licensure requirements for adoption. *Journal of Nursing Regulation, 2*(3), 19–22.

National Council of State Boards of Nursing. (1996). National council begins revising models for nursing regulation. *Issues: A Newsletter of the National Council of State Boards of Nursing, 17*(3), 3.

National Council of State Boards of Nursing. (2007). The joint statement on delegation developed by the American Nurses Association and the National Council of State Boards of Nursing. Retrieved from https://www.ncsbn.org/Delegation_joint_statement_NCSBN-ANA.pdf

National Council of State Boards of Nursing. (2010). Your state board of nursing works for you: A health care consumer's guide [Fact sheet]. Retrieved from https://www.ncsbn.org/A_Health_Care_Consumers_Guide.pdf

National Council of State Boards of Nursing. (2011a). State and territorial boards of nursing: What every nurse needs to know. Retrieved from https://www.ncsbn.org/What_Every_Nurse_Needs_to_Know.pdf

National Council of State Boards of Nursing. (2011b). *What you need to know about nursing licensure and boards of nursing.* Chicago, IL: Author.

National Council of State Boards of Nursing. (2016a). About NCSBN. Retrieved from https://www.ncsbn.org/about.htm

National Council of State Boards of Nursing. (2016b). Contact a board of nursing. Retrieved from https://www.ncsbn.org/contact-bon.htm

National Council of State Boards of Nursing. (2016c). Delegation. Retrieved from https://www.ncsbn.org/1625.htm

National Council of State Boards of Nursing. (2016d). Guiding principles of nursing regulation: Adopted by the 2007 NCSBN Delegate Assembly. Retrieved from https://www.ncsbn.org/Guiding_Principles.pdf

National Council State Boards of Nursing. (2016e). Licensure. Retrieved from https://www.ncsbn.org/licensure.htm

National Council of State Boards of Nursing. (2016f). Licensure compacts. Retrieved from https://www.ncsbn.org/compacts.htm

National Council of State Boards of Nursing. (2016g). National guidelines for nursing delegation. *Journal of Nursing Regulation, 7*(1), 5–14.

National Council of State Boards of Nursing. (2016h). NCSBN model act. Retrieved from https://www.ncsbn.org/14_Model_Act_0914.pdf

National Council of State Boards of Nursing. (2016i). NCSBN model rules. Retrieved from https://www.ncsbn.org/14_Model_Rules_0914.pdf

National Council of State Boards of Nursing. (2016j). Nurse licensure compact: Frequently asked questions [Fact sheet]. Retrieved from https://www.ncsbn.org/NLC_FAQ.pdf

National Council of State Boards of Nursing. (2016k). Nurse practice act, rules & regulations. Retrieved from http://www.ncsbn.org/nurse-practice-act.htm

National Council of State Boards of Nursing. (2016l). Nurse licensure compact: Five reasons to endorse the NLC. Retrieved from https://www.ncsbn.org/Reasons_to_Endorse.pdf

National Council of State Boards of Nursing. (2016m). What every nurse needs to know. Retrieved from https://www.ncsbn.org/What_Every_Nurse_Needs_to_Know.pdf

National Council of State Boards of Nursing. (2016n). What nurses need to know. Retrieved from https://www.ncsbn.org/NLC_What_Nurses_Need_to_Know.pdf

New Hampshire Board of Nursing. (2016). Nurse licensure compact: Frequently asked questions. Retrieved from https://www.nh.gov/nursing/faq/nurse-licensure-compact.htm

Nurse Licensure Compact Administrators. (2014). *Articles of organization of the Nurse Licensure Compact Administrators.* Retrieved from https://wwww.ncsbn.org/AOO_2014.pdf

Ridenour, J. (2011). Nurse Licensure Compact myths & facts. Retrieved from https://www.ncsbn.org/201106_NLC_JRidenour.pdf

Roberts, M. M. (1954). *American nursing: History and interpretation.* New York, NY: Macmillan.

Russell, K. (2012). Nurse practice acts guide and govern nursing practice. *Journal of Nursing Regulation, 3*(3), 36–42.

Schmitt, K., & Shimberg, B. (1996). *Demystifying occupational and professional regulation: Answers to questions you may have been afraid to ask.* Lexington, KY: Council on Licensure, Enforcement and Regulation.

The Joint Commission. (2016a). Accreditation. Retrieved from http://www.jointcommission.org/accreditation/accreditation_main.aspx

The Joint Commission. (2016b). Certification. Retrieved from http://www.jointcommission.org/certification/certification_main.aspx

UNC-TV. (2012). North Carolina nurses: A century of caring [Documentary]. Retrieved from http://www.unctv.org/content/ncnurses

Understanding the NCLEX-RN

Judith A. Halstead

LEARNING OUTCOMES

After reading this chapter you will be able to:

- Explain the purpose of the licensure examination (NCLEX-RN) for registered nurses.
- Describe how the NCLEX-RN is developed and validated.
- Analyze the components of the NCLEX-RN test plan.
- Discuss the computer adaptive testing (CAT) format, including the benefits of this form of testing.
- Understand the various types of questions on the NCLEX-RN.
- Develop strategies to assist in preparing to take the NCLEX-RN.

Introduction

As students prepare to graduate from their prelicensure nursing program, thoughts turn naturally to two major events in their professional lives—acquiring their first position as a registered nurse and passing the registered

---

The editors wish to acknowledge the contributions of Lillia Loriz and Lucy B. Trice to the previous edition of this chapter.

nurse licensure examination. For many students, taking the licensure examination can be a stressful event; after all, one cannot practice as a registered nurse without passing the examination. However, with proper preparation, much can be done to raise self-confidence levels and decrease the normal feelings of anxiety and stress associated with taking the examination.

The purpose of this chapter is to provide an overview of the **National Council Licensure Examination for Registered Nurses (NCLEX-RN)** examination and strategies on how to best prepare to take the examination. A brief overview of the purpose of the examination and how it is developed and validated as a reflection on current RN practice is provided, followed by a discussion of the examination, content areas, and the types of test questions found on the examination. Finally, strategies on how to prepare and take the examination are included.

> **KEY TERM**
>
> **National Council Licensing Examination for Registered Nurses (NCLEX–RN):** This examination must be taken by all graduates of diploma, associate degree, and baccalaureate degree nursing programs prior to a license being issued. Successful completion of the examination is a requirement for practice as a registered nurse.

Purpose of the NCLEX-RN

The **National Council of State Boards of Nursing (NCSBN)** is the professional nursing regulatory body given the task of providing a means to ensure that those who are licensed to practice as registered nurses are "safe" in terms of their knowledge base. The NCSBN performs this function by developing and providing an examination that those educated as registered nurses through diploma, associate degree, and baccalaureate degree programs must successfully complete in order to receive a license to practice nursing. This test is the National Council Licensure Examination for Registered Nurses, more commonly known as the NCLEX-RN. The NCSBN performs the same function for those educated as practical nurses, through the National Council Licensure Examination for Practical Nurses or NCLEX-PN.

> **KEY TERM**
>
> **National Council of State Boards of Nursing (NCSBN):** The nursing regulatory body given the task of providing a means to ensure that those who are licensed to practice as nurses are "safe" in terms of their knowledge base.

The need for a means of ensuring that all nurses who have graduated from a nursing program have a minimal level of competency was recognized as early as 1867 in England; however, this notion did not take root in the United States until 1896 (Kelly & Joel, 1996). In the early days of U.S. nursing education, nursing schools were designed to meet the individual needs of the hospitals housing the programs. Some schools of nursing existed in full-spectrum hospitals, which offered a wide variety of services including medical, surgical, obstetric, and pediatric care. Others were associated with hospitals offering specialized care only, such as psychiatric and children's hospitals. Nurses graduating from schools associated with full-spectrum hospitals had a different skill set from those educated in single specialty hospitals. Additionally, many of those practicing as nurses had no formal training at all but could call themselves nurses because there were no legal restrictions on their representing themselves as such (Kalisch & Kalisch, 2004).

This wide disparity in the skills of those calling themselves nurses was the impetus for the movement to license nurses. The movement began in the United States in the early part of the 20th century, and by 1923, every state had instituted a form of licensure known as permissive licensure. Licensure was not required, hence the term *permissive*. The rules were voluntary and basically provided a means for licensure to be permitted but not required. In each state, requirements for licensure included educational requirements, rules for examinations, as well as provision for revocation of the license (Kalisch & Kalisch, 1995). Although this type of licensure was not mandatory, it was required in order to use the title "registered nurse." Licensure did not become universally mandatory in all 50 states until the middle of the 20th century.

The purpose of all activities associated with nursing licensure is to address safety for the public who are the recipients of nursing care. Licensing examinations for entry-level nurses and practical nurses are measures of *minimal* safety in practice. They do not indicate that the individual who has passed these examinations and obtained a license has an exceptional amount of knowledge, but rather that he or she has the minimal amount believed necessary for "safe" practice. The nursing profession has a duty to protect the public from unsafe care, and the NCLEX-RN is one measure designed to accomplish this task. Chapter 3 further discusses the concept and implications of licensure for registered nurses.

Nursing programs must be approved for operation by their state board of nursing for their graduates to be granted permission by the NCSBN to take the NCLEX-RN. State boards of nursing have a responsibility for reviewing the performance of the school's graduates on the licensure examination. The success of first-time test takers in particular is tracked, and it is possible for schools to be put on probation or have their state board of nursing approval revoked if the NCLEX-RN success rate of their graduates falls below the accepted range stipulated by the particular state's board of nursing.

Development of the NCLEX-RN

Since the establishment of an examination process to ensure basic safety of RN practice, the test itself has gradually evolved from an examination that was state administered and specific to an individual state's requirements to the one nationally normed and universal computerized examination that today's graduates experience. Long gone are the days when nursing graduates had the opportunity to take the examination only during two specified times of the year and were required to travel to large, centralized testing sites to sit with hundreds of other test takers to complete the test by paper and pencil. The examination typically required 2 full days of testing.

KEY TERM

Computer adaptive testing (CAT): An interactive testing format used on the NCLEX-RN to adjust the type of question and level of testing difficulty based on the test taker's previous response. In the NCLEX-RN examination, the testing continues until the student either achieves a consistent level of test item difficulty that indicates a satisfactory performance level and passing of the examination, does not achieve a consistent level of testing difficulty required to indicate a satisfactory performance level and thus fails the examination, or completes all of the test items on the examination or time expires on the test.

Today, the NCLEX-RN **computer adaptive testing (CAT)** format is nationally established by the NCSBN and adopted by all U.S. states and its territories. After completing an application process and receiving approval to take the examination, graduates of nursing programs can arrange to take the examination at local testing centers at a time and place that is largely convenient to their individual schedules. The time that is allowed to take the examination does not exceed 6 hours and frequently requires less time, depending upon the performance of the test taker. Once graduates have obtained the results of their NCLEX-RN indicating that they have passed the examination, they are eligible to apply for licensure as a registered nurse in any state of their choosing.

The last major change in the NCLEX-RN testing format was the conversion to the CAT in 1994. This represents the first time the NCLEX-RN was available to test takers in a computerized format. Although the content was the same as in the previous paper-and-pencil format, the CAT format brought about a number of changes. Although one did not need sophisticated computer skills to take the test, having the test appear on a screen rather than on a piece of paper represented a significant change in test-taking practices. Perhaps the greatest change in terms of the format for many graduates, however, was that one could no longer go back and forth from a current question to an earlier question. Each question must be answered before the test will progress to displaying another question. This particular change has effectively eliminated any ability for one question to inadvertently provide a clue to a previously answered question. Furthermore, once a test question has been answered and entered, it is not possible to return to the question to change the answer. The CAT format is discussed in more detail later in this chapter.

The advent of the computerized NCLEX-RN brought about several other changes in the overall process. As previously mentioned, the test can now be taken as soon as permission is granted for the individual by the appropriate state board of nursing and an appointment is made at any of the many sites administering the test throughout the country. New graduates may sit for the examination within 6 weeks of completing requirements for their nursing degree. Additionally, new graduates can take the examination at any authorized testing site, regardless of where they wish to be licensed initially. The test results are mailed to the candidate from the respective state board of nursing approximately 1 month from the date of testing. Finally, should the need to retest arise, the waiting time is a minimum of 45 days (or longer depending on the state board of nursing/regulatory body) rather than the previous mandatory 6-month retest waiting time. The actual amount of time between retesting is set by the individual state boards of nursing. The candidate bulletin explaining the test plan, how to register for the examination, and other pertinent details about the examination are available online at https://www.ncsbn.org. Initially, with the conversion to the CAT the structure of the test questions themselves did not change from the paper-and-pencil test; they retained the multiple-choice format. However, the testing format has now evolved so the examination currently includes a number of other testing formats in addition to the standard multiple-choice testing option. These formats include multiple response, fill-in-the-blank/calculations, hot spots, exhibits, and drag and drop/ordered response items. Each of these testing formats will be discussed in detail later in this chapter.

Future Areas of Development for the NCLEX-RN

Just as the knowledge explosion in health care continues to drive changes in nursing practice, it will also necessitate changes in NCLEX-RN test content as well as methods of testing in order to verify minimal competence to practice. Every 3 years, the NCSBN conducts a job analysis study that explores the entry-level skills and knowledge needed by beginning nurses. The NCSBN is responsible for preparing a licensing examination that is psychometrically sound and valid, as well as legally defensible. The triennial job analysis studies assist the NCSBN in doing this; the process used for conducting the triennial job analysis can be found on the NCSBN website at http://www.ncsbn.org (NCSBN, 2016b).

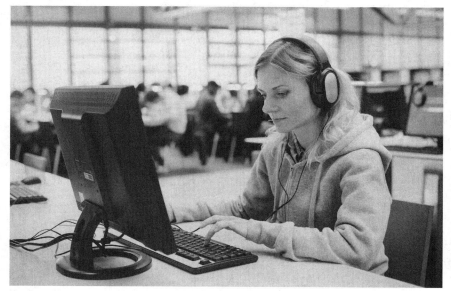

Nursing student taking a computerized test.
© Ditty_about_summer/Shutterstock

Further, the growth in culturally diverse patient populations mandates that concepts related to cultural competence be included in the curriculum of nursing programs and that minimal competence in this area be addressed in the licensing examination (Fitzpatrick, 2007). Another issue that continues to be debated within the profession is the question of differentiated practice and whether separate licensure examinations should exist for graduates of different educational programs.

Most recently another development in the administration of the NCLEX-RN occurred when Canada adopted the NCLEX-RN to serve as the national licensure examination for graduates of Canadian nursing programs. This marks the first time that the NCLEX-RN was adopted for use in another country. **Contemporary Practice Highlight 4-1** provides additional information on this historic event.

Components of the NCLEX-RN Test Plan

The NCSBN is responsible for the development of the NCLEX-RN exam. As previously discussed, the examination is developed from an analysis of the job functions performed by selected entry-level nurses in the first year of employment.

CONTEMPORARY PRACTICE HIGHLIGHT 4–1

NCSBN NCLEX–RN USED TO GRANT CANADIAN RN LICENSURE

Historically, the NCLEX-RN has been offered only to nursing graduates for the purposes of domestic licensure, i.e., to those nursing graduates who wished to become licensed to practice nursing in the United States. This changed in November 2014 when the NCSBN opened the examination to graduates of Canadian nursing schools for purposes of achieving licensure to practice as an RN in Canada. The NCLEX-RN can now be taken to be licensed as an RN for those who wish to practice in Alberta, British Columbia, Manitoba, New Brunswick, Newfoundland and Labrador, Northwest Territories and Nunavut, Nova Scotia, Ontario, Prince Edward Island, and Saskatchewan. The Canadian nursing regulatory body, the Canadian Council of Registered Nurse Regulators (CCRNR), worked collaboratively with the NCSBN to plan and implement the use of the NCLEX-RN in Canada. The CCRNR was seeking a means by which to introduce an examination process in Canada that used the latest in technology, provided enhanced test security, and allowed for year-round national delivery of a licensing exam to graduates of Canadian schools. This is the first time that the NCLEX-RN has been adopted by another country to allow for RN licensure to practice in that country.

Data from National Council of State Boards of Nursing. (2014). NCSBN opens registration for NCLEX in Canada. News Release 10-22-14. Retrieved from https://www.ncsbn.org/6655.htm

The 2016 NCLEX-RN **test plan** was developed from the 2014 job analysis study (NCSBN, 2015). The current test plan can be obtained at https://www.ncsbn.org/testplans.htm. Students are encouraged to go to the NCSBN website and obtain a copy of the test plan because it provides a framework for the development of test items and can be used by students as they organize their study materials and begin their preparation for taking the examination.

The test plan is organized around a client needs framework consisting of four main categories, providing a structure within which nursing actions and competencies can be tested. The term *client* is used interchangeably with the terms *patient* or *resident* because this encompasses a broader population for nursing care. This framework also focuses on clients in all care settings and across all age groups.

In addition to the client needs framework, there are integrated processes that are considered fundamental to nursing practice and integrated for testing throughout the categories of the client needs framework; these processes can be tested in relation to any client or any setting. The five categories of integrated processes are Nursing Process; Caring; Communication and Documentation; Teaching/Learning; and Culture and Spirituality (NCSBN, 2016b, p. 5). Definitions for each of these processes can be found in the most current NCLEX test plan, which is available for downloading from the NCSBN website. The implications for the learner are that it is essential to be competent in understanding the integrated processes and applying the principles and concepts related to using the nursing process; developing mutually collaborative, respectful, and trusting relationships with clients; communicating, verbally and nonverbally, with clients, families, and other healthcare providers and accurately documenting these interactions; teaching clients and their families/significant others in the care of all clients in any setting; and considering the uniqueness of all clients in their beliefs and preferences when providing care.

Framework of Client Needs

The client needs framework is divided into four major client needs categories; two of the categories are further divided into subcategories (see **Box 4-1**). Each of these categories is described in the following sections; for a complete and detailed description of each category, please see the most current NCLEX-RN test plan available at the NCSBN website.

Safe and Effective Care Environment

The nurse is responsible for promoting the achievement of client outcomes by directing and providing nursing care in a care setting in a manner that protects

---

**BOX 4-1   CATEGORIES AND SUBCATEG-
ORIES OF NCLEX-RN TEST PLAN**

Safe and Effective Care Environment
• Management of Care
• Safety and Infection Control
Health Promotion and Maintenance
Psychosocial Integrity
Physiological Integrity
• Basic Care and Comfort
• Pharmacological and Parenteral Therapies
• Reduction of Risk Potential
• Physiological Adaptation

Data from National Council of State Boards of Nursing.
(2016a). 2016 NCLEX® examination candidate bulletin.
Retrieved from https://www.ncsbn.org/089900_2016_
Bulletin_Proof3.pdf

---

clients, family/significant others, and other healthcare providers (NCSBN, 2016b, p. 6). This category is further divided into Management of Care and Safety and Infection Control. Management of Care addresses concepts related to providing and directing nursing care in a healthcare delivery setting that is designed to protect patients, family, and other healthcare personnel; this subcategory accounts for approximately 17–23 percent of the test plan (NCSBN, 2016b, p. 5). Management of care can include, but is not limited to, such nursing responsibilities as prioritizing client care, delegating and supervising care, making appropriate referrals to community resources, maintaining client confidentiality, and providing and participating in staff education.

Safety and Infection Control is focused on health and environmental hazards (NCSBN, 2016b, p. 7) in the care setting and constitutes approximately 9–15 percent of the test plan (p. 5). Safety issues, for both the patient and the nurse, have gained increasing importance, and the NCLEX-RN test plan reflects this change in emphasis. Examples of content areas that may be addressed in this subcategory include surgical asepsis, safe use of medical devices and restraints, handling infectious materials, and emergency response planning, to name just a few topics.

Health Promotion and Maintenance

This category addresses incorporating concepts from growth and development and the prevention and early detection of health problems into the provision of nursing care, as well as nursing strategies designed to promote the achievement of optimal client health (NCSBN, 2016b, p. 7). Approximately 6–12 percent of the test plan is devoted to health promotion and maintenance activities (NCSBN, 2016b, p. 5). Throughout this content area, the candidate is expected to demonstrate knowledge related to providing care to individuals across the life span (e.g., care of the pregnant client and newborn, elder care); physical assessment skills; providing adequate education to meet the needs of the client, family, or significant other (e.g., lifestyle choices, sexually transmitted diseases, self-care activities); and anticipating and preventing potential future health problems through health promotion (e.g., immunizations) and screening activities.

Psychosocial Integrity

The Psychosocial Integrity category is a broadly encompassing category that addresses content areas related to promoting and supporting the "emotional, mental and social well-being of the client and family/significant others experiencing stressful events, as well as clients with acute or chronic mental illness" (NCSBN, 2016b, p. 7). Throughout this content area, the candidate should be able to demonstrate the ability to assess clients and families at risk of mental health problems, substance abuse, provide care to clients in a variety of crisis situations, provide end-of-life care, support for grief and loss, incorporate client stress management techniques, and use therapeutic communication, to name a few examples of the broadness of this category. This category accounts for approximately 6–12 percent of the test plan (NCSBN, 2016b, p. 5).

Physiological Integrity

As a single category, physiological integrity accounts for the largest percentage of the total test plan, ranging anywhere from 38–62 percent (NCSBN, 2016b, p. 5). The category topics are focused on nursing care that is related to safely meeting the client's activities of daily living; providing safe administration of medications; decreasing the potential for client complications; and managing the nursing care of clients with acute, chronic, and/or life-threatening health problems (NCSBN, 2016b, p. 8).

This category is further divided into four subcategories: Basic Care and Comfort, Pharmacological and Parenteral Therapies, Reduction of Risk Potential, and Physiological Adaptation. The subcategory of Basic Care and Comfort, 6–12 percent of the test plan (NCSBN, 2016b, p. 5), addresses knowledge and competencies related to performing basic nursing skills, including, but not limited to, monitoring vital signs, height and weight, hydration status, and application and removal of orthopedic devices.

The subcategory of Pharmacological and Parenteral Therapies includes all aspects of nursing care related to safe medication administration such as basic dosage calculations; medication administration via all routes, including parenteral; monitoring client responses and outcomes related to medication administration; administration of blood products; total parenteral nutrition; and client and family education regarding medications. In addition, the basic information regarding common medications, their mechanism of action, uses and contraindications, and drug interactions is also part of this subcategory. This subcategory accounts for approximately 12 to 18 percent of the total test plan (NCSBN, 2016b, p. 5).

The subcategory of Reduction of Risk Potential, accounting for 9–15 percent of the test plan (NCSBN, 2016b, p. 5), is related to decreasing the likelihood of the client developing complications from existing health problems or care received. Monitoring the patient for complications is an important nursing responsibility that is addressed in this category, as is the nursing care related to preparing the client for diagnostic tests and surgical procedures, monitoring the patient following the procedures, and understanding the implications of laboratory values to client care.

The final subcategory for this section is Physiological Adaptation, which is related to providing nursing care to clients who are acutely or chronically ill or experiencing life-threatening health problems (NCSBN, 2016b, p. 8). This category constitutes 11–17 percent of the test plan (NCSBN, 2016b, p. 5). Such health problems as fluid and electrolyte imbalances, hemodynamic instabilities, and medical emergencies, as well as other physiological alterations, are addressed in this category.

The content area information that is provided in the NCLEX test plan framework can help students determine how to most effectively plan and use their study time. Students can also use this information to actively seek learning experiences in the final semesters of their nursing program to ensure that they are developing the necessary knowledge and competencies in all areas of nursing practice to be successful on the examination.

Computer Adaptive Testing

Computer adaptive testing (CAT) is a method of computerized testing that adapts to the test taker's responses on test items and alters the level of complexity of subsequent test items based upon previous item responses. As the test taker answers each question, the CAT will adjust subsequent test items to the level of the test taker's knowledge and abilities (as demonstrated by answers on previous items) until, ultimately, the test taker either demonstrates satisfactory performance at the level designated for passing the examination or demonstrates unsatisfactory performance on the examination, as evidenced by the inability to consistently reach and accurately respond to items at a preset level of complexity, thus failing the examination (Lavin & Rosario-Sim, 2013). This is the format in which all candidates for the NCLEX take the examination.

Taking an examination that is administered via the CAT format requires that test candidates understand certain concepts about the administration of the test. First, it is important to understand that all questions must be answered in the order they appear on the computer screen; candidates cannot go back and forth between test items. The candidate can take as long as needed to read and respond to each question; however, the question must be answered before progressing to the next test item. Second, candidates should plan their time spent on each test item, so as to allow enough time to answer the maximum number of questions (265) in the maximum allowed time (6 hours), should that be necessary. If uncertain of an answer, the candidate should make a best guess based on critical reasoning skills and then move on to the next item.

Third, as previously indicated, CAT testing does not allow the candidate to return to an item once an answer has been submitted. The difficulty of the test items is adjusted as the candidate answers the items and demonstrates proficiency in various areas. Essentially, the candidate will be tested at a certain level of difficulty, and if he or she correctly responds to that specific item, the next test item generated by the CAT program is again at that level. After the candidate is again successful at this level, the next item generated will then be at a higher level of difficulty; if the candidate is unsuccessful at answering that item correctly, the level of difficulty for the next item will be lower. The goal is to determine when the candidate remains at a consistent level of ability. The ability estimate is based on the percentage of test items answered correctly and the difficulty of the items that were administered. The test will automatically stop when either the test bank is exhausted (the candidate answered 265 questions), the test length is reached (6 hours for the NCLEX-RN), or the ability level is estimated with sufficient accuracy (Lavin & Rosario-Sim, 2013).

The Passing Standard

The passing standard is the minimum level of ability required for safe and effective entry-level nursing practice. In order to pass the NCLEX-RN exam, the candidate must perform above the passing standard.

The passing standard is evaluated once every 3 years and adjusted accordingly. The NCSBN board of directors makes this determination based on information gathered during that period of time. The information used by the board includes results of surveys, performance of past graduates, and past passing standards. Standard-setting surveys and exercises are conducted to determine the passing standard and what that standard would mean. In addition, the board of directors reviews the historical record of the passing standard since the implementation of CAT and correlates these findings with summaries of candidate performance. All these factors are considered as decisions are made in order to determine the passing standard. Once this passing standard is set, all candidates must perform above this standard in order to pass the NCLEX-RN examination. The current passing standard is scheduled to be in effect until March 31, 2019, when it will be reevaluated by the NCSBN board of directors (NCSBN, 2016b).

Types of Questions on the NCLEX-RN Examination

As mentioned earlier, the NCLEX-RN examination uses a variety of test item formats. Many of the questions are multiple choice; however, alternate item formats are also used and include multiple response, fill-in-the blank (calculations), hot spots, charts/exhibits, drag and drop/ordered response, audio items, and graphics.

Multiple-choice items are the most common test items on the examination. For these items, the candidate is presented with a question or clinical situation in the question's stem and then asked to select the one best answer from a list of four possible options. **Box 4-2** provides an example of a traditional multiple-choice item.

Multiple-response questions present the candidate with a question, followed by a list of possible responses. The candidate is asked to select all options that apply, allowing for more than one correct response. The candidate must select *all* of the appropriate responses for the item to be answered correctly. **Box 4-3** provides an example of a multiple-answer/multiple-response test item.

BOX 4-2   MULTIPLE-CHOICE TEST ITEM

Which of the following neurological assessments would the nurse conduct to evaluate the patient's cerebellar function?

1. Abdominal reflex
2. Romberg test
3. Glasgow coma scale
4. Babinski test

Answer: 2

BOX 4-3   MULTIPLE-RESPONSE ITEM

The nurse is providing post-mortem care for a client. Which of the following interventions would be appropriate for the nurse to complete prior to allowing the family to see the client? Select all that apply.

1. Clean and reposition the client's body.
2. Call the physician to verify the time of death.
3. Provide sterile gloves to family members.
4. Freshen the bed linens and pull covers to the client's shoulders.

Answer: 1, 4

Fill-in-the-blank items present a question and then ask the candidate to type in a response. Most commonly, the fill-in-the-blank items represent drug dosage calculation problems or situations in which the candidate is required to calculate the client's intake/output record. The candidate is expected to calculate the response without the benefit of potential answers from which to choose. A drop-down calculator is provided to assist with calculations; it can be found by clicking on the calculator button located at the bottom right side of the computer screen. **Box 4-4** provides an example of a fill-in-the-blank test item.

Hot spots present candidates with a question and a diagram or figure. The candidate needs to use the mouse to identify and select an area on the diagram/figure, then click on the left mouse button in order to indicate an answer. Hot spot questions are frequently used to ask candidates to select appropriate areas to auscultate heart, lung, and abdominal sounds. **Box 4-5** provides an example of a "hot spot" test item.

Chart/exhibit items present the candidate with a scenario and a chart or exhibit that contains information required to answer the question. The exhibit may be in the form of a table, graph, or diagram. For example, an exhibit may provide the candidate with a listing of a client's arterial blood gas values, to enable the candidate to respond to a question about the client's physiological status. **Box 4-6** provides an example of an exhibit question asking the test taker to identify a cardiac rhythm.

Drag and drop/ordered response test items present the candidate with a question and a list of options that the candidate is required to sequence, prioritize, or rank order to answer the question. In this type of test format, the unordered options appear on the left side of the computer screen. The candidate must use the mouse to click and drag the options to the right side of the screen, placing them in the appropriate order, and then confirm completion of that test item to record the answer. **Box 4-7** provides an example of a sequencing test item.

BOX 4-4   FILL-IN-THE-BLANK ITEM

A patient has an order for sodium phenobarbital 60 milligrams intramuscularly every 8 hours. The nurse has a vial that reads sodium phenobarbital 100 milligrams/2 milliliters. How many milliliters will the nurse need to administer?

1. Provide a numeric answer:

_____ milliliters

Answer: 1.2

BOX 4–5   HOT SPOT TEST ITEM

Place an X over the anatomical location where the nurse would auscultate bronchial breath sounds.

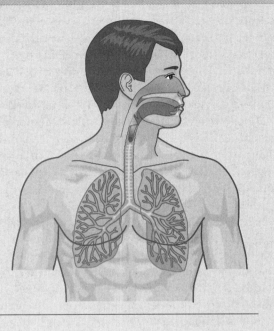

BOX 4–6   EXHIBIT TEST ITEM

How would the nurse interpret this cardiac rhythm?

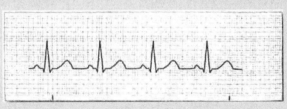

Reproduced from *Arrhythmia Recognition: The Art of Interpretation*, courtesy of Tomas B. Garcia, MD.

Answer: Sinus bradycardia

Audio test items require the candidate to listen to a short audio clip and then answer a test question based upon the scenario contained in the clip. *Graphic* test items have options that depict graphics for answers instead of text.

BOX 4–7 DRAG AND DROP/ORDERED RESPONSE TEST ITEM

This question will require you to use the mouse to place the responses in a correct sequence of actions based on the situation.

A patient has just been admitted to the hospital to receive treatment for an exacerbation of his COPD. In which order should the nurse complete the following sequence of nursing actions?

1. Place allergy band on patient arm.
2. Order patient meals and procedures.
3. Complete the patient assessment.
4. Call the healthcare provider to obtain admission orders.

Answer: 3, 1, 4, 2

Preparing for the NCLEX-RN

There are multiple ways to prepare for taking the NCLEX-RN. The most important point is actually having a plan for preparation and implementing it prior to graduation. Students should become familiar with the NCLEX-RN test plan early in their program and use it to guide their study throughout the curriculum (Pressler & Kenner, 2012). It is also important that candidates select a method of review and preparation that will work best for them. Learning styles differ from individual to individual; some learn best visually, others prefer an auditory approach. Some prefer to study in isolation, whereas others find group study work to be most effective. Regardless of the preparation method chosen, all students will benefit by reviewing and preparing for the NCLEX, even those students who have performed consistently well in school. It is the student's responsibility to take preparation for the NCLEX seriously; lack of preparation can lead to failure of the examination and a delay in becoming licensed as an RN.

How to go about reviewing for the NCLEX is up to the individual. There are many well-written NCLEX review books on the market. Most of these books use the NCLEX-RN test plan as a framework for organizing their content and categorizing their test items. They also may have an accompanying CD with computerized test questions that have been written using all of the various test item formats used on the NCLEX. Candidates should review and select the book that they find most helpful; it is especially helpful to select a book that provides rationale for right and wrong answers and offers questions in all of the testing formats used on the NCLEX.

In addition to review books, there are a variety of computerized and online test review products. These products can help candidates get a sense of what it is like to take a test with the CAT format. There are also formal review programs that are offered over various lengths of time. These review programs may be offered by the school of nursing or potential employers. Faculty may be helpful in assisting candidates to evaluate the worthiness of any given review product (Pressler & Kenner, 2012). A good rule of thumb is that what has worked for a candidate in the past in terms of preparing for a test will probably work best when preparing for the NCLEX-RN, so students shouldn't abandon or change previously proven methods of helpful study. Although how to structure and plan the review is an individual preference, the following guidelines may be helpful when preparing to take the NCLEX-RN. Attending to a solid knowledge base, enhancing test-taking skills, and managing anxiety can help students perform their best on the NCLEX (Simon, McGinniss, & Krauss, 2013). **Box 4-8** summarizes these preparation tips.

- *Conduct a self-assessment:* Students should begin their preparation by reviewing the NCLEX test plan and assessing their knowledge base and readiness to take the examination. This self-assessment is ideally conducted before the final semesters of the nursing program, so that the student has time to seek learning experiences that will help them to strengthen their knowledge base in areas they feel less confident about. Students should identify the content areas they know well, the areas that they know less well, and those that they may not have studied for a while. When preparing for the NCLEX-RN, students will want to spend more time reviewing areas that they are not comfortable with or that they have not reviewed recently. Many nursing programs provide students with the opportunity to take commercially prepared NCLEX "readiness" tests that predict the likelihood of passing the licensing examination. Students should take these tests, and their results, seriously and use them as a self-assessment guide for developing their study plans.
- *Develop a timetable for review and preparation:* After completing the self-assessment, it is important to look at the volume of material to be reviewed and the amount of time that exists before scheduling to take the test. A timetable

---

BOX 4-8 TIPS ON PREPARING FOR THE NCLEX-RN

- Conduct a self-assessment of readiness to take the NCLEX-RN.
- Develop a timetable to guide preparation.
- Become familiar with the NCLEX-RN test plan.
- Know the test item formats used on the NCLEX-RN.
- Practice answering test questions.
- Enroll in an NCLEX-RN review course.
- Hone test-taking skills and take steps to reduce test-taking anxiety.

should be developed that allows for consistent and steady progression through the review process. The important thing to remember is that a timetable should be set that provides the opportunity for a thorough review and fosters the self-discipline to actually do the review. Students should not wait until they graduate before they begin their review; as stated previously, beginning the review while still in school can help identify areas where additional learning experiences, especially in the clinical setting, will help increase knowledge of the content. Students who think they lack the self-discipline to adhere to a review schedule, may find it helpful to commit to a study partner who will help keep them on their review schedule. Some students also may benefit from participating in small study groups.

■ *Become familiar with the NCLEX-RN test plan:* Students should be familiar with the NCLEX-RN test plan prior to beginning to review for the examination. When reviewing, it is important to remember to focus on concepts and fundamental processes, not factual information. A complete and up-to-date description of the test plan is always available for downloading from the NCSBN website at https://www.ncsbn.org/testplans.htm.

■ *Know the test item formats used on the NCLEX-RN:* Just as knowing the test plan around which the NCLEX-RN is organized is important, knowing what type of questions to expect is also important. The format of the question often drives how to study. For example, in a typical, one-answer-only, multiple-choice question, the correct answer must be recognized and selected from among the options provided. However, in fill-in-the-blank and hot spot questions, it is necessary to be able to critically reason and supply the answer without prompting or validation from a list of options. Students should develop a review plan that includes practice with answering the various test item formats included on the NCLEX.

■ *Practice answering test questions:* Just as knowing the types of questions to expect is important, practice in answering various types of questions is equally valuable. As discussed previously, there are many sources of practice questions similar to those on the NCLEX-RN. An important part of taking the practice questions is developing an understanding of the rationale of why the correct answer is correct and why the wrong answers are wrong. Examining the rationale for all correct and wrong answers helps students to develop insight into the context in which the questions are posed, as well as what words in the stem of the question are important to note before choosing an answer. Words or phrases such as *first, first step, next step, best represents, priority action,* or *primary reason* often indicate which of the answer options is the "best" choice, even though all of the answers might actually represent correct actions that could be taken in the situation posed in the question.

■ *Enroll in NCLEX-RN review courses:* There are many review courses available, ranging in length of time and format, including online offerings (Lavin & Rosario-Sim, 2013). The advantage to review courses is that they organize the content and provide a structured approach for students to follow as they conduct their review. These courses are designed to cover content that is common to all types of nursing programs. They are not meant to teach content, but rather to review it. Students should pay particular attention to content that they have had more difficulty understanding during their nursing program, as well as any new content covered in the review, and plan to study these areas in more depth following the review course.

The downside to review courses is that they can be expensive and are usually offered at specific times that may not be convenient. Characteristics of a good review course include competent and current faculty, comprehensiveness, opportunities to answer test questions throughout the review, a comprehensive computerized examination to assist with self-assessment prior to the course and/or provide a measure of how prepared one is for the NCLEX-RN exam following completion of the course, and a guarantee that the course may be repeated at least once free of charge, if unsuccessful in passing the NCLEX-RN.

■ *Hone test-taking skills:* It is important to spend time honing test-taking skills, especially if the student has previously experienced difficulty taking tests. There are books that can help with enhancing test-taking skills, and most colleges and universities housing nursing programs have academic support services to assist in test-taking skills.

Another area to consider is test anxiety. Students who have experienced test anxiety in the past should prepare to address it prior to taking the NCLEX-RN as well. Most colleges and universities offer support for students in this area. Finally, students who have any kind of documented disability for which they need to seek an accommodation will want to investigate obtaining the accommodation for taking the NCLEX-RN as well. In general, students who needed accommodation for a disability during their nursing program, particularly with test-taking, will want to make that known when applying to take the NCLEX-RN. With a high-stakes test such as the NCLEX, students who require accommodations should not be tempted to forego those accommodations when taking this examination. Testing accommodations must be requested through the regulatory body (state board of nursing) before applying to take the NCLEX. Arrangements for accommodations take additional time to process, so students should allow a minimum of 60 days in advance for processing of any request for accommodations.

Taking the NCLEX-RN

There are obviously significant consequences to taking the NCLEX-RN. If graduates pass the NCLEX, they become eligible to receive their license to practice as registered nurses and are on their way to transitioning from school to practice and a wonderful career filled with new and fulfilling experiences. However, if the examination is not passed, graduates will not be able to practice as registered nurses until they are able to pass the examination. In addition, taking the examination in an unfamiliar environment with people one does not know can be stressful. For these reasons, for many candidates the anxiety level associated with the examination experience can be very high. It is important that students feel confident in their preparation for the examination. Following the preparation tips presented in this chapter can help increase feelings of self-confidence and decrease any feelings of anxiety.

Students should plan to take the examination within 3 months of graduation, as evidence exists that the chance of failure increases the longer the graduate delays taking the examination (Lavin & Rosario-Sim, 2013; Serenbus, 2016), and securing licensure early will increase employment opportunities. In many instances employers may not hire a new RN graduate until the licensing examination has been passed. Waiting until the license has been granted can actually benefit the graduate as this allows for more time to prepare for taking the exam, rather than trying to study and cope with orientation to a new position simultaneously.

In anticipation of taking the examination, candidates should mentally prepare to take the maximum number of questions (265) and plan to pace themselves accordingly when taking the test. A pace of allowing 1–2 minutes per test question is a comfortable pace, with 1 minute being the average amount of time spent on a question. It is also important for candidates to remember that it is not possible to tell how well they are doing on the examination based on the length of time that the test is administered; the test may be passed within either a short or long testing period.

In addition to preparing for the test, there are other strategies that can be used to help put oneself at ease prior to taking the test. For example, conducting a practice run to the testing facility prior to the testing day can help relieve anxiety on the day of the test. Know the address and location of the testing facility and the best route to take to travel there, including typical traffic patterns to be anticipated on the day of the test. To arrive on time and unrushed, allow plenty of time to arrive at the testing site on the day of the examination.

During the final few days before the examination, the focus should be on obtaining plenty of rest and engaging in only brief periods of review time. Scheduling some time for relaxation to enjoy favorite pastimes is another good strategy to minimize anxiety.

On the day of the examination wear comfortable clothes and allow time to have a nutritious breakfast, including protein. Candidates should plan to arrive at the testing site 30 minutes before the scheduled testing time and should also be sure they have all necessary identification required to be allowed to take the test. Snacks may be brought to the test site and left in the locker provided, to be accessed during break periods. During the examination, two brief optional break periods are automatically provided to the candidates and snacks may be eaten during those times. The first optional break is offered 2 hours into the testing time, and the second optionally scheduled break is offered 3.5 hours into the testing time (NCSBN, 2016a). Although breaks are considered optional, it is important for candidates to take the breaks as scheduled, because not taking them can affect concentration.

Following the test, results will be available about 6 weeks after the date of testing. Some state boards of nursing will make scores available within 48 hours of testing for an additional fee.

Summary

This chapter has presented some basic information regarding the NCLEX-RN examination. The purpose of the NCLEX-RN and how it was developed were discussed. This chapter also provided a discussion of the components of the NCLEX-RN test plan to help candidates organize their preparation for the examination. Finally, a section on the types of questions found on the NCLEX-RN and how to prepare for the examination was included. The information provided in this chapter can help graduates prepare for a successful NCLEX-RN examination experience.

Reflective Practice Questions

1. Consider your own plans for preparing to take the NCLEX-RN. Are you satisfied with the steps that you have taken to date? What else can you do to develop and implement a plan that will support your success on the examination?

2. Conduct a self-assessment of your areas of strengths and areas that need improvement related to taking the NCLEX-RN. What learning experiences can you capitalize on in your remaining time in your nursing program to assist you in your preparation for the examination?

3. Do you think the job analysis process as it is currently conducted is a satisfactory method of determining the content that should be on the NCLEX-RN? What are the benefits of this methodology? Are there any inherent limitations?

References

Fitzpatrick, J. (2007). Cultural competence in nursing education revisited. *Nursing Education Perspectives, 28*(1), 5.

Kalisch, P. A., & Kalisch, B. J. (1995). *American nursing: A history* (3rd ed.). Philadelphia, PA: Lippincott Williams & Wilkins.

Kalisch, P. A., & Kalisch, B. J. (2004). *American nursing: A history* (4th ed.). Philadelphia, PA: Lippincott Williams & Wilkins.

Kelly, L., & Joel, L. (1996). *The nursing experience: Trends, challenges, and transitions* (3rd ed.). New York, NY: McGraw-Hill.

Lavin, J., & Rosario-Sim, M. (2013). Understanding the NCLEX: How to increase success on the revised 2013 examination. *Nursing Education Perspectives, 34*(3), 196–198.

National Council of State Boards of Nursing. (2014). NCSBN opens registration for NCLEX in Canada. News Release 10-22-14. Retrieved from https://www.ncsbn.org/6655.htm

National Council of State Boards of Nursing. (2015). 2014 RN practice analysis: Linking the NCLEX-RN examination to practice - U.S. and Canada (Vol. 62). Retrieved from https://www.ncsbn.org/7109.htm

National Council of State Boards of Nursing. (2016a). *2016 NCLEX® examination candidate bulletin.* Retrieved from https://www.ncsbn.org/089900_2016_Bulletin_Proof3.pdf

National Council of State Boards of Nursing. (2016b). *Test plan for the National Council Licensure Examination for Registered Nurses.* Retrieved from https://www.ncsbn.org/2016_RN_DetTestPlan_Educator.pdf

Pressler, J., & Kenner, C. (2012). Supporting student success on the NCLEX-RN. *Nurse Educator, 37*(3), 94–96.

Serenbus, J. F. (2016). First-time pass rates: A comprehensive program approach. *Journal of Nursing Regulation, 6*(4), 38–44.

Simon, E., McGinniss, S., & Krauss, B. (2013). Predictor variables for NCLEX-RN readiness exam performance. *Nursing Education Perspectives, 14*(1), 18–24.

Professional Nursing Organizations

Judith A. Halstead

LEARNING OUTCOMES

After reading this chapter you will be able to:

- Describe the purposes of professional nursing organizations.
- Analyze the importance of matching the mission of the organization with the members' expectations.
- Describe at least three different professional nursing organizations and their missions.
- Identify three member benefits associated with professional nursing organizations.
- Explain how nursing organizations advocate for nursing and quality patient care in the political arena.
- Consider individual career plans and the function of professional nursing organizations in advancing career development.

The editors wish to acknowledge the contributions of Karen Peddicord to the previous edition of this chapter.

Introduction

One of the characteristics of a profession is the existence of a professional culture that fosters the values and ethos of the profession among its members. This professional culture is commonly nurtured and maintained through the actions of the profession's organizations (Matthews, 2012). Professional organizations are developed to collectively advocate on behalf of their members and other constituents, publicly representing the core values of the nursing profession to others.

Nursing's first professional organization was founded in 1893 as the American Society of Superintendents of Training Schools for Nurses; today this organization is known as the National League for Nursing. Three years later, in 1896, a second nursing organization was founded, the Associated Alumnae of Trained Nurses of the United States and Canada, which evolved into the American Nurses Association (ANA). In 1899 these two nursing organizations were joined by a third organization, the International Council of Nurses, the first international professional nursing organization. Today, these historic and venerable nursing organizations remain vibrant and influential in nursing and health care and are now joined by more than 100 national professional nursing organizations, as well as growing numbers of international nursing organizations (Matthews, 2012). Together, these professional organizations constitute the "voice of nursing" in a variety of professional, political, regulatory, clinical, and educational matters.

> **KEY TERM**
>
> **Professional nursing organization:** A collective entity of nurse members that has as its purpose enhancement of some element of patient care or the nursing profession.

> **KEY TERM**
>
> **Membership:** The state of being a member or person in a group, in this case, a professional nursing organization.

This chapter provides an overview of **professional nursing organizations**, describing the various types of nursing organizations and the purposes they serve in advancing the nursing profession. This chapter also provides information about the many types of professional nursing organizations that exist and describes the benefits of **membership** for individual nurses, the profession, and the public. Specific information about a select number of professional nursing organizations is provided. How professional nursing organizations can serve as a vehicle for the career development of the individual nurse, beginning in nursing school, is also presented. Motivating factors for joining nursing organizations are addressed.

The Nature of Professional Nursing Organizations

Professional nursing organizations are an effective means by which the nursing profession can influence healthcare policy, represent and protect the interests of nurses, provide continuing education opportunities for nurses, and advocate for the highest quality care possible to the public. The many professional nursing organizations provide a variety of foci to match the interests of nurse members. For example, the

ANA is the largest of all the U.S. professional nursing organizations, representing the nursing profession and interests of 3.4 million nurses. The ANA's stated mission is "nurses advancing our profession to improve the health of all" (ANA, 2016a).

In contrast, there are many specialty nursing organizations that support the interests of nurses who practice in specific clinical environments. Examples of such specialty organizations include the Oncology Nursing Society (ONS), the Emergency Nurses Association (ENA), and the American Association of Critical-Care Nurses (AACN). There are also professional nursing organizations that are focused on specific roles of nurses. Examples of these include the American College of Nurse Midwives (ACNM), the American Association of Colleges of Nursing, the National League for Nursing (NLN), the National Association of Clinical Nurse Specialists (NACNS), and the American Organization of Nurse Executives (AONE). The Nursing Organization Alliance (www.nursing-alliance.org) is a coalition of 64 nursing organizations that collaboratively address issues of interest to nursing. Although it is not a comprehensive listing of all nursing organizations, a review of their membership list can provide the reader with an understanding of the many different types of professional nursing organizations and the diversity of their missions.

The Mission and Impact of Professional Nursing Organizations

Professional nursing organizations provide the opportunity for nursing as a profession to influence nursing practice, nursing education, health policy, and healthcare standards. There are multiple facets to these membership organizations that contribute to changes in the profession and provide a collective means by which nurses can be involved in shaping healthcare policy. Individual membership in nursing organizations also helps nurses stay current about issues that affect their specific practice area and nursing role. Participating in professional organizations can facilitate leadership development, develop skill in collaboration, provide networking opportunities for each member, and potentially result in career advancement. **Box 5-1** summarizes the types of mission focus that professional nursing organizations can have.

To fulfill their mission, nursing organizations further the development of nursing **standards of practice**, expand the body of knowledge through research and evidence-based practice, and promote nurses' general welfare in the workplace. Nursing organizations also provide **continuing nursing education**, foster the continued development of nursing as a profession, and serve as legislative and political advocates for nurses and those served by nurses. The organizations may be local, regional, national, or international in scope. Many national and international nursing

> **KEY TERM**
> **Standards of practice:** The criteria against which professional practice is measured.

> **KEY TERM**
> **Continuing nursing education:** Ongoing education that nurses take part in after they have achieved basic preparation and licensure.

BOX 5-1 MISSION FOCUS OF PROFESSIONAL NURSING ORGANIZATIONS

- Nursing as a profession
- Clinical specialties role function (e.g., nurse educator, administrator, researcher)
- Collective bargaining
- Political advocacy and lobbying
- Healthcare policy

---

organizations have local or regional affiliates or chapters, making it possible for members to participate in and attend organization-sponsored events in their community. Sigma Theta Tau International Nursing Honor Society (STTI) is an example of an international nursing organization with a presence in over 85 countries with approximately 500 chapters worldwide.

The organization's mission statement provides insight into the purpose and objectives of the organization. For individual nurses who are seeking a professional organization that corresponds with their interests, examining the organization's mission statement is a first step in determining if the organization is a potential match.

Mission Statements

Each professional organization has a mission statement, which indicates the organization's primary purpose(s) and drives the development of the organization's strategic plan and priority goals for that specific organization. For example, the AACN has as part of its mission statement, "Acute and critical care nurses rely on AACN for expert knowledge and the influence to fulfill their promise to patients and their families. AACN drives excellence because nothing less is acceptable" (AACN, 2016). It follows that one of AACN's high-priority activities is meeting the continuing education needs of its members who practice in acute and critical care environments. The National Student Nurses Association (NSNA) has as its mission "to mentor students preparing for initial licensure as registered nurses, and to convey the standards, ethics, and skills that students will need as responsible and accountable leaders and members of the profession" (NSNA, 2016). This statement makes it clear what the NSNA's priority goals are so that members understand that they can expect to gain information to help them take the first steps toward professional practice and leadership. **Contemporary Practice Highlight 5-1** provides additional information about NSNA.

When deciding which professional organization(s) to join, each nurse must determine whether his or her reasons for professional membership match the stated mission of the organization (see **Box 5-2**). If there is not a similarity in objectives, the member can be disappointed and not perceive any value in belonging to the organization. It can be helpful to have conversations with other nurses in

CONTEMPORARY PRACTICE HIGHLIGHT 5-1

NATIONAL STUDENT NURSES ASSOCIATION

The National Student Nurses Association (NSNA) was founded in 1952 as a nonprofit organization with a purpose of promoting the professional development of nursing students in diploma, associate, baccalaureate, and generic graduate nursing student programs. Today the NSNA has grown to have over 60,000 members in all 50 states, the District of Columbia, Guam, Puerto Rico, and the U.S. Virgin Islands. The NSNA is led by a national board of directors consisting of nursing students elected from member schools who have chapters. Many nursing leaders begin their professional leadership development by joining their school chapter of the NSNA as students and serving as leaders within the organization. The experience they gain as leaders in their student organization provides them with the opportunity to develop foundational leadership skills that they can continue to develop as they transition from the student role to the role as a practicing nurse. More information about NSNA and membership benefits and opportunities can be found at www.nsna.org.

BOX 5-2   REASONS FOR JOINING PROFESSIONAL ORGANIZATIONS

- Advocate for the profession
- Participate in continuing education programs
- Lobby for changes in healthcare policy
- Pursue networking opportunities
- Stay current in clinical specialty or role
- Develop leadership skills
- Access resources to support career development

---

the workplace to determine which professional organizations they belong to and for what reasons. Most of the professional nursing organization websites have abundant information about not only the mission of the organization but also strategic direction, recent activities, and member benefits (Greggs-McQuilkin, 2005). This information is very useful in finding the best match to support the nurse's own career objectives.

Professional Nursing Organizations with Clinical, Political, and Regulatory Focus

Nursing provides many professional career options representing many opportunities for individuals to specialize. Career options are widely diversified not only by these many specialty opportunities but also by role functions. For example, there are nurse researchers, nurse educators, nursing care providers, clinical nurse specialists, nurse practitioners, nurse informaticists, and administrators, to name just a few. Overlaid upon each of these role functions is usually at least one, or perhaps more, clinical foci. This section provides an overview of the many types of nursing organizations in existence, including those with a clinical, political, and regulatory focus.

There are professional nursing organizations whose primary mission is to support distinctive nursing role functions. The NACNS, the American Association of Nurse Anesthetists, National Association of School Nurses, the National Nursing Staff Development Organization, the NLN, and the American Association of Nurse Attorneys are just a few of the nursing organizations that support a specific role function within the profession. The NSNA created to support nursing students in their role as learners has state chapter affiliates with local chapters established within schools of nursing. For nurses whose primary role is focused on nursing research, there are several regionally organized nursing research societies—the Southern Nursing Research Society, Midwest Nursing Research Society, Western Nursing Research Society, and Eastern Nursing Research Society—with a purpose of promoting nursing research. There are also nursing organizations that support both a role within a given clinical focus, including the National Association of Nurse Practitioners in Women's Health, the National Association of Pediatric Nurse Practitioners, and the American Pediatric Surgical Nurses Association.

Clinical Focus

Many nursing organizations are structured around a particular clinical specialty area and include within their mission political, advocacy, regulatory, and professional purposes related to the clinical area. Examples of clinically focused professional organizations include American Psychiatric Nurses Association, Society for Vascular Nursing, Academy of Medical-Surgical Nurses, and National Association of Orthopaedic Nurses. Part of the mission of a **nursing specialty organization** is to enhance the health of patients in their care.

> **KEY TERM**
>
> **Nursing specialty organization:** A professional nursing organization that has a particular clinical focus.

Connection to a clinical specialty organization ensures up-to-date practice information for the specific population of patients that the nurse cares for, helping him or her to optimize the quality of care delivered. To fulfill this purpose, the nursing organizations may create a wide variety of practice and educational resources. These resources can take many forms including standards of practice, evidence-based practice guidelines, research projects, protocols, educational seminars, and publications such as practice and scholarly journals. Many of these educational resources have migrated to online formats and webinars in an effort to promote wide dissemination of the resources to members, reduce cost to the members and/or their organization, and provide easy and timely access for busy nursing professionals with difficult scheduling needs. Continuing nursing education is often included in the resources to assist members in maintaining needed contact hours for licensure and specialty credentialing. A few organizations, such as the ONS and the AACN, offer specialty credentialing known as **certification** in their respective specialty, signifying the nurse has achieved a level of excellence in practice. **Box 5-3** summarizes the types of professional resources provided by organizations to their members.

> **KEY TERM**
>
> **Certification:** A designation earned by a person to ensure that he or she is qualified to perform a task or job.

Political Focus

Nursing as a profession has a responsibility to society, with a specific aim to improve the health of the nation. Professional nursing organizations fulfill the obligation of nursing to support improved health outcomes in national and global environments in several different ways. Many international and national organizations support work at the state level through local chapters, sections, or some form of alliance. In the United States, the ANA is the largest professional nursing organization that represents the views and needs of its members in various policymaking arenas. All nurses can become members of the ANA through membership in their state nursing associations.

Through ANA's political and legislative program, the organization has taken action on such issues as adequate reimbursement for healthcare services, access to health care, and appropriate nurse staffing ratios. The ANA also has programs focused on the health and safety of the individual nurse and nursing profession. The ANA "Healthy Nurse" and "Healthy Nurse, Healthy Nation" programs promote health habits such as sleep, physical exercise, managing stress, getting screenings, and living smoke-free lifestyles for nurses. See Chapter 12 for more information on the importance of caring for oneself by promoting a healthy lifestyle.

BOX 5-3   TYPES OF PRACTICE AND EDUCATIONAL RESOURCES FROM PROFESSIONAL NURSING ORGANIZATIONS

- Standards of practice
- Policy (position) statements
- Evidence-based practice guidelines
- Research project priorities and protocols
- Grant funding
- Safe and healthy work environments

- Health maintenance programs for nurses
- Practice and scholarly journals
- Conferences, seminars, webinars
- Continuing nursing education credits
- Specialty credentialing (certification)

Box 5-4 lists some of the areas in which ANA has recently presented congressional testimony on behalf of the nursing profession. A complete listing of policy and advocacy activities can be found on the ANA website at www.nursingworld.org. State nursing associations also engage in policy and advocacy activities at the state government level, thus allowing nurses to influence legislation related to nursing and health care in their own states.

Regulatory Focus

Specialty organizations also have a responsibility to support regulatory efforts in the areas of both healthcare reform and professional practice for the purposes of protecting the public's health and safety. For example, the National Council of State Boards of Nursing is a primary regulatory body in nursing. NCSBN is a not-for-profit, independent organization governed by a board of directors and a delegate assembly representing 59 member boards of nursing, which include the 50 states, the District of Columbia, and four U.S. territories—American Samoa, Guam, the Northern Mariana Islands, and the Virgin Islands. Some states have separate boards of nursing for RNs and LPN/VNs, which brings the total of NCSBN member boards to 59.

The purpose of the NCSBN is to provide an organization "through which boards of nursing act and counsel together on matters of common interest and concern affecting public health, safety and welfare, including the development of nursing licensure examinations" (NCSBN, 2016). NCSBN develops the NCLEX-RN and NCLEX-PN examinations and therefore has a large role in the regulation of nursing licensure in the United States. The NCSBN also provides resources for boards of nursing to support them in their roles of regulating nursing education and practice in their respective states and territories. Additionally, the NCSBN is a leader in providing national expertise to regulatory issues that affect nursing practice such as telehealth and interstate practice (NCSBN, 2016). See Chapter 4 for more information about the NCLEX-RN examination and Chapter 3 about nursing licensure.

BOX 5-4   AMERICAN NURSES ASSOCIATION POLITICAL ADVOCACY ACTIONS

- Health and Environment
- Healthcare Reform
- Registered Nurse Immigration
- Nurse Workforce Development Program (Title VIII) Funding

- Safe Patient Handling
- School-Based Health Centers

Data from American Nurses Association. (2016b). Policies and advocacy. Retrieved from http://nursingworld.org/MainMenu Categories/Policy-Advocacy

Professional Organization Membership and Involvement

Nurses represent the largest number of healthcare workers in the United States, and as such, have the potential to wield significant influence in shaping healthcare reform in this country. Historically, however, the voice of nursing in these national discussions has not been representative of the numbers of nurses in the profession, and the potential for nursing's contributions to advancing the health of the nation has not been realized (Ashton, 2012). Concerns about the lack of nursing representation on national healthcare boards has led to an initiative to secure the placement of 10,000 nurses on national boards by the year 2020 (see **Contemporary Practice Highlight 5-2**).

Addressing the concern about the lack of nursing leadership in health care, the Institute of Medicine (IOM) *Future of Nursing* report (2011) called for the nursing workforce to be prepared to lead change in health care. The IOM report specifically recommended that professional nursing organizations assume a role in developing nurse leaders by providing mentoring and leadership development programs and providing opportunities to develop leadership skills by assuming leadership roles within the organizations.

All nurses are expected to be leaders and the nursing profession needs to consider strategies by which to build the leadership capacity of nurses, including new graduates (Galuska, 2012; Scott & Miles, 2013). One strategy is to encourage membership in professional nursing organizations. Individual nurses can assume responsibility for developing their own leadership competencies by becoming members of professional nursing organizations and taking advantage of volunteer opportunities to become involved in the organization's activities (Galuska, 2012; Ross, Fitzpatrick,

---

CONTEMPORARY PRACTICE HIGHLIGHT 5-2

10,000 NURSES BY 2020 NATIONAL INITIATIVE

The Nurses on Boards Coalition is an initiative that includes representation from national nursing and other interested organizations who have joined together to increase the presence of nurses on health-related boards in corporations and nonprofit organizations. Launched in 2014, the coalition aims to place 10,000 nurses by the year 2020 on a variety of boards and commissions that focus on health-related topics. Achieving this goal would increase nursing's presence and leadership on influential decision-making bodies. The ultimate goal of the initiative is to "improve the health of communities and the nation through the service of nurses on boards and other bodies."

Data from Nurses on Board Coalition. (2016). 10,000 nurses by 2020. Retrieved from http://www.nurses onboardscoalition.org

Click, Krouse, & Clavelle, 2014). A study by Catallo, Spalding, and Haghiri-Vijeh (2014) demonstrated that professional nursing organizations can play a key role in engaging nurses in nursing and healthcare policy issues.

If nurses are not represented in national and international discussions related to health care, someone else would surely speak for them. The involvement of professional nursing organizations in all aspects of health care and political forums ensures that nurses represent the interests of nurses. By being a member of a professional organization, not only are nurses supporting the ability of professional associations to participate in these important forums, but in some cases, the individual nurse has the opportunity to provide specific testimony and be the voice at the table. Nurses can be called on to provide expert information on anything related to practice and the profession. An example is testifying in the local or national legislature on a specific health issue, such as universal access to care.

There are a number of activities in which a nurse can become involved as a member of an organization. Task forces and workgroups, leadership positions, and liaison and authorship opportunities are some common examples of contributions that nurses can make to an organization, at the same time developing their own leadership competencies.

Task Forces and Work Groups

Many times, professional associations need members with specific expertise to represent them in groups external to the organization, as well as groups or task forces within the organization. These small groups of expert members may develop standards of practice for a specialty, for example. They may also create evidence-based guidelines for practice or develop a position statement. Depending on the structure of governance within the organization, designated small groups may be advisory panels that make recommendations for the strategic direction of the association. In any of these situations, members have the opportunity to play a key role in setting practice or direction for the organization, and in many instances, the nursing profession. The members in these groups also have the advantage of networking with other experts in the field through their participation in these activities and becoming a nationally or internationally known expert in the field over time.

Leadership

Members of a professional organization have abundant leadership opportunities. Often, nursing organizations are seeking volunteer members for a myriad of positions. Organizations need volunteer members to help plan events such as annual or regional meetings or to review abstracts or grant submissions. Chair positions are available for task forces and committees at both the national and local levels. Participating initially at the local level is an excellent way to become involved and to learn more about the organization. Such involvement can then naturally lead to participation at the state and national level. Members can progress from local or chapter leaders to eventually becoming a member of the board of directors. Although time consuming, leadership activities provide tremendous opportunity for recognition and also become very important for creating future career opportunities.

Liaison Activity

Frequently, nursing organizations require someone with a specific expertise to represent their particular interest to other organizations. For example, the APRN Consensus and Licensure, Accreditation, Certification, Education (LACE) initiatives were developed through the involvement of liaisons from numerous nursing organizations. Liaison activity often extends beyond nursing associations to other healthcare-related entities. The March of Dimes, for example, may request representation from Association of Women's Health, Obstetric, and Neonatal Nurses (AWHONN) or ACNM on issues related to prevention of preterm labor or standards of care for mothers with preterm labor. The possibilities are as diverse as the healthcare environment; leadership opportunities for members of professional nursing organizations are considerable.

Authorship Opportunities

Nursing organizations provide many resources, including professional journals, to their members and others. These professional journals provide opportunities for nurses to author manuscripts. Authors submit their manuscripts to editors for publication in the journals. Depending on the intended purpose of the journal, these manuscripts may be original research or practice related. Members are often solicited to author textbooks, monographs, and position statements as well. Educational resources created by a professional nursing organization are most often written by a membership group, and this is an opportunity for new authors to be mentored in publishing. The writing opportunities are many for members who choose to share their practice innovations and new research findings.

Summary

A large number of professional nursing associations exist that are aligned with many important purposes within the nursing profession, including clinical, political, and regulatory foci. There is a nursing organization to meet the needs and interests of any individual nurse, and these organizations can be matched to specialty, role function, or nursing in general, as is the case with the ANA.

Professional nursing organizations provide many important functions that sustain the profession and provide opportunities for professional development. Membership in professional organizations offer many benefits including professional journals, continuing education, certification, networking, specialty standards, and leadership development. Organizations also provide input to active political forums and represent their members' views in various healthcare and political arenas. It is imperative that nurses participate actively in their nursing organization to ensure the best for themselves as a profession and the best health outcomes for their patients.

Reflective Practice Questions

1. Select a professional nursing organization that you are interested in joining following graduation. How does the organization's mission support your philosophy of nursing care and your own professional development needs?
2. What motivates you to join a professional organization? What would you consider to be some of the barriers that might lead you to not pursue organizational membership?
3. How does nurses' participation in professional nursing and other healthcare organizations benefit patient care?

References

American Association of Critical-Care Nurses. (2016). Mission statement. Retrieved from www.aacn.org

American Nurses Association. (2016a). Mission statement. Retrieved from http://nursingworld.org/FunctionalMenuCategories/AboutANA

American Nurses Association. (2016b). Policies and advocacy. Retrieved from http://nursingworld.org/MainMenuCategories/Policy-Advocacy

Ashton, K. (2012). Nurse educators and the future of nursing. *Journal of Continuing Education in Nursing, 43*(3), 113–116. doi: 10.3928/00220124-20120116-02

Catallo, C., Spalding, K., & Haghiri-Vijeh, R. (2014). Nursing professional organizations: What are they doing to engage nurses in health policy? *SAGE Open, 4*(4). doi: 10.1177/2158244014560534

Galuska, L. (2012). Cultivating nursing leadership for our envisioned future. *Advances in Nursing Science, 35*(4), 333–345. doi: 10.1097/ANS.Ob013e318271d2cd

Greggs-McQuilkin, D. (2005). Why join a professional nursing organization? *Nursing, 35,* 19.

Institute of Medicine. (2011). *The future of nursing: Leading change, advancing health.* Washington, DC: National Academies Press.

Matthews, J. (2012). Role of professional organizations in advocating for the nursing profession. *Online Journal of Issues in Nursing, 17*(1), manuscript 3. doi: 10.3912/OJIN.Vol17No01Man03.

National Council of State Boards of Nursing. (2016). *About NCSBN.* Retrieved from https://www.ncsbn.org/about.htm

National Student Nurses Association. (2016). *About us.* Retrieved from http://www.nsna.org/AboutUs.aspx

Nurses on Board Coalition. (2016). 10,000 nurses by 2020. Retrieved from http://www.nursesonboardscoalition.org

Ross, E., Fitzpatrick, J., Click, E., Krouse, H., & Clavelle, J. (2014). Transformational leadership practices of nurse leaders in professional nursing associations. *Journal of Nursing Administration, 44*(4), 201–216. doi: 10.1097/NNA0000000000000058

Scott, E., & Miles, J. (2013). Advancing leadership capacity in nursing. *Nursing Administration Quarterly, 37*(1), 77–82. doi: 10.1097/NAQ.0b013e3182751998

Transitions in Nursing: Future of Nursing and Transition to Practice

Monique Ridosh

LEARNING OUTCOMES

After reading this chapter you will be able to:

- Discuss the changes and challenges affecting the future of nursing in practice, education, and research.
- Discuss the linkage of change events in practice, education, and research.
- Understand the transition from education to practice.
- Define competence in nursing practice.
- Describe the knowledge, skills, and attitudes required for the transition into professional nursing practice.
- Discuss strategies to enhance the transition experience.
- Describe key elements to be considered when selecting a future work environment.
- Create a strategic plan for your own future career pathway.

The editors wish to acknowledge the contributions of Ellen Wathen and Pamela B. Koob to the previous edition of this chapter.

Introduction

Changes and challenges facing the future of nursing in practice and education are described in the beginning of this chapter. A discussion follows regarding issues that nurses face during the transition experience into practice. Strategies will be offered to help the nurse acclimate and ease this potentially challenging time entering new practice environments.

Future Pathway for Nursing Practice

The future of nursing practice is being transformed by multiple complex factors including consumer demands, data-driven initiatives for quality and safety, constant change at a rapid pace, and the need for universal access to care. Care must be safe, effective, patient centered, timely, efficient, and equitable. The responsibility of ensuring that these practice initiatives are realized in all types of healthcare settings is critical for nurses. Safety and quality are at the core of every strategic plan for the future. The current and future healthcare environments are driven by the trend toward public reporting and increased scrutiny. Nursing executives, leaders, and consumers are making quality and safety a top priority. This chapter reviews four aspects of transition into nursing: key trends influencing nursing practice, education, and research; standards for practice; changes in the nursing role; and the guiding principles for future patient care delivery.

Key Trends Influencing Nursing Practice, Education, and Research

Changing Sociodemographics for Nurses

The demographic profile of the nursing profession as well as the public is rapidly changing. Most nurses are over 40 years of age (approximately 70 percent). According to the National Workforce Survey of Registered Nurses the majority of nurses continue to be White (83 percent); only about 19 percent are from other races or ethnicity, with Hispanic at 3 percent, African American at 6 percent, or Asian at 6 percent (Budden, Zhong, Moulton, & Cimiotti, 2013). Of the 2.8 million nurses licensed in the United States, 55 percent have a bachelor's degree or higher (U.S. Department of Health and Human Services, 2013). An annual increase of 86.3 percent of registered nurses (RNs) have obtained their bachelor's since 2009 and the number of graduates with master's and/or doctoral degrees has increased by 67 percent from 2007 to 2011 (U.S. Department of Health and Human Services, 2013). Although a recent increase in graduate degrees have been awarded, nurse educator shortages worsen. Faculty vacancy rates are about 6.9 percent and according to a *Special Survey on Vacant Faculty Positions* (Li & Fang, 2014) a total of 1,236 faculty vacancies were identified from 714 nursing schools (80.0 percent response rate). In a recent report from the AACN (2015), *2014–2015 Enrollment and Graduations in Baccalaureate and Graduate Programs in Nursing*, 68,938 qualified applicants were turned away due to faculty shortage, lack of clinical sites and preceptors, classroom space, and finances. A barrier to the faculty shortage is the competitive salary offered in practice settings for the advanced practice registered nurse (APRN).

Evolving Nurse Roles

Clinical environments are increasingly complex. New graduates and experienced nurses require continued skill development in communication, financial management, and outcomes management. Nurses have opportunities to participate in organizational educational programs for professional development. Examples are research conferences offering continuing education credits, inservice programs, or interdisciplinary grand rounds. Hospitals are investing in new graduate nurse traineeships or residency programs to further develop the expertise of new nurses lasting anywhere from 3 months to a year. These programs provide a combination of didactic instruction pertinent to a specialty area and supportive mentorship to increase retention of new nurses. As the demand for quality and safety becomes ever more intense, so too will the demand for a highly skilled faculty and nursing workforce. It is imperative that undergraduate and graduate nursing curricula and continued nursing education programs focus strongly on these skills and **competencies** for future nurses.

> **KEY TERM**
> **Competencies:** Measurable levels of knowledge, skills, and attitudes required to perform in a professional role.

Nurses must also be knowledgeable regarding accreditation criteria such as core measurement data. Nurses can play a role in multidisciplinary programs to design measurement tools regarding patient and nursing **satisfaction** surveys, which are useful to target areas of improvement.

> **KEY TERM**
> **Satisfaction:** A measure of the quality of a service or organization based on consumer or employee perceptions. Satisfaction ratings provide outcome measurement, contributing to consumerism and improvement processes to increase productivity and retention.

As health care continues to change rapidly, the need for changes in our traditional nursing roles has never been more apparent. Traditional models of health care have focused on curing illness. Today, however, health care must be client directed, and nurses will be at the forefront of changes that will provide high-quality, cost-effective care for the betterment of the client, family, and community.

Nurse practitioners are becoming the comprehensive primary care practitioners of U.S. health care. The United States has seen an increased emphasis on primary care where nurse practitioners provide a cost-effective alternative along with other interprofessional health providers. Increases in two models of care, the medical home and nurse-managed health centers, are designed to address the current and future primary care provider shortage (Auerbach et al., 2013). This trend in models of care has been paralleled by an increase in APRN and physician assistant (PA) programs. The care management involved in primary care has become the basis of their practices. The Doctor of Nursing Practice (DNP) programs are also an opportunity to advance nursing knowledge and practice to improve the health of the nation. *The Essentials of Doctoral Education for Advanced Nursing Practice* (AACN, 2006) outlines the competencies for DNP programs. The DNP curriculum and educational standards and the measurement of client outcomes must be maintained as a **benchmark** of quality for the future of nursing education and practice.

Evidence-based nursing practice (discussed in more detail in Chapter 10) is developing as a practice standard globally. The gap between published research and translating these findings into practice is recognized as a critical issue for the future of nursing. Using evidence to guide clinical practice is challenging in an environment with competing demands for time, resources, and budget limitations. Obtaining awards for grant funding to conduct studies and support researcher salaries and consultants are further challenges. Creating structures and support for nurses in hospitals, schools, and community organizations to use evidence in practice will promote excellent client outcomes.

Standards for Practice

The American Nurses Association (ANA) outlines standards for practice to guide professional development for the future of nursing. Standards include evaluating the quality and effectiveness of care, evaluating one's own practice and adherence to professional standards, maintaining currency in education, contributing to professional development of others, acting ethically, working collaboratively, and using evidence and research for practice. The American Organization of Nurse Executives (AONE) developed guiding principles for future care delivery. These principles were developed based on complexity of technology in healthcare environment, growth of persons with chronic health conditions in our aging population, diversity of patients served, and variety of delivery settings (AONE, 2010). Principles can be found online (AONE, 2010).

In 1983, the American Academy of Nursing's (AAN's) Taskforce on Nursing Practice in Hospitals conducted a study to determine common variables in hospitals that were influential in recruiting and retaining excellent nurses. Forty-one of the 163 organizations shared characteristics that became "Forces of Magnetism" in these "Magnet" organizations. The American Nurses Credentialing Center (ANCC, 2015a) developed a Magnet designation in 1990. This designation has currently evolved into a recognition program to acknowledge organizations providing nursing excellence. The program is a mechanism to benchmark excellence for consumers and professionals. The Magnet program is based on research regarding quality indicators and standards of practice. The program can be viewed as a framework for dissemination of best practice strategies to be used by nursing professionals.

The five components of the framework model including transformational leadership, structural empowerment, exemplary professional practice, new knowledge including innovation and improvements, and empirical quality results (ANCC, 2015b) are described in **Box 6-1**.

This Magnet model uses outcome measurement and documentation. As healthcare reform evolves, magnetism contributes to the success of organizations. It provides direction for organizations to survive in the climate of nursing shortages and to maintain excellent patient outcomes by integrating practice and research as described in the examples in **Box 6-2**.

Knowledge, Skills, and Attitudes (KSA)

As nurses enter practice they are expected to practice safely within a healthcare system. The Quality and Safety Education for Nurses (QSEN) Institute has spearheaded a national initiative to delineate competencies and resources to guide curricula. Competencies for prelicensure nursing students include patient-centered care, functioning within collaborative interprofessional teams, integrating evidence-based practice

---

BOX 6-1 COMPONENTS OF THE MAGNET MODEL

1. *Transformational leadership* is essential to the success of today's nurse administrator. A transformational leader will prepare nurses for future challenges. The mindset of this leader must be that of a futurist to prepare the organization to be engaged in the change process. Organizations today are revising their strategic plans and creating new visions to meet the demands of the future.

2. *Structural empowerment* refers to the development of new structures and processes that will engage the organization to meet goals and desired outcomes. Innovative programs such as Transforming Care at the Bedside (TCAB), an initiative led by the Robert Wood Johnson Foundation and the Institute for Health Care Improvement, created a framework for change on medical/surgical units in four categories: safe and reliable care, vitality and teamwork, patient-centered care, and value-added care processes.

3. *Exemplary professional practice* is considered the "essence" of a Magnet organization. Professional practice is demonstrated by nurses applying new knowledge and evidence in practice. Nurses are engaged in practice councils and shared governance to act as change agents.

4. *New knowledge, innovation, and improvements* incorporate all prior components of leadership, empowerment, and exemplary practice to produce new models of care. This component is the application of existing and new evidence to contribute to the body of nursing knowledge.

5. *Empirical quality results* focus on outcome measurements. Organizations must be accountable for producing results versus simply changing structure and processes. Quantitative benchmarking will occur in areas of clinical outcomes related to nursing, workforce outcomes, patient and consumer outcomes, and organizational outcomes. The question now is, "What difference have you made?" (ANCC, 2015b).

BOX 6-2   EXAMPLES OF STRATEGIES TO INTEGRATE PRACTICE AND RESEARCH

- Establish forums for presentation and discussion of research topics such as monthly research grand rounds and journal clubs.
- Create professional practice council with specific goal to review and update evidence-based practice protocols.
- Support yearly research conference attendance for all nurses.
- Create mentorship opportunities for nurses in practice environments to conduct research.

- Identify funding to support research consultation and support in health system budgets.
- Support presentations of outcomes research at local, regional, and national conferences.
- Create collaborative research initiatives with members from academic and nurse practice environments.
- Establish interprofessional teams to facilitate and support research in practice environments.

---

with patient/family values, continuous quality improvement, minimizing risk of harm to patients and providers, and using informatics to support care (Cronenwett, 2012). In 2012, the Robert Wood Johnson Foundation and the American Colleges of Nursing expanded the QSEN initiative to create graduate-level competencies. The goal for QSEN is to provide information for nurses to continuously improve the quality and safety of the patient care environment. **Table 6-1** provides a general description of the six competencies for prelicensure (QSEN, 2014), which were adapted from the Institute of Medicine. A full description of these competencies is available on the QSEN website at http://www.qsen.org.

Nursing students begin to build this competency skill set throughout their educational experiences, particularly in the semesters immediately prior to graduation, as they synthesize all they have learned in their final clinical learning experiences. It is during this time that students should make every effort to further strengthen their knowledge base by working collaboratively with faculty and preceptors to seek out individual clinical experiences and learning outcomes they may not previously have had the opportunity to acquire.

Cognitive Knowledge Base

Nursing students are expected to integrate the knowledge they gain in the classroom into the patient care they provide in the clinical setting (www.QSEN.org). While in coursework, nursing students are likely to be provided with content related to illnesses and health problems including associated signs and symptoms, outcomes, and potential complications. Case study exemplars may also be provided for discussion and to stimulate critical thinking. Clinical learning experiences essentially provide opportunities to apply what is learned in the coursework. To increase the focus on developing competency in quality and patient safety, as called for in the

TABLE 6-1 QUALITY AND SAFETY COMPETENCIES

Competencies	Defining Characteristics
Patient-Centered Care	Nurses should use the patient's needs, preferences, and values as the central focus when developing the plan of care.
Teamwork and Collaboration	Nurses should work as part of a team to effectively execute the patient-driven plan of care.
Evidence-Based Practice	Nurses should use evidence-based data in conjunction with patient preferences and values to implement the plan of care.
Quality Improvement	Nurses should be involved in the continual monitoring of patient data to determine areas for process improvement.
Safety	Nurses should ensure patient safety by providing patient care in accordance with organizational policies.
Informatics	Nurses should use technology as available to support the safe implementation of patient care.

Data from QSEN Institute. (2014). Pre-licensure KSAs. Retrieved from http://qsen.org/competencies/pre-licensure-ksas

QSEN initiative, students must go beyond acquiring this fundamental cognitive knowledge base. For example, preparation for clinical learning experiences can include a review of the current best practices related to quality and safety for their patients' diagnoses and treatment plans (QSEN, 2014). This review of best practices can also be used to guide the development of patients' plans of care and shared with other nursing students during pre- or postconferences. Nursing students can also compare and contrast what the literature supports as recommendations for patient care and what they actually find being practiced within the clinical setting. These are just a few examples of how students can best use their clinical experiences to increase their knowledge base and prepare for transition into the "real" world of practice.

Psychomotor Skills

Nursing students learn how to perform many psychomotor skills throughout their education; as they master these skills they should always be focused on safety for the patient (QSEN, 2014). It is important for students to assume responsibility for actively seeking out opportunities to enhance the development of their psychomotor skills. In addition to learning the skills required to perform the procedure, these repeated experiences allow students to learn the nuances of patient care that cannot be found in textbooks or institutional policies. Nursing students are better served by having the opportunity to perform the same skills as often as possible in different patient care settings. This practice will help nursing students to become more comfortable in their skills for these procedures and also gain the necessary confidence to perform new procedures in complex settings, thus easing their transition from student to practitioner upon graduation.

Professional Values and Attitudes

Acquiring and demonstrating the values and attitudes of a professional are critical competencies for the new nurse. Some of these values and attitudes include demonstrating integrity, open communication, mutual respect of others, engaging in collaboration and teamwork, and understanding and acknowledging one's own strengths and limitations (www.QSEN.org). As one means of easing the transition from student to practicing nurse, nursing students can engage in self-reflection about strengths and weaknesses and then clearly communicate their self-identified learning needs to faculty and preceptors. Students and practicing nurses alike should seek and be open to constructive criticism from others.

In addition, the healthcare team is becoming more culturally diverse and consists of professionals with different levels of experience across varied age groups. Respect for cultural and generational differences among the healthcare team is of paramount importance in the work environment; misunderstandings among team members can divert needed attention away from patient care and adversely affect patient safety. Developing an understanding and appreciation of these workforce generational and cultural differences now, while still in nursing school, can greatly facilitate how quickly the new nurse becomes an accepted and skilled member of the healthcare team in the work environment.

Changes in the Nursing Role

Porter-O'Grady and Malloch (2014) compare the old healthcare paradigm with the new. Hospital-based nursing was the hallmark of nursing in years past. Today, most procedures are done on an outpatient or overnight basis. Care models are designed to bring the center of care to the client's community. Telehealth, school clinics, and mobile vans that travel to schools and nursing homes are commonplace. Hierarchical management is no longer the norm as organizational decision making flows in all directions (Porter-O'Grady & Malloch, 2014). Technology, miniaturization, and globalization have altered how we practice and do business. Today nurses at all levels of the organizational structure are involved in decentralized budgeting, shared governance, and strategic planning. Focus has moved from "sick care" to health care and promotion, prevention, and continuity of care. Cost containment is always important, but patient satisfaction and caregiver/agency accountability are vital. Documentation has moved from being written to being electronically recorded.

Thus, nurses are challenged to provide high-quality, cost-effective, and efficient care in a more complex environment with scarcer resources. Nurses are in a unique position to redefine the role of nursing to positively influence health care in this country as well as internationally. Nursing professionals can make a tremendous difference in preventing and controlling disease as well as improving outcomes and deceasing mortalities for those who have a chronic illness. Acting as change agents requires nurses to be active participants in health prevention as well as making it known publicly who nurses are and what nurses do.

Transition from Education to Practice

Nurses enter practice in a variety of ways and settings in the healthcare environment. At various levels of entry to practice, careers are filled with periods of transition. Entry to practice occurs when meeting minimum competency to practice in the new role. Whether the chosen educational program was at the associate, bachelor's, or master's level, entry to practice in a new profession requires lifelong learning. The transition experience is a process over time that includes stages of acquiring skills, gaining confidence and competence in the practice role with new levels of responsibilities. An awareness of where nurses are in the process can help them move through the experience in a way that achieves successful transition (Poronsky, 2013). Difficulties in the transition experience of graduates in residency programs were studied through interviews and were characterized by "role changes, lack of confidence, workload, fears, and orientation issues" (Fink, Krugman, Casey, & Goode, 2008).

Caring for human lives is an enormous responsibility that can lead to feeling overwhelmed, frustrated, and fatigued. Words of encouragement and reassurances from preceptors and other experienced nurses that these feelings are quite normal will help new graduates as they assume their new responsibilities. Nursing students and new graduates typically want to know and be able to do everything the job entails immediately upon graduation. Although it is not comfortable to feel inexperienced in a role that has responsibilities with such high human stakes, it is unrealistic to expect to be able to automatically function as expertly as those with years of nursing experience. With the passage of time and an ever-growing body of experience, the requisite knowledge and skills needed to function as competent nurses will develop and build. When beginning clinical practice, the novice nurse should be asking questions and aligning with a mentor or other experienced nurses for guidance and support.

New nurses can progress by talking to their preceptor, a mentor, their manager, and other experienced nurses. These individuals can assist the graduate nurses in identifying the positive aspects of their new role and setting realistic expectations and goals. At the very beginning of accepting a new position, the new graduate should take steps to identify and incorporate self-care activities into his or her lifestyle, as one means of coping with work-related stressors (see Chapter 12). These strategies can be as simple as daily exercise, healthy eating, and scheduled leisure activities. Networking with other new graduates under the guidance of an experienced nurse can also assist new graduates in realizing their feelings are normal.

The Transition Model (Anderson, Goodman, & Schlossberg, 2012) explains the process and suggests coping strategies for adults in transition. Three major components of the model are (a) approaching transition (identification and process), (b) taking stock of coping resources, and (c) taking charge. In approaching transition an awareness of the nature of the transition and assessment of whether you are *moving in, through,* or *out of* the transition is indicated. Taking stock of coping resources can be guided by identifying the person's **S**ituation, **S**elf, **S**upport, and **S**trategies (4Ss). Taking charge involves strengthening resources (Anderson, Goodman & Scholossberg, 2012). **Figure 6-1** further explains the components of the 4S model as a reflection activity.

Having support systems in place can be an effective strategy for coping with role transition. New graduates should seek out the individual(s) with whom they feel most comfortable sharing their thoughts or asking questions. Preceptors and mentors can be effective members of the support system. Additional members of a new graduate's support system can be faculty, other experienced nurses, clinical educators, nurse managers, peers and discussion groups, and professional organizations.

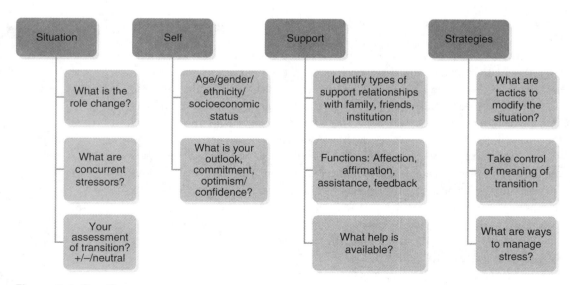

Figure 6-1 The 4Ss.
Data from Anderson, M., Goodman, J., & Schlossberg, N. (2012). *Counseling adults in transition: Linking Schlossberg's theory with practice in a diverse world* (4th ed.). New York, NY: Springer.

Role Transition

Studies conducted on national samples of new nurses support the need for transition to practice programs in the workplace beyond traditional orientation. Organizations have experienced a high turnover rate within the first year of practice for new nurses, which has both financial and patient safety implications. Additionally, in a time of nursing shortage, new nurses' satisfaction with employment and development to competent level of practice are essential to ensure an adequate workforce for the future. In an effort to prepare nursing students for a successful **role transition**, nursing faculty have incorporated experiential learning experiences into nursing curricula that focus on specific competencies required for practice in today's complex healthcare settings.

> **KEY TERM**
> **Role transition:** A process within the transition experience related to formation of a new identity as an independent provider of care. Assimilation to the new role requires both personal and institutional support.

These competencies include a focus on patient-centered care, teamwork and collaboration, evidence-based practice, quality improvement, safety, and informatics (Cronenwett, 2012). These competencies are elaborated in this chapter. Nursing students share the responsibility with their faculty to seek out learning experiences that will provide opportunities to acquire a foundation in each of these competency areas. The experiences that faculty and preceptors share serve as resources for nursing students as they enter the workforce. As nursing students' transition into their roles as RNs and advanced practitioners, these competencies serve as a blueprint for their success in the nursing profession.

From Novice to Advanced Beginner

When new graduates at any level enter the workforce, they may feel that they are expected to know "everything" in order to provide nursing care to their patients. This is an unrealistic expectation for a **novice** practitioner; actually, it is an unrealistic expectation for any practitioner because the complexity of nursing practice means

> **KEY TERM**
> **Novice:** Someone who has no experience with a given situation (Benner, 1984).

that all nurses are continually in a learning role to stay current and competent. Most new graduates have the benefit of an orientation period in their new position. The usual goals for these orientation periods include reviewing regulatory and institutional policies, nursing policies and responsibilities, patient care equipment and technology, and role expectations. Orientation programs are addressed at further length later in this chapter. Although the nature and length of the orientation period vary among institutions, new graduates must remember that the orientation period was established to facilitate their role transition and is designed to provide them with the opportunity to work alongside an experienced nurse as they assume their patient care responsibilities. The primary role of this experienced nurse, who may be termed a **preceptor** or

> **KEY TERM**
> **Preceptor:** An experienced nurse who facilitates and evaluates student learning in the clinical area over a specified time period of time (Billings & Halstead, 2013, p. 327).

Mentor: Someone who develops a long-term relationship with a mentee, without assessment or evaluation (Huybrecht et al., 2011).

Advanced beginner: Someone who has limited experience with a given situation (Benner, 1984).

Competent: Someone with 2 to 3 years of experience who is consciously aware of a given situation in its individual parts and can develop a long-range action plan (Benner, 1984).

Proficient: Someone with the experience to see a given situation in wholes rather than individual parts, who can analyze the situation and determine whether the typical picture is not materializing, and who can determine what needs to be revised within the plan of care in response (Benner, 1984).

Expert: Someone with the vast experience to intuitively assess a given situation and accurately target the problem area without being distracted by other unrelated symptoms (Benner, 1984).

mentor, is to explain the organization's policies and procedures, assist with assimilation into the culture of the organization, provide guidance in clinical decision making, and, in general, be available to answer questions. It is important for the new graduate to maximize the opportunities the orientation period provides and fully capitalize upon the assistance and learning experiences that are formally provided by the organization during this time frame.

Why do new graduates feel insecure within their role as a nurse? Some of these feelings of insecurity are based on their limited patient experience in the clinical setting. Nurses new to the profession need time and experience to fortify and expand their skill set. Benner (1984) explained the skills acquisition concept in her outline of the five stages of nursing proficiency in her book, *From Novice to Expert: Excellence and Power in Clinical Nursing Practice*. The five stages of skills acquisition are novice, **advanced beginner**, **competent**, **proficient**, and **expert**. Benner applied the Dreyfus model of skills acquisition to nursing (**Table 6-2**). As novice nurses gain experience, they are better able to analyze patient situations and use their past patient encounters to respond with appropriate interventions. The goal is to eventually be able to draw upon their past experiences to analyze patient problems, foresee potential complications, and intervene with preventative care.

Nursing students and new graduates are considered novices because they have very little experience in assuming responsibility for patient care in various clinical situations. Throughout their nursing education, in both the classroom and the clinical setting, students are provided with a set of guidelines to follow for providing care to their patients in selected situations. Even though these sets of guidelines assist nursing students in providing patient care, their inexperience leaves these novices with the inability to adapt or modify their provision of care based on variances within the patients' actual conditions.

With time and experience novices become what Benner (1984) refers to as advanced beginners—those nurses who have limited patient experiences but can recognize the similarities between current patient care situations and past patient care experiences. Most graduate nurses enter the workforce as novices, because they are faced with many patient care situations that they have never before experienced. They find that each patient brings a new and individualized variation to what may have been a seemingly familiar clinical

TABLE 6-2 DREYFUS MODEL APPLIED TO NURSING

Stages	Performance Characteristics
Novice	No experiences Rules-oriented behaviors
Advanced Beginner	Prior limited experiences Recognition-based behaviors
Competent	2–3 years of experience Mastery, organization skills
Proficient	Experience-based abilities Perceptions of the whole
Expert	Experience-based intuitions Accurately targets problems

Data from Benner, P. (1984). *From novice to expert: Excellence and power in clinical nursing practice.* Menlo Park, CA: Addison-Wesley.

scenario. Newly graduated nurses need to file away experiences that vary from the norm for future referencing as they learn how to adapt in situations based on these past patient encounters.

To summarize, new graduates will inevitably face some challenges as they transition from the role of the student to the role of a professional nurse. However, skill sets and strategies that nursing students develop and use while still in their nursing program assist in this transition.

Preparing for Transition into Practice

The Orientation Period

In most institutions, nurses can expect a detailed orientation when they are first hired. During the interview process, it is appropriate to ask about the length and type of orientation period that will be provided. The formalized orientation after graduation acquaints new nurses with their role responsibilities and expectations, emphasizes policies related to the safe delivery of patient care, provides opportunity to demonstrate psychomotor skills and learn new skills required for the position, and familiarizes them with available resources within the institution. During this formal orientation period, new graduates are also assigned to work with experienced nurses who have the responsibility for providing and overseeing patient care experiences that promote the acquisition of additional knowledge and skills. In addition, these experienced nurses provide information about the nursing unit layout, location of equipment, unit-based responsibilities, how patient assignments are posted, when meal breaks are taken, how report is given between shifts, and how staff communicates within the shift (i.e., phones, text, etc.)—in general, orienting the new nurse to the expectations related to the daily routine of the unit.

Healthcare institutions may provide both agency orientation and nursing department orientation sessions. The agency orientation may include information for all new employees, such as benefits, confidentiality, fire and electrical safety, and emergency preparedness. Nursing department orientation may include information specifically for the job role, such as medication safety and nursing policies, and hands-on practice with patient care equipment. The agency orientation may be 1 to 2 days in length. Nursing department orientation typically can range anywhere from 4 weeks for nonintensive care units to several months for intensive care units. In some cases, the period of orientation may be adjusted depending on how quickly the new nurse acclimates to the role responsibilities.

Preceptor's Role in Orientation

Many institutions use the preceptor model in their orientation programs to assist in the orientation of new nurses. Preceptors are experienced nurses who are assigned to new graduates for the length of their orientation period. Orientation programs provide good support for the preceptor model by sharing work and patient assignment schedules with the new graduate and allocating time to provide assessment, evaluation, and feedback (Blegen et al., 2015).

Mentor's Role in Orientation

Mentors differ from preceptors in that serving as a mentor is not an assigned role, nor does it exist for a specified period of time as does the preceptor role (i.e., the length of new graduate orientation). Mentors are experienced nurses who form a professional long-term relationship with a mentee without formal assessment or evaluation (Huybrecht et al., 2011). Mentors are viewed as role models who provide advice and guidance on patient care issues as well as professional development issues. A mentor–mentee relationship will last as long as it is mutually beneficial to both parties.

Nursing students should explore which healthcare institutions provide a mentoring program or foster professional mentoring relationships. They should ask for the specifics of the program—how mentors are selected, what training mentors receive, how long the program has been in existence, how many nurses have participated, whether the program has been evaluated by both mentors and mentees, and whether a summary of these evaluations is available for review.

Having a professional mentor can be very helpful to the new graduate during role transition. Above all, a mentor should be someone who is a good listener and conveys interest in the new graduate's professional growth, someone to whom the new graduate can turn for guidance with career issues and concerns. For some new graduates, former faculty may continue to serve as mentors; others may find mentors in the institution in which they are employed or through professional organization activities. Seeking a mentor is a proactive strategy for managing the stress of a new role and is one strategy that all new graduates should seriously consider to help them cope with the "reality shock" that has been inevitably associated with becoming an RN.

Current evidence from study of Transition to Practice training programs suggest structured established programs can increase job satisfaction, reduce work stress, and decrease turnover (Spector et al., 2015). When nurses enter a new practice role in their careers they should seek employers who support advanced training in the form of residencies or fellowships with specific characteristics described in **Box 6-3**.

BOX 6-3 CHARACTERISTICS OF RESIDENCIES OR FELLOWSHIPS FOR NEW PRACTICE ROLES

- **Agency support:** Support is needed from managers and coworkers. Agency infrastructure should include a formal policy that outlines the curriculum and criteria of the residency or fellowship.
- **Time commitment:** Minimum of 6 months in program length.
- **Preceptorship:** One or more preceptors should be appointed to mentor the new nurse. The preceptor and new nurse should establish mutual goals and have regularly scheduled time for evaluation and exchange.
- **Skills checklist and curriculum:** Individualized to the new nurse, the area of specialty, and the assigned clinical area. Practice outcomes and guidelines from specific professional organizations should be included, where appropriate.
- **Include QSEN, The Joint Commission, and other competencies for the specialty area:** Competencies such as communication, safety, informatics, electronic health record system, quality improvement, chain of command, governance, evidence-based practice, and clinical reasoning should be included in a competency checklist for the preceptorship.
- **Feedback and shared reflections:** Preceptors, new nurses, and managers should have time to learn, obtain feedback, and share. A scheduled open-group forum with other new nurses is often a comfortable environment for exchange.
- **Leadership and professional development:** Opportunities to build and grow in management, negotiation, safe delegation, and fiscal skills should be included in the curriculum. The preceptor and new nurse should develop a plan for professional development.
- **Interprofessional practice:** The work environment should include open exchange between the new nurse and interprofessional team members to improve patient care and encourage family involvement.

Maximizing the Benefits of Student Intern/Extern/ Residency/Fellowship Programs

Students may want to consider seeking opportunities to gain additional clinical experiences in programs designed to allow them to work under the direct supervision of an experienced nurse. Multiple opportunities exist through intern, extern, residency, and fellowship programs developed at many healthcare institutions to meet the experience and learning needs of nursing students. Nursing students may find that the additional experiences offered through these programs will ease the transition to their new role of professional nurse because they offer an opportunity to perfect and expand their skill set. In addition, many students elect to accept intern/extern positions at institutions where they hope to practice as RNs upon graduation, thus providing them with an opportunity to become familiar with the institution's culture and policies.

There are some subtle differences in extern and intern positions. *Extern programs* are usually offered when nursing students have limited clinical experience and wish to gain more hands-on patient encounters under the direct supervision of RNs. Externs working alongside RNs are able to gain insights into the many roles nurses fulfill during their shifts. Extern programs offer an opportunity for nursing students to develop skill with specific tasks within their limited skill set, become more confident in these skills and their role in patient care delivery, and feel less fearful of making mistakes.

Intern and residency programs may be offered during the last semester of nursing school or as part of the new nurse orientation. These programs offer nursing students entering practice the opportunity to develop their prioritization, time-management, and critical thinking skills as they take a full patient assignment under the direct supervision of RNs. The goal of the intern and residency programs is to ease students and graduate nurses into the real world of nursing, with all the complexities and decisions to be made for a full caseload of patients. As a result, these student nurses may feel more prepared for their role as RNs.

Another advantage of participating in intern and extern programs is that many nursing students are hired as graduate nurses based on the relationships they build with the manager and nursing staff within these programs. Managers and staff nurses are able to examine the nursing students' potential during their extern and intern programs prior to graduation and determine their preference for hiring them based on their performance. In turn, nursing students can also use the extern and intern programs to determine if the healthcare institution is where they wish to work upon graduation and in what area.

With the clinical experiences provided in the extern and intern programs, students may have a smoother transition to the nurse role. Nursing students not only have been able to improve their skill set within these programs but also have been able to increase their confidence levels related to skills performance. Employers benefit from higher retention rates, which may indicate that new nurses experience greater job satisfaction after graduation due in part to participating in these programs.

Fellowship opportunities are available for new graduates or experienced RNs wishing to obtain specialty training in clinical areas such as critical care, oncology, or emergency nursing practice.

New nurse graduates need to realize that they will continue to consult frequently with their preceptors and other experienced healthcare professionals for advice and guidance even after their orientation phase has ended. New nurse graduates should assume their new role with the understanding that they have shared responsibility for identifying their learning needs. For example, in orientation they may be asked to complete a skill set checklist to identify what skills they have performed previously and feel competent in, what skills they have limited experience with, and what skills they have never performed. The preceptor supervising their orientation will review this list and verify competence in the performance of all skills. It is important that novice nurses be honest when expressing their comfort level with various patient care experiences so that the preceptor can seek out appropriate opportunities to help them further develop their decision-making skills. As novices, they also need to be open to constructive feedback related to their nursing skills so that they can continue to improve in the role. Participating regularly in continuing education offerings that are made available by the institution or through professional organizations is another strategy that can boost a new graduate's safe performance.

Guiding Principles for Future Patient Care Delivery

Work Environment

When seeking their first position after graduation, what should nursing students look for in the work environment? What are some of the key characteristics of a good work environment? For instance, do the nurses have varied levels of experience or are they all new graduates? What is the mix of the other healthcare workers and how do they get along? Do nurses have a voice in their practice or are all the decisions made at the administrative level and passed down to staff? Multigenerational differences can influence the nature of the work environment, as can the governance structure and the presence of collective bargaining units. Work environment elements are briefly addressed in the sections that follow.

Multigenerational Workforces

The generational composition of healthcare work environments is increasingly diverse. Being aware of the generational differences and differing core values and beliefs held among healthcare team members is an important element in promoting a cohesive working environment. There are typically four generations in the current workforce; these generations and some key strategies for workplace collaboration are listed in **Table 6-3**. Life events during the formative years for those born in these generations molded the characteristics they exhibit in the

TABLE 6-3 FOUR GENERATIONS IN THE WORK ENVIRONMENT

Generation	Workplace Collaboration
Silents or Veterans (1925–1945)	Acknowledge their experience. Assist them to value differences. Keep these nurses productive.
Baby Boomers (1946–1964)	Embrace diversity. Consider how traditional rules of management and leadership can be adapted.
Generation X (1965–1980)	Encourage work-life balance. Give meaningful responsibilities that are fast-paced and suit their style. Consider benefits that include flexible shifts and hours.
Generation Y or Millennials (1980–2000)	Pair nurses who are experts in technology with other veteran nurses. In turn, veteran nurses share best practices. Communication is often preferred with technology such as text, Snapchat, and Twitter.

work environment. Veterans lived through the economic hardship and experience of World War II and the Great Depression. Baby Boomers were born in the postwar era in a period of prosperity and lived to work. Generation Xers grew up in a time that valued personal growth or individualism, not as a part of a team. Millennials were raised in the midst of terrorism and increasing violence in the world around them. They value peer relationships and are adaptable to change.

Each generation brings positive elements to the working environment. Being aware of and respecting the differences in other generations will enhance the communication and teamwork on the healthcare team. Nurses and other healthcare workers must find a way to make their diversity a positive influence in their working relationships. Communication and conflict resolution are conducive to promoting a positive work environment for all. Finding value in each other's contributions and demonstrating respect for each other despite these differences can lead to a strong team caring for patients and their families (Hendricks & Cope, 2013). As new nurse graduates enter the workforce they must be aware of and sensitive to these differences in values and beliefs, and strive for open communication and mutual respect among all members of the team.

Governance Structures

How are nursing decisions made? Who is fundamental in creating and implementing these changes? Is nursing empowered to be proactive in making policy changes to meet the future needs of patients and staff? Knowing who makes the decisions related to patient care should be an important element of the work environment for graduate nurses. If nurses wish to work in a patient care unit where they make the decisions on how the care is provided, then a shared governance structure will be more inviting. If they are satisfied with the administrators of the healthcare institution directing their methods of care delivery, then a centralized governance structure may be more appealing.

Shared Governance

Models demonstrating staff nurse involvement at the decision-making level in nursing are referred to as shared governance models. The organizational structure of such organizations is relatively flat as compared to the more typical hierarchal design. The patient care unit is the central location where decisions are made, partnering nursing staff with management. Within shared governance structures, nursing staff have control of their work environments with shared power, autonomy, and accountability to make patient care decisions or changes within their nursing practice. Nursing management is charged with providing the nursing staff with the necessary resources to change practice standards and policy that affect patient care delivery. Despite the variations of the shared governance models that exist in multiple healthcare institutions, the core element of autonomy should be evident in nursing practice. Staff nurses must know that they have the power to change nurse practice environments.

Examples of shared governance include creating nursing councils (or committees) for practice, research, quality, education, and recruitment and retention. Council membership consists of nursing representatives from patient care units who meet on a regular basis to assess the need for changes in practice. These nursing representatives are charged with collecting evidence-based data to support changes and recommend policy changes. Nursing representatives share these decisions with their colleagues within their patient care unit and seek feedback. This communication between the council representatives and the nurses on the patient care units is essential for the success of shared governance.

Another example of shared governance would be the use of collaborative teams for systems improvement. Continual process improvement is standard in the healthcare environment, and nursing plays a key role due to nurses' direct patient contact. Nurses see firsthand what issues affect patient care and can collect the necessary data for evaluation. Nurses are asked to serve on the teams with other healthcare workers and administrative staff to analyze patient care data and provide recommendations on proposed changes in patient care delivery.

For example, nurses on a patient care safety team could lead to prevention of catheter-associated urinary tract infection (CAUTI) by identifying gaps in the current practice and collect and analyze data supporting the appropriate use of indwelling urinary catheters. The nurses could then assist with the policy development, education plan for the nursing staff, and the timeline for implementing the change in practice to reduce CAUTI through fewer use of catheters, timely removal, and evidence-based protocol for insertion, maintenance, and post-removal care (tool available online [ANA, n.d.]).

Whether or not a future employer has a shared governance structure can be a vitally important consideration to new graduates when selecting a position. How policy decisions that affect nursing practice are made in the organization is an important question to ask in the interview process.

Collective Bargaining

According to the ANA Bill of Rights "nurses have the right to negotiate the conditions of their employment, either as individuals or collectively, in all practice settings" (ANA, 2016b). The ANA is nursing's professional organization that works to advocate and support the rights of nurses in the workplace. "The ANA advances the nursing profession by fostering high standards of nursing practice, promoting a safe and ethical work environment, bolstering the health and wellness of nurses, and advocating on health care issues that affect nurses and the public" (ANA, 2016a). Since 1946, the ANA has supported collective bargaining as a means to seek solutions for nursing shortages. More recently a new approach within systems focuses on using shared governance structures as a means to give nurses more voice in their overall practice (Porter-O'Grady, 2012).

In a collective bargaining structure, nurses may worry about the impact of strikes on the delivery of patient care. Nursing students must consider their options regarding whether they want to work within an environment that is unionized.

Critical Thinking/Problem Solving

The art of **critical thinking** and problem solving is one of the most important skills for nursing students to master. Critical thinking is characterized by habits of the mind and skills of the nurse. Habits of the mind include confidence, contextual perspective, creativity; flexibility, inquisitiveness, intellectual integrity, intuition, open mindedness, perseverance, and reflection. Skills include analyzing, discriminating, logical reasoning, applying standards, information seeking, predicting, and transforming knowledge (Scheffer & Rubenfeld, 2000).

> **KEY TERM**
> **Critical thinking:** A systematic process of assessing, grouping, and evaluating data to determine the best plan of action for each patient care issue.

Nursing students have limited time in most clinical settings and frequently do not have the opportunity to see the outcomes of the clinical decisions being made by the experienced nurses with a multipatient case load.

What can nursing students do to prepare themselves for making critical patient care decisions? The first step is to develop a good foundational knowledge base, such as that acquired through the nursing curriculum, as a starting point for the decision-making process. What are more difficult to prepare for, however, are the clinical variations and complications in patients that can affect treatment protocols and nursing care. Asking "why" questions of other more experienced practitioners is vital to the student and novice nurse's understandings of the rationale for clinical decisions made in patient care situations. Asking "why" questions of nursing faculty and experienced nurses in the clinical setting prompts these experienced nurses to "think out loud" and share their expertise about how and why clinical decisions are made.

Again, nursing students should assume responsibility for obtaining as many hands-on clinical experiences as possible, even if they have already had multiple patients with similar admitting diagnoses. Patients with identical diagnoses will have individualized differences from which students can learn. For example, will a patient undergoing a cholecystectomy with a history of diabetes receive a different postoperative plan of care than a patient without diabetes? How does the history of diabetes affect medication administration issues, postoperative incision care, and postoperative infection rates? What if the patient with diabetes has nausea and vomiting postoperatively? How does this affect their dietary intake and insulin administration?

When nursing students are preparing for their clinical experiences, they should ask themselves "why" questions. For instance, why are specific tests being ordered, were the test results normal or abnormal, and how do these results affect the patient? Or what medications are ordered, what conditions are the medications used for, and why are these medications ordered for this particular patient? Nursing students can practice asking themselves "why" questions by reviewing the exercises provided within this chapter (**Box 6-4**). These types of exercises are also an excellent means of preparing for the NCLEX-RN examination. Additional activities are discussed in the prioritization section of this chapter.

BOX 6-4   CRITICAL THINKING EXERCISE

You can develop your critical thinking skills either by yourself or with a group of your peers with this exercise. First, review your patient's clinical data. Then ask yourself and/or your peers the following questions:

- What clinical signs are being exhibited by the patient and is there any reason to be alarmed?
- Which data are considered normal?
- Which data are considered abnormal? Why?
- Which data abnormalities are pertinent for the provider to be notified about immediately? Why? What would happen if these data were not called to the attention of the provider immediately?

- Which abnormalities can you wait to notify the provider about (i.e., provider can review the data on patient rounds during the current shift)? Why?

These crucial "why" questions will assist you with your critical thinking skills and patient care decisions as you "think out loud" and seek answers to the "why" questions. Develop the habit of approaching all of your patient care assignments in this manner.

Data from Etheridge, S. (2007). Learning to think like a nurse: Stories from new nurse graduates. *Journal of Continuing Education in Nursing, 38*(1), 24–30.

Guiding Principles for Patient Care Delivery

Time Management/Organization

All new nurses need to possess time management and organizational skills. Seldom is the patient's plan of care managed and directed by the nurse without revisions or interruptions. These alterations can be caused by changes in patients' conditions, tests being performed without preset schedules, new patient admissions, patient discharges, emergencies (e.g., code blue, seizures, patient falls), unanticipated delays in supplies and equipment, and interruptions from other healthcare providers and family members. Nursing students not only need to learn how to organize their responsibilities for patient care and manage time effectively, they also need to learn to be flexible and comfortable with adapting to unexpected changes in their work plan. Developing these skills while still in nursing school will help students make the transition to caring for multiple patients in practice.

The standard principles of time management can be taught, but the method of implementing these principles into the work environment is individualized rather than uniform. Each nursing student needs to find a method of time management that works for them and consistently seek experiences to develop those skills. Observing how other nursing students and experienced nurses organize their responsibilities can be very helpful, as can asking experienced nurses why they organize their work in certain ways. Discussing various time-management methods with nursing faculty can provide additional insight and another voice of experience.

A time-management system does not need to be complex. For example, it can be as easy as A-B-C. Nursing students can review the responsibilities for the patients in their care and then categorize these tasks as an A (must be done), a B (should be done), or a C (could be done). The A responsibilities are priority interventions such as suctioning a tracheostomy and ensuring the patient has a clear airway. B responsibilities have a lower priority than the A responsibilities but are still important; for example, taking the patient's vital signs every 4 hours. The C responsibilities are less vital to patient care and can be postponed to a later time on the current or later shifts, such as changing a postoperative dressing on a stable patient. The important point is that the nursing student consciously considers means by which to develop his or her time-management skills and organize the delivery of patient care.

Delegation

Safe delegation of nursing care to other care providers is a key responsibility of the RN. Nursing students usually deliver the majority of their assigned patients' care during their clinical assignments and therefore do not have much opportunity to develop their delegation skills. When nursing students graduate and assume their first nursing position, they quickly learn the importance of being able to function as a leader and member of the healthcare team. Nurses need to be able to effectively delegate tasks to appropriate team members.

How do new nurses learn what they can delegate and who they can delegate to? Who is responsible for the delegation of patient care? A first step to learning about the act of delegation for nursing students is to understand the legal responsibilities associated with the process. Observing the amount of delegation occurring in their clinical settings by their preceptors can also be a good initial learning experience for students.

Delegation is defined as "transferring to a competent individual authority to perform a selected nursing task in a selected situation" (National Council of State Boards of Nursing [NCSBN], 1995, p. 1). The five rights of delegation are listed in **Box 6-5** (Henderson et al., 2006; NCSBN, 1995). These five rights of delegation outline the RN's legal responsibilities associated with delegation.

> **KEY TERM**
>
> **Delegation:** The transfer of the performance of a selected nursing task in a selected situation to a competent individual authority (National Council of State Boards of Nursing, 1995).

The delegation of patient care is based on state nurse practice acts and healthcare institutions' job descriptions. Each state's nurse practice act addresses the RN's responsibility for delegation. The RN who is delegating patient care must know what responsibilities are in the other healthcare provider's job description. For instance, can a nursing assistant insert a urethral catheter or change a dressing over a postoperative incision? If the RN delegates patient care duties to other healthcare workers and those duties are not allowed within their job description, then the RN can be held liable for inappropriate delegation. The healthcare worker to whom duties are being delegated is also responsible for informing others if the duties being delegated are not within his or her job description. If the healthcare worker performs the delegated duties despite being aware that the duties are not within the job description, then the healthcare worker can also be held responsible and liable. Delegation is an important skill for nursing students to learn to use because it will be essential in their professional practice after graduation.

BOX 6-5 FIVE RIGHTS OF DELEGATION

1. Identify the right task to delegate.
2. Identify the right circumstances for delegation.
3. Select the right person for delegation.
4. Use the right direction and communication when delegating.
5. Identify the right supervision and evaluation.

Modified from American Nurses Association, & National Council of State Boards of Nursing. (n.d.). Joint statement of delegation. Retrieved from https://www.ncsbn.org /Delegation_joint_statement_NCSBN-ANA.pdf

National guidelines were recently developed by two expert panels convened by the NCSBN to standardize the delegation process. A delegation model (available at http://www.ncsbn.org) delineates responsibilities of employers/nurse leaders, licensed nurses, and delegatees. Nursing students can learn how to effectively delegate within a team by reviewing the National Guidelines for Nursing Delegation (NCSBN, 2016) and following a decision tree when planning care. The process includes four steps: (a) assessment and planning; (b) communication; (c) surveillance and supervision; and (d) evaluation and feedback. In the assessment and planning step, it is important to understand the rules and scope of practice of the delegatee, assess client needs and competence of assistive personnel to ensure match, and to identify if appropriate supervision is available. Two-way communication between the nurse and assistive personnel is necessary to complete the second step. Surveillance and supervision involves monitoring of performance and compliance with standards of practice and institutional policies. The final step is to evaluate and provide feedback which ensures a reflection of activity and outcome to guide future delegation.

Prioritization

The ability to prioritize patient care needs in any setting is one of the most important skills that nursing students can practice and is a skill they will be expected to demonstrate in clinical practice. The challenge for students and novice nurses, of course, is to identify which patient care needs demand immediate attention and which can wait. Nursing students should seek opportunities to observe how experienced nurses prioritize care not only for one patient, but also between patients, asking "why" questions as appropriate to understand rationale for decision making. For example, the nurse call light is on for two patients, one who has a tracheostomy and one who needs to be assessed for pain. Does the nurse see the patient who could be in respiratory distress first? What would the nurse consider when making this decision? Maintaining an open airway is always a priority but perhaps the patient with the tracheostomy is calling for help to be repositioned and the other patient is experiencing great pain. More information is needed to make the correct decision. This is a simplified example of a situation which requires clinical decision making, yet one that illustrates nurses are called upon frequently to meet important and competing patient demands and must be able to prioritize the order in which they will respond.

Prioritization begins with differentiating abnormal or relevant findings from normal and it takes the novice nurse time to develop this skill. There are exercises, however, that nursing students can incorporate into their study to learn how to prioritize safely and appropriately. **Case Study 6-1** illustrates activities requiring prioritization. Further highlighting the importance of critical thinking skills in prioritizing patient care, **Contemporary Practice Highlight 6-1** provides a scenario that presents some of the simultaneous nursing care decisions that are very typically required in an acute care healthcare setting.

CASE STUDY 6-1
PRIORITIZING PATIENT AND FAMILY NEEDS

You are working on a pediatric critical care floor and just received the morning report. Your assignment includes two patients. One is a 1-year-old patient with Down syndrome who needs gastric tube feedings and oxygen by nasal cannula. The other is a 12-year-old girl who has a large abdominal incision, drainage tubes, and requires mechanical ventilation. A family member of the 12-year-old patient walks up to you and says she needs your help immediately to secure an endotracheal tube connected to a ventilator. The 1-year-old just woke up, is irritable, crying, and alone in the room in a crib. The monitor in the 1-year-old's room is alarming and you determine his oxygen saturation rate is not showing. Another nurse's patient adjacent to your patients has an IV pump alarming, that patient's nurse asked you to "watch" when she is not at the bedside since he is on a Dopamine drip. You must prioritize who and what you will address first.

Which situation does in fact need your immediate attention? What should you consider in making your decision? What nursing assessment and interventions are necessary to address these patient and family needs? Rank these tasks in order of importance. Take a moment to brainstorm all solutions and their rationale. When in a real life clinical decision-making situation, you will need to make these decisions quickly. Practicing scenarios like these will give you the opportunity to develop critical thinking skills that will better enable you to identify solutions in the future.

Now that you have taken a moment to think, let us review the case. While maintaining an airway, a priority leads you to see the patient on the ventilator first, that patient was accompanied and not in respiratory distress—the tape on the tube was loose. The patient on the cardiac drip could potentially go into arrest if medication abruptly stopped flowing due to the pump not operating properly and needed to be reset and restarted at the appropriate rate. The 1-year-old was irritable but breathing. He needed consoling and reconnection of his oxygen saturation monitor. After assessing all three situations and obtaining more information you must evaluate your resources and reprioritize. Is there someone you can delegate the routine care of the infant? Is there a respiratory therapist available to check and replace tape on the endotracheal tube? What do you need to address the pump with the medication drip? It is most important to troubleshoot the pump of the cardiac medication and alert the nurse assigned to that patient.

Seek opportunities in your clinical experiences to identify immediate care needs you must prioritize. Practice your critical thinking skills and review information with your nursing instructor, preceptor, or mentor. Making the right decisions about prioritization takes practice and engagement with others in the practice environment, many times involving a charge nurse. Think about how you can intentionally practice and support your colleagues in your clinical practice environments to make the best decisions about prioritizing care.

CONTEMPORARY PRACTICE HIGHLIGHT 6-1

EFFECTIVE PRIORITIZATION OF PATIENT CARE WHEN DELEGATING CARE

Expanding on the case study, the routine care of the 1-year-old may be a task you consider delegating. In this Contemporary Practice Highlight, we review the steps of how to make that decision. Accessing the Decision Tree developed by the NCSBN as previously cited, follow the path to delegate or not to delegate to nursing assistive personnel.

Step 1: Assessment and Planning

The following questions must be answered before proceeding to next step.

Are there any rules or laws that support delegation? If yes, is the task of calming an irritable 1-year-old who is on a monitor in the scope of practice of the delegating nurse? If yes, is the delegating nurse competent to make the decision about delegating? If yes, is the task consistent with all of the criteria for delegation to assistive personnel, such as it is routine care that does not involve ongoing assessment, interpretation, and intervention (e.g., troubleshooting a cardiac medication pump). Does the nursing assistive personnel have the appropriate knowledge, skills, and abilities to accept the delegation? Is the delegatee trained on how to replace an oxygen saturation monitor lead? Does the delegatee have the capacity to meet needs of the patient? Are there policies or procedures in place for this task? Is appropriate supervision available? If any of the answers are no then you cannot proceed to delegate.

Step 2: Communication

Communication between the nurse and the assistive personnel must be a two-way process. As the nurse communicates need to comfort the 1-year-old and replace the lead for the monitor the nurse should ensure the assistive personnel has understood and has the opportunity to ask questions. If the patient for example is inconsolable within a few minutes is further assessment needed by the nurse? Does the assistive personnel have enough information to perform any additional tasks prior to additional communication with the nurse? If the monitor lead is not reconnected or not working the assistive personnel needs to communicate that to the nurse within an appropriate timeframe.

Step 3: Surveillance and Supervision

In this step the nurse is responsible for monitoring performance and ensuring compliance. Does the assistive personnel complete the task of comforting the patient and reconnecting the monitor lead to ensure proper monitoring of oxygen saturation? Was additional assessment necessary once the saturation monitor was replaced? Did the assistive personnel report a low saturation and need for further intervention to prevent patient's condition worsening?

CONTEMPORARY PRACTICE HIGHLIGHT 6–1 (*continued*)

Step 4: Evaluation and Feedback

Evaluation of the effectiveness of the delegation is in important last step. Review of the entire process may identify issues which can be prevented in the future. For example, was the communication effective? Did the assistive personnel know what to do if a low saturation rate was detected once reconnected? Was appropriate feedback provided on the performance of the task? Was there anything that could change in future delegation of the same or similar task?

This Contemporary Practice Highlight was an example of a common task that could be delegated to assistive personnel but also could have serious consequences if not done properly and a patient would not be reconnected to a monitor and would be at risk for undetected desaturation episode without monitoring. Another consequence could be if the assistive personnel provided additional care in comforting the child such as attempting to feed when the patient does not eat by mouth. Communication between the nurse and the assistive personnel must be two-way and must include every step to ensure patient safety at all times.

Summary

This chapter has summarized key issues for the future transformation of nursing practice, education, and research. Nursing professionals have a major role to play in improving care outcomes through the application of evidence-based care and emphasis on quality and safety.

Some of the challenges nursing students face were discussed regarding transition from the role of student to the role of RN. Strategies for acquiring the necessary experiences that will help new nurses successfully make this transition were highlighted. Assuming responsibility for their own learning and being proactive in seeking out needed learning experiences are two of the best strategies that nursing students can employ to help prepare themselves for practice in the real world. Graduating and entering the practice environment as a nurse is an exciting time in your new career. Use your time wisely before graduating to prepare yourself for this transition, take stock and take charge of your experience. Seek mentors, develop your support systems, and find the right work environment for you. Welcome to the nursing profession!

Reflective Practice Questions

1. You are on a multidisciplinary team that is developing a patient satisfaction survey for completion at discharge. What questions do you feel reflect the most critical aspects of patient satisfaction that are a direct result of nursing care?

2. In the next 5 years, approximately 340,000 nurses are expected to retire from the profession. Many nurses have already worked 30 to 40 years. What educational and care delivery models will capitalize on the collaboration of experienced nurses with new graduates to enhance nursing excellence? As a new graduate, what type of mentorship are you seeking? What will you contribute back to your mentor?

3. How much more education do you feel you need in nursing? Where do you see yourself in the profession in 5 years? Ten years? Have you thought about getting a master's degree in nursing or becoming a nurse practitioner, nurse anesthetist, or other advanced practice nurse? Where would you start with your plan and how would you accomplish this?

4. How do we enhance research skills in our current nursing workforce? How should we engage senior nurse researchers in the patient care environment with other nurses and healthcare professionals?

5. You are working with a nursing technician who tells you she is allowed to change dressings and apply antibiotic ointment to wounds. You consult the job description for nursing technicians to determine if this task can be delegated. What do you think you will find? Is the nursing technician allowed to change dressings? Is the nursing technician allowed to apply antibiotic ointment? Is this antibiotic ointment considered a medication? Depending on your state laws and institutional guidelines, what is your response to the nursing technician?

6. You are seeking a job as a registered nurse and have narrowed it down to two hospitals on the West Coast. Both hospitals state that they have shared governance structures, and similar wages, professional development programs, and benefits. One hospital is unionized and the other is not. What other questions do you need to have answered before making your final decision between the two hospitals?

7. Consider your own nursing practice development needs as you prepare to graduate. What additional learning experiences will be most helpful to you? How do you plan to acquire these experiences?

References

American Association of Colleges of Nursing. (2006). The essentials of doctoral education for advanced nursing practice. Retrieved from http://www.aacn.nche.edu/dnp/Essentials.pdf

American Association of Colleges of Nursing. (2015). *2014–2015 enrollment and graduations in baccalaureate and graduate programs in nursing.* Washington, DC: Author.

American Nurses Association. (n.d.). Streamlined evidence-based RN tool: Catheter associated urinary tract infection (CAUTI) prevention. Retrieved from http://nursingworld.org/CAUTI-Tool

American Nurses Association. (2016a). About ANA. Retrieved from http://nursingworld.org/aboutana

American Nurses Association. (2016b). Nurses bill of rights. Retrieved from http://www.nursingworld.org/NursesBillofRights

American Nurses Association, & National Council of State Boards of Nursing. (n.d.). Joint statement of delegation. Retrieved from https://www.ncsbn.org/Delegation_joint_statement_NCSBN-ANA.pdf

American Nurses Credentialing Center. (2015a). *History of the Magnet program.* Retrieved from http://www.nursecredentialing.org/Magnet/ProgramOverview/HistoryoftheMagnetProgram

American Nurses Credentialing Center. (2015b). *Magnet model.* Retrieved from http://www.nursecredentialing.org/Magnet/NewMagnetModel.aspx

American Organization of Nurse Executives. (2010). AONE guiding principles for future patient care delivery toolkit. Retrieved from http://www.aone.org/resources/future-patient-care.pdf

Anderson, M., Goodman, J., & Schlossberg, N. (2012). *Counseling adults in transition: Linking Schlossberg's theory with practice in a diverse world* (4th ed.). New York, NY: Springer. Retrieved from http://www.eblib.com

Auerbach, D. I., Chen, P. G., Friedberg, M. W., Reid, R., Lau, C., Buerhaus, P. I., & Mehrotra, A. (2013). Nurse-managed health centers and patient-centered medical homes could mitigate expected primary care physician shortage. *Health Affairs, 32*(11), 1933–1941.

Benner, P. (1984). *From novice to expert: Excellence and power in clinical nursing practice.* Menlo Park, CA: Addison-Wesley.

Billings, D. M., & Halstead, J. A. (2013). *Teaching in nursing: A guide for faculty.* Amsterdam, The Netherlands: Elsevier Health Sciences.

Blegen, M. A., Spector, N., Ulrich, B. T., Lynn, M. R., Barnsteiner, J., & Silvestre, J. (2015). Preceptor support in hospital transition to practice programs. *Journal of Nursing Administration, 45*(12), 642–649.

Budden, J. S., Zhong, E. H., Moulton, P., & Cimiotti, J. P. (2013). Highlights of the National Workforce Survey of Registered Nurses. *Journal of Nursing Regulation, 4*(2), 5–14.

Cronenwett, L. (2012). A national initiative: Quality and Safety Education for Nurses (QSEN). In G. Sherwood, & J. Barnsteiner (Eds.), *Quality and safety in nursing: A competency approach to improving outcomes.* Chichester, West Sussex; Ames, Iowa: Wiley-Blackwell.

Etheridge, S. (2007). Learning to think like a nurse: Stories from new nurse graduates. *Journal of Continuing Education in Nursing, 38*(1), 24–30.

Fink, R., Krugman, M., Casey, K., & Goode, C. (2008). The graduate nurse experience: Qualitative residency program outcomes. *Journal of Nursing Administration, 38*(7/8), 341–348.

Henderson, D., Sealover, P., Sharrer, V., Fusner, S., Jones, S., & Sweet, S. (2006). Nursing EDGE: Evaluating delegation guidelines in education. *International Journal of Nursing Education Scholarship, 3*(1), Article 15. Retrieved from http://www.bepress.com/ijnes/vol3/iss1/art15

Hendricks, J. M., & Cope, V. C. (2013). Generational diversity: What nurse managers need to know. *Journal of Advanced Nursing, 69*(3), 717–725.

Huybrecht, S., Loeckx, W., Quaeyhaegens, Y., De Tobel, D., & Mistiaen, W. (2011). Mentoring in nursing education: Perceived characteristics of mentors and the consequences of mentorship. *Nurse Education Today, 31*(3), 274–278.

Li, Y., & Fang, D. (2014). Special survey on vacant faculty positions. Washington, DC: American Association of Colleges of Nursing. Retrieved from http://www.aacn.nche .edu/leading-initiatives/research-data/vacancy14.pdf

Maslow, A. (1968). *Toward a psychology of being.* Princeton, NJ: Van Nostrand.

National Council of State Boards of Nursing. (1995). Delegation: Concepts and decision-making process. *National Council Position Paper.* Retrieved from https://nursing.iowa.gov/sites /default/files/media/delegation1.pdf

National Council of State Boards of Nursing. (2016). National guidelines for nursing delegation. *Journal of Nursing Regulation, 7*(1), 5–14.

Poronsky, C. B. (2013). Exploring the transition from registered nurse to family nurse practitioner. *Journal of Professional Nursing, 29*(6), 350–358.

Porter-O'Grady, T. (2012). Reframing knowledge work: Shared governance in the postdigital age. *Creative Nursing, 18*(4), 152–159.

Porter-O'Grady, T., & Malloch, K. (2014). *Quantum leadership: Building better partnerships for sustainable health.* Burlington, MA: Jones & Bartlett Learning.

QSEN Institute. (2014). Pre-licensure KSAs. Retrieved from http://qsen.org/competencies /pre-licensure-ksas

Scheffer, B. K., & Rubenfeld, M. G. (2000). A consensus statement on critical thinking in nursing. *Journal of Nursing Education, 39*(8), 352–359.

Spector, N., Blegen, M. A., Silvestre, J., Barnsteiner, J., Lynn, M. R., Ulrich, B., . . . Alexander, M. (2015). Transition to practice study in hospital settings. *Journal of Nursing Regulation, 5*(4), 24–38.

U.S. Department of Health and Human Services. (2013). *The US nursing workforce: Trends in supply and education.* Rockville, MD: Author. Retrieved from http://bhpr.hrsa.gov /healthworkforce/supplydemand/nursing/nursingworkforce/nursingworkforcefull report.pdf

Unit II

The *Environment* and *Nursing* Practice

Interprofessional Issues: Collaboration and Collegiality

Deanna L. Reising and Rebecca A. Feather

LEARNING OUTCOMES

After reading this chapter you will be able to:

- Discuss the importance of interprofessional collegiality.
- Describe ways that individuals in different health professions can work together to improve patient outcomes.
- Define the importance of interprofessional collaboration.
- List the core competencies for interprofessional collaboration.
- Examine the significance of collegiality and collaboration in advancing patient-centered care.
- Identify the role of the leader in the interprofessional team.
- Explain the role of the nurse as a part of the interprofessional team.
- Evaluate how to know when conflict resolution has occurred among interprofessional team members.
- Describe the value of interprofessional education.

The editors wish to acknowledge the contributions of Pamela B. Koob to the previous edition of this chapter.

Introduction

The planning and delivering of patient care is the responsibility of multiple professionals. Nurses and other healthcare professionals are uniquely prepared to manage certain aspects of patient care. Through interprofessional collaboration and collegiality, patients can benefit from higher levels of care coordination, better satisfaction, improved health outcomes, and decreased cost of care. The purpose of this chapter is to describe the key aspects of the nursing role as a member of the interprofessional healthcare team. The chapter also defines the core competencies expected of nurses as they partner with the interprofessional team to improve the care of patients.

KEY TERM

Collaboration: Working jointly with other healthcare professionals in a collegial manner. A process whereby healthcare professionals work together to improve patient/client outcomes (ANA, 2015b).

KEY TERM

Collegiality: Sharing authority and responsibility to reach a prescribed goal or outcome. Power and responsibility are shared, and mutual respect and collaboration are desired (AACN, 2016).

KEY TERM

Communication: "All the cognitive, affective and behavioral responses that can be used to convey a message to another person" (Watson, 1979, p. 33). Communication can be verbal, such as through one's words, how these words are expressed, the tone used in expressing these words, and their pace, clarity, timing, and relevance. Communication can also be nonverbal, where words are not used, but meanings or expressions are communicated via body language, facial expressions, and the use of touch, space, and/or sound. Communication can be varied through the aspect of one's culture as well.

Professional Collaboration and Collegiality

Collaboration is specifically noted by the American Nurses Association (ANA) in its standards of professional performance, *Nursing: Scope and Standards of Practice* (2015b). The standards refer to the expected performance and behaviors of a professional nurse. Collaboration, as a standard of professional performance, requires the nurse to partner with all stakeholders, including the healthcare consumer and other professionals, to advocate for positive patient outcomes and high-quality care. This collaboration involves the use of effective group dynamics and conflict management to build successful healthcare teams. A necessary precursor to collaboration, **collegiality** involves sharing knowledge and skills, giving constructive feedback, improving and enhancing practice, and contributing to and supporting learning within the work environment (American Association of Critical-Care Nurses [AACN], 2016).

Further, the standard of practice delineating the nurse's role in coordination of care assumes collaboration and collegiality in relationship with other healthcare team members. Further, the standard on effective **communication** is a key prerequisite to collaboration, collegiality, and coordination of care (ANA, 2015b). Collaboration at the direct practice level is beneficial to the individual healthcare consumer, but the *ANA Code of Ethics for Nurses* also calls for collaboration at the health policy level to promote health diplomacy and reduce health disparities (ANA, 2015a).

Collaboration is intrinsic and vital to success in nursing practice today. When one works collaboratively, there is an implication that there is cooperation with other healthcare professionals and that a team effort is involved in this work. Further, working collaboratively implies an even distribution of power.

A team that works collaboratively is nonhierarchical. Power is shared and each individual's input is valued equally. In such cases, titles and roles are insignificant. Everyone's voice is important and is heard. As a nurse, you will be involved in many such team efforts. In fact, you will often be placed in charge of a team or be designated as the leader of a particular group. Thus, it is vital that you learn to work collaboratively and respectfully with others (Kearney-Nunnery, 2012).

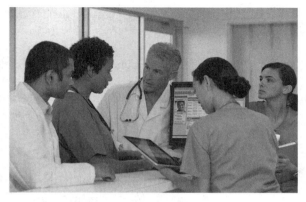

Interprofessional collaborative practice team discussing patient care.
© Ariel Skelley/Blend Images/Getty

Historical Context of Collaboration

In 1992, the ANA defined collaboration as follows: "Collaboration means a collegial working relationship with another healthcare provider in the provision of (to supply) patient care. Collaborative practice requires the discussion of patient diagnosis, and cooperation in the management and delivery of care. Each collaborator is available to the other for consultation either in person or by a communication device, but need not be physically present on the premises at the time the actions are performed. The patient-designated healthcare provider is responsible for the overall direction and management of patient care" (p. 117).

Later, in 1998, the ANA released an executive summary related to collaboration as an intrinsic part of nursing. In the document, they wrote the following points (p. 1):

- "Intrinsic to nursing is the collaborative process: nurses and physicians working together and independently assessing, diagnosing, and caring for consumers by preparing patient histories, conducting physical and psychosocial assessments, and reviewing and discussing their cases with other health professions to determine the changing health status of each client."
- "To provide effective and comprehensive care, nurses, physicians, and other healthcare professionals must collaborate with each other. No group can claim total authority over the other."
- "Each profession exhibits different areas of professional competence that, when combined together, provide a continuum of care that the consumer has come to expect."

Although organizations such as the National Academies of Practice have long called for more collaboration across healthcare disciplines to affect policy, research around failure-to-rescue began to highlight the issues with barriers related to ineffective communication and collaboration (Johnston et al., 2015). As a result, regulatory bodies have set standards for communication. The Joint Commission has published a guide for communication (2009) and has a separate safety goal on improving staff communication in its National Patient Safety Goals (2015). Interventions and tools such as Situation-Background-Assessment-Recommendation (SBAR), Early Warning Systems (EWS), and Rapid Response Teams (RRTs) have been designed to promote better team communication and collaboration.

In a similar time frame, the Institute of Medicine (IOM) published reports about avoidable patient harm and deaths. In the seminal report *To Err is Human* (2000), experts in health care concluded that there were a tremendous number of medical errors causing human suffering and that collaborative interventions were a method to reduce these medical errors. Since then, the IOM (2003) has called for health professions educators to train future healthcare providers on how to work in interdisciplinary teams that would foster these collaborative interventions.

Today, collaborative practice is embedded in initiatives for patient care. A key initiative is patient-centered care. In the late 1980s and early 1990s, extensive research was conducted through interviews with thousands of patients, family members, and professional healthcare staff to uncover the experience of health care. The purpose of this research was to assist healthcare providers in understanding how they could improve care from the patient perspective. As a result, seven dimensions of patient-centered care emerged, with an eighth dimension added at a later date (Picker Institute, 2013). **Box 7-1** lists what are now called the Picker Principles of Patient-Centered Care.

Collaboration and interprofessional relationships are also included as criteria for The Magnet® Recognition Program. Magnet® is a designation awarded by the American Nurses Credentialing Center (ANCC) that recognizes organizations that demonstrate

---

BOX 7-1   PICKER PRINCIPLES OF PATIENT-CENTERED CARE

- Respect for patients' values, preferences, and expressed needs
- Coordination and integration of care
- Information, communication, and education
- Physical comfort
- Emotional support and alleviation of fear and anxiety

- Involvement of family and friends
- Transition and continuity
- Access to care

Data from Picker Institute. (2013). *Principles of patient-centered care.* Retrieved from http://pickerinstitute.org /about/picker-principles

nursing excellence and high-quality patient care. The Magnet Model is based on research conducted in the 1980s by McClure, Poulin, Sovie, and Wandelt (1983). In this groundbreaking research, the "magnet effect" was characterized as one that had structures and processes to support nursing leadership, staff nurse autonomy and authority, and the ability to attract and retain nurses. From the research, 14 Forces of Magnetism were extracted and source statements were written for each force. Even early in the Magnet process, Interdisciplinary Relationships were identified as one of the 14 Forces of Magnetism that organizations must exemplify to receive Magnet designation. In 2008, the 14 Forces of Magnetism were consolidated into five Magnet Model components and Interdisciplinary Relationships was merged into the component Exemplary Professional Practice (ANCC, 2015).

Core Competencies for Interprofessional Collaborative Practice

In 2011, an expert panel representing the professional organizations from nursing, medicine, pharmacy, osteopathic medicine, dentistry, and public health developed a comprehensive set of core competencies for **interprofessional collaborative practice** (Interprofessional Education Collaborative Expert Panel [IPECEP], 2011). Although specifically targeting the 2003 IOM report on health professions education, the competencies are meant to address competency development across the career of healthcare professionals.

> **KEY TERM**
> **Interprofessional collaborative practice:** "When multiple health workers from different professional backgrounds work together with patients, families, carers [sic], and communities to deliver the highest quality of care" (WHO, 2010, p. 13).

The expert panel developed four competency domains for interprofessional collaborative practice. The Interprofessional Education Collaborative (IPEC) competencies are found in **Box 7-2**.

Each domain has associated competency statements that further identify the skill set for the interprofessional collaborator. The emergence of interprofessional collaborative initiatives is not solely limited to the United States. Canada and the United Kingdom have organizations, Canadian Interprofessional Health Collaborative ([CIHC], 2010) and Centre for the Advancement of Interprofessional Education ([CAIPE], 2011) respectively, which are working toward similar interprofessional collaborative goals as the IPECEP panel in the United States.

Interprofessional collaborative practice is the focus of a national coordinating center housed at the University of Minnesota, the National Center for Interprofessional Practice and Education (National Center for IPPE). The National Center for IPPE is funded by the Health Resources and Services Administration (HRSA), the Josiah Macy Jr. Foundation, the Robert Wood Johnson Foundation, and the Gordon and Betty Moore Foundation. The purpose of the center is to support "incubator" sites that test the outcomes of interprofessional collaboratives. These outcomes are

---

BOX 7-2   INTERPROFESSIONAL EDUCATION COLLABORATIVE CORE COMPETENCIES

- Values/Ethics for Interprofessional Practice: "Work with individuals of other professions to maintain a climate of mutual respect and shared values" (p. 19).
- Roles/Responsibilities: "Use the knowledge of one's own role and those of other professions to appropriately assess and address the healthcare needs of the patients and populations served" (p. 21).
- Interprofessional Communication: "Communicate with patients, families, communities, and other health professionals in a responsive and responsible manner that supports a team

approach to the maintenance of health and the treatment of disease" (p. 23).
- Teams and Teamwork: "Apply relationship-building values and the principles of team dynamics to perform effectively in different team roles to plan and deliver patient-/population-centered care that is safe, timely, efficient, effective, and equitable" (p. 25).

Data from Interprofessional Education Collaborative. (2011). *Core competencies for interprofessional collaborative practice.* Retrieved from http://www.aacn.nche.edu/education-resources/ipecreport.pdf

---

associated with the Institute of Healthcare Improvement's ([IHI], 2016) "Triple Aim," which seeks to (a) improve the patient experience, (b) improve the health of populations, and (c) reduce the per capita cost of care. The National Center for IPPE seeks to create a partnership between practice and education to affect the Triple Aim and to improve collaborative practice for the benefit of patients.

Interprofessional Education

There are numerous examples that show the benefits of students being exposed to interprofessional education (IPE) and interprofessional teams that function well together. Such practices can take place in courses that highlight IPE by placing students in clinical settings where they observe and work with other professional disciplines. This allows the nursing student to learn about the way patient care occurs in areas and departments they do not typically interact with on a daily basis. As a result, students learn about collaboration from highly functioning teams, which may also lead them to desire a more interprofessional approach to learning. It is important for nursing and all health science students to possess the skills needed to work in a collegial and collaborative environment once they are out in the workforce. In order for this to occur, the beginning steps must take place in academia. Students must be encouraged to be change agents and continually improve the healthcare process (Cuff et al., 2014).

The University of Toronto developed an IPE curriculum and program that prepares health professions students as interprofessional collaborative care providers ready for entry to practice. The framework consists of learning experiences across the curriculum that include exposure (introduction), immersion (development), and competence (entry to practice). Experiences include the knowledge, skills, and attitudes that are built upon at each successive encounter, resulting in a provider who is competent in collaboration and communications skills (University of Toronto, n.d.).

Several universities are developing and integrating IPE programs in their curricula. Virginia Commonwealth University (VCU) provides interprofessional training in the context of the critical care environment to nursing and medical students and also offer IPE courses on mindfulness, quality and safety, and geriatrics (VCU, 2015). Building on the University of Toronto framework, nursing and medical students at Indiana University in Bloomington engage in formal team training using TeamSTEPPS from the Agency for Healthcare Research and Quality (AHRQ). TeamSTEPPS methodology is discussed later in this chapter. Using IPEC competencies and best practices from TeamSTEPPS, roles, interprofessional communication, and teamwork are developed over a 2-year period using standardized patients, simulations, and direct practice (Feather, Carr, Reising, & Garletts, 2016; Reising, Carr, Shea, & King, 2011). **Contemporary Practice Highlights 7-1** and **7-2** are additional examples of interprofessional education learning experiences involving nursing students, medical students, and other health profession students.

Healthcare Outcomes Related to Interprofessional Collaboration

The Cochrane Collaboration contains a community of experts that provides systematic reviews of primary research in the area of healthcare and is often used by healthcare experts in determining evidence-based practice (Cochrane Collaboration, 2015). In 2008, the first Cochrane Review on the healthcare outcomes of IPE was published. In 2013, this review was updated to include studies published between 2006 and 2011. Of the 15 studies published between 2006 and 2011 that met review criteria, 7 studies found that IPE had positive outcomes (professional practice and/or patient care), 4 of the studies had positive and neutral (mixed) outcomes, and 4 studies reported no impact on practice or care (Reeves, Perrier, Goldman, Freeth, & Zwarenstein, 2013). **Box 7-3** highlights the positive outcomes found in the 2013 Cochrane review.

Some experts are calling for an extension of the outcomes of the "Triple Aim" to the "Quadruple Aim." This fourth aim advances the outcome of improving the caregiver's experience and postulates a link between caregiver experience and the rest of the aims in the Triple Aim (Bodenheimer & Sinsky, 2014). Supporting this theory is a study conducted by Helfrich et al. (2014) where burnout was the outcome measure. The intervention involved a team-based care approach and found that in a Veterans Administration (VA) medical home environment, team-based care was associated with lower burnout.

CONTEMPORARY PRACTICE HIGHLIGHT 7-1

APPLICATION OF THE WHO FRAMEWORK FOR ACTION ON INTERPROFESSIONAL EDUCATION AND COLLABORATIVE PRACTICE

In the WHO framework described earlier, there is a clear link between how health professions students are educated for collaboration and their impact on improving health outcomes. The National Center for IPPE asserts that health professions students can have an impact on the IHI Triple Aim while also learning with, from, and about one another (IHI, 2016; National Center for IPPE, 2015). In an example of one project that demonstrates how education and practice interweave to improve patients' outcomes, Indiana University schools of nursing and medicine in Bloomington, Indiana have created student "navigator" teams. The purpose of these teams is to work with the Integrated Care Management department at Indiana University Health Bloomington Hospital, specifically the transitional care nurse manager, to increase the number of home visits to patients who are at high risk for readmission after an acute care discharge. These student teams, consisting of senior bachelor in science in nursing (BSN) students and second-year medical students, follow up with patients in the home to determine what difficulties patients and families may be having with regard to managing their care and to secure additional resources if necessary.

Student teams have increased the capacity of the Transitional Care Program and have worked collaboratively to, for example:

- Detect increases in weight in heart failure patients
- Ensure that healthy meals are available for the patient
- Determine issues with regard to medication safety and compliance
- Secure necessary resources such as weight scales and telehealth for patients

The student navigator teams have improved patient outcomes and decreased the cost of care by reducing readmissions to the hospital, direct effects on the IHI Triple Aim. The model advances a continuity of care healthcare model, where students engage in direct collaboration with one another to improve patient care.

In another example at the same university, nursing, medical, speech language pathology, and social work students work collaboratively to coach patients to meet patient-centered goals. Student teams participate in training on motivational interviewing and health coaching to assist patients in setting goals to realize their health potential. Significant gains were made in patient weight management, decreased A1c levels, increased activity levels and exercise, reduced smoking to better control hypertension and diabetes, and decreased patient risks for stroke and cardiovascular disease.

The activities reported here were supported (in part) by the Josiah Macy Jr. Foundation.

THE RICHMOND HEALTH AND WELLNESS PROGRAM: AN EXAMPLE OF PRACTICE-BASED INTERPROFESSIONAL EDUCATION

The Richmond Health and Wellness Program (RHWP) at Virginia Commonwealth University is an example of a project that demonstrates community-based IPE through healthcare delivery. Developed by faculty from the schools of nursing, pharmacy, medicine, and social work, RHWP provides care coordination and health promotion to low-income, urban, older and disabled adults residing in high-rise apartment buildings across greater Richmond. The goal is to improve the health and well-being of the residents and decrease emergent healthcare use while also providing a rich environment for interprofessional, community-based learning for students and faculty.

In the model, a team of students from each discipline are supervised by licensed clinical faculty as they collaborate with the residents to identify and overcome barriers related to social determinants of health that affect their wellness. One distinctive aspect of the program is that the interactions with the residents occur at their place of residence. By interacting with the community members in their places of residence, the residents are viewed less as patients and more as community members who are empowered to work to overcome their own challenges. Through meeting with the individuals in community rooms and occasional home visits, the students truly learn the individuals' perspectives on health and their lives and use that enhanced understanding to provide more patient-centered care.

Another unique aspect of the program is the modeling of interprofessional practice by the team of faculty. Students are not placed in teams with the expectation that they implicitly understand how to work collaboratively or leverage the skill sets of their peers. Instead, the faculty team routinely models appropriate communication, care plan development, and discipline-specific deferral points throughout the experience. Perhaps the most striking example of this collaboration is the addition to the program of mental health services through the department of psychology in collaboration with the psych-mental health students from the school of nursing in order to fill an unmet need identified by the residents themselves and the housing building managers. The faculty work with the community to build the team each individual needs and in doing so exemplify competent interprofessional practice.

Finally, the rich learning environment helps students master core content for their professional practice. Although students are taught and evaluated on geriatric concepts and communication techniques in the classroom, through RHWP, they apply this material in interprofessional teams, integrating learning that shapes future practice while also appreciating how reliant healthcare providers are on each other. For example, students use motivational interviewing techniques to spur positive behavior change in the individuals. Practice in this type of model underscores the team role supporting behavior change while also ensuring teams are not haphazardly brought together with unrealistic expectations.

(*continues*)

CONTEMPORARY PRACTICE HIGHLIGHT 7-2 (*continued*)

Additionally, the program includes 30-minute didactic sessions that are delivered on site at the housing building at the start of clinic days to emphasize key geriatric and interprofessional principles from the classroom. Students are then able to directly translate this knowledge to the clinical encounters during their team sessions with the residents.

RHWP represents a well-organized, community-based IPE student model that fosters transdisciplinary and interprofessional collaboration. Through preceptor modeling, students learn about shared leadership and effective collaboration. In addition, the applied, community-embedded nature of the program bolsters classroom learning and helps students better understand their patients' perspectives on health and illness, ensuring a better prepared workforce of health professionals that can deliver competent, population-focused health services. Most important, the program has had a positive impact on students, faculty, community members, and the underserved community as a whole.

Highlight contributed by Kelechi Unegbu-Ogbonna, Pamela Parsons, and Alan Dow. The activities reported here were supported (in part) by the Josiah Macy Jr. Foundation.

BOX 7-3   COCHRANE REVIEW: POSITIVE OUTCOMES OF INTERPROFESSIONAL EDUCATION

Patient Care
- Improved diabetes care
- Improved emergency care patient satisfaction
- Reduced emergency care error rates
- Improved management of care in domestic violence cases

Professional Practice
- Improved emergency care culture
- Increased collaborative team behavior in emergency care and the operating room
- Improved mental health practitioner competencies in the delivery of care

Data from Reeves, S., Perrier, L, Goldman, J., Freeth, D., & Zwarenstein, M. (2013). Interprofessional education: Effects on professional practice and healthcare outcomes (update). *Cochrane Database of Systematic Reviews*, 3. doi: 10.1002/14651858.CD002213.pub3

The Patient Protection and Affordable Care Act (PPACA), enacted on March 23, 2010, was a primary driver in HRSA's decision to fund the National Center for Interprofessional Practice and Education. As care models become more integrated through reimbursement and other financial incentives, collaborative care will determine how effective the new delivery system will be. Without collaborative care, the systems will remain fragmented and costly and continue to put patients at risk for medical errors (IOM, 2015).

Collaborative Practice Models

Accomplishing collaboration begins with developing and organizing a collaborative team consisting of different professionals from the healthcare arena. Anyone involved with patient care should be involved or represented on the team. The team requires administrative support to become successful and everyone on the team buying into the concept and process of the team. Collaboration requires special resources, including dedicated technological structures that specifically facilitate collaboration and education (Stuart & Triola, 2015; World Health Organization [WHO], 2010). Teams that work together collaboratively provide greater diversity and a broad range of expertise. Research has shown that such teams do save money and they also improve efficiency and prevent errors (WHO, 2010).

In 2010, WHO advanced a Framework for Action on Interprofessional Education and Collaborative Practice (see **Figure 7-1**). The framework demonstrates how to transform local health needs into improved health outcomes using both IPE and collaborative practice.

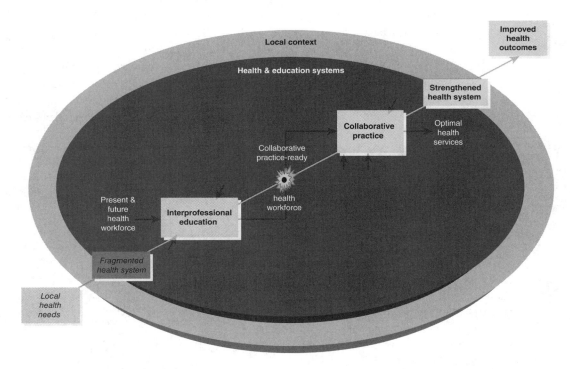

Figure 7-1 Health and education systems.

Specific actions have also been recommended by WHO (2010) to advance collaborative practice for improved health outcomes, working environment, and health professional satisfaction (see **Box 7-4**).

In an example of collaboration for improved health outcomes, the Patient-Centered Primary Care Collaborative (PCPCC) was established in 2006 to advance primary care (PCPCC, 2015a). In a key initiative, the collaborative developed the medical home model, which is philosophically grounded in team-based care, a primary feature of collaborative care. Working from the Agency for Healthcare Research and Quality, the PCPCC medical home model includes these concepts: patient centered, comprehensive, coordinated, accessible, and committed to quality and safety. Consistent with similar research, the medical home model reports better support and communication, stronger relationships with providers, and time saving (PCPCC, 2015b).

The collaborative practice model advanced by IPEC also recognizes the importance of patient- and family-centered care as an outcome of interprofessional practice. As with the WHO model, the IPEC model identifies a learning continuum that begins with health professions education. Achieving IPEC competencies is done within a focus on patient-centered care and population health (IPEC, 2011).

Those who develop collaborative models have emphasized the importance of structured education in a novice-to-expert approach (Benner, 1982). One method used to teach basic team and collaboration skills is TeamSTEPPS. Developed by the Department of Defense (DoD) and the Agency for Healthcare Research and Quality, TeamSTEPPS training focuses on evidence-based teamwork skills that are used to improve patient care (AHRQ, 2015a). Teamwork skills include team leadership, situation monitoring, mutual support, communication, and teamwork improvement. Several tools are introduced that are used in many organizations today such

---

BOX 7-4   ACTIONS TO ADVANCE COLLABORATIVE PRACTICE FOR IMPROVED HEALTH OUTCOMES

- Structure processes that promote shared decision making, regular communication, and community involvement.
- Design a built environment that promotes, fosters, and extends interprofessional collaborative practice both within and across service agencies.
- Develop personnel policies that recognize and support collaborative practice and offer fair and equitable remuneration models.
- Develop a delivery model that allows adequate time and space for staff to focus on

interprofessional collaboration and delivery of care.
- Develop governance models that establish teamwork and shared responsibility for healthcare service delivery between team members as the normative practice.

Data from World Health Organization. (2010). *Framework for action on interprofessional education & collaborative practice.* Geneva, Switzerland: Author. Retrieved from http://apps.who.int/iris/bitstream/10665/70185/1/WHO_HRH_HPN_10.3_eng.pdf?ua=1

as SBAR, huddles, and debriefing (AHRQ, 2015b). TeamSTEPPS provides practical skills that can be practiced to improve teamwork and collaboration.

The Nurse as a Collaborator and Team Leader

Nurses collaborate with many other healthcare professionals to provide the highest quality care to the patient. Nurses have collaborated on many patient care issues, including policy changes to improve patient care, ethical issues concerning patients, financial concerns of the patient, and a variety of other issues pertinent to the profession and the delivery of high-quality patient care. The primary goal of nurses is to provide the best and highest quality care to all patients, regardless of their race, religion, ethnicity, gender, sexual orientation, or ability to pay.

Collaboration allows and promotes autonomy, professionalism, self-confidence, and improved patient outcomes. Nurses who are functioning as team leaders have the opportunity to bring about improved patient outcomes as they share information with other healthcare professionals about clients. Professional nurses who participate in collaboration and active problem solving can use insights obtained from other professional healthcare workers to enhance and provide excellent client care.

There are definite benefits to working collaboratively with others. Such benefits include improved patient care, which is more patient centered; better educated patients; patient involvement in decision making; overall improved quality; cost savings; decreased lengths of stay; and the emergence of collegial relationships. Working together in a collaborative fashion improves the work environment as well. Typically, in work environments where there are collegiality and collaboration, there is increased job satisfaction and decreased turnover in nursing staff (Karanikola et al., 2014). Thus, there are advantages to such partnerships for the nurse, patient, team members, and the involved institutions of care.

To function collaboratively, it is vital that nurses have excellent communication skills. Further, there needs to be mutual respect and trust among those working together collaboratively. Nursing professionals need to be able to accept constructive criticism in a professional manner, as well as provide it to others in a constructive communication style.

Nurses must also be able to negotiate and make collaborative decisions. Combining the prerequisite clinical skills, knowledge, and expertise, decision making is part of the repertoire of a nursing professional. In a collaborative environment, decision making is a team effort. This requires trust, respect, consideration of others' opinions, and clinical expertise. It is important to remember that the patient is always the first priority. Keeping this in mind, working collaboratively with others is focused in the right direction.

Another important aspect of working collaboratively and collegially is conflict management. Role conflict can easily occur when working in a team. Individuals can all have different expectations and goals that may not be consistent with those of other team members. If expectations differ from one or several team members' expectations, role conflict can occur. It is important to keep an open mind, engage in mutual respect and trust with your team colleagues, explore barriers that may be present or perhaps invisible, and discuss each other's beliefs and experiences to reach compromises that enhance the quality of patient care. Nursing professionals are expected to have the skills, education, and experience to resolve conflicts in a professional and respectful manner. Ensuring shared leadership within a team can help reduce conflict or promote a healthy approach to managing conflict (Mitchell et al., 2012).

There are many times when the nurse might assume the role of team leader. These situations involve patient care conferences and quality improvement activities within formal and informal group settings. Nurses, in their role as coordinator of care, often find themselves in the best position to organize and lead teams of providers to promote optimal individual patient and population health outcomes. For example, for an individual patient, nurses may coordinate care among physicians and respiratory therapists to ensure proper oxygenation. On a larger scale, nurses may lead a team that produces a protocol for successful oxygen weaning to be used on all patients on oxygen therapy. Having essential leadership skills to guide teams is a necessary capability for all nurses.

Summary

The healthcare setting is changing daily with vast opportunities and needs for interprofessional healthcare teams. In today's healthcare environment, the population is aging and persons with chronic health conditions are increasingly common. In hospitals, nursing homes, and home health settings, the acuity level of the clients requires that nurses, physicians, social workers, dietitians, psychologists, and other healthcare professionals work together to provide the best, highest quality care. The collaborative practice model will enhance and improve client outcomes while decreasing or sustaining costs. As the government and healthcare institutions strive to reduce costs and yet improve patient outcomes, nurses must function as collaborators and interprofessional healthcare team members.

The National Institutes of Health (NIH) represent all disciplines of healthcare providers collaborating to achieve improved public health of the nation. The mission of the NIH is to improve the health and quality of life of all citizens. Nursing professionals have a major role to play in reaching this goal. Today clients are more knowledgeable and they seek a more holistic form of healthcare delivery. Working with others in a collegial and collaborative fashion is vital to safe, client-driven, and cost-effective care. Nurses must be educated and prepared to be active participants on the healthcare team with the client, the client's family, and a variety of other healthcare professionals.

Reflective Practice Questions

1. After reading this chapter, how do you perceive your nursing student role as a collaborator on the healthcare team?
2. Have you been a member of a collaborative team or an observer? What issues, if any, did you see regarding the sharing or lack of sharing of power? How was this or could this have been better resolved?
3. Review the collaborative practice model described in this chapter. Is there anything you feel does not "fit" or anything that you as a professional nurse would add?
4. Describe a healthcare situation that involved role conflict or decision making on your part. What was the most difficult aspect of your role? How did you handle the situation? What would you have done differently?

References

Agency for Healthcare Research and Quality. (2015a). *TeamSTEPPS®: Strategies and tools to enhance performance and patient safety*. Retrieved from http://www.ahrq.gov /professionals/education/curriculum-tools/teamstepps/index.html

Agency for Healthcare Research and Quality. (2015b). *TeamSTEPPS fundamentals course: Module 1*. Retrieved from http://www.ahrq.gov/professionals/education/curriculum-tools /teamstepps/instructor/fundamentals/module1/m1evidencebase.html

American Association of Critical-Care Nurses. (2016). *Standards for acute and critical care nursing practice*. Retrieved from http://www.aacn.org/wd/practice/content/standards.for .acute.and.ccnursing.practice.pcms?menu=

American Nurses Association. (1992). *House of delegates report: 1992 convention. Las Vegas, Nevada*. Kansas City, MO: Author.

American Nurses Association. (1998). Collaboration and independent practice: Ongoing issues for nursing. *Trends and Issues, 3*(5). Retrieved from http://www.nursingworld.org /DocumentVault/NTI/Vol3No5May1998.aspx

American Nurses Association. (2015a). *Code of ethics for nurses with interpretive statements*. Silver Spring, MD: Author.

American Nurses Association. (2015b). *Nursing: Scope and standards of practice* (3rd ed.). Silver Spring, MD: Author.

American Nurses Credentialing Center. (2015). *Announcing a new model for ANCC's Magnet Recognition program®*. Retrieved from http://www.nursecredentialing.org/MagnetModel

Benner, P. (1982). From novice to expert. *American Journal of Nursing, 82*(3), 402–407.

Bodenheimer, T., & Sinsky, C. (2014). From triple to quadruple aim: Care of the patient requires care of the provider. *Annals of Family Medicine, 12*(6), 573–576. doi: 10.1370/afm.1713

Canadian Interprofessional Health Collaborative. (2010). *A national interprofessional competency framework*. Retrieved from http://www.cihc.ca/files/CIHC_IPCompeten- cies_Feb1210.pdf

Centre for the Advancement of Interprofessional Education. (2011). *The definition and principles of interprofessional education*. Retrieved from http://caipe.org.uk/about-us /the-definition-and-principles-of-interprofessional-education/

Cochrane Collaboration. (2015). *What is Cochrane evidence and how can it help you?*. Retrieved from http://www.cochrane.org/what-is-cochrane-evidence

Cuff, P., Schmitt, M., Zierler, B., Cox, M., Maeseneer, J., Maine, L., . . .Thibault, G. (2014). Interprofessional education for collaborative practice: views from a global forum workshop. *Journal of Interprofessional Care, 28*(1), 2–4.

Feather, R. A., Carr, D. E., Reising, D. L., & Garletts, D. (2016). Team-based learning for nursing and medical students: Focus group results from an interprofessional education project. *Nurse Educator, 41*(4), E1–E5. doi:10.1097/NNE.0000000000000240

Helfrich, C. D., Dolan, E. D., Simonetti, J., Reid, R. J., Joos, S., Wakefield, B. J., . . . Nelson, K. (2014). Elements of team-based care in a patient-centered medical home are associated with lower burnout among VA primary care employees. *Journal of General Internal Medicine, 29*(Suppl. 2), 659–666. doi: 10.1007/s11606-013-2702-z

Institute of Healthcare Improvement. (2016). *The IHI Triple Aim initiative.* Retrieved from http://www.ihi.org/engage/initiatives/tripleaim/Pages/default.aspx

Institute of Medicine. (2000). *To err is human: Building a safer health system.* Washington, DC: National Academy Press.

Institute of Medicine. (2003). *Health professions education: A bridge to quality.* Washington, DC: National Academies Press.

Institute of Medicine. (2015). *Measuring the impact of interprofessional practice and patient outcomes.* Washington, DC: National Academies Press.

Interprofessional Education Collaborative. (2011). *Core competencies for interprofessional collaborative practice.* Retrieved from http://www.aacn.nche.edu/education-resources /ipecreport.pdf

Johnston, M. J., Arora, S., King, D., Bouras, G., Almoudaris, A. M., Davis, R., & Darzi, A. (2015). A systematic review to identify the factors that affect failure to rescue and escalation of care in surgery. *Surgery, 157*(4), 752–763.

Karanikola, M. N. K., Albarran, J. W., Drigo, E., Giannakopoulou, M., Kalafati, M., Mpouzika, M., . . . Papathanassoglou, E. D. E. (2014). Moral distress, autonomy and nurse-physician collaboration among intensive care units in Italy. *Journal of Nursing Management, 22*(4), 472–484. doi: 10.1111/jonm.12046

Kearney-Nunnery, R. (2012). *Advancing your career: Concepts of professional nursing* (5th ed.). Philadelphia, PA: F.A. Davis.

McClure, M. L., Poulin, M., Sovie, M., & Wandelt, M. (1983). *Magnet hospitals: Attraction and retention of professional nurses.* Kansas City, MO: American Nurses Association.

Mitchell, P., Wynia, M., Golden, R. G., McNellis, B., Okun, S., Webb, C. E., . . . Von Kohorn, I. (2012). Core principles & values of effective team-based health care. Retrieved from https://www.nationalahec.org/pdfs/vsrt-team-based-care-principles-values.pdf

National Center for Interprofessional Practice and Education. (2015). *Connecting.* Retrieved from https://nexusipe.org/connecting

Patient-Centered Primary Care Collaborative. (2015a). About us. Washington, DC: Author. Retrieved from https://www.pcpcc.org/about/

Patient-Centered Primary Care Collaborative. (2015b). Defining the medical home. Washington, DC: Author. Retrieved from https://www.pcpcc.org/about/medical-home

Picker Institute. (2013). *Principles of patient-centered care.* Retrieved from http:// pickerinstitute.org/about/picker-principles

Reeves, S., Perrier, L., Goldman, J., Freeth, D., & Zwarenstein, M. (2013). Interprofessional education: Effects on professional practice and healthcare outcomes (update). *Cochrane Database of Systematic Reviews, 3.* doi: 10.1002/14651858.CD002213.pub3

Reising, D. L., Carr, D. E., Shea, R. A., & King, J. M. (2011). Comparison of communication outcomes in traditional versus simulation strategies in nursing and medical students. *Nursing Education Perspectives, 32*(5), 323–327.

Stuart, G. & Triola, M. (2015). *Enhancing health professions education through technology: Building a continuously learning health system.* New York: Josiah Macy Jr. Foundation.

The Joint Commission. (2009). *The Joint Commission guide to improving staff communication.* Oakbrook Terrace, IL: Author.

The Joint Commission. (2015). *2015 hospital national patient safety goals.* Retrieved from. http://www.jointcommission.org/assets/1/6/2015_hap_npsg_er.pdf

University of Toronto. (n.d.). *A framework for the development of interprofessional education values and core competencies.* Retrieved from http://www.ipe.utoronto.ca /interprofessional-education-curriculum

Virginia Commonwealth University. (2015). *Educational programs.* Retrieved from http:// ipe.vcu.edu/educational-programs

Watson, J. (1979). *Nursing: The philosophy and science of nursing.* Boston, MA: Little Brown.

World Health Organization. (2010). *Framework for action on interprofessional education & collaborative practice.* Geneva, Switzerland: Author. Retrieved from http://apps.who.int /iris/bitstream/10665/70185/1/WHO_HRH_HPN_10.3_eng.pdf?ua=1

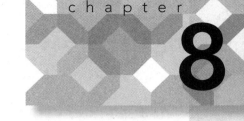

The Culture of Safety

Patricia Ebright

LEARNING OUTCOMES

After reading this chapter you will be able to:

- Describe the historical evolution of the current focus and approach toward patient safety in health care.
- Describe components of a framework for work in complex environments.
- Explain the relationship among human factors, work complexity, and the evolution of adverse events in health care.
- Identify critical components of an effective culture of safety.
- Identify the challenges in moving toward an improved culture of safety in health care.
- Apply research findings on nursing work complexity to designing safer practice environments.
- Describe the new accountabilities in the approach to patient safety for healthcare leaders, educators, and practitioners.

History of the Patient Safety Movement

The nursing profession has a rich history of developing standards, education, and approaches to nursing care that reflects an emphasis on **patient safety** and quality. Therefore, it cannot be said that before the release of the Institute of Medicine report (IOM, 2000) on **medical error** and patient safety, nurses were not aware of incidents where patients may have been injured or killed by mistakes in the application or omission of medical interventions. Starting in the early 1980s, however, a series of events leading up to the IOM report drew attention to the injuries and deaths resulting from medical error. Eichhorn (2013) reviewed the important contributions of the Anesthesia Patient Safety Foundation starting in 1984 for improvement of perioperative patient safety. In addition, several other activities preceded the current focus and extraordinary shift in approach to patient safety in health care. These activities included reports of findings from physician studies on the large numbers of preventable disabling injuries and deaths identified from medical records in the 1990s (e.g., Leape, 1994); regulatory and legislative activities led by The Joint Commission (TJC, 2016b) requiring hospital compliance with monitoring, investigation, and reporting of errors; and the creation of national organizations focused on patient safety (e.g., the National Patient Safety Foundation in 1998 and the National Quality Forum in 1999).

Most healthcare providers and consumers were not aware of the magnitude of the problem of medical errors until the IOM report was published in 2000. According to this report, tens of thousands of Americans die each year from errors in medical care and hundreds of thousands are injured, or almost injured, during their care. The IOM report served as a wake-up call that more needed to be done to prevent harm to patients and to improve quality of care. Some leaders in the healthcare industry realized that traditional approaches to safety and quality would no longer be sufficient to respond to the improvements necessary based on the outcomes reported in the IOM report. For example, in *Crossing the Quality Chasm: A New Health System for the 21st Century* (IOM, 2001), the authors called for fundamental change in the healthcare system focused on six goals for improvement (see **Box 8-1**).

Influenced and led by recommendations from subsequent IOM committee reports that were focused specifically on safety, healthcare leaders searched for solutions from industries other than health care. This search resulted in the adoption of strategies used by other industries such as the airline, aerospace, and nuclear industries to prevent high-stakes failures and reduce the harm resulting from error. Learning from expert resources outside health care, a major change in thinking occurred as to why healthcare errors happen, the role of the individual in error generation, and the roles that healthcare providers and leaders play in increasing and sustaining patient safety.

Healthcare leaders learned that to make sustainable improvements in patient safety, their focus had to switch from individual healthcare providers and workers to the

---

BOX 8-1   INSTITUTE OF MEDICINE GOALS FOR HEALTH CARE

Health care should be:

Safe: Patients should not be harmed by care that is intended to help them.

Effective: Care should be based on scientific knowledge and offered to all who could benefit and not to those not likely to benefit.

Patient-centered: Care should be respectful of and responsive to individual patient preferences, needs, and values.

Timely: Waits, and sometimes harmful delays in care, should be reduced for both those who receive care and those who give care.

Efficient: Care should be given without wasting equipment, supplies, ideas, and energy.

Equitable: Care should not vary in quality because of personal characteristics such as gender, ethnicity, geographic location, and socioeconomic status.

Data from Institute of Medicine. (2001). *Crossing the quality chasm: A new health system for the 21st century.* Washington, DC: National Academy Press.

---

complex systems in which they work, and to the complexity as well as limitations within the individuals themselves. The new focus for understanding error turned from the traditional approach to patient safety that demanded perfect individual performance in imperfect situations, to understanding the imperfect situations in which imperfect performers work. This shift in focus from the individual to the multiple complex systems and processes throughout an organization has been a formidable challenge that healthcare leaders, including nurses, have been addressing since 2000.

Although numerous regulatory and legislative efforts have been established to move the healthcare industry forward with respect to safety and quality, changing an industry **safety culture** from one that has been characterized as a "blame" culture to a "nonblame" culture has been much more difficult than originally anticipated. How we respond to errors and to those involved, what we expect from those involved, what we do to learn from errors, and even how we plan and design to prevent or limit future errors reflects the degree to which we have shifted our emphasis from individuals to systems for making improvements in safety. Healthcare organizations vary in their growth toward the recommendations set forth by the IOM reports. Legislative and regulatory efforts continue to move the safety and quality work forward.

KEY TERM

Complex systems: Systems in which work includes both cognitive and physical demands and is characterized by dynamism, large numbers of parts and connectedness between parts, high uncertainty, and risk (Woods, Dekker, Cook, Johannesen, & Sarter, 2010).

KEY TERM

Safety culture: The product of individual and group beliefs, values, attitudes, perceptions, competencies, and patterns of behavior that determine the organization's commitment to quality and patient safety (TJC, 2016b).

Regulatory and Legislative Focus on Patient Safety

Legislative action and changes in the focus of accrediting bodies since 2000 reflect the important impact of the IOM reports. In response to the IOM reports, at least 22 states initiated a medical error **reporting system** in an effort to improve patient safety by 2005. And in July 2005, Congress overwhelmingly voted to pass the Patient Safety and Quality Improvement Act. This legislation was designed to encourage states to participate in a national medical error database, and it protects the confidentiality of individuals who report errors and the organizations involved in the errors. Starting with Minnesota in 2003 (Minnesota Department of Health, 2007), individual states have continued to enact legislation to require healthcare organizational reporting of serious errors and public disclosure. Additional national efforts to share knowledge regarding best practices through state and organizational alliances have begun to demonstrate progress in the effort to decrease harm to patients (U.S. Department of Health and Human Services, 2015). **Contemporary Practice Highlight 8-1** identifies other organizations and agencies that have initiated changes in criteria, standards, and funding priorities in response to the increased emphasis on improving patient safety.

> **KEY TERM**
>
> **Reporting system:** A system for blame-free reporting of a system or process failure or the results of proactive risk assessments (TJC, 2016b).

The remainder of this chapter describes the new approach to patient safety and quality that health care has taken to make improvements based on learning from

---

CONTEMPORARY PRACTICE HIGHLIGHT 8-1

FOCUSING ON PATIENT SAFETY

Since 2003, The Joint Commission (2016a) has published annual updated lists of Patient Safety Goals that healthcare organizations must achieve to receive successful accreditation review. The Institute for Healthcare Improvement (IHI) has sponsored multiple clinically focused improvement initiatives to jumpstart realization of patient outcomes through specific quality and safety guidelines that have resulted in thousands of lives saved. Numerous national and also international agencies and organizations include quality- and safety-related web-based educational and resource information for healthcare providers, patients and consumers, policymakers, and researchers. The following organizations have responded since the 2000 IOM report with expanded efforts to improve patient safety and maintain excellent web resources: National Patient Safety Foundation (NPSF), Agency for Healthcare Research and Quality (AHRQ), Department of Health and Human Services (DHHS), Centers for Disease Control and Prevention (CDC), Center for Medicare and Medicaid Services (CMS), IHI, Institute for Safe Medication Practices (ISMP), Quality and Safety Education for Nurses (QSEN), and the World Health Organization (WHO).

other industries and the implications this new approach has for nursing practice. The cultural changes needed to move these new approaches forward are an important focus of the ongoing efforts because patient safety depends on changes in practice and accountabilities at all levels of healthcare organizations, including regulatory, legislative, and consumer groups.

Core Concepts in the Post IOM Report Approach to Patient Safety

Human factors science is focused on human performance, the interaction of humans in different situations, and its application to errors in healthcare environments and with technology. Healthcare and human factors researchers have developed a framework to understand patient safety based on work by Reason (1990) to explain how things go wrong in healthcare situations (Woods et al., 2010). One major hypothesis of this approach is that events are not the result of a single failure of an unreliable component (such as an individual) but rather the result of multiple failures in the intended defenses of a system. Researchers propose that progress toward improving patient safety can occur only when five principles that underlie productive work toward improving safety are appreciated by the providers in a healthcare system (see **Box 8-2**).

> **KEY TERM**
> **Human factors:** Human factors (ergonomics) is the scientific discipline concerned with the understanding of interactions among humans and other elements of a system and the profession that applies theory, principles, data, and other methods to the design in order to optimize human well-being and overall system performance (Human Factors and Ergonomics Society, 2016).

Using Reason's Swiss Cheese Model to Explain Failure

According to Reason (1990), **layers of defense** exist at all levels of an organization and provide boundaries around which decisions are developed and implemented. Typical healthcare organizational defenses include, but are not limited to, policies and procedures, standard care guidelines, chain of command processes for communication and decisions, budget and resource allocations, report and hand-off mechanisms, competency standards, and technology. **Latent conditions**, or **gaps**, are discontinuities in the layers of defenses in the work environment. For example, a gap exists when a specific patient situation does not exactly fit a policy and procedure for medication administration (an institutional boundary related to rules) and following the policy or procedure would not be in the best interest of the patient. Another example of an existing gap is the lack of available personnel on a busy unit for one specific shift (an institutional boundary related

> **KEY TERM**
> **Layers of defense:** Organizational safeguards in place to prevent anticipated injury, damage, or failure (Reason, 1990).

> **KEY TERM**
> **Latent conditions:** Error-producing factors like poor design, gaps in supervision, undetected system failures, lack of training, and the like arising from the decision-making levels (blunt end) of organizations that combine with active failures to result in adverse events (Reason, 1997).

> **KEY TERM**
> **Gaps:** Another term for latent conditions or error-producing factors (Woods et al., 2010.).

BOX 8-2   PRINCIPLES FOR IMPROVING PATIENT SAFETY

1. Safety is made and broken in systems, not by individuals. Adverse events result from the way work is designed and the interaction of components of the system.
2. Progress on safety begins with understanding technical work. Our current understanding of real work is naïve and incomplete, leading to the development of performance rules that are impossible to apply in a complex, heterogeneous, and rapidly changing world.
3. Progress in safety depends on understanding how technical and organizational factors play out in real work.
4. Productive discussions of safety avoid confounding failure with error. Failure results from a breakdown in systems, whereas error is usually assigned to humans and relates to a social process for attributing cause.

5. Safety is dynamic and not static; it is constantly renegotiated. Complex, ever-changing systems require that people change and adapt constantly. However, adaptation is often based on inadequate information and only partly successful. Understanding this dynamic is the foundation for understanding safety. Increasing complexity makes safety harder to achieve.
6. Trade-offs are at the core of safety. Complex work environments will always be characterized by uncertainty, discontinuities, and missing information. Understanding how people cope with these challenges will increase understanding of safety.

Data from Woods, D., & Cook, R. I. (1998). *Characteristics of patient safety: Five principles that underlie productive work.* Chicago, IL: CtL.

---

to budget) that does not provide enough staff with the necessary competencies and experience required to provide care for the unit's number and acuity level of patients.

Neither of these situations represents an overt failure in itself, but each constitutes a type of gap or latent condition that threatens the continuity of care and, when combined with other gaps, may lead to a **near-miss event**—any process variation that did not affect the outcome but for which a recurrence carries a significant chance of a serious adverse outcome—or **adverse event**—a patient safety event that resulted in harm to a patient (TJC, 2016b). Adverse events may result from acts of commission or omission (e.g., administration of the wrong medication, failure to make a timely diagnosis or institute the appropriate therapeutic intervention, adverse reactions or negative outcomes of treatment, etc.). Some examples of more common adverse events include patient falls, medication errors, procedural errors/complications, completed suicides, parasuicidal behaviors (attempts/gestures/threats), and missing patient events.

KEY TERM

Near-miss event: Also known as "close call," "no harm," or "good catch." A patient safety event that did not cause harm as defined by the term sentinel event (TJC, 2016b).

KEY TERM

Adverse event: A patient safety event that resulted in harm to a patient (TJC, 2016b).

Active failures are errors and violations caused by acts performed by workers (e.g., nurses) closest to the sharp end of the system (e.g., patient care) that affect system safety most directly (Reason, 1997). What we have learned over the past 20 years in safety is that most active failures are consequences of latent conditions and not principal causes of accidents (Reason). For example, using a situation discussed previously, inadequate staffing (system gap or latent condition) for a specific shift may result in a nurse who is responding to time pressures to bypass checking all patient identifiers (active failure) before administering the wrong medication. The latent condition of inadequate staffing was one of the contributors to the error.

Sometimes system gaps (or latent conditions) have been around for a very long time and go unrecognized by the organization. They have become part of the "routine" work. As a result, implementation of new processes may unintentionally disrupt the effectiveness of existing bridges, as well as create new gaps in the system. For example, introduction of time-consuming processes surrounding one new technology that requires increased nurse monitoring and treatment of the patient, as well as maintenance of the technology, may cause disruptions in other aspects of patient care that lead to decision **trade-offs** (decision resolutions that involve conflicting choices between highly unlikely but highly undesirable events and highly likely but less catastrophic ones). Trade-offs are made by nurses and other healthcare providers between interacting or conflicting goals, between values or costs placed on different possible outcomes or courses of action, and between the risks of different errors (Woods et al., 2010) and more serious adverse patient outcomes. Again, using the

situation discussed previously, the nurse who administered the wrong medication to a patient was dealing with time pressures that required decisions about multiple and competing work requirements. She trusted that the medication was the correct drug, dosage, route, and time for that patient and didn't follow all checks because she had retrieved it from that patient's medication supply. She was then able to more rapidly respond to another nurse's request for help in another room. She "traded off" doing a complete check to be responsive to the need of another colleague and patient. Nurses and other direct care practitioners in current healthcare environments demonstrate resilience every day by anticipating and recognizing, and then coping with or bridging, multiple gaps. Examples are nurses who increase their "checking" of the care provided by the technician with whom they have not previously worked rather than rely on reported information, or nurses who develop their own sophisticated system of readily available handwritten notes to track medication and treatments every shift. Bridging gaps is not exclusive to nurses. Other examples of bridging gaps include physicians who always look for the "reliable, competent" nurse with whom they have worked before to discuss patient status rather than risk receiving unreliable information from nurses they do not know.

Leape and Berwick (2005) explained that health care lags behind other industries in safety because of its reliance on individual performance as the key to improvement. Other industries have reduced errors by understanding that people do make mistakes in changing environments and that the way to be safer is to design systems so that it is difficult to make a mistake and easy to recover from mistakes that do occur. And in fact, human factors researchers champion the individual as the resilient factor and solution for reaching safety in complex systems and as an essential participant in efforts that have the potential for making progress in patient safety.

Complexity of Work at Point of Care Delivery (the Sharp End)

A major barrier to making progress in safety is the failure to find out what lies behind attributions of error (Woods et al., 2010). Researchers argue that understanding how people anticipate, detect, and bridge gaps in real work contexts is necessary for making improvements in patient safety. Healthcare workers actually create safety daily in the presence of multiple latent conditions or gaps and are the resilient factor for preventing accidents in complex systems (Woods et al., 2010).

> **KEY TERM**
> **Sharp end:** Frontline personnel at the operations point of the organization; for example, at the point of patient care in a healthcare organization (Woods et al., 2010).

> **KEY TERM**
> **Blunt end:** Levels of strategic and other top-level decision-making persons or groups in an organization that affect the work at the point of care delivery (the sharp end) (Woods et al., 2010).

Nurses and other healthcare workers at the point of care delivery (the **sharp end**) are involved in constantly evolving situations. Supported, and constrained, by organizational resources and layers of defense from above (the **blunt end**), healthcare workers continuously manage workloads using their knowledge, immediate perceptions, and own goals to handle situations in the presence of multiple goal conflicts, obstacles, hazards, ambiguous and inadequate or missing data, and behaviors (the system complexities on the left side of the model) surrounding care situations. For example, unpredictability, missing knowledge, clumsy technology, and constant change are a few of the multiple features of the current healthcare environment that confront healthcare practitioners. To prevent things from going wrong, practitioners act by anticipating, reacting, accommodating, adapting, and coping (the worker resiliency on the right side of the model) to bridge gaps constantly while compromising among multiple competing goals to make trade-off decisions in the midst of a changing environment.

The cognitive work required in complex work environments can be very demanding and despite best efforts, can result in decisions leading to adverse events. Woods et al. (2010) described four characteristic dimensions of complex environments that increase problem-solving demands and difficulty: dynamism, large numbers of parts and connectedness between parts, high uncertainty, and risk. In research on

---

BOX 8-3   COMPLEX WORK ENVIRONMENTS: CHARACTERISTICS THAT INFLUENCE DECISION MAKING

- Time pressures
- High stakes
- Inadequate information
- Ill-defined goals
- Poorly defined procedures
- Dynamic conditions

- Teamwork
- Stress

Reproduced from Klein, G. (1998). *Sources of power: How people make decisions.* Cambridge, MA: Massachusetts Institute of Technology.

---

complexity of work and decision making, Klein (1998) identified common characteristics across different types of occupations and industries that influence decision making (see **Box 8-3**). These common characteristics include time pressures, high stakes, inadequate information (missing, ambiguous, or erroneous), ill-defined goals, poorly defined procedures, dynamic conditions, people working in teams, and stress. Using knowledge, paying attention to shifts in current situational states, and balancing interacting and sometimes conflicting goals, workers in complex worlds make decisions and act, creating and actually increasing safety most of the time.

Human Limitations and Complexity

Human factors explain why we cannot expect perfect performance in complex work environments. An important aspect in developing an understanding about getting the best performance within the complexity described earlier is an explicit acceptance of the simple fact that humans are limited in the amount of information and complexity of tasks they are able to manage effectively and safely. Human beings are not perfect. Researchers report that during situations with multiple tasks, human limitations result from a variety of factors that affect cognitive function in dynamic evolving situations, the management of workload in time, and the control of attention (Woods et al., 2010). Humans demonstrate limitations related to memory capacity, attention span, distractions, biases, physical capability, and performance in the presence of fatigue, negative emotions, and/or illness.

Woods et al. (2010) identified two major human performance problems related to changes in attentional dynamics during certain situations—loss of situation awareness and fixation. **Loss of situation awareness** refers to failure to maintain accurate tracking of the multiple and changing interactions between parts of processes or systems. Maintaining situation awareness in complex situations would represent the ability to scrutinize and refine expectations based on new information and/or contextual aspects of a situation,

KEY TERM

Loss of situation awareness: Failure to maintain accurate tracking of the multiple processes or systems in time (Woods et al., 2010).

KEY TERM
Mindfulness: The ability to scrutinize and refine expectations based on new information and/or contextual aspects of a situation (Langer, 1989).

KEY TERM
Fixation: Failure to revise the assessment of a situation as new information becomes available (Woods et al., 2010).

KEY TERM
Sensemaking: The ability to reconstruct and interpret incoming information anew in ambiguous, complex, and evolving situations (Klein et al., 1987).

KEY TERM
Slips and lapses: Execution failures or "errors which result from some failure in the execution and/or storage of an action sequence, regardless of whether or not the plan which guided them was adequate to achieve its objective" (Reason, 1990, p. 9).

KEY TERM
Mistakes: Planning failures—"deficiencies or failures in the judgmental and/or inferential processes involved in the selection of an object or in the specification of the means to achieve it" (Reason, 1990, p. 9).

or to demonstrate what Langer and Piper (1987) defined as **mindfulness**. **Fixation** refers to failure to revise the assessment of a situation as new information becomes available. Avoiding fixation in complex situations is desirable. If individuals avoid fixation, they are demonstrating **sensemaking**, or the ability to reconstruct and interpret incoming information anew in ambiguous, complex, and evolving situations (Klein, Moon, & Hoffman, 2006). Nurses and other healthcare providers are constantly taking in new information in clinical care settings that require that they demonstrate sensemaking to accurately interpret the meaning of the information and the impact it will have on decisions they need to make about patient care.

Fallibility is part of the human condition. Reason (1990) described three basic error types that are uniquely human and complicate human performance given the best of situations. **Slips and lapses** (execution errors) are defined as "errors which result from some failure in the execution and/or storage of an action sequence, regardless of whether or not the plan which guided them was adequate to achieve its objective" (p. 9). A simple example might be when you inadvertently place an ointment instead of toothpaste on your toothbrush, having grabbed the wrong tube. These are reflex skills that go awry because of unconscious error. Any break in a routine or distraction can precipitate a slip. Reason states that the differences between slips and lapses are that slips are usually observable events whereas lapses may involve only memory and be evident only to the person experiencing the lapses. Both slips and lapses generally occur during the performance of a routine skill or behavior.

Mistakes (planning failures) occur when there are "deficiencies or failures in the judgmental and/or inferential processes involved in the selection of an object or in the specification of the means to achieve it" (Reason, 1990, p. 9). Mistakes occur in situations related to a new or unfamiliar situation or a lack of understanding of the problem caused by limited availability of information. Mistakes generally occur after identification of a problem situation.

In addition to these specific human factors, other contributors that may affect human performance are the following: environmental factors including heat, cold, noise, visual stimuli, motion, distractions, and lighting; physiologic factors including fatigue, sleep loss, alcohol, drugs, and illness; and psychological factors including competing activities and emotional states such as boredom, fear, anxiety, frustration, and anger. Given the characteristics of complex work environments within health care and the variety of factors represented by the sharp end/blunt end model, it is reasonable to expect that human limitations would further complicate a healthcare practitioner's ability to maintain mindfulness and demonstrate continuous sense-making in every situation. For example, nurses and other healthcare practitioners who are distracted frequently during work may not be able to maintain an accurate, complete, and updated picture of the current work environment and patient situations. Healthcare environments have been referred to as "environments prone to distraction." It is the failure to appreciate the contribution of complexity in our healthcare environments and human limitations of practitioners that remains one of the largest barriers in efforts to improve patient safety.

Hindsight Bias and Blame

Before the IOM released its report in 2000, traditional healthcare review of adverse events or accidents usually started at the point of the accident and included only investigation of the person(s) and details surrounding the immediate outcome. Monitoring focused on the actions and expertise of the persons involved in the outcome and on the effects and errors that followed. In the past, remedial action was directed most often toward the staff person involved in the adverse event. Although the approach to adverse event investigation has moved to a broader search for possible latent conditions or gaps, what continue to be underappreciated in many investigative reviews are the multiple environmental latent conditions, or gaps, that enabled the immediate situation characteristics to arise. This is due in part to the hindsight bias that characterizes all reviews of accidents.

Hindsight bias is the natural tendency for humans looking back from an accident to consistently overstate what could have been anticipated in foresight and to see only a simplified path of decision making related to the specific accident (Woods et al., 2010). What is lost in hindsight are all of the complex human and environmental factors and unavoidable trade-offs that contributed to the experience of the person involved in the actual situation. As a result of using hindsight bias, people close to adverse events are often counseled, inflexible policies and procedures remain or are rewritten to increase enforcement, and realistic alternative plans for dealing with the effect of the complexity in future situations may not even be considered.

> **KEY TERM**
>
> **Hindsight bias:** The natural tendency for humans looking back from an accident to consistently overstate what could have been anticipated in foresight and to see only a simplified path of decision making related to the specific accident (Woods et al., 2010).

Failure to recognize the paralyzing impact of hindsight bias in the aftermath of an accident may be one of the largest barriers to making system improvements that could prevent future accidents. Lost as a result of hindsight bias is important learning about system gaps that could be redesigned and eliminated from the organization. In addition, hindsight bias competes with a focus on potential system supports that might be appropriate to implement given normal human limitations that contributed to the event. Direction is also needed for increasing individual resiliency for responding to future similar complex situations.

Patient Safety Culture

Clear awareness of the effect of hindsight bias on learning and purposeful efforts toward avoiding the tendency to simplify explanations after near-miss and adverse events are core organizational behaviors that represent a patient safety culture for improving and providing safe patient care. These and additional characteristics of effective patient safety cultures that are essential for learning from near-miss and adverse events are listed in **Box 8-4**.

One of the most difficult aspects of health care's shift to the new approach to patient safety has been consistent application of the nonpunitive method to accident investigation. The traditional focus on the individual as the object of blame at the point of the adverse event has been a formidable target for change. Contributors to this difficulty are our human tendency for hindsight bias, as well as the catastrophic human suffering that may occur as a result of some medical adverse events. Woods et al. (2010) maintain that attribution of error after the fact is a process of social judgment rather than an objective conclusion that separates us from the event and enables us to move past it quickly, thinking we have figured out what caused the event. Unfortunately, this reaction diverts us from the very thing that will help to prevent future events—learning about what enabled it to occur in the first place and what could be done to prevent the possibility of later occurrences.

In acknowledging human limitations we have had to change our expectations about healthcare worker accountabilities related to patient safety. Whereas we used to expect that individual nurses and other healthcare providers would perform

---

BOX 8-4   CHARACTERISTICS OF EFFECTIVE PATIENT SAFETY CULTURES

- Acknowledgement of human limitations
- Awareness of the effect of hindsight bias on learning
- Avoidance of the tendency to simplify explanations of near-miss and adverse events
- Commitment on the part of management to nonpunitive problem-solving approaches to accident investigation and modeling of these approaches

- Facilitation of open communication and involvement of front-line workers for learning and problem solving
- Design of formal systems of follow-up, communication, and training after new learning and before intended changes are developed and implemented

Data from Cooper, M. D. (2000). Towards a model of safety culture. *Safety Science, 36*, 111–136.

perfectly in all situations, we now know that the complexity of healthcare work prevents what we might define as perfect performance in all situations. New areas of accountabilities for patient safety that must be accepted by healthcare providers, including nurses, include speaking up about barriers to safe care practices, sharing stories about details of what happened surrounding a near-miss or adverse event, demonstrating nonblame and supportive behaviors with coworkers after an event, and participating in problem solving to improve systems to prevent future events. Unless there was intent by the individual worker to cause harm, there is no place for blame in event investigation. Even an adverse event involving an inexperienced worker or a poorly performing worker is most often the result of system inadequacies that allowed the worker to be present in the situation in the first place. Managing poor performance is critical to patient safety but should be managed proactively and separately from investigations of near-miss and adverse events.

As a result of the discomfort that healthcare managers and leaders feel with nonblame and nonpunitive language, alternative approaches have arisen to guide them through decision making regarding follow-up actions after near-miss and adverse events. An effort to balance no blame and accountability has character-ized the second decade of patient safety efforts while continuing to emphasize the importance of systems influences resulting in error (Wachter & Pronovost, 2009). One such approach is Just Culture (2016). The Just Culture philosophy supports human fallibility as a reason for medical adverse events but also balances distinc-tions among systems failure, reckless conduct, and at-risk behavior. Just Culture algorithms, if used properly, offer a consistent organizational process and approach for application of a nonpunitive response to adverse events.

Research on Nursing Work Complexity

To understand human performance in complex systems that results in failure or adverse events in healthcare situations, researchers must focus on studying the function of the system in which healthcare providers are embedded, including complexities and hazards at the sharp end, how providers cope with system gaps, and how system gaps are created or avoided through operational changes (Woods et al., 2010). This section presents research on nursing work and descriptions of factors characteristic of nursing work environments, factors that influence regis-tered nurse (RN) decision making, and RN strategies for managing workflow in providing patient care.

A comprehensive search of the literature in 2000 revealed no research focused on both the complexity of the healthcare system and its relationship to nurses' work in actual situations. Using frameworks developed by human performance researchers, nurse researchers have subsequently conducted studies to describe registered nurse work (e.g., Ebright, Patterson, Chalko, & Render, 2003; Ebright,

Urden, Patterson, & Chalko, 2004; Kalisch & Xie, 2014; Potter et al., 2005; Sitterding, Ebright, Broome, Patterson, & Wuchner, 2014).

Guided by the sharp end/blunt end framework, Ebright et al. (2003) conducted a study of RNs working on acute care units in one large urban healthcare facility. The purpose of the study was to identify contributors to work complexity, strategies used to manage complexity for desired outcomes, and factors affecting cognitive work leading to clinical and workload management decisions. Data were collected through direct observations of individual RNs working on nine different units, followed by individual interviews using **cognitive task analysis** techniques. Analyses of the data resulted in descriptive data that included numbers of interruptions, sources of interruptions, travel patterns, types of clinical care provided, and the types of knowledge, cues, and other factors that influenced specific decision making during the situations observed. Recording all activities of an individual nurse in sequence, thereby avoiding limitation of the data by using preselected categories, provided rich representations of the actual complex flow of RN work. **Figure 8-1** represents the sharp end of the sharp end/blunt end framework with consistently recurring patterns of work complexities, work strategies, and influencers of decision making identified across nine different RNs and units studied.

> **KEY TERM**
>
> **Cognitive task analysis:** A technique for interview data collection and analysis to describe the cognitive work and influencing factors surrounding situations that led to and resulted in decisions.

Contributors to work complexity patterns included missing equipment, interruptions, and waiting for access to needed systems and resources. RNs reported lack of time to complete interventions that were judged necessary to reach desired outcomes and inconsistencies in how information was communicated or could be relied on for access if needed. RN patterns of work strategies included anticipating or forward thinking, proactively monitoring patient status to detect early warning signals, strategic delegation, and hand-off decisions to maintain flow of workload. RNs used individually constructed workflow sheets to track and document care (memory aid). Results showed that RNs implement a cognitive strategy for moving on to other activities to prevent down time when not able to complete something because of waiting for processes or inability to access resources (**stacking**).

> **KEY TERM**
>
> **Stacking:** A cognitive decision-making strategy for dealing with multiple care delivery requirements, including a mental list of to-be-done tasks and a strategy for preventing error and/or minimizing bad outcomes (Sitterding & Ebright, 2015).

Potter et al. (2005) described the cognitive work of seven RNs on an acute care unit from direct observation and interview. The researchers found the average number of stacked activities across RN lists of activities to be completed over one shift to be 11, with the maximum number of activities for an RN at any one time to be 16. Ebright and colleagues have modified their original definition of stacking to include the cognitive work of stacking that includes the organizing and reprioritizing of activities as situations in care or workflow evolve. This definition is similar to the cognitive work in sensemaking of immediate

Coordinating Knowledge, Mindset, and Goals

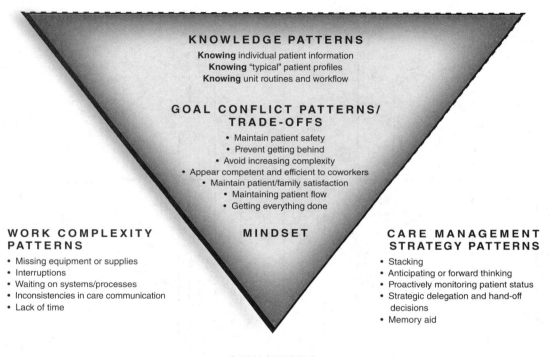

Figure 8-1 RN work at the sharp end.

and changing situations. Ebright et al. (2003) found several factors that influenced RN decision making during patient care, as represented in Figure 8-1. Two major categories of factors were knowledge considered in the decision making and goal conflicts that arose in the midst of providing care. Three patterns of knowledge were identified: knowledge about individual patients, typical patient disease profiles, and unit workflow routines. The patterns of goal conflict (simultaneous and sometimes competing goals attempted but difficult to reach in a timely or as expected manner) were the following: maintaining patient safety, preventing getting behind, avoiding increasing complexity, appearing competent and efficient to patients/families and coworkers, and maintaining patient/family satisfaction. Having to choose work on one goal at the expense of another is when nurses make trade-offs, as discussed earlier.

Figure 8-2 represents one individual RN's work over a period of 7 hours. The data were collected by directly observing the nurse and recording all activities in

Nursing Work
"and the invisible part...mindfulness and sensemaking"

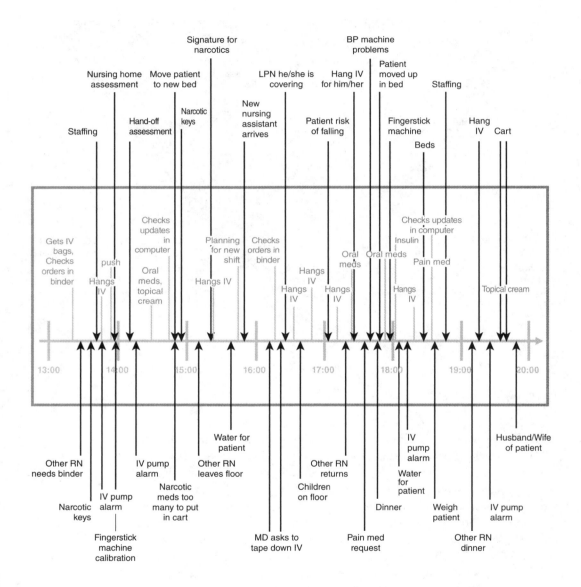

Figure 8–2 RN work complexity.
Reproduced from Patterson, E. (2003). *Nursing work complexity.*

sequence, including interrupting and medication administration during that time period. The unpredictability and obvious lack of linearity in being able to complete even one medication administration task without interruption is apparent. The important contribution of this representation is that it demonstrates to those who are not nurses or no longer work at the sharp end that it is in the midst of this complex environment that nurses strive to maintain mindfulness and continuous sensemaking as they do their best to provide safe care.

Using cognitive task analysis techniques to collect detailed stories from nurses with less than 1 year of experience about actual near-miss and/or adverse events resulted in similar data regarding the factors contributing to RN work complexity and the multiple influencers of decision making (Ebright et al., 2004). In addition, common characteristics surrounding the events were identified across RN participants and situations. For example, in all cases the RNs were anticipating, getting ready for, or performing some procedure or activity for the very first time since starting work on the unit. Distraction, anxiety, or both seemed to be a factor contributing to the near-miss or adverse event, even if the event was not related to the "first time" performance. In all cases, the RNs described being time constrained and feeling pressured to complete, or get ready for, some activity. In a majority of the cases, some type of handoff of patient information was judged incomplete or not as helpful as it could have been. And the social pressure to perform well, whether self-imposed or originating from other RNs, was a factor influencing decision making in the majority of cases.

The researchers concluded that increasing knowledge about the complexities of actual work situations involving newer RNs and what puts them at risk for error is essential. Clinical unit strategies for managing RN anxiety generated from social pressure to perform well and/or from anticipation of performance of new activities would be a place to start for supporting new nurses.

Research reports related to nursing work in subsequent years has supported earlier findings and extended understanding of the essential and yet invisible cognitive work of nursing (e.g., Sitterding et al., 2014; Sitterding & Ebright, 2015) as well as negative outcomes of nurse work in complex systems (e.g., Kalisch & Xie, 2014).

Implications of the Post IOM Report Approach to Patient Safety

Healthcare Organizations

Given the new learning about complexity and human factors, and the futility of patient safety improvement efforts that focus on only individuals without consideration of the complex systems in which they work, most healthcare organizations are involved in major efforts to change. Making decisions that result in safe care in all situations requires practitioners who are supported by systems that account for human limitations and operations decision makers who understand work at the sharp end and how changes will affect that work. Improvement in patient safety will occur only through an effective culture of safety that is characterized by encouragement of open and honest communication about failures and learning from the reporting and investigations that follow. Creating and maintaining these characteristics is difficult given our traditional approaches to failure. **Box 8-5** identifies some of the current activities and efforts by healthcare organizations to move toward safer environments.

The accountability in practice for RNs is no longer to perform perfectly in imperfect situations. We have learned that perfection is not possible in most situations. However, given our new approach, the new accountabilities for RNs are to identify barriers to providing safe patient care and proactively engage patients and significant other caregivers in assessment, planning, and care delivery, speak up about near misses and adverse events, participate in problem solving for system changes or gap elimination, and keep up to date on required educational offerings about changes, new processes, procedures, and technologies. Examples of initiatives for process improvement and risk reduction in complex healthcare situations involving RNs include clearer identification and attention to high alert medications (Institute for Healthcare Improvement [IHI], 2016); adoption of standards and templates for effective and efficient communication like SBAR

BOX 8-5 HEALTHCARE ORGANIZATIONAL EFFORTS TO CREATE SAFER CARE ENVIRONMENTS

- Identify and reduce system gaps that contribute to complexity.
- Redesign physical structures, technology, and process and procedural designs to streamline real work at the point of care and account for human limitations.
- Increase access to real-time information to support decision making through better use of informatics technology.
- Develop nonpunitive error reporting structures to encourage practitioners to speak up about near-miss and adverse events.
- Develop formal disclosure processes and patient/family supports for informing about adverse event occurrences.
- Develop formal processes for support of practitioners involved in adverse events.
- Implement leadership activities to increase leaders' understanding of work and their visibility to sharp end workers to build trust in openness and learning.
- Educate employees throughout the organization from board of directors and throughout about human factors and system failure.
- Increase patient/family engagement programs in care and safety quality efforts.

(Situation, Background, Assessment, Recommendation) across disciplines (IHI, 2016); and simple rules of engagement for difficult or challenging conversations like the challenge rule (American College of Emergency Physicians, 2016). Although these specific techniques will change over time as healthcare environments, technology, regulations, providers, and healthcare consumer needs change, the new accountabilities for RNs will continue. For managers and administrators, the new accountabilities are to facilitate an environment where open and honest communication is encouraged, rewarded, and used in improving systems of care and to involve sharp-end workers in designing and implementing change. Despite these necessary steps, overcoming the tendency to blame and engage in hindsight bias, along with the legal and economic challenges inherent in publicly reporting adverse events, will continue to be formidable obstacles as health care moves forward in efforts to improve safety.

Nursing Education

Nursing education programs have begun to redesign curricula based on the learning about complex systems, advances in technology, and the changing role of the nurse in health care. Essential knowledge for RNs to perform successfully in healthcare settings is that which prepares them as knowledge workers, system thinkers, complex system managers, and team members/leaders. The knowledge that enables RN performance in each of these roles is necessary for a most critical aspect of RN functioning based on research that describes stacking in their work.

Stacking, or the essential yet invisible cognitive decision making that results in RNs organizing and prioritizing activities (the decisions about what to do and when to do it), depends on nurses' ability to access relevant information, maintain situation awareness or mindfulness in the midst of unpredictability, and manage with accurate sensemaking as situations change. Although the healthcare organizations in which students or RNs work have some responsibility for designing supports into processes and systems, the constantly changing patient status and human behaviors of practitioners and patients/families will always demand the nurse have the knowledge and skills for managing and adapting to this complexity for safe patient outcomes. **Box 8-6** contains proposed content and teaching/learning strategies considered to be important for incorporation into nursing education curricula to facilitate student acquisition of the requisite knowledge and skills for managing complexity in the healthcare environment. **Contemporary Practice Highlight 8-2** provides information about Quality and Safety Education for Nurses (QSEN), an initiative dedicated to increasing the nursing profession's commitment to patient safety and quality.

BOX 8-6   PROPOSED NURSING CURRICULUM: COMPLEX SYSTEM CONTENT AND TEACHING/LEARNING STRATEGIES

- Complex system theory content
- Creative teaching/learning strategies for understanding complex system characteristics
- Simulations representing multiple contextual demands and challenges
- Stacking and stacking management principles and content to guide decisions and strategies about workflow
- Clinical debriefings that incorporate workload management strategies as well as individual patient case studies
- Conversations about and modeling of a culture of open and honest communication about:

  - System complexity contributions to near misses and errors in student/faculty clinical experiences
  - Realistic expectations of novice abilities in managing complex healthcare environments
  - Student/novice accountability and communication skills for seeking assistance in new and/or uncomfortable experiences
- Behavioral competencies for effective team membership and team leadership
- Communication strategies for effective engagement of patients and family caregivers

---

CONTEMPORARY PRACTICE HIGHLIGHT 8-2

QUALITY AND SAFETY EDUCATION FOR NURSES

Quality and Safety Education for Nurses (QSEN) is an initiative funded by the Robert Wood Johnson Foundation with the goal of fostering commitment to the IOM-recommended quality and safety competencies within the nursing profession. One of the QSEN's priority actions has been to define and disseminate quality and safety competencies for nursing. These competencies and further information about QSEN's goals and activities can be found at http://www.qsen.org.

In addition to curricular implications resulting from learning about patient safety, there are new accountabilities for nursing faculty who teach and work with students in healthcare organizations. These include speaking up about system complexity in clinical settings to the appropriate person in charge of operations, role modeling for students' appropriate communication strategies leading to system improvements, and role modeling nonblame language and the search for learning following near-miss and adverse events.

Summary

Several key events in the healthcare industry including legislative and regulatory factors have led to the current focus on patient safety in health care. One overall framework guiding post-IOM report patient safety initiatives and adapted from the work of James Reason provides a context for understanding the evolution of failure in health care despite our best intentions and focus on quality and safety. The sharp end/blunt end model explains work in complex systems, the contribution of complex environmental and human limitations on cognitive work, and the resulting decision making at the point of patient care.

Developing an effective patient safety culture has become the goal of healthcare institutions across the United States and the world. Yet a huge challenge to these efforts is the traditional healthcare approach to medical error that includes the hindsight bias reaction of simplifying situations surrounding an adverse event. Recent research findings on the complexity of nursing work describe contributors to the complex work of nursing, strategies that nurses use to deal with the complexity, and the factors that influence decision making at the point of care. As a result of the new approach to patient safety, organizations, nursing educators, and nurses all have new accountabilities for making improvements in patient safety.

Reflective Practice Questions

1. What factors were found to contribute to nursing work complexity in recent research on nursing work? What factors in your work environment contribute to work complexity?
2. Think of an adverse event involving a nurse or nurses in your workplace. You may or may not have been involved in the event. Were your RN colleagues' verbal and/or non-verbal reactions to the event reflective of an effective safety culture as described in this chapter?
3. In the adverse event you recalled in question two, what human factors contributed to the adverse event?
4. In the recalled event from question two, what work process or system design change might decrease the risk of the adverse event happening again?
5. Describe what you personally are accountable for in relation to improvement after awareness of an adverse event. What could you have contributed or did you contribute to learning from the event described in question two?

References

American College of Emergency Physicians. (2016, June 1). *The two-challenge rule.* Retrieved from https://www.acep.org/membership/sections/quality-improvement ---patient-safety-section/04---the-two-challenge-rule/

Cooper, M. D. (2000). Towards a model of safety culture. *Safety Science, 36,* 111–136.

Ebright, R., Patterson, E., Chalko, B., & Render, M. (2003). Understanding the complexity of registered nurse work in acute care settings. *Journal of Nursing Administration, 33*(12), 630–638.

Ebright, R., Urden, L., Patterson, E., & Chalko, B. (2004). Themes surrounding novice nurse near-miss and adverse event situations. *Journal of Nursing Administration, 34*(11), 531–538.

Eichhorn, H. J. (2013). Review article: Practical current issues in perioperative patient safety. *Canadian Journal of Anesthesia, 60,* 111–118. doi: 10.1007/s12630-012-9852-z

Human Factors and Ergonomics Society. (2016). About HFES. Retrieved from www.hfes .org/web/AboutHFES/about.html

Institute for Healthcare Improvement. (2016). *SBAR toolkit.* Retrieved from http://www.ihi .org/resources/Pages/Tools/SBARToolkit.aspx

Institute of Medicine. (2000). *To err is human: Building a safer health system.* Washington, DC: National Academy Press.

Institute of Medicine. (2001). *Crossing the quality chasm: A new health system for the 21st century.* Washington, DC: National Academy Press.

Just Culture. (2016). The Just Culture Community. Retrieved from http://legacy.justculture.org

Kalisch, B. J., & Xie, B. (2014). Errors of omission: Missed nursing care. *Western Journal of Nursing Research, 36*(7), 875–890. doi: 10.1177/0193945914531859

Klein, G. (1998). *Sources of power: How people make decisions.* Cambridge, MA: Massachusetts Institute of Technology.

Klein, G., Moon, B., & Hoffman, R. F. (2006). Making sense of sensemaking I: Alternative perspectives. *IEEE Intelligent Systems, 21*(4), 70–73.

Langer, E. J. (1989). *Mindfulness.* Reading, MA: Addison-Wesley.

Langer, E. J., & Piper, A. (1987). The prevention of mindlessness. *Journal of Personality and Social Psychology, 53,* 280–287.

Leape, L. (1994). Error in medicine. *Journal of the American Medical Association, 272,* 1851–1857.

Leape, L. L., & Berwick, D. M. (2005). Five years after to err is human: What have we learned? *Journal of the American Medical Association, 293,* 2384–2390.

Minnesota Department of Health. (2007). *Background on Minnesota's adverse health events reporting law.* Retrieved from http://www.health.state.mn.us/patientsafety/ae/background.html

Potter, P., Wolf, L., Boxerman, S., Grayson, D., Sledge, J., Dunagan, C., & Evanoff, B. (2005). Understanding the cognitive work of nursing in the acute care environment. *Journal of Nursing Administration, 35*(7/8), 327–335.

Reason, J. (1990). *Human error.* Cambridge, MA: Cambridge University Press.

Reason, J. (1997). *Managing the risks of organizational accidents.* Burlington, VT: Ashgate.

Sitterding, M. C., & Ebright, P. (2015). Information overload: A framework for explaining the issues and creating solutions. In M.C. Sitterding & M. Broome (Eds.), *Information overload* (pp. 11–33). Silver Spring, MD: American Nurses Association.

Sitterding, M. C., Ebright, P., Broome, M., Patterson, E., & Wuchner, S. (2014). Situation awareness and interruption handling during medication administration. *Western Journal of Nursing Research,* 36(7):891–916. doi: 10.1177/0193945914533426

The Joint Commission. (2016a). *2016 patient safety goals.* Retrieved from http://www .jointcommission.org/standards_information/npsgs.aspx

The Joint Commission. (2016b). *Patient safety systems (PS)*. Retrieved from https://www
.jointcommission.org/assets/1/18/PSC_for_Web.pdf

U.S. Department of Health and Human Services. (2015, December 1). New HHS data shows
major strides made in patient safety, leading to improved care and savings. Retrieved
from http://www.hhs.gov/about/news/2015/12/01/national-patient-safety-efforts-save
-lives-and-costs.html#

Wachter, R. M. & Pronovost, P. J. (2009). Balancing "no blame" with accountability in patient
safety. *New England Journal of Medicine*, 361, 1401–1406.

Woods, D. D., & Cook, R. I. (1998). *Characteristics of patient safety: Five principles that
underlie productive work*. Chicago, IL: CtL.

Woods, D. D., Dekker, S., Cook, R., Johannesen, L., & Sarter, N. (2010). *Behind human error*
(2nd ed.). Burlington, VT: Ashgate.

Quality and Performance Outcomes in Healthcare Systems

Catherine Dingley

LEARNING OUTCOMES

After reading this chapter you will be able to:

- Define performance outcomes and what effect they have on nursing practice and healthcare delivery systems.
- Define quality in health care.
- Discuss historical and societal factors that have led to the emphasis on quality outcome measures in health care.
- Explain the effects of regulatory and accreditation agencies in improving performance outcomes of health care.
- Define core performance measures.
- Describe nursing performance indicators and discuss how they are "nursing sensitive."
- List different agencies that have developed nursing performance outcomes and what measurement tools are used to determine these outcomes.
- Analyze how pay-for-performance and reimbursement plans may affect the quality of health care.
- Describe how vulnerable populations are at risk for poor health outcomes.

The editors wish to acknowledge the contributions of Beverly S. Farmer to the previous edition of this chapter.

Introduction

In today's world of changing healthcare delivery systems, managed care, medical homes, and the Affordable Care Act, the nursing profession has been called to transform the delivery of the client's care to coordinate with specific care delivery systems. Critical thinking and care decisions in partnership with clients and their families are vital to address health outcomes within today's complex delivery system models. Concurrently, public interest in and demand for improved performance outcomes have proliferated in the last decade.

This chapter focuses on performance indicators and how public and regulatory organizations use these indicators as predictors of healthcare quality. Quality outcomes and measures are complex and are measured by federal and private agencies. This chapter examines specific measurements and the various agencies that are concerned with healthcare quality. There is not one consistent measurement tool or organization that has all the answers. The history of why performance measures are considered such an important part of healthcare measurement is explored as well as how other industry standards have helped define healthcare quality. Healthcare indicators and nursing-specific indictors are presented to analyze the correlation of nursing quality care measures with improved quality outcomes.

Performance Outcomes

A recent study estimates approximately 440,000 Americans die each year from preventable hospital errors (Makary & Daniel, 2016), making medical errors the third leading cause of death in the United States. In the 2000 landmark report, *To Err Is Human: Building a Safer Health System*, the Institute of Medicine reported between 44,000 and 98,000 Americans died each year as a result of preventable medical errors. At that time, medical errors were the eighth leading cause of death in the United States. The report described the U.S. healthcare system as fractured, prone to errors, and detrimental to safe patient care. As consumers and the public become more aware of these statistics, the increased demand for improvement has become critical to the healthcare industry. Consumers no longer tolerate complacency in healthcare improvements. **Performance outcomes** are the measure of a quality organization. Performance outcomes can measure an organization's performance or client care outcomes, depending on the measurement tool. Within healthcare organizations, performance outcomes that are nurse sensitive have become an important determinant in the quality of the organization.

Standards and outcomes can be developed and made available in a variety of ways. Standards can be developed and used by

TABLE 9-1 EXAMPLES OF HEALTHCARE OUTCOMES QUALITY MEASURES	
Measure	Example
Mortality	Infant death rate
Physiologic measures	Blood pressure
Clinical events	Stroke
Symptoms	Difficulty breathing
Functional measures	Walking a designated distance

public regulatory processes or through private voluntary processes. These standards may determine licensure, such as with CMS, or accreditations through The Joint Commission. Standards measure consistency and uniformity and set expectations of performance. The process of developing standards can set the expectations for the organizations and health professionals that are affected by the standards. The publication and dissemination of standards help healthcare consumers to set expectations as well. Expectations for performance play an important role in establishing norms and facilitating improvements in outcomes. Examples of healthcare outcomes are shown in **Table 9-1**.

Health care is rapidly changing. One of the reasons for these changes is the continually expanding proliferation of information. Information that in the past was either not measured or not made public has become easily accessible to the general public. Information is easily accessible and can assist patients in selecting a provider. As an example, patients can use publicly available information to select a surgeon by reviewing the statistics of the number and types of surgeries performed, what percentage of patients developed postoperative infections, or how many patients had other complications. The public can use the Internet or printed material to find and compare hospitals within a given area to determine which has the best outcomes for a given diagnosis or which quality awards have been given to a particular hospital. Consumers must learn how to navigate and interpret information related to quality of care and performance indicators to make informed decisions.

Defining Quality

The public does not routinely choose a restaurant because it just satisfies the customer. Many people look for a restaurant that has a competitive advantage such as great service, better prices, delicious food, or better than expected ambiance.

The same strategies can be used for people when choosing a healthcare provider or hospital. Some use the argument that third-party payers have more choice than an individual, but it does not take long for a physician or healthcare organization with poor performance outcomes to become highlighted and not be chosen by the third-party payer. It is easy for a person to use the Internet to find information about a physician or hospital. This is a much newer concept to the business of health care than to other businesses, which have been compared publicly for many years. New tools and resources for assessing and improving healthcare quality are available, and others continue to be rapidly developed (see **Sidebar 9-1**).

Consumers want quality. A frequently used definition of quality is "meeting or exceeding the customers' expectations." For some people high-quality health care means seeing their doctor or nurse practitioner right away, being treated courteously by the staff, and having the provider spend time with them (see **Sidebar 9-2**). Although these things are important, clinical performance measures should be the most important outcome measure when determining whether a healthcare professional or organization is a provider of quality health care.

Measuring quality through performance outcomes is one way to determine quality in health care. There are many agencies, organizations, and individuals that measure healthcare quality; there is no one way to determine the quality of healthcare. Becoming aware of how data are collected, analyzed, and reported is a key aspect of using quality measures to make informed decisions.

The Institute of Medicine defines quality as the degree to which health services for individuals and populations increase the likelihood of desired health outcomes and are consistent with current professional knowledge (Lohr, 1990). Good quality means providing clients with appropriate services in a technically competent manner, with good communication, shared decision making, and cultural sensitivity.

In today's healthcare environment, the meticulous collection and meaningful portrayal of relevant quality data and information are equally vital to healthcare organizations, practitioners, purchasers, and the public. It is through the use of reliable performance data that healthcare organizations and individual practitioners are able to determine priority areas for quality improvement, and purchasers and consumers can make informed decisions about accessing and purchasing healthcare services. Data access and quality vary by organization, department, and unit and are important considerations. Examples of data sources include clinical data usually accessed through the medical record, administrative data such as billing records, operational data such as staffing and staff mix, and survey data such as patient satisfaction and employee engagement. Given the complex nature of health care, a set of measures derived from multiple data sources will likely provide a more comprehensive view of quality of care (see **Sidebar 9-3**). Measures of quality are used for multiple purposes: to drive quality improvement, for public accountability, to inform consumer decisions, and to pay for performance. Patient care outcomes are dependent upon the entire healthcare team working together; however, nurses are particularly concerned with indicators that reflect nursing care. The following section explains the historical evolution of quality measures in health care. Understanding the historical perspective and challenges will help to formulate a more consistent national strategy for performance data needs and improvements in the future.

> ### SIDEBAR 9-3
>
> The National Quality Strategy was first published in March 2011 and is led by the Agency for Healthcare Research and Quality on behalf of the U.S. Department of Health and Human Services. Established as part of the Affordable Care Act, the National Quality Strategy serves as a catalyst and compass for a nationwide focus on quality improvement efforts and approach to measuring quality. The National Quality Strategy is guided by three aims to provide better, more affordable care for individuals and the community.
>
> Reproduced from Agency for Healthcare Research and Quality. (n.d.). Working for quality: Achieving better health and health care for all Americans. Retrieved from http://www.ahrq.gov/workingforquality/

The History of Quality Measures in Health Care

Quality is not a new concept. From early civilization it has been important to the survival of humans. Plato has even been credited with inventing the term *quality*. The modern quality movement began in the United States during the late 1920s with the work of Walter Shewhart. He provided great insight into the collection, analysis, and presentation of data in the quality discipline. Shewhart developed control charts that provide a statistical basis for separating variation. In the 1950s Japan emerged as an economic power in response to the emphasis on quality in the writings of W. Edwards Deming, Joseph Juran, and Armand Feigenbaum. Deming advocated improving the system rather than criticizing workers when things went wrong as well as focusing on the processes that needed to be improved. He is also credited with creating the Deming Cycle (Plan-Do-Study-Act). Joseph Juran was instrumental in introducing the quality trilogy of quality planning, quality control, and quality improvement. Juran's focus was on improving the current system. Feigenbaum is credited with the concept of Total Quality Management (TQM).

In the early 1980s the United States recognized and put into practice the works of Deming, Juran, and Feigenbaum. The concepts of these early scholars were embraced by the manufacturing industry, but the healthcare industry did not initially visualize the impact that could be made on health care. During the 1990s, healthcare organizations finally began applying these authors' principles.

Another innovation in quality was Six Sigma, a set of practices perfected by Bill Smith at Motorola in 1986. Six Sigma manages process variations that cause defects and systematically works toward managing variations to eliminate the defects. Bill Smith did not invent Six Sigma; rather he applied methodologies that had been available since the 1920s developed by pioneers like Shewhart, Deming, Juran, Isikawa, and others. The tools used in Six Sigma programs are actually a subset of the quality disciplines that have been used for quality control, TQM, and Zero Defects. Many prominent healthcare organizations have adopted the Six Sigma tools as their approach for quality improvement and innovation. Many other individuals have contributed to the knowledge of **quality management**. Although each has provided distinct knowledge to the study of quality, there is a consistent link throughout their contributions and ideas.

> **KEY TERM**
>
> **Quality management:** A method for ensuring that all the activities necessary to design, develop, and implement a product or service are effective and efficient with respect to the system and its performance.

Regulatory and Accrediting Agencies

There are many regulatory and accrediting bodies that drive the use of performance outcomes within health care. These bodies share many similarities in the defining of performance outcomes, but the methods of measurement or the process for collecting information may be different. Understanding the purpose and the focus of these organizations makes it easier to interpret the information and use it appropriately. The following sections highlight the areas of focus for the primary regulatory and accrediting agencies.

Center for Medicare and Medicaid Services

The **Center for Medicare and Medicaid Services (CMS)** is a U.S. federal agency that administers Medicare, Medicaid, and the State Children's Health Insurance Program. It provides information for health professionals, regional governments, and consumers in regard to how an organization meets the standards set by the CMS. The CMS has a set of rules and regulations that contains the minimum health and safety requirements that hospitals must meet to participate in the Medicare and Medicaid programs. These rules are known as the Conditions of Participation, and every healthcare organization must meet these guidelines in order to be reimbursed for care provided to Medicare clients.

> **KEY TERM**
>
> **Center for Medicare and Medicaid Services (CMS):** A U.S. federal agency that administers Medicare, Medicaid, and the State Children's Health Insurance Program. It provides information for healthcare professionals, regional governments, and consumers in regard to how an organization meets the standards set by the agency itself.

The CMS gives deemed status to some accrediting agencies, which certifies that the accreditation meets the standards set forth by the CMS. In order for a healthcare organization to participate in and receive payment from the Medicare or Medicaid programs, it must meet the eligibility requirements for program participation, including a certification of compliance with the Conditions of Participation, or standards, set forth in federal regulations. This certification is based on a survey conducted by a state agency on behalf of CMS. However, if a national accrediting organization has and enforces standards that meet or exceed the federal Conditions of Participation, CMS may grant the accrediting organization "deeming" authority and deem each accredited healthcare organization as meeting Medicare and Medicaid certification requirements. The accredited healthcare organization would then have deemed status and would not be subject to Medicare's survey and certification process.

CMS works in conjunction with the Hospital Quality Alliance (HQA), a public–private collaboration on hospital performance measurement and reporting. This collaboration includes the American Hospital Association, the Federation of American Hospitals, and the Association of American Medical Colleges. It is supported by the **Agency for Healthcare Research and Quality (AHRQ)**, CMS, and other organizations such as the National Quality Forum (NQF), The Joint Commission, the American Medical Association, the Consumer-Purchaser Disclosure Project, the AFL-CIO, AARP, and the U.S. Chamber of Commerce (see **Contemporary Practice Highlight 9-1**). Through this initiative, a robust, prioritized, and standardized set of hospital quality measures has been refined for use in voluntary public reporting. As the first step, Hospital Compare, a website/web-based tool, was developed to publicly report valid, credible, and user-friendly information about the quality of care delivered in the nation's hospitals (CMS, n.d.).

> **KEY TERM**
>
> **Agency for Healthcare Research and Quality (AHRQ):** The health services research arm of the U.S. Department of Health and Human Services, complementing the biomedical research mission of its sister agency, the National Institutes of Health. It is a home to research centers that specialize in major areas of healthcare research such as quality improvement and patient safety, outcomes and effectiveness of care, clinical practice and technology assessment, and healthcare organization and delivery systems.

State Departments of Health

State departments of health regulate healthcare organizations in each state. State health departments have the responsibility of overseeing all healthcare organizations to ensure the public that health care is safe and that organizations follow the conditions outlined by CMS. State health departments also monitor the quality of care and have processes that facilitate public reporting of complaints regarding safety and quality. Representatives from the state health department may conduct an inspection based on a reported event.

States also license healthcare workers including physicians, nurses, and pharmacists. Many state health departments collect and provide performance information about specific healthcare providers or organizations. This information is then made available to the public. For an example of information from a

AGENCY FOR HEALTHCARE RESEARCH AND QUALITY

Not only are regulatory and accrediting bodies involved in patient safety and quality, but many government and private sector organizations also have a clear interest in the performance outcomes of healthcare organizations. One such organization is the Agency for Healthcare Research and Quality (AHRQ). The goal of AHRQ is to improve the health and health care of all Americans by supporting and conducting research that provides evidence-based information on healthcare outcomes, quality, cost, use, and access to care. In addition, the AHRQ works with a wide variety of partners to ensure that the results of research are brought to the point of care and available for use by federal, state, and local policymakers.

Historically, clinicians have relied primarily on traditional biomedical measures, such as the results of laboratory tests, to determine whether a health intervention is necessary and whether it is successful. Researchers have discovered, however, that when they use only these measures, they miss many of the outcomes that matter most to patients. Hence, outcomes research also measures how clients function, their experiences with care, and quality of life.

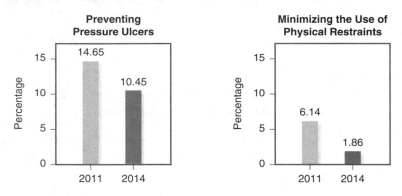

Figure 9-1 Example data from a Quality Improvement Organizations report.
Data from Quality Improvement Organizations. (2014). Raising the bar: IPRO's Medicare quality improvement report for New York State (2011-2014). Retrieved from http://ipro.org/wp-content/uploads/2014/08/QIO_Report_2014_07_24_v1.pdf

state quality report card from New York's Quality Improvement Organization (QIO), see **Figure 9-1**.

The Joint Commission

The Joint Commission, an independent, not-for-profit organization, evaluates and accredits nearly 15,000 healthcare organizations and programs in the United States. Its standards focus not simply on an organization's ability to provide safe, high-quality care but on its actual performance. Standards set forth performance expectations for activities that affect the safety and quality of patient care. If an organization does the right things and does them well, there is a strong likelihood that its clients will experience good outcomes. The Joint Commission develops its standards in consultation with healthcare experts, providers, measurement experts, purchasers, and consumers. The results of the survey for accreditation may be accessed on The Joint Commission website at http://www.jointcommission.org and The Joint Commission Quality Check® at http://www.qualitycheck.org/qualityreport.aspx?hcoid=479835.

For clinicians and clients, outcomes research provides evidence about benefits, risks, and results of treatments so they can make more informed decisions. For example, one group of researchers studied the outcomes of clients with pneumonia, a common cause of hospitalization in elderly people. They developed a way for clinicians to determine which patients with pneumonia can be treated safely at home, an option that not only reduces Medicare costs but also is preferred by many clients and their families. In areas such as cancer, where cure may be an elusive goal, outcomes research has provided information to help patients make choices that will improve their quality of life.

Outcomes researchers can identify potentially effective strategies they can implement to improve the quality and value of care. AHRQ-sponsored outcomes studies, for example, have shown that even when treatments are known to be effective, many people who could benefit from them are not getting them. Beta-blocker medication, given after myocardial infarction, can reduce mortality; blood-thinning medication can prevent strokes; and thrombolytic ("clot-buster") therapy given immediately after a heart attack can reduce the damage from the attack. Yet in each case, some eligible clients are not getting these treatments (see **Sidebar 9-4**). By identifying and addressing the barriers to better care—for example, through development of a tool to help providers know which clients with suspected myocardial infarction will benefit from thrombolytic treatment—AHRQ (2014) researchers have helped translate these findings into practical strategies to improve care at the bedside.

The Institute for Healthcare Improvement

The **Institute for Healthcare Improvement (IHI)** is a not-for-profit organization leading the improvement of health care throughout the world. IHI was founded in 1991 and is based in Cambridge, Massachusetts. IHI's work is funded primarily

SIDEBAR 9-4
Some eligible clients are still not receiving the treatment that has been demonstrated in AHRQ studies to be the most effective.

KEY TERM
Institute of Healthcare Improvement (IHI): A not-for-profit organization seeking to improve health care around the world. IHI's work is funded primarily through fee-based program offerings and services, and also through the support of a group of foundations, companies, and individuals. It conducted the 5 Million Lives Campaign.

through their own fee-based program offerings and services and also through the generous contributions of a distinguished group of foundations, companies, and individuals (IHI, 2016b).

The IHI's 5 Million Lives Campaign targeted a reduction of 5 million instances of harm from December 2006 through December 2008. The campaign continued the six interventions of the 100,000 Lives Campaign and added six more. The campaign's aim was to support the reduction of medical harm, defined as "unintended physical injury resulting from or contributed to by medical care (including the absence of indicated medical treatment), that requires additional monitoring, treatment, or hospitalization, or that results in death" (McCannon, Hackbarth, & Griffith, 2007). The goal of a reduction of five million incidents of harm in 2 years is based on an estimate that 40 to 50 incidents occur per 100 admissions, for a total of 15 million incidents of medical harm each year in the United States. Participants in the 5 Million Lives Campaign made exciting progress since the launch of the 100,000 Lives Campaign in December 2004 (McCannon et al., 2007). Hospitals across the United States made unprecedented commitments to quality and patient safety, with many demonstrating impressive results. At its formal close in December 2008, the campaign celebrated the enrollment of 4,050 hospitals, with more than 2,000 facilities pursuing each of the campaign's 12 interventions to reduce infection, surgical complication, medication errors, and other forms of unreliable care in facilities. Eight states enrolled 100 percent of their hospitals and 18 states enrolled over 90 percent of their hospitals in the campaign (IHI, 2016a). **Box 9-1** shows the initiatives of this campaign.

The **Leapfrog Group** was formed in 1998. A group of large employers came together to discuss how they could work together to use their ability to purchase health care to have an influence on its quality and affordability. They recognized that there were problems in the healthcare marketplace. Employers were spending billions of dollars on health care for their employees with no way of assessing its quality or comparing healthcare providers. The founders realized they could take "leaps" forward with their employees, retirees, and families by rewarding hospitals that implement significant improvements in quality and safety. Funding to set up Leapfrog came from the Business Roundtable (BRT) and the Leapfrog Group was officially launched in November 2000. Leapfrog is supported by the BRT, The Robert Wood Johnson Foundation, Leapfrog members, and others (see **Sidebar 9-5**).

KEY TERM

Leapfrog Group: A voluntary program aimed at mobilizing employer purchasing power to alert the U.S. health industry on "leaps" in healthcare safety, quality, and customer value so they will be recognized and rewarded. Among other initiatives, Leapfrog works with its employer members to encourage transparency and easy access to healthcare information as well as providing rewards for hospitals that have a proven record of high-quality care.

SIDEBAR 9-5

Healthcare providers are faced with an increasingly challenging regulatory environment. They need to demonstrate their quality of care to The Joint Commission and CMS, as well as to a range of pay-for-performance and quality improvement initiatives such as the Leapfrog Hospital Rewards Program and the American Heart Association's Get with the Guidelines program.

BOX 9-1   INSTITUTE FOR HEALTHCARE IMPROVEMENT CAMPAIGN INITIATIVES

1. **Deploy Rapid Response Teams** ... at the first sign of patient decline
2. **Deliver Reliable, Evidence-Based Care for Acute Myocardial Infarction** ... to prevent deaths from heart attack
3. **Prevent Adverse Drug Events (ADEs)** ... by implementing medication reconciliation
4. **Prevent Central Line Infections** ... by implementing a series of interdependent, scientifically grounded steps
5. **Prevent Surgical Site Infections** ... by reliably delivering the correct perioperative antibiotics at the proper time
6. **Prevent Ventilator-Associated Pneumonia** ... by implementing a series of interdependent, scientifically grounded steps
7. **Prevent Harm from High-Alert Medications** ... starting with a focus on anticoagulants, sedatives, narcotics, and insulin
8. **Reduce Surgical Complications** ... by reliably implementing all of the changes in care recommended by SCIP, the Surgical Care Improvement Project
9. **Prevent Pressure Ulcers** ... by reliably using science-based guidelines for their prevention
10. **Reduce Methicillin-Resistant *Staphylococcus aureus* (MRSA) infection** ... by reliably implementing scientifically proven infection control practices
11. **Deliver Reliable, Evidence-Based Care for Congestive Heart Failure** ... to avoid readmissions
12. **Get Boards on Board** ... by defining and spreading the best-known leveraged processes for hospital Boards of Directors, so that they can become far more effective in accelerating organizational progress toward safe care

Modified from Institute for Healthcare Improvement. (2016a). 5 Million Lives Campaign overview. Retrieved from http://www.ihi.org/Engage/Initiatives/Completed/5MillionLivesCampaign/Pages/default.aspx

The Hospital Quality Initiative (HQI), like other CMS quality initiatives, consists of many facets. Its goals are to improve the care provided by the nation's hospitals and to provide quality information to consumers and others. CMS has several efforts in progress to provide hospital quality information to consumers and others and improve the care provided by the nation's hospitals. These activities build upon previous CMS and QIO efforts on behalf of Medicare beneficiaries and other adults to promote the best medical practices associated with certain clinical conditions. One way that these outcomes are reported is through the **core measures**. These measures represent wide agreement from CMS, the hospital industry, and public sector stakeholders such as The Joint Commission, the NQF, and the AHRQ. The hospital quality measures currently listed on Hospital Compare have gone through years of extensive testing for validity and reliability by CMS and the QIOs,

> **KEY TERM**
>
> **Core measures:** Used to measure the quality of care provided by a hospital and its providers for clients with a specific diagnosis such as heart failure, pneumonia, or acute myocardial infarction. These measures are determined by the Center for Medicare and Medicaid Services, The Joint Commission, and the American Hospital Association, and provide a basis for value-based purchasing of healthcare services.

The Joint Commission, the HQA, and researchers. The hospital quality measures are also endorsed by the NQF, a national standards-setting entity.

Core Measures

In 2001, the **Institute of Medicine (IOM)** released *Crossing the Quality Chasm: A New Health System for the 21st Century*. This landmark report put the spotlight on the issue of poor healthcare quality. The report called for changes to our healthcare system and for collaboration between government and the medical community. Thus in 2003 Congress enacted the Medicare Modernization Act and in 2005 the Deficit Reduction Act, both containing provisions that call upon hospitals to report clinical care data measuring performance. In 2003 hospitals began publishing their performance data on 21 clinical quality measures of care provided to patients admitted for myocardial infarction, heart failure, pneumonia, and surgical care infection prevention. Each hospital submits data to CMS to receive a score for each of these measures, which represents the percentage of cases in which the hospital provided the recommended care. CMS then publishes hospitals' performance data each quarter. This allows the public and payers to observe how a hospital is performing relative to other hospitals and helps to facilitate value-based purchasing. Hospital Value-Based Purchasing (VBP) links Medicare payment to a value-based system to improve healthcare quality, including the quality of care provided in the inpatient hospital setting. Participating hospitals are paid for care services based on the quality of care, not just quantity of the services they provide. Congress authorized Inpatient Hospital VBP in Section 3001(a) of the Affordable Care Act. The program uses the hospital quality data reporting infrastructure developed for the Hospital Inpatient Quality Reporting (IQR) Program, which was authorized by Section 501(b) of the Medicare Prescription Drug, Improvement, and Modernization Act of 2003.

All of the Hospital Core Quality Measures used by The Joint Commission and CMS are endorsed by the NQF (see **Sidebar 9-6**). These measures are also used for the Hospital Quality Alliance: Improving Care through Information initiative, a voluntary public reporting initiative led by the American Hospital Association, the Federation of American Hospitals, and the Association of American Medical Colleges. This initiative is supported by The Joint Commission, CMS, NQF, AHRQ, AFL-CIO, and AARP (formerly American Association of Retired Persons).

Currently, Hospital Core Quality Measure sets exist for acute myocardial infarction, heart failure, pneumonia, and Surgical Care Improvement Project (the surgical infection prevention measures were transitioned into SCIP). In addition, The Joint Commission has core measure sets for pregnancy and related conditions and children's asthma care.

CMS, along with its sister agency, AHRQ, developed a standardized survey of patient perspectives of their hospital care, known as Hospital Consumer Assessment of Healthcare Providers and Systems (HCAHPS). Information from this survey is publicly reported on Hospital Compare. Public reporting of standardized measures on patients' perspectives of the quality of hospital care will encourage consumers and their providers to discuss their care and make more informed decisions on how to get the best hospital care, as well as increase the public accountability of hospitals.

Improving the Quality of Care

Nurses are well suited to lead and participate in performance improvement efforts, as they interact with patients and families in multiple settings and provide care management across the continuum of health (Kronick, 2014). Understanding how to improve performance indicators begins with a foundation of continuous quality improvement (CQI). CQI is a framework for improvement that continuously assesses the various aspects of care delivery and asks questions such as "How are we doing?" and "How can we improve and provide more effective, efficient care in a timely manner?" A CQI framework should include the systematic assessment of current practices, a plan to implement improvements, and a clear goal with a vision of the desired outcome.

CQI initiatives should focus on the combination of "Structure, Process, Outcomes" (Donabedian, 1980). "Structure" includes physical space and buildings, human resources such as staff, and financial and technological resources. Structural components are usually easily observed and measured and can focus on items such as the number, mix, and adequacy of staff, equipment, and space. "Process" focuses on activities, tasks, and workflow that achieve specific results and outcomes. Activities related to diagnosing and treating patients, communication and interpersonal collaboration, and medication reconciliation are all examples of processes. The results and effects of care processes on the health of patients and families represent "Outcomes." Measures such as knowledge, quality of life, satisfaction with care, health behaviors, and clinical indicators are examples of outcomes and can represent a change in patient health status due to specific interventions.

A number of quality improvement models have been used in healthcare organizations. Two of the most common are the IHI Model for Improvement and the Toyota Lean Model.

IHI Model for Improvement

The Plan-Do-Study-Act cycle, commonly known as PDSA, is the foundation for improvement initiatives in the IHI Model. PDSA consists of a series of steps that focus on goal setting, team building, planning, and testing possible improvement interventions. PDSA, also known as the Deming Wheel, was developed by Dr. W. Edward Deming (1993) and used in a number of industrial settings.

The PDSA cycle includes:

- Plan: Establish the purpose/goals of the improvement project. Identify metrics of success. Develop the steps and actions of the plan.
- Do: Implement the plan, put it into action.
- Study: Evaluate the plan's progress, success, and how it can be improved. Measure and monitor the outcomes of the plan.
- Act: Make adjustments to the plan, goals, and processes as needed, based on what has been learned in the "Study" phase. Integrate what has been learned by the entire cycle.

The entire process is cyclical in nature and can be repeated over and over in a continual process of improvement. Often the PDSA initiative is implemented on a smaller scale in the first cycle and then expanded out to include more units, departments, or across the organization.

Toyota Lean Model

Based on the Toyota production system, the Lean Model has been applied increasingly in health care over the last 10 years. The primary focus of the Lean Model is to eliminate waste in a system by applying manufacturing-based approaches. Improving quality of care in healthcare organizations is accomplished by streamlining value-added activities (as identified by customers), eliminating nonvalue-added activities, and mapping and monitoring processes from start to finish.

"Lean" quality improvement projects strive to eliminate waste (of time and resources), improve the workflow, decrease delays in care, apply evidence for decision making, and empower and motivate staff to develop and sustain the improvements. Improvement teams are established and include a variety of stakeholders and one or two members who have little knowledge of the problem and can serve as "fresh eyes." A series of work meetings known as rapid improvement events (RIEs) are used to assess the problem, identify areas and strategies for improvement, and make significant changes in a short time frame.

Nursing Performance Measures

Nurses, as the principal caregivers in any healthcare system, directly and profoundly affect the lives of clients and are critical to the quality of care they receive. Client acuity and shorter lengths of stay, the shortage of qualified nurses, changing technology, and expansion of public and community health services must be addressed in the context of quality care. Higher client expectations have produced a greater demand for quality, and mounting financial pressures require nursing to examine the balance of quality and cost (see **Sidebar 9-7**).

Nursing care is critical to the quality of client care and the success of any healthcare delivery system. Given the importance of nursing care, standardized nursing care performance measures is a major factor in healthcare quality improvement and work system performance. The importance of such measures is intensified by ongoing challenges to provide nursing staff that is educated and experienced in each specialty. Furthermore, as new ways to deliver client-centered care are developed, standardized ways to measure the performance of care delivered by healthcare teams will be essential to evaluating the effectiveness of these new practices. The following section describes specific initiatives to measure nursing performance.

National Database of Nursing Quality Indicators

In 1994, the American Nurses Association (ANA) launched the Safety & Quality Initiative to explore and identify the empirical linkages between nursing care and patient outcomes (see **Sidebar 9-8**). The Nursing Care Report Card for Acute Care (ANA, 1995) proposed 21 measures of hospital performance with an established or theoretical link to the availability and quality of nursing services in acute care settings. Since the initial creation of these early nursing indicators, extensive work and research have been conducted to further develop indicators that are sensitive to nursing care.

Nursing-sensitive indicators from **National Database of Nursing Quality Indicators (NDNQI)** reflect the structure, process, and outcomes of nursing care (see **Table 9-2**). The structure of nursing care is indicated by the supply of nursing staff, the skill level of the nursing staff, and the education/certification of nursing staff. Process indicators measure aspects of nursing care such as assessment, intervention, and RN job satisfaction.

Client outcomes that are determined to be nursing sensitive are those that improve if there is a greater quantity or quality of nursing care (e.g., pressure ulcers, falls, and intravenous infiltrations).

Some client outcomes are more highly related to other aspects of institutional care, such as medical decisions and institutional policies (e.g., frequency of primary C-sections, cardiac failure), and are not considered "nursing sensitive."

TABLE 9-2 NURSING-SENSITIVE INDICATORS FROM NDNQI

Indicator	Sub-indicator	Measure(s)
Nursing Hours per Patient Day[1,2]	a. Registered Nurses (RN) b. Licensed Practical/Vocational Nurses (LPN/LVN) c. Unlicensed Assistive Personnel (UAP)	Structure
Patient Falls[1,2]		Process & Outcome
Patient Falls with Injury[1,2]	a. Injury Level	Process & Outcome
Pediatric Pain Assessment, Intervention, Reassessment (AIR) Cycle		Process
Pediatric Peripheral Intravenous Infiltration Rate		Outcome
Pressure Ulcer Prevalence[1]	a. Community Acquired b. Hospital Acquired c. Unit Acquired	Process & Outcome
Psychiatric Physical/Sexual Assault Rate		Outcome
Restraint Prevalence[2]		Outcome
RN Education/Certification		Structure
RN Satisfaction Survey Options[1,3]	a. Job Satisfaction Scales b. Job Satisfaction Scales – Short Form c. Practice Environment Scale (PES)[2]	Process & Outcome
Skill Mix: Percent of total nursing hours supplied by[1,2]	a. RNs b. LPN/LVNs c. UAP d. % of total nursing hours supplied by Agency Staff	Structure
Voluntary Nurse Turnover[2]		Structure
Nurse Vacancy Rate		Structure

| Nosocomial Infections (Pending for 2007) a. Urinary catheter-associated urinary tract infection (UTI)[2] b. Central line catheter–associated blood stream infection (CABSI)[1,2] c. Ventilator-associated pneumonia (VAP)[2] | Outcome |

[1] Original ANA Nursing-Sensitive Indicator

[2] NQF Endorsed Nursing-Sensitive Indicator "NQF-15"

[3] The RN Survey is annual, whereas the other indicators are quarterly

Reproduced from Montalvo, I. (2007). The National Database of Nursing Quality Indicators® (NDNQI®). *Online Journal of Issues in Nursing, 12*(3), Manuscript 2. doi: 10.3912/OJIN.Vol12No03Man02. *Online Journal of Issues in Nursing* by American Nurses Association. Reproduced with permission of American Nurses Association.

The NQF is a not-for-profit membership organization created to develop and implement a national strategy for healthcare quality measurement and reporting (see **Table 9-3**). A shared sense of urgency about the impact of healthcare quality on patient outcomes, workforce productivity, and healthcare costs prompted leaders in the public and private sectors to create the NQF as a mechanism to bring about national change. NQF (2007) is leading an effort to understand more fully the extent to which nurses contribute to improved patient safety and healthcare outcomes and promote nursing care quality.

Nursing is the largest healthcare profession in the United States, with nurses serving as the principal caregivers in hospitals and other institutional care settings. Nursing time constitutes the single largest operational expense in any healthcare delivery system (see **Sidebar 9-9**). Therefore, considering nursing as an organized service and nurses as individual caregivers are critical to optimal healthcare system performance. The NQF (2007) has endorsed 15 nurse-sensitive measures through its formal Consensus Development Process. This was the first set of national standardized performance measures to assess the extent to which nurses in acute care hospitals contribute to client safety, healthcare quality, and a professional work environment. These consensus standards can be used by consumers to assess the quality of nursing care in hospitals, and they can be used by providers to identify opportunities for improvement of critical outcomes and processes of care. Furthermore, these standards are used by purchasers to create incentives and reward hospitals for better performance.

> **SIDEBAR 9-9**
> Nursing is the largest healthcare profession in the United States. Nursing constitutes the largest operational expense in any healthcare system.

TABLE 9-3 NQF 15 NATIONAL VOLUNTARY CONSENSUS STANDARDS FOR NURSING-SENSITIVE CARE

Category	Measure
Patient-Centered Outcome Measures	1. Death among surgical inpatients with treatable serious complications (failure to rescue) 2. Pressure ulcer prevalence 3. Fall prevalence 4. Falls with injury 5. Restraint prevalence (vest and limb only) 6. Urinary catheter-associated urinary tract infections for intensive care unit (ICU) patients 7. Central line catheter-associated bloodstream infection rate for ICU and high-risk nursery (HRN) 8. Ventilator-associated pneumonia for ICU and HRN
Nursing-Centered Intervention Measures	9. Smoking cessation counseling for acute myocardial infarction 10. Smoking cessation counseling for heart failure 11. Smoking cessation counseling for pneumonia
System-Centered Measures	12. Skill mix 13. Nursing care hours per patient day 14. Practice environment scale-nursing work index 15. Voluntary turnover

Reproduced from National Quality Forum. (2004). National voluntary consensus standards for nursing-sensitive care: An initial performance measurement set. A consensus report. Washington, DC: Author. Retrieved from http://www.qualityforum.org /Publications/2004/10/National_Voluntary_Consensus_Standards_for_Nursing-Sensitive_Care__An_Initial_Performance _Measure_Set.aspx. Copyright © 2004 National Quality Forum.

American Nursing Credentialing Center Magnet Recognition Program

KEY TERM

Magnet status: The Magnet Recognition Program, established by the American Nurses Credentialing Center in 1993, recognizes healthcare organizations that demonstrate excellence in nursing practice and adherence to national standards for the organization and delivery of nursing services.

Another measure of nursing performance is **Magnet status**. The Magnet designation is awarded by the American Nursing Credentialing Center (ANCC) Magnet Recognition Program (2008) to a healthcare organization that has demonstrated an environment of excellence for nursing practice and client care (see **Sidebar 9-10**). Research shows that Magnet hospitals have better client outcomes and a higher level of client and nurse satisfaction compared to non-Magnet hospitals. To achieve this status of excellence, a team of professionals with experience in quality indicators, nursing administration, and nursing care evaluates a hospital's nursing services, clinical outcomes, and client care delivery systems. **Table 9-4** provides examples of NQF consensus standards and measures with nursing-sensitive care.

There are 14 Forces of Magnetism™, originally identified more than 25 years ago, that must be achieved by an organization prior to becoming designated a magnet hospital. The ANCC developed the new Magnet Model based on five model components. The model provides a new perspective on the sources of evidence that demonstrates a work environment supportive of excellence in nursing practice (ANCC, 2008). Magnet recognition involves the entire hospital but the focus is on nursing care and nursing satisfaction. Refer to Chapter 6 for more information about the components of the Magnet Model and examples of nursing strategies to maintain excellent outcomes.

Cost and Performance

As healthcare costs continue to rise the government is exploring ways to reward those individuals and organizations that are consistent in having positive performance outcomes. **Pay-for-performance** strategies for achieving systemwide improvements in healthcare quality and patient safety have been introduced into the healthcare arena as a strategy to reward good performance outcomes. It promotes structured incentives

for practitioners and providers to achieve benchmarks of performance. The hope is that by offering positive rewards—both for reaching thresholds of performance and for making continuous strides in improving the quality of health care—high-quality health care will be delivered on a consistent basis. This approach acknowledges the reality that financial rewards are among the most powerful tools for bringing about behavior change.

The Patient Protection and Affordable Care Act of 2010 developed several Medicare programs intended to improve healthcare quality, using pay-for-performance payment strategies to put financial pressure on medical providers. In these programs, reimbursement is based on performance on measures related to care processes, patient satisfaction scores, and/or specified patient outcomes. The rationale behind pay-for-performance is the result of a real problem: Payment for medical services, particularly by the large government health programs, does not reflect value or benefit for patients.

However, pay-for-performance programs operate in a complex reimbursement environment that often creates barriers to reaching the goal of consistent, high-quality care for all patients. For example, payment systems frequently do not recognize the nuances of care delivery, nor do they always pay fairly for important aspects of care, such as activities that support patient education, continuity of care, or integration of services. Such policies and programs must be credible, minimize unintended

TABLE 9-4 EXAMPLES OF NQF CONSENSUS STANDARDS AND MEASURES WITH NURSING-SENSITIVE CARE

Measure	Examples of Nursing Care, Preventive Care, and Reporting
Examples of Patient-Centered Outcome Measures	
Pressure ulcer	• A thorough skin examination is performed by the RN upon admission. • All existing pressure ulcers are measured in size and documented. • Patient is placed on skin protocols. • Referral is made to a wound care specialist.
Falls	• Fall-risk assessments are completed at admission and monitored continuously. • Fall-risk patients are placed on fall precautions. • All falls are documented and reported to the primary provider. • Once a fall occurs, fall precautions are strictly adhered to prevent further falls.
Falls with injuries	• Documentation and reporting to the primary provider is done. • The fall is discussed with the patient's family members, as appropriate. • Quality team members review the incident to explore "lessons learned" and advise nurses on care strategies to prevent further falls.
Death of a surgical inpatient with a treatable serious complication (i.e., failure to rescue)	• The incident will be reviewed by a multidisciplinary quality team. • The following will be reviewed: failure to recognize symptoms of deterioration, time taken to report to the surgeon and emergency response team, time taken to respond to the complications, and how protocols were followed. • "Lessons learned" will be shared by the quality team with the physicians and nurses.
Examples of Nursing-Centered Intervention Measures	
Smoking cessation counseling for a patient who experienced a myocardial infarction	• On the admission assessment or at the earliest time the patient is stable, documentation of smoking history is completed by the RN. Data are recorded on number of years smoked, how many cigarettes smoked per day, and the number of times the patient has attempted to quit. • Nursing assessment includes asking the patient if they are contemplating, interested in, or desire to quit smoking. • Counseling strategies include exploring options for smoking cessation assistance programs such as professional organizations, group classes, medications to assist in cessation, and online resources. • Discharge planning should include discussing referral to cardiac rehab counseling where maintenance of smoking cessation support can occur.

Measure	Examples of Nursing Care, Preventive Care, and Reporting
Examples of System-Centered Measures	
Nursing unit-based skill mix of patient-care providers	• Each nursing unit or care area documents the number of nurse technicians/aides, licensed professional nurses, and RNs per shift and per patient.
Hours of nursing care provided per patient day	• This data is compared to standards and followed closely in relationship to deviation from standard benchmarks such as an increase in falls, pressure ulcers, and hospital-associated infections.

negative consequences, and most importantly, be transparent and attentive to ethical considerations. It is important to recognize as well that non-financial incentives can also drive positive behavior changes.

As pay-for-performance programs continue to develop, it will be important to determine the effectiveness of these programs in ensuring quality and cost-effective health care. The broad-scale implementation and success of these programs must coincide with the timely creation and deployment of an electronic health infrastructure that facilitates the collection, transmittal, and analyses of the performance data that will drive these programs. The design of these programs and ongoing efforts to evaluate their effectiveness should eventually provide the bases for understanding how best to use financial and other incentives to leverage continuous improvement in the safety and quality of health care (see **Sidebar 9-11**).

Alignment of payment program incentives to support the provision of safe, high-quality care is a complex undertaking, for it must simultaneously achieve fair reimbursement for necessary services, promote desired behavior change, and avoid unintended consequences. In the end, payment policies and programs must work to the advantage of the client and support the provision of client-centered care.

Quality of Care and Vulnerable Populations

The United States can be described as a country of diversity that includes different vulnerable populations including ethnic minority groups, low-income groups, frail elderly living with multiple chronic health conditions, and immigrants (see **Sidebar 9-12**). A wide range of disparities in education and

SIDEBAR 9-11
Further research is needed on pay-for-performance programs. The design of these programs and ongoing efforts to evaluate their effectiveness should eventually provide the bases for understanding how best to use financial and other incentives to leverage continuous improvement in the safety and quality of health care.

SIDEBAR 9-12
Vulnerable populations include the uninsured, the poor, the working poor who do not receive adequate health benefits, and the underinsured. Economic, social, and political issues of vulnerable populations need to be addressed in the healthcare system and delivery models. Vulnerable populations often receive little preventive care, resulting in them seeking care in a health crisis and experiencing poor outcomes.

income levels associated with vulnerable populations affect access to health care and opportunities for health-promotion activities. The changing ethnic composition of the United States creates a demand for a healthcare system that is more responsive to minorities and the needs of the vulnerable. Hispanics, Muslims, and Asians are among the minority ethnic and religious groups whose presence is noticeably increasing in the United States. There is a growing demand for healthcare providers who speak languages other than English and understand the health needs of a multiethnic society.

In the 21st century, ethnic minorities are estimated to make up 28.2 percent of the U.S. population, expected to climb to 37 percent by the year 2025 (U.S. Census Bureau, 2014). The economic, social, and political issues that result from these growing populations will affect these groups' access to health care and services that are affordable. Healthcare personnel, especially in nursing, also need to become more diversified to meet the health needs of the growing body of people with diverse ethnic backgrounds requiring care.

Vulnerable populations include the uninsured, the working poor who do not receive adequate health benefits, and the underinsured. Over one third of the U.S. public is uninsured or underinsured. These groups receive less than adequate health care, often receiving too little too late. Limited access to preventive care often results in crisis visits to emergency rooms and urgent care centers. The underserved often receive little primary prevention or continuity of care for chronic conditions. The underserved also often receive their health care from the public sector and through local, state, and federal funding. This places a great strain on healthcare services in communities, adding to the burden of disease costs.

The inequitable distribution of wealth is a contributing factor to the uneven distribution of health care. Many Americans living in poverty are the victims of social and environmental harms such as drug addiction, acquired immunodeficiency syndrome (AIDS), crime, and chronic illness. Infants born from mothers with substance disorders can also suffer from addiction and low birth weight with consequential mental and physical problems. The need for health services for vulnerable populations is strongly tied to the poor economic conditions of the communities in which they reside. All of these factors result in disparities in health outcomes for vulnerable populations as they often experience higher morbidity and mortality and worse quality of life than other groups with similar health conditions.

Summary

Nursing must become more transparent in the performance outcomes that are specific to nursing care and translated at the bedside to improved client outcomes. Measurement of outcomes profoundly affects healthcare delivery and reimbursement. The measurement of performance outcomes of nursing care through organizations such as NQF and ANCC's Magnet demonstrate the importance of public perspective of direct care. Both the state and federal government use data from organizations to compare individual practitioners and organizations on a variety of quality of care performance indicators.

As performance outcomes become more refined and there is more consensus in the methodology of the data collection, even more emphasis will be placed on these outcomes. Choice of healthcare providers will be based on the clinical performance outcomes. In the past there has been a strong emphasis on financial outcomes and while these outcomes continue to be a driving force in healthcare, more emphasis is now placed on safety and the clinical outcomes of clients. It is important to note that the financial and clinical outcomes are not mutually exclusive. More and more organizations are realizing better financial outcomes as the performance outcomes improve in patient care.

Reflective Practice Questions

1. Recollect a client you have cared for who experienced a myocardial infarction. How did the Core Quality Measures translate at the bedside for nursing care and overall healthcare toward better outcomes for this client?
2. Compare and contrast the different agencies that are driving the use of performance outcomes in health care.
3. How does having magnet status at a hospital affect client performance outcomes? How does magnet status affect the autonomy and satisfaction of nurses?
4. Do you agree or disagree with the concept of *pay-for-performance*? Give rationale to support your stand.

References

Agency for Healthcare Research and Quality. (2014). The outcome of outcomes research at AHCPR: Recommendations December 2014. Retrieved from http://www.ahrq.gov/research/findings/final-reports/outcomes-research/recommendations.html

Agency for Healthcare Research and Quality. (n.d.). Working for quality: Achieving better health and health care for all Americans. Retrieved from http://www.ahrq.gov/workingforquality/

American Nurses Association. (1995). *Nursings report card for acute care*. Washington, DC: American Nurses Publishing.

American Nurses Credentialing Center. (2008). Overview of ANCC Magnet Recognition Program®: New model. Retrieved from http://www.nursecredentialing.org/documents/magnet/newmodelbrochure.aspx

Centers for Medicare & Medicaid Services. (n.d.). Hospital compare. Retrieved from https://www.cms.gov/Medicare/Quality-Initiatives-Patient-Assessment-Instruments/HospitalQualityInits/HospitalCompare.html

Deming, W. E. (1993). *The new economics.* Cambridge, MA: MIT Press.

Donabedian, A. (1980). *Explorations in quality assessment and monitoring: Vol. 1. The definition of quality and approaches to its assessment.* Ann Arbor, MI: Health Administration Press.

Institute for Healthcare Improvement. (2016a). 5 Million Lives Campaign overview. Retrieved from http://www.ihi.org/Engage/Initiatives/Completed/5MillionLivesCampaign/Pages/default.aspx

Institute for Healthcare Improvement. (2016b). About us. Retrieved from http://www.ihi.org/about/Pages/default.aspx

Institute of Medicine. (2000). *To err is human: Building a safer health system.* Washington, DC: National Academy Press.

Institute of Medicine. (2001). *Crossing the quality chasm: A new health system for the 21st century.* Washington, DC: National Academy Press.

Kronick, R. (2014). Patient safety: The Agency for Healthcare Research and Quality's ongoing commitment. *Journal of Nursing Care Quality, 29*(3), 195–199.

Lohr, K. (Ed.). (1990). *Medicare: A strategy for quality assurance* (Vol. 1). Washington, DC: National Academy Press.

Makary, M., & Daniel, M. (2016, May 3). Medical error—the third leading cause of death in the U.S. *BMJ, 353.* doi: 10.1136/bmj.i2139.

McCannon, C., Hackbarth, A., & Griffin, F. (2007). Miles to go: an introduction to the 5 Million Lives Campaign. *Joint Commission Journal on Quality and Patient Safety, 33*(8), 477–484.

Montalvo, I. (2007). The National Database of Nursing Quality Indicators® (NDNQI®). *Online Journal of Issues in Nursing, 12*(3), Manuscript 2. doi: 10.3912/OJIN.Vol12No03Man02

National Quality Forum. (2004). National voluntary consensus standards for nursing-sensitive care: An initial performance measurement set. A consensus report. Washington, DC: Author. Retrieved from http://www.qualityforum.org/Publications/2004/10/National_Voluntary_Consensus_Standards_for_Nursing-Sensitive_Care__An_Initial_Performance_Measure_Set.aspx

National Quality Forum. (2007). Tracking NQF-endorsed consensus standards for nursing-sensitive care. Retrieved from http://www.qualityforum.org/Publications/2007/07/Tracking_NQF-Endorsed%C2%AE_Consensus_Standards_for_Nursing-Sensitive_Care__A_15-Month_Study.aspx

Quality Improvement Organizations. (2014). *Raising the bar: IPRO's Medicare quality improvement report for New York state (2011–2014).* Retrieved from http://ipro.org/wp-content/uploads/2014/08/QIO_Report_2014_07_24_v1.pdf

The Joint Commission. (n.d.). The Joint Commission Quality Check®. Retrieved from http://www.qualitycheck.org/qualityreport.aspx?hcoid=479835

U.S. Census Bureau. (2014). U.S. Census Bureau national characteristics. Retrieved from http://www.census.gov/popest/data/national/asrh/2014/

Evidence-Based Nursing Practice

Susan Sheriff and Gayle Roux

LEARNING OUTCOMES

After reading this chapter you will be able to:

- Describe evidence-based healthcare, evidence-based practice (EBP), and evidence-based nursing (EBN).
- Understand the components and benefits of EBP.
- Discuss the process and key steps of EBP.
- Describe the principles of evidence to guide clinical practice in EBN.
- Describe the levels of evidence and critically appraise research findings.
- Understand the process of application of research in practice.
- Use specific clinical examples to apply research evidence.

Introduction

The purpose of this chapter is to explore the background, history, process, and applications of **evidence-based practice (EBP)**. Examples of data sources for EBP in contemporary practice are included. The role of the nurse in applying research findings to practice is examined, and implications for nursing

---

The editors wish to acknowledge the contributions of Mary Reid Nichols and Nena R. Harris to the previous edition of this chapter.

Evidence–based practice (EBP):
The process of problem solving using the best research evidence in clinical decision making for patient care. It is a combination of a systematic search for and critical appraisal of the most relevant research available to answer a specific clinical question, with the clinician's own clinical expertise and patient values and preferences included (Melnyk & Fineout-Overholt, 2015).

education, research, and practice are also addressed. EBP is foundational for excellent clinical practice, the development of guidelines, and making decisions about diagnostic testing and changes in treatments or procedures (Melnyk, Fineout-Overholt, Gallagher-Ford, & Kaplan, 2012). EBP begins with a clinical question (e.g., "What is the best way to reduce the severity of neonatal lung disease? In men and women admitted to the intensive care unit, do earplugs or headphones improve self-perceived quality of sleep?"). EBP changes practice by the identification and evaluation of the best research available to answer the question (e.g., "Prenatal steroids reduce the severity of neonatal lung disease. Headphones improve self-perceived quality of sleep in men and women in the intensive care unit." Higgins & Green, 2011).

Despite sufficient data linking EBP with improved clinical outcomes, many clinicians have yet to adopt these principles into their practice. Research supports that EBP promotes improved health care and better health outcomes, but it is not the standard of care that is consistently practiced by healthcare workers in the United States (Melnyk & Fineout-Overholt, 2015). Nurses need to be continually asking themselves, "How do I know what specific evidence will benefit patient care?"

What Are Evidence-Based Health Care, Evidence-Based Practice, and Evidence-Based Nursing?

Evidence-based health care, conducted with caring and with an awareness of the patient and family's preferences and values, helps nurses and other healthcare providers to make better clinical decisions that ensure optimal patient outcomes (Melnyk et al., 2012). The goal of evidence-based health delivery of care is high-quality care with cost restraint. *Evidence-based practice* is a problem-solving approach to clinical care that incorporates the diligent use of current best evidence from well-designed studies and clinical expertise. The types of evidence used to inform practice changes can be scientific research or systematic reviews, and they can also include nonresearch evidence such as accrediting agency requirements and quality improvement projects. *Evidence-based nursing* is the clinical decision-making process by nurses that is a combination and integration of the best research evidence.

Melnyk and Fineout-Overholt (2015) reported EBP is based on clinical decision making that includes the patient's clinical state, the specific clinical setting, and the patient's circumstances. EBP is a lifelong problem-solving approach to the delivery of health care that integrates the best evidence from well-designed studies and integrates it with a patient's preferences and values and a clinician's expertise (Melnyk & Fineout-Overholt, 2015). Research findings indicate that the implementation of EBP leads to better patient care, improved clinical outcomes, decreased health care costs, and assists policy-making organizations in attaining high safety and reliability (Melnyk et al., 2012). Each clinician is required to solve clinical problems, and the goal is that research evidence will be used to guide clinical practice. Evidence can be derived from published research findings or clinicians can personally conduct research. For the clinician, conducting research may involve conducting a small clinical study to develop clinical protocols or it could mean assisting with larger clinical trials that test the efficacy of a clinical protocol on a large number of patients. Research evidence is the basis for implementing change in nursing practice, which also correlates with the nursing process. Winters and Echeverri (2012) described steps nurses can use to change nursing practice using research by starting with a clinical question, searching for evidence, and translating the evidence to the bedside.

EBP refers to clinical decisions based on the best research evidence, such as that found in a **randomized controlled trial (RCT)**, and is considered to be foundational evidence for best practice; however, EBP also includes clinical expertise and patient values (Makic, Rauen, Jones, & Fisk, 2015). EBP uses a hierarchy of evidence (from 1 = highest level of evidence to 5 = lowest level of evidence) to guide decision making; this hierarchy is discussed later in this chapter. Brown and Ecoff (2011) indicated

> **KEY TERM**
>
> **Randomized controlled trial (RCT):** Experimental research that is the strongest design to support a cause and effect relationship. Subjects are randomly assigned to a treatment group or a control group.

that the newest developments in EBP updates and continuing education are based on the results of the latest RCTs where significant statistical results from research findings are the basis for practice guidelines.

EBP, supported empirically by RCTs, is best used to answer what specific treatment will work best for a specific condition. An example of EBP is the well-known and ground-breaking zidovudine (AZT) efficacy and safety clinical trial during which it was found that all human immunodeficiency virus (HIV)-infected pregnant women who received AZT during pregnancy did not transmit HIV to their fetus (Stevens & Lyall, 2014). Melnyk and Fineout-Overholt (2015) have identified four essential components of EBP that are foundational to evidence-based clinical decision making (see **Box 10-1**).

Every day, nurses are required to make clinical judgments about patient care interventions. During the process of delivering patient care, nurses must rely on EBPs from appropriate medication administration to best practices for discharged patients. If the hospital supports EBPs, there must be a culture that provides nurses answers while delivering patient care. Nurses cite a lack of time

BOX 10-1   COMPONENTS OF EVIDENCE-BASED PRACTICE

- Research evidence, evidence-based theories, expert opinions
- Evidence obtained from patient assessment, physical exam, availability of resources
- Clinical expertise and experience
- Patient preferences and values

Data from Melnyk, B. M., & Fineout-Overholt, E. (2015). *Evidence-based practice in nursing and healthcare: A guide to best practice* (3rd ed.). Philadelphia, PA: Lippincott.

and limited resources as major barriers to accomplishing this task. Resources must be provided that nurses can readily access for decision making and appropriate nursing interventions. Nurse clinicians need to understand, use, and apply the concept of EBP in order to provide excellent patient care. Excellent patient care is based on research evidence and can be used to create clinical guidelines to standardize patient care (Melnyk & Fineout-Overholt, 2015). In addition, nurses need to obtain and keep current with the most up-to-date information about new research findings and to maintain professional competence. EBP is becoming more evident in clinical practice and in clinical education (Balshem et al., 2011; Krugman, 2011; Linton & Prasun, 2013). With the increased emphasis on EBP, contemporary nursing education now focuses on an exploration of evidence from RCTs as well as from other naturalistic studies where concepts are explored in the context of clinical management of patients (Taylor, 2011). Nurse clinicians at the bedside are in an excellent position to contribute to nursing knowledge and improve patient care by identifying clinical problems, collecting data for nursing research studies, and then applying research findings in the clinical care setting (Keough, Stevenson, Martinovich, Young, & Tanabe, 2011).

As a result of methodologically rigorous review of the best evidence on a specific topic, evidence-based clinical practice guidelines have been developed to guide clinical practice. This has improved quality of care, provided a more streamlined patient care process, and improved patient outcomes (Melnyk & Fineout-Overholt, 2015). For example, Cochrane used the findings from thousands of low-birth-weight and preterm infants that resulted in infant mortality as an exemplar for EBP. Based on supporting evidence from RCTs, it was concluded by the meta-analysis that prenatal steroids reduce the severity of neonatal lung disease in high-risk women and reduce preterm infant mortality from 50 percent to 30 percent (Gupta, Prasanth, Chen, & Yeh, 2012). The clinical application of EBP has five benefits (see **Box 10-2**).

BOX 10-2   BENEFITS OF EVIDENCE-BASED PRACTICE

1. Foundation for practice guidelines, diagnostic testing, and changes in treatments or procedures
2. Eliminates unnecessary treatment or procedures
3. Evaluates research findings to find treatments or procedures that are effective and/or are cost effective
4. Helps to standardize care
5. Assists with evaluating clinical outcomes

History and Background of Evidence-Based Practice

Florence Nightingale (1859/1957) is acknowledged as the first nursing researcher as she applied evidence to practice in the 19th century. *Notes on Nursing*, originally published in 1859, was an early version of EBP. Nightingale's method was to rigorously monitor all nursing care for the effectiveness of patient outcomes. From the mid-19th century until the mid-20th century, however, clinical decisions were primarily based on expert opinion and clinical experience. In the 1960s, a British epidemiologist, Dr. Archie Cochrane, was responsible for introducing the notion of EBP, asserting that effective patient care required empirically based interventions. Beginning in 1972, Cochrane's publications were critical of the medical profession because there were few **systematic reviews** of evidence for making healthcare policy and clinical patient care decisions (Enkin, 2012). Cochrane believed that only RCTs were sufficient evidence for making medical decisions (Higgins & Green, 2011). Until his death in 1988, Cochrane was a staunch advocate for EBP and as a result had a profound influence on how modern patient care and healthcare policy decisions are made.

> **KEY TERM**
>
> **Systematic reviews:** Summaries of evidence obtained by researchers on a specific topic or clinical problem. They use a rigorous step-by-step process to identify, synthesize, and evaluate research studies to answer a specific clinical question and to make conclusions about best evidence.

The Process of Evidence-Based Practice

Melnyk and Fineout-Overholt (2015) identified five key steps of EBP. A systematic step-by-step approach can be used to examine the "burning clinical question" and follow the evidence to make a clinical decision and evaluate the change.

The following section provides an example of using the PICOT steps (see **Box 10-3**) with the clinical question regarding best practices to prevent unplanned pregnancies in adolescent women. PICOT stands for population, intervention, comparison

---

BOX 10–3 PICOT FORMAT

P Patient population (i.e., adolescent women)
I Intervention of interest. (i.e., abstinence education or oral contraceptives)
C Comparison intervention (i.e., abstinence or oral contraceptives)
O Outcome (i.e., pregnancy prevention)
T Time. (i.e., to determine which intervention can reduce adolescent pregnancy)

Data from Melnyk, B. M., & Fineout-Overholt, E. (2015). *Evidence-based practice in nursing and healthcare: A guide to best practice* (3rd ed.). Philadelphia, PA: Lippincott.

---

intervention, outcome, and time (Echevarria & Walker, 2014). The PICOT format is used to answer the following questions:

1. Who are the patients, clients, or individuals of a particular age, gender, community, or group (e.g., adolescent women)?
2. What interventions have answered the specific clinical question (e.g., abstinence education)?
3. Is there a comparison with another intervention (e.g., oral contraceptives)?
4. What are the consequences of the intervention (e.g., pregnancy prevention)?
5. How much time does it take to demonstrate the clinical outcomes?

The search for best evidence (Guyatt et al., 2011) is achieved by conducting systematic reviews or meta-analyses on empirical evidence (see **Contemporary Practice Highlight 10-1**). The evidence is evaluated by the type of evidence and ranges from highest (level 1 evidence) to lowest (level 7 evidence). The seven levels of evidence known as the rating system for the hierarchy of evidence is shown in **Box 10-4**.

KEY TERM

Evidence-based nursing (EBN):
Clinical decision making by nurses that is a combination and integration of the best research evidence; it also includes the nurse's clinical expertise and patient values and preferences about a specific type of care.

Evidence-Based Nursing

Evidence-based nursing (EBN) is at the core of the knowledge base for professional nursing practice. EBN uses EBP to make clinical decisions and improve nursing practice. EBN encompasses a broader approach than EBP. EBN is more than research utilization; it includes EBN skills needed for clinical decisions grounded in evidence. These skills are listed in **Box 10-5**.

EBN, based on the nursing model of decision making and clinical judgment, is central to the knowledge base for nursing practice. Nursing decisions are often based on the effectiveness of nursing interventions that can sometimes, but not always, be evaluated only by RCTs (Fawcett, 2012). The nursing practice model is based on empirical evidence and the evaluation of clinical practice and its effects on the patient

CLINICAL ISSUES AND EVIDENCE-BASED PRACTICE QUESTIONS

Marciano, Merlin, Bessen, and Street (2014) report that 20 percent of healthcare practices are not evidenced-based. This is an alarming percentage of healthcare practices that are not based on evidence, but rather tradition and ritual. The following examples highlight contemporary nursing practices and the current research findings on these topics.

NASOGASTIC TUBE PLACEMENT

Issues
- Gastric feeding is the most preferred route of tube feeding, but correct placement of nasogastric (NG) tubes is critical for patient safety.
- Improper placement of NG tubes used for feeding may lead to serious complications including aspiration pneumonia or even death of the patient.

Examples of Clinical Questions
- What are the best methods for measuring the tube length to result in proper placement of the NG tube?
- What is the most frequently used method to measure correct length of the NG tube?
- What is the evidence for previous methods which have traditionally been used for placement of NG tubes in adults?
- Can the best external anatomical landmarks for positioning NG tubes in adults be determined?

Research Evidence
- The nose-to-ear-to-xiphisternum method should no longer be taught in nursing programs or used in practice (de Oliveira Santos, Woith, de Freitas, & Zeferino, 2016).

WOUND CARE

Issues
- Evidence for the best cleaning agents for acute or chronic wounds
- Effectiveness of normal saline versus other solutions for wound cleaning

Examples of Clinical Questions
- When cleansing wounds, can the cleansing agents be cytotoxic to tissues and cause destruction of healthy cells?
- Is tap water as effective as other cleansing agents for wound cleansing?
- Is there any evidence that tap water to cleanse acute wounds in adults increases or reduces infection?
- Can antiseptic solutions hinder the healing process of wounds?

Research Evidence
- The use of tap water to cleanse acute wounds in adults was not associated with a statistically significant difference in infection when compared to saline. Antiseptic solutions can impede the healing process (Moscati, Mayrose, Reardon, Janicke, & Jehle, 2007).

(continues)

CONTEMPORARY PRACTICE HIGHLIGHT 10-1 (*continued*)

PRACTICE GUIDELINES

It is important for nurses to utilize extensive resources and be committed to life-long learning to ensure practice procedures are based on evidence. Various ways to keep current include joining journal clubs, participating in webinars and professional meetings, forming liaisons with librarians who will assist in literature reviews, and ensuring the policies used in your agency are documented with the latest research evidence. Consider joining the policy and procedure committee at your agency to establish and update evidence-based procedures. Formulating interprofessional committees is effective in bringing varied scientific fields together to review the best evidence for practice guidelines.

BOX 10-4   RATING SYSTEM FOR HIERARCHY OF EVIDENCE

Level 1 evidence: Systematic review or meta-analysis of all RCTs, or EBP
Level 2 evidence: Obtained from at least one well-designed RCT
Level 3 evidence: Obtained from a well-designed **controlled trial** without randomization
Level 4 evidence: Obtained from well-designed case-control and cohort studies without randomization
Level 5 evidence: Obtained from systematic reviews of descriptive and qualitative studies
Level 6 evidence: Obtained from a single descriptive or qualitative study
Level 7 evidence: Obtained from the opinion of authorities and/or reports of expert committees

Data from Harris, R. P., Helfand, M., Woolf, S. H., Lohr, K. N., Mulrow, C. D., Teutsch, S. M., & Atkins, D. (2001). Current methods of the U.S. Preventative Services Task Force: A review of the methods. *American Journal of Preventive Services, 20*(Suppl. 3), 21–35; Guyatt, G., Oxman, A. D., Akl, E. A., Kunz, R., Vist, G., Brozek, J., . . . Schünemann, H. J. (2011). GRADE guidelines: 1. Introduction—GRADE evidence profiles and summary of findings tables. *Journal of Clinical Epidemiology, 64*(4), 383–394. doi:10.1016/j.jclinepi.2010.04.026

BOX 10-5   EVIDENCE-BASED NURSING SKILLS

1. Define the patient problem.
2. Determine the information needed by searching the literature.
3. Select the best evidence.
4. Categorize the evidence.
5. Synthesize clinical application.
6. Determine the balance between advantages and disadvantages.
7. Implement and evaluate clinical decision based on patient values.

or client. The best evidence in nursing incorporates relevant clinical research and also focuses on the safety, effectiveness, and cost-effectiveness of nursing interventions. EBN also takes into consideration available resources, accurate ways to measure nursing interventions, the strength of cause-and-effect relationships, and the perceived meaning of the patient's experiences (Brown, 2014). EBN follows the principles of EBP and includes the four elements of evidence-based decision making for nursing care: best research evidence, clinical expertise, patient preferences in their specific situation, and available resources for nursing assessment and interventions (Brown, 2014). EBN additionally considers ethical and cultural aspects, psychosocial issues, and family considerations in clinical care decisions (Fawcett, 2012). During the late 1970s, research utilization was found in much of the nursing literature. Melnyk and Fineout-Overholt (2015) described research utilization as using "research findings in all aspects of one's work as a registered nurse" (p. 19). Thus, EBN is the clinical decision making by nurses that is a culmination of the best practice evidence.

> **KEY TERM**
> **Controlled trial:** Research in which there is a treatment group and a group that does not receive the treatment (control group) so that comparisons can be made about the effectiveness of an intervention on a specific health issue and health outcome.

The following example helps clarify the differences between EBP and EBN. Several RCTs may offer evidence that use of tap water for wound cleansing is as effective as using normal saline (Fernandez & Griffiths, 2012). EBP would take account of the evidence that the use of tap water to cleanse acute wounds reduces infection and that several randomized controlled studies concluded that there was no difference in the infection and healing rates in wounds cleansed with tap water compared with other solutions (Fernandez & Griffiths, 2012). However, EBN will also take into consideration the impact of this intervention on each individual, the family caregivers (e.g., Is using tap water uncomfortable compared to normal saline in wound cleansing?), and economics both in the hospital and at home (e.g., Which method of wound cleansing is more cost effective?) and evaluate the effectiveness and patient acceptance of the treatment as well as outcomes associated with quality of life (similar outcomes as far as wound healing and infection rates). In summary, EBP uses RCTs to decide the effectiveness of a treatment, whereas EBN applies the evidence to establish clinical practice guidelines that help to standardize patient care leading to optimal, cost-effective patient care (Melnyk & Fineout-Overholt, 2015).

As interprofessional research teams are formed, a spirit of questioning of current practice and how to improve patient outcomes in the healthcare setting is generated. EBN helps nurses ask important clinical questions, differentiate between strong and weak research evidence, clearly understand research study results, sort out the risks and benefits of clinical management options, and apply specific evidence to individual patients to improve clinical outcomes (Brown, 2014). As stated earlier, the strongest research evidence comes from the systematic reviews and **meta-analyses** of RCTs.

> **KEY TERM**
> **Meta-analyses:** The summarizations of the results of several quantitative studies critically reviewed, synthesized, and evaluated to answer a specific clinical question about the effectiveness of an intervention across multiple studies in different settings.

Descriptive studies: Research conducted in order to describe characteristics of selected variables or a certain phenomenon.

Qualitative studies: Descriptive research in which variables are not quantified numerically to describe a phenomenon of interest. Qualitative research is used to examine subjective human experience by using non-statistical methods of analysis (Borbasi & Jackson, 2012). It is associated with naturalistic inquiry, which explores the complex experience of human beings.

The outcomes of the evidence-based research should be disseminated and incorporated into practice. When RCTs are not available, evidence from nonrandomized **descriptive studies** and **qualitative studies** as well as expert opinions and evidence-based theories may guide clinical decisions (Melnyk & Fineout-Overholt, 2015).

Applying Research Findings to Practice

Published models can be applied to improve clinical decision making. In order for nurses to operate in an evidence-based manner, they need to be aware of how to introduce, develop, and evaluate EBP. The Iowa model offers practical advice for nurses in practice. The Iowa model focuses on an organized process for use of research, along with other types of evidence, for nursing practice. Since its origin in 1994, it has been continually referenced in nursing journal articles and extensively used in clinical research programs (Doody & Doody, 2011). This model allows nurses to focus on knowledge and problem-focused triggers, leading staff to question current practice. The Iowa model initiates with forming a team that includes all interested stakeholders. The process of changing a specific area of practice is conducted by specialist staff team members who can provide input and support and discuss the practicality of the proposed change. Evidence is retrieved through electronic databases such as CINAHL, Medline, Cochrane, and National Institute for Health and Clinical Excellence, using key terms. To grade the evidence, the team will address quality areas of the individual research and the strength of the body of evidence overall. After a review of the literature, the team members set recommendations for practice. The type and strength of evidence used in practice needs to be clear and based on the consistency of replicated studies. For the Iowa model to be effective, clinical agencies need social and organizational support and value placed on the integration of evidence into practice and the application of research findings. This can be achieved through in-service education, audit, and feedback provided by team members. Evaluation should be carried out at different periods during and following the intervention. Evaluation is critical to determine if the outcomes identified in the research actually occur in practice.

Also, in addition to the levels of research evidence discussed earlier, evidence is evaluated by the quality of the study—good, fair, or poor—and the net benefit to the patient—substantial, moderate, small, or negative. Recommendations for application of research findings and guidelines are based on the U.S. Preventive Services Task Force's list of the strength of recommendations (see **Contemporary Practice Highlight 10-2**).

CONTEMPORARY PRACTICE HIGHLIGHT 10-2

EXAMPLES OF LEVEL 1 EVIDENCE: LIKELY RELIABLE EVIDENCE

The research studies described here provide examples of Level 1 evidence based on the analysis and evaluation of the studies. Review the study examples and answer the following questions in your practice:

- Based on this level of evidence, how might you change your practice for each of these studies?
- How would you implement this information in education programs for community members with asthma?
- What type of education and suicide assessment should be used for a patient with depression who has been on selective serotonin reuptake inhibitors (SSRIs) for 1 week?
  - *Research studies:* Anticholinergics reduce asthma-related hospital admission (Rodrigo & Castro-Rodriguez, 2005). This was based on 32 RCTs that included 3,611

patients and 10 trials that included 1,786 children and adolescents.
- *The practice implications:* Multiple doses of inhaled ipratropium (an anticholinergic) compared to beta2-agonists may reduce the rate of hospital admissions in adults and children with moderate to severe asthma.
- *Research studies:* SSRIs have onset efficacy for depression as early as 1 to 6 weeks (Taylor, Freemantle, Geddes, & Bhagwagar, 2006). Based on 28 RCTs with a total of 5,872 patients.
- *The practice implications:* There is no significant advantage of SSRIs at 1 week; however, after 2–6 weeks, there was a 79 percent increased chance of remission of depression among those receiving an SSRI compared with those receiving placebo.

Clinical Application Examples

The scientific literature for nursing as well as other health disciplines has dramatically increased the current body of knowledge in the last few years. The state of the science can be examined in the literature and reviewed for the level of evidence for clinical application. The following are a few key examples in various nursing specialty fields where evidence is substantiating a change in the way nurses practice. Clarke (2014) found that skin-to-skin contact between mother and baby at birth reduces crying, improves mother–baby interaction, keeps baby warmer, and helps women breastfeed successfully. This may be characterized as Level 2 evidence (likely effective) and was based on the analysis of 1,925 mother–baby pairs in at least two clinical trials with more benefits demonstrated than adverse effects. This intervention would be *strongly recommended* because there is good evidence of improved health outcomes and the benefits outweigh harm.

Erhardt, Rice, Troszak, and Zhu (2016) and Lee et al. (2012) found that the use of helmets resulted in a 63–88 percent reduction in head and facial injuries in bicyclists of all ages involved in all types of crashes including those involved with motor vehicles. Although the conclusions were based on five well-conducted **case-control studies**, not RCTs, this evidence supports the consideration to *strongly recommend* (good evidence of improved health outcomes, benefits outweigh harm) the application of research findings to clinical practice through safety education on helmet use for individuals and communities.

Lee et al. (2012) assessed interventions designed to prevent the incidence of falls in elderly people (either living in the community or in institutional or hospital care). Based on 21,668 subjects, the authors concluded that interventions to prevent falls are likely to be effective and are now available; however, less is known about their effectiveness in preventing fall-related injuries from clinical trials. This would likely be a *recommended* intervention (fair evidence of improved health outcomes, benefits outweigh harm).

From Clinical Questions to Evidence

Gallin and Ognibene (2012) noted that clinical questions provide the basis for research, and research provides a way to evaluate the effectiveness and safety of clinical practice. Research starts with a clinical question about a clinical problem from everyday clinical practice, patient care practices, interventions, and cost-effective high-quality care (see **Contemporary Practice Highlight 10-3**). Additionally, social issues can influence research questions based on gender, race, poverty, and healthcare disparities. These research questions translate into research aims or purposes for a research study with two primary criteria: clinical significance and a gap in current knowledge (National Institutes of Health, www.nih.gov). Priorities for funding in nursing research can be found within the National Institute of Nursing Research (NINR) pathways, and health promotion and disease prevention objectives in *Healthy People 2020* (U.S. Department of Health and Human Services, n.d.).

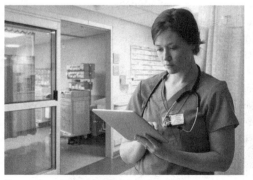

Nurse using a tablet to collect and store data.
© Blend Images - Jose Luis Pelaez Inc/Brand X Pictures/Getty

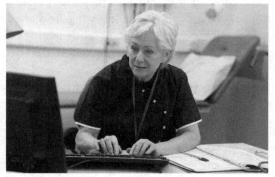

Nurse using technology to conduct research.
© Monkey Business Images/Shutterstock

> ### CONTEMPORARY PRACTICE HIGHLIGHT 10-3
>
> #### CLINICAL QUESTIONS IN WOMEN'S HEALTH
>
> Lowdermilk (2012) listed recent systematic reviews from the Cochrane Database and included various topical issues in women's health as examples of researchable clinical questions. These questions included evidence-based care for topics including, but not limited to, feeding schedules for preterm infants, self-management interventions for women with eating disorders, and effectiveness of screening for intimate partner (Lowdermilk, 2012). Women's health questions are critical for nursing science as women have not been as well represented as men in research.
>
> Reflect on various clinical situations you experienced in your childbearing and family clinical courses. Select several questions and consider the following:
>
> - Did you observe or participate in various practices that you thought might be based on tradition rather than evidence?
> - Do you have a passion for this clinical issue that would continually motivate you?
> - How would you establish what is already known on this clinical question?
> - Is this clinical question consistent with the research priorities of the NINR?
> - How would you motivate other nurses, physicians, and interprofessional colleagues to become involved on your research team on the investigation of this clinical question?
> - What would it cost to investigate this clinical question?
> - What is the involvement level from the patients and families that you consider is important in order to obtain their experiences on the clinical question?

Implications for Education, Research, and Practice

The goal for nursing science and nursing knowledge is that EBP become part of the professional culture of nursing through education, research, and practice. Translational research focuses on translating or applying the research findings from basic/preclinical studies to human studies and treatment trials. Translation of research findings to the patient and community so that evidence is adopted to improve health outcomes is the end goal of research. The translational research movement is about 2 decades old in the United States. The term "bench to bedside" captures the practical mindedness of research and the value placed on deliverables leading to improved assessment, treatment, and prevention. Translation science emphasizes bridging research findings from the bench to the bedside. A further challenge in addition to translation of findings to the bedside is the need to move from emphasizing disciplinary-focused research to tackling research and "burning clinical questions" with an interprofessional team approach.

Nursing Education

Informatics is a required skill in nursing education for professional access to well-designed research. Information literacy is an essential component of EBP because it enhances the nurse's ability to use the best available research literature to ensure optimal patient outcomes. Undergraduate nursing education programs continue to implement improved course outcomes that will focus on incorporating research evidence to guide clinical practice (Niven, Roy, Schaefer, Gasquoine, & Ward, 2013). Memorization of rote facts needs to be replaced with teaching the critical thinking skills required for contemporary clinical situations because evidence-based teaching prepares clinicians for EBN (Oja, 2011). Students and new graduates need to have high-level thinking capabilities to ensure patient safety and high-quality patient care (Oja, 2011).

Focusing on advanced degrees in nursing is key to preparing nurses for research and leadership in clinical practice. Nurses with advanced degrees (master of science in nursing [MSN], doctor of nursing practice [DNP], and doctor of philosophy in nursing [PhD]) will be better prepared to influence patients, other nurses, and interprofessional team members, and the healthcare system. Advanced practice registered nurses (APRNs) are also in a position to help in the design and implementation of clinical nursing research that provides the basis for the development of evidence-based clinical practice guidelines and protocols. Gerrish et al. (2011) contends that APRNs can facilitate EBP as a solution to bridge the gaps among education, research, and practice. Continuing education programs for practicing clinicians also will increasingly be focused on EBP and EBN, which optimally will guide professional practice.

Nursing Research

Currey, Considine, and Khaw (2011) urged all nurses to be involved in research, either as consumers of research or as participants involved in the research process itself. Clinicians at the bedside are well positioned to contribute to the nursing profession's body of knowledge and enhance nursing care by identifying nursing clinical questions worthy of research, being involved in data collection for nursing studies, and applying research findings to clinical care. Nurse scientists, APRNs, and nurse clinicians need to work collaboratively to develop, implement, and evaluate carefully designed clinical research (Currey et al., 2011). Increasing knowledge and skills associated with the EBP process provides nurse clinicians with the tools required to maintain ownership of their practices and help to transform health care.

Nursing Practice

Melnyk, Gallagher-Ford, & Fineout-Overholt (2014) described the application of clinical practice guidelines (CPGs) as being an additional expected outcome of EBP.

CPGs or **clinical care protocols** reflect the most up-to-date practice based on evidence and knowledge; the goal is to have the latest scientific knowledge available to clinicians (Gerrish et al., 2011). Although there is a plethora of research demonstrating well-designed clinical intervention research, few research findings are effectively implemented in the clinical setting (Gallin & Ognibene, 2012).

Health care is reported to be in crisis and in need of change (Institute of Medicine [IOM], 2001). The report emphasized that a fundamental change in the current healthcare system is needed to close the gap between practice and patient care quality. The IOM recommended a redesign of the healthcare system that includes policymakers, healthcare leaders, clinicians, regulators, and informed consumers working in collaborative teams. Implementation of EBP in teams and strengthening clinical information systems is needed to improve the overall quality of health care (Spruce, Van Wicklin, Hicks, Conner, & Dunn, 2014). Better clinical decisions and improved patient outcomes can be realized by health care that is evidence-based and provided in a caring context. Additionally, Fineout-Overholt, Melnyk, and Shultz (2011) stressed that the key elements of a best practice culture are EBP mentors, partnerships between academic and clinical settings, well-designed research and resources, and administrative support, all of which will foster the acceleration and adoption of EBP in education and clinical settings.

> **KEY TERM**
>
> **Clinical care protocols:** Clinical practice guidelines (CPGs) that reflect the most up-to-date practice based on evidence for reference and knowledge with the goal of having the latest scientific knowledge available to clinicians to make decisions about care. Elements include systematic literature review and the consensus of expert decision makers and consumers who consider the evidence and make recommendations.

Summary

This chapter has explored EBP and EBN including the background, key steps, components, and benefits. Additionally, this chapter described methods of incorporating EBP into clinical decision making. Information was provided on the application of EBP in clinical practice and how to access and evaluate appropriate clinically relevant research literature. Nurses must be proficient in skills on how to access resources for a literature search and to evaluate research-based evidence. Information was highlighted on how to understand the levels of evidence and how to evaluate the effects of interventions on patient outcomes.

Nursing students, clinicians, interprofessional team members, agency personnel, and faculty can lead practice innovations supported by EBP. As professional nurses navigate through the clinical practice arena, each clinical decision will be based not only on the best research evidence available but also on professional experience and the client or patient values and preferences. The goal of using evidence to guide nursing practice must be based on the realization that there can be a significant improvement in healthcare outcomes when EBN care is used (Currey et al., 2011; Fineout-Overholt et al., 2011). It is critical that nurses continually question what they do and remember that EBN can improve patient safety, quality, cost, and the effectiveness of health care.

Reflective Practice Questions

1. Using a model such as the Iowa model, how can a nurse make EBP more focused and acceptable to other nurses and interprofessional clinicians to successfully integrate research findings into practice?
2. How does the nursing clinician use research evidence in clinical practice in specific specialty areas?
3. How can you align support and resources for EBP from the clinical agency where you work?
4. What types of professional organizations could you join that would be a resource for EBP strategies where you work?

References

Balshem, H., Helfand, M., Schünemann, H. J., Oxman, A. D., Kunz, R., Brozek, J., & Guyatt, G. H. (2011). GRADE guidelines: 3. rating the quality of evidence. *Journal of Clinical Epidemiology, 64*(4), 401–406. doi: 10.1016/j.jclinepi.2010.07.015

Borbasi, S., & Jackson, D. (2012). *Navigating the maze of research.* Chatswood, Sydney, Australia: Mosby Elsevier.

Brown, C., & Ecoff, L. (2011). A systematic approach to the inclusion of evidence in healthcare design. *Health Environments Research & Design Journal, 4*(2), 7–16.

Brown, S. J. (2014*). Evidence-based nursing: The research-practice connection* (3rd ed.). Burlington, MA: Jones & Bartlett Learning.

Clarke, J. (2014). The first embrace: Skin-to- skin contact between mother and baby just after birth has immense benefits, argues Jenny Clarke (reflections). *Nursing Standard, 29*(4), 26.

Currey, J., Considine, J., & Khaw, D. (2011). Clinical nurse research consultant: A clinical and academic role to advance practice and the discipline of nursing. *Journal of Advanced Nursing, 67*(10), 2275–2283. doi: 10.1111/j.1365-2648.2011.05687.x

De Oliveira Santos, S. C. V., Woith, W., de Freitas, M. I. P., & Zeferino, E. B. B. (2016). Methods to determine the internal length of nasogastric feeding tubes: An integrative review. *International Journal of Nursing Studies, 61,* 95–103.

Doody, C. & Doody, O. (2011). Introducing evidence into nursing practice: Using the IOWA model. *British Journal of Nursing, 20*(11), 661–664.

Echevarria. I. M., & Walker, S. (2014). To make your case, start with a PICOT question. *Nursing, 44*(2), 18–19.

Enkin, M. (2012). Current overviews of research evidence from controlled trials in midwifery obstetrics. *Journal of Obstetricians and Gynecologists of Canada, 9,* 23–33.

Erhardt, T., Rice, T., Troszak, L., & Zhu, M. (2016). Motorcycle helmet type and the risk of head injury and neck injury during motorcycle collisions in California. *Accident; Analysis and Prevention, 86,* 23. doi: 10.1016/j.aap.2015.10.004

Fawcett, J. (2012). Thoughts about evidence-based nursing practice. *Nursing Science Quarterly, 25*(2), 199–200. doi: 10.1177/0894318412437967

Fernandez, R., & Griffiths, R. (2012). Water for wound cleansing. *Cochrane Database of Systematic Reviews, 2,* CD003861. doi: 10.1002/14651858.CD003861.pub3

Fineout-Overholt, E., Melnyk, B. M., & Shultz, A. (2011). Transforming health care from inside out: Advancing evidence-based practice in the 21st century. *Journal of Professional Nursing, 21*(6), 335–344.

Gallin, J. I., & Ognibene, F. P. (2012). *Principles and practice of clinical research* (3rd ed.). London: Elsevier/Academic Press.

Gerrish, K., McDonnell, A., Nolan, M., Guillaume, L., Kirshbaum, M., & Tod, A. (2011). The role of advanced practice nurses in knowledge brokering as a means of promoting evidence-based practice among clinical nurses. *Journal of Advanced Nursing, 67*(9), 2004–2014. doi: 10.1111/j.1365-2648.2011.05642.x

Gupta, S., Prasanth, K., Chen, C.-M., & Yeh, T. F. (2012). Postnatal corticosteroids for prevention and treatment of chronic lung disease in the preterm newborn. *International Journal of Pediatrics.* http://doi.org/10.1155/2012/315642

Guyatt, G., Oxman, A. D., Akl, E. A., Kunz, R., Vist, G., Brozek, J., . . . Schünemann, H. J. (2011). GRADE guidelines: 1. Introduction—GRADE evidence profiles and summary of findings tables. *Journal of Clinical Epidemiology, 64*(4), 383–394. doi: 10.1016/j.jclinepi.2010.04.026

Harris, R. P., Helfand, M., Woolf, S. H., Lohr, K. N., Mulrow, C. D., Teutsch, S. M., & Atkins, D. (2001). Current methods of the U.S. Preventive Services Task Force: A review of the methods. *American Journal of Preventive Services, 20*(Suppl. 3), 21–35.

Higgins, J. P. T., & Green, S. (Eds.). (2011). *Handbook for systematic reviews of interventions* (Ver. 5.1.0). Cochrane Collaboration.

Institute of Medicine. (2001). *Crossing the quality chasm: A new health system for the 21st century.* Washington, DC: National Academy Press.

Keough, V., Stevenson, A., Martinovich, Z., Young, R., & Tanabe, P. (2011). Nurse practitioner certification and practice settings: Implications for education and practice. *Journal of Nursing Scholarship, 43*(2), 195–202.

Krugman, M. (2011). Evidence-based practice. *Journal for Nurses in Staff Development, 27*(6), 310–312. doi: 10.1097/NND.0b013e31823866ac

Lee, H., Chang, K., Tsauo, J., Hung, J., Huang, Y., & Lin, S. (2012). Effects of a multifactorial fall prevention program on fall incidence and physical function in community-dwelling elderly with risk of fall. *Archives of Physical Medicine and Rehabilitation.* doi: 10.1016/j.apmr.2012.11.037

Linton, M. J., & Prasun, M. A. (2013). Evidence-based practice: Collaboration between education and nursing management. *Journal of Nursing Management, 21*(1), 5–16. doi: 10.1111/j.1365-2834.2012.01440.x

Lowdermilk, D. L. (2012). *Maternity & women's health care* (10th ed.). St. Louis, MO: Mosby.

Makic, M. B, Rauen, C., Jones, K., & Fisk, A. C. (2015). Continuing to challenge practice to be evidence based. *Critical Care Nurse, 35*(2), 39–50.

Marciano N. J., Merlin T. L., Bessen T., & Street J. M. (2014). To what extent are current guidelines for cutaneous melanoma follow up based on scientific evidence? *International Journal of Clinical Practice, 68*(6), 761–770.

Melnyk, B. M., & Fineout-Overholt, E. (2015). *Evidence-based practice in nursing and healthcare: A guide to best practice* (3rd ed.). Philadelphia, PA: Lippincott.

Melnyk, B. M., Fineout-Overholt, E., Gallagher-Ford, L., & Kaplan, L. (2012). The state of evidence-based practice in US nurses: Critical implications for nurse leaders and educators. *Journal of Nursing Administration, 42*(9), 410–417.

Melnyk, B. M., Gallagher-Ford, L., & Fineout-Overholt, E. (2014). The establishment of evidence-based practice competencies for practicing registered nurses and advanced practice nurses in real-world clinical settings: Proficiencies to improve healthcare quality, reliability, patient outcomes, and costs. *Worldviews on Evidence-Based Nursing, 11*(1), 5–15.

Moscati R. M., Mayrose J., Reardon R. F., Janicke D. M., & Jehle D. V. (2007). A multicenter comparison of tap water versus sterile saline for wound irrigation. *Academic Emergency Medicine, 14*(5), 404–409.

Nightingale, F. (1957). *Notes on nursing: What it is and what it is not.* Philadelphia, PA: Lippincott. (Originally published 1859.)

Niven, E., Roy, D. E., Schaefer, B. A., Gasquoine, S. E., & Ward, F. A. (2013). Making research real: Embedding a longitudinal study in a taught research course for undergraduate nursing students. *Nurse Education Today, 33*(1), 64–68. http://dx.doi.org/10.1016/j.nedt.2011.10.024

Oja, K. (2011). Using problem-based learning in the clinical setting to improve nursing students' critical thinking: An evidence review. *Journal of Nursing Education, 50*(3), 145–151. doi: 10.3928/01484834-20101230-10

Rodrigo, G. J., & Castro-Rodriguez, J. A. (2005). Anticholinergics in the treatment of children and adults with acute asthma: A systematic review with meta-analysis. *Thorax, 60*(0), 740–746.

Spruce, L, Van Wicklin, S. A., Hicks, R. W., Conner, R., & Dunn, D. (2014). Introducing AORN's new model for evidence rating. *AORN, 99*(2), 243–255.

Stevens, J., & Lyall, H. (2014). Mother to child transmission of HIV: What works and how much is enough? *Journal of Infection, 69*, S56–S62. doi: 10.1016/j.jinf.2014.07.018

Taylor, C., (2011*). Fundamentals of nursing: The art and science of nursing care* (7th ed.). Philadelphia, PA: Wolters Kluwer Health/Lippincott Williams & Wilkins.

Taylor, M. J., Freemantle, N., Geddes, J. R., & Bhagwagar, Z. (2006). Early onset of selective serotonin reuptake inhibitor antidepressant action: Systematic review and meta-analysis. *Archives of General Psychiatry, 63*(11), 1217–1223.

U.S. Department of Health and Human Services, Office of Disease Prevention and Health Promotion. (n.d.). Healthy People 2020. Retrieved from https://www.healthypeople.gov

Winters, C. A., & Echeverri, R. (2012). Teaching strategies to support evidence-based practice. *Critical Care Nurse, 32*(3), 49–54.

chapter 11

Nursing and Disaster Preparedness

Janice Springer

LEARNING OUTCOMES

After reading this chapter you will be able to:

- Identify two resources for information on potential contaminants from chemical, biological, radiation, nuclear, or explosive events.
- Discuss two possible roles of nurses in preparedness for a natural disaster.
- Review the role of the public health nurse in emergency planning and response activities.
- Identify the essential branches of the Incident Command System.
- Recognize when use of personal protective equipment (PPE) and decontamination are required for staff, client, or public safety.
- Discuss health education practices that increase preparedness for a family to survive emergencies.

Introduction

Since the beginning of the 21st century, the world has experienced many events that have caused multiple agencies including health professionals to engage in **disaster preparedness** activities. The events of September 11, 2001, the emergence of new infectious diseases such as severe acute respiratory syndrome (SARS) in 2003, H1N1 (2009), Ebola (2014), and natural

The editors wish to acknowledge the contributions of Kristi L. Lewis to the previous edition of this chapter.

disasters such as the Indian Ocean tsunami in 2004, Hurricanes Katrina (2005) and Sandy (2012), and the Fukushima trilogy of earthquake/tsunami/nuclear plant breach (2011), all have brought attention to the need for better planning to prevent such events and control the aftermath. Although events that have resulted in high morbidity and mortality are not new, it is important to note that not until after the events of September 11 did the medical community in the United States realize that they were not prepared for terrorist attacks. In December 2003, Homeland Security Presidential Directive 8 (Federal Emergency Management Agency [FEMA], 2015) was released by President George W. Bush to set the national preparedness strategy. This directive was organized as an all-hazards framework to guide preparedness activities from the local to the national level. Hurricane Katrina in 2005 served to reinforce the need for extensive planning and preparation for natural disasters.

Disaster preparedness activities are operational at local, state, and federal levels. One of the main target audiences for being involved in creating awareness, building education, training, and drills is healthcare professionals. Training and education are necessary to prepare the current and future workforce for developing, disseminating, and evaluating such activities in addition to responding in the time of need. Universities and colleges offer courses in emergency planning and response. Many offer certificate, undergraduate, and graduate-level degree programs to help expand the knowledge base. In response to the events of September 11, the Association of American Medical Colleges (AAMC) made recommendations that U.S. medical schools should educate students on emergency planning and response activities as part of their education curriculum to ensure that events would be well coordinated.

Public health nurses (PHNs) have long been active in disaster preparedness activities from planning and execution phases to the follow-up post-disaster. PHNs can support "population-based practice like rapid needs assessments of communities impacted by the incident, population-based triage, mass dispensing of preventive or curative therapies, community education, providing care or managing shelters for displaced populations and, of course, provision of ongoing continuity in essential public health services" (Association of Public Health Nurses, 2014, p. 4).

Nurses in hospitals, acute care clinics, and mental health facilities have taken on a significantly enhanced role in the last decade. Disaster preparedness activities at all levels should involve more than the public health workforce and are not just the role of public health professionals. Healthcare providers, individuals, and institutions use an all-hazards strategy of planning for disaster, surge capacity, decontamination, and more. Nurses in all settings should play a part in disaster preparedness activities in their organization and know their role in response (see **Sidebar 11-1**).

The purpose of this chapter is to provide an overview of the specific topic areas within disaster preparedness and the role of nursing. This chapter focuses on emergency planning and response as it relates to nursing professionals; it is divided into topics of types of disaster, including natural and caused by humans; Incident Command System; personal preparedness; and the disaster cycle. Mass causalities, triage, the psychological impact, and the role of the nurse in planning and assisting with such emergencies also will be discussed.

SIDEBAR 11-1
Disaster preparedness and response requires collaboration from many disciplines including public health, medicine, public administration, social work, psychology, public planning, emergency management, and the private sector as well as nursing.

Definitions Within Disaster

- **Disaster.** In the dictionary it is defined as "a calamitous event, especially one occurring suddenly and causing great loss of life, damage, or hardship, as a flood, airplane crash, or business failure" (Dictionary.com, n.d.). As the CDC (2015a) explains, "From the standpoint of public health, a disaster is defined on the basis of its consequences on health and health services. A disaster is a serious disruption of the functioning of society, causing widespread human, material, or environmental losses that exceeds the local capacity to respond, and calls for external assistance."
- **All-Hazards.** "The spectrum of all types of hazards including accidents, technological events, natural disasters, terrorist attacks, warfare, and chemical, biological including pandemic influenza, radiological, nuclear, or explosive events" (Blanchard, 2008, p. 18).
- **Vulnerabilities.** Vulnerability is the condition determined by physical, social, economic, and environmental factors or processes, which increase the susceptibility of a community to the impact of hazards (United Nations International Strategy for Disaster Reduction [UNISDR], 2009).
- **Risk.** The word "risk" has two distinctive connotations: in popular usage. The emphasis is usually placed on the concept of chance or possibility, such as in "the risk of an accident," whereas in technical settings the emphasis is usually placed on the consequences, in terms of "potential losses" for some particular cause, place, or period. It can be noted that people do not necessarily share the same perceptions of the significance and underlying causes of different risks (UNISDR, 2009).
- **Disaster Nursing.** In a position statement, the International Council of Nurses (ICN) describes the value of nurse involvement in disasters as: "Nurses with their technical skills and knowledge of epidemiology, physiology, pharmacology, cultural-familial structures, and psychosocial issues can assist in disaster preparedness programs, as well as during

disasters. Nurses, as team members, can play a strategic role cooperating with health and social disciplines, government bodies, community groups, and non-governmental agencies, including humanitarian organizations" (ICN, 2006, p. 2)

SIDEBAR 11-2

Natural disasters may include tornadoes, hurricanes, floods, fires, drought, blizzards or ice storms, earthquakes, extreme heat events, avalanches, tsunamis, volcanos, wildfires, and other natural events (Abrams & Pacific Northwest Annual Conference Disaster Response Team, 2009).

- **Natural Disasters.** Natural disasters have always occurred, causing extensive destruction and mass casualties. Natural disasters and severe weather can occur in any place with little, if any, warning (see **Sidebar 11-2**). Climate change may be contributing to an increase in frequency or severity of natural disasters (Field, Barros, Stocker, & Dahe, 2012).

Incident Command System

Whether in the realm of public health such as a local health department, school district, occupational health or home care, or in a hospital system, every nurse should be familiar with the Incident Command System (ICS), known as Hospital Incident Command System (HICS) in the hospital. Incident command came from the profession of firefighting as a strategy to manage the response operation, chains of authority, communications, and role clarity (FEMA, 2004). It lies in a subset of strategies within the National Incident Management System (NIMS) (FEMA, 2015). In 2006, federal funding began as a strategy to encourage all sectors of disaster response to integrate ICS into their structures. This system is arranged across four primary roles of Operations, Logistics, Planning, and Finance. The leaders of these sections report up to the incident commander and down to their branch chiefs. **Figure 11-1** is a sample of the typical format of an ICS structure. This is expandable and contractible depending upon the size of the incident. Nurses' roles often fall into Operations, representing the health lead inside the event. Nurses could also manage the safety officer role in some settings. In some situations, the safety officer functions something like an occupational health advisor, ensuring that health and safety support is offered in daily briefings, doing site visits for hazard analysis, and keeping abreast of risks to responders. Free training in ICS is available at http://www.fema.gov. Everyone in a leadership role from incident commander to branch section chiefs should have education, training, and practice to be most effective using ICS.

How Bad Is It?

There are multiple methods for anticipating, such as for a hurricane, or evaluating, after a tornado, how destructive a disaster event was or might be.

The Fujita or Fujita-Pearson Scale rates tornado intensity (see **Table 11-1**). The Fujita scale was developed and implemented by Dr. Ted Fujita and Dr. Greg Forbes. It is used after the event and includes analysis of scope and depth of damage to structures and impact on the environment to determine the strength of the tornado.

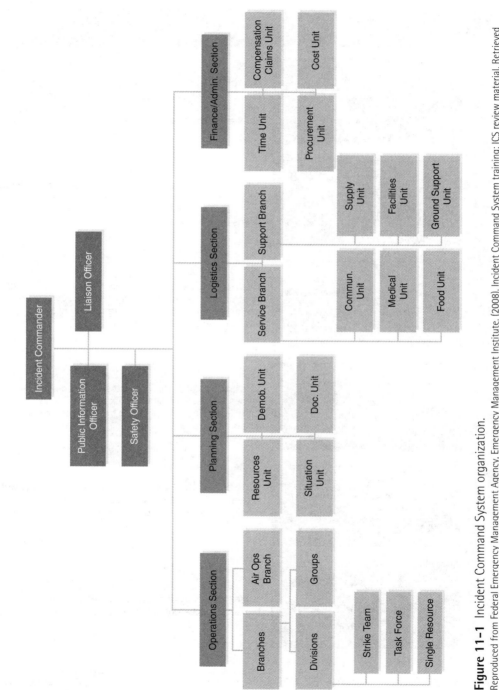

Figure 11-1 Incident Command System organization.

TABLE 11-1 ENHANCED FUJITA TORNADO SCALE

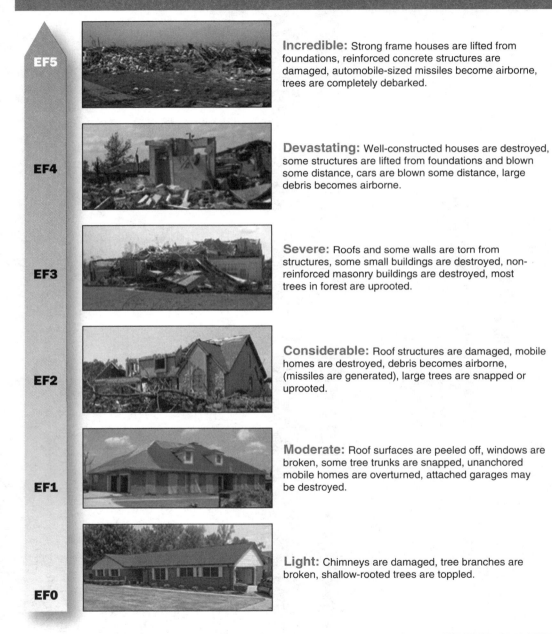

EF5

Incredible: Strong frame houses are lifted from foundations, reinforced concrete structures are damaged, automobile-sized missiles become airborne, trees are completely debarked.

EF4

Devastating: Well-constructed houses are destroyed, some structures are lifted from foundations and blown some distance, cars are blown some distance, large debris becomes airborne.

EF3

Severe: Roofs and some walls are torn from structures, some small buildings are destroyed, non-reinforced masonry buildings are destroyed, most trees in forest are uprooted.

EF2

Considerable: Roof structures are damaged, mobile homes are destroyed, debris becomes airborne, (missiles are generated), large trees are snapped or uprooted.

EF1

Moderate: Roof surfaces are peeled off, windows are broken, some tree trunks are snapped, unanchored mobile homes are overturned, attached garages may be destroyed.

EF0

Light: Chimneys are damaged, tree branches are broken, shallow-rooted trees are toppled.

Reproduced from Federal Emergency Management Agency. (2011). *Tornado outbreak of 2011 in Alabama, Georgia, Mississippi, Tennessee, and Missouri: EF scale summary.* Retrieved from http://www.fema.gov/media-library-data/20130726-1827-25045 -7585/tornado_mat_app_e_508.pdf

The hurricane scale is determined by wind speed. The Saffir-Simpson Hurricane Wind Scale demonstrates the range of wind and destruction predictable (see **Table 11-2**).

TABLE 11-2 SAFFIR-SIMPSON HURRICANE WIND SCALE

Category	Sustained Winds	Types of Damage Due to Hurricane Winds
1	74–95 mph 64–82 kt 119–153 km/h	**Very dangerous winds will produce some damage.** Well-constructed frame homes could have damage to roof, shingles, vinyl siding, and gutters. Large branches of trees will snap and shallowly rooted trees may be toppled. Extensive damage to power lines and poles likely will result in power outages that could last a few to several days.
2	96–110 mph 83–95 kt 154–177 km/h	**Extremely dangerous winds will cause extensive damage.** Well-constructed frame homes could sustain major roof and siding damage. Many shallowly rooted trees will be snapped or uprooted and block numerous roads. Near-total power loss is expected with outages that could last from several days to weeks.
3 (major)	111–129 mph 96–112 kt 178–208 km/h	**Devastating damage will occur.** Well-built framed homes may incur major damage or removal of roof decking and gable ends. Many trees will be snapped or uprooted, blocking numerous roads. Electricity and water will be unavailable for several days to weeks after the storm passes.
4 (major)	130–156 mph 113–136 kt 209–251 km/h	**Catastrophic damage will occur.** Well-built framed homes can sustain severe damage with loss of most of the roof structure and/or some exterior walls. Most trees will be snapped or uprooted and power poles downed. Fallen trees and power poles will isolate residential areas. Power outages will last weeks to possibly months. Most of the area will be uninhabitable for weeks or months.
5 (major)	157 mph or higher 137 kt or higher 252 km/h or higher	**Catastrophic damage will occur.** A high percentage of framed homes will be destroyed, with total roof failure and wall collapse. Fallen trees and power poles will isolate residential areas. Power outages will last for weeks to possibly months. Most of the area will be uninhabitable for weeks or months.

Reproduced from National Hurricane Center, & National Oceanic and Atmospheric Administration. (n.d.). Saffir-Simpson Hurricane Wind Scale. Retrieved from http://www.nhc.noaa.gov/aboutsshws.php

This can be tracked ahead of the storm and informs planners about the projected wind speeds on landfall. There is some correlation between the wind speed of the hurricane and the predictable scope of destruction on arrival, but it is not as absolute as the Fujita scale. A level I hurricane may sound as if it is "smaller" or "less of a problem" than a level III, but the other circumstances such as how low the elevation is where it hits, accompanying rain events, and fragility of the infrastructure (such as levees or dams) can lead to significant destruction no matter what the level predicted.

Some international communities classify disasters according to the magnitude of the disaster in relation to the ability of the agency or community to respond:

1. *Level I:* If the organization, agency, or community is able to contain the event and respond effectively using its own resources.
2. *Level II:* If the disaster requires assistance from external sources, but these can be obtained from nearby agencies.
3. *Level III:* If the disaster is of a magnitude that exceeds the capacity of the local community or region and requires assistance from state-level or even federal assets. (Office of Disaster Preparedness and Management, 2013)

Severe weather can include extreme heat during the summer months and extreme cold during the winter months, which may lead to ice and snowstorms. Both natural disasters and severe weather result in secondary conditions or effects that can cause or pose a health threat. Examples of a secondary effect would include a power outage from a storm or mold from a flood.

Earthquakes are an example of a natural disaster that can result in extensive destruction and mass casualties. Many feel that earthquakes are rare and that only certain geographical locations in the United States (like California) are prone to having an earthquake. According to current scientific understanding, the New Madrid seismic zone of the central United States (which includes Arkansas, Missouri, Tennessee, and Kentucky) is capable of producing significantly damaging earthquakes in the near future, perhaps sometime prior to 2035 (Central United States Earthquake Consortium [CUSEC], 2015).

There is a 40 percent chance of a major earthquake in the Coos Bay, Oregon region during the next 50 years (Goldfinger et al., 2012). According to the U.S. Geological Survey (2012), which provides scientific information about the natural hazards that threaten lives, that earthquake could approach the intensity of the Tohoku quake that devastated Japan in March 2011. This area is known as the Cascadia subduction zone, and such an event could include tsunami, mass evacuations, and significant numbers of deceased and injured, affecting nursing care in multiple settings (Jones, 2006).

Tornadoes are another type of natural disaster that has led to the need for better emergency planning and more resources in response. During a 4-day period from April 25 to 28, 2011, more than 200 tornados occurred in five states. Ultimately 338 people died (CDC, 2012; National Oceanic and Atmospheric Administration [NOAA], 2011). Each year within the United States there are approximately 1,200 tornados (National Severe Storms Laboratory [NSSL], 2015). Systems for aggregating the numbers of injuries and deaths directly attributable to tornados and other natural disasters are in development by the CDC (2014a; see **Sidebar 11-3**). Tornadoes can arise quickly with little warning and within minutes can cause severe destruction and loss of life. Although injuries can occur during the actual event, most occur in the days and weeks after the tornado. Such injuries are related to postevent cleanup activities including stepping on nails, broken glass, and other debris (CDC, 2014a).

> **SIDEBAR 11-3**
> Community education on the importance of following safety warnings is key. "Each year flooding kills more individuals than tornados, lightning, and hail" (NOAA, 2016).

Although tornadoes can occur with little warning, hurricanes often can be detected early, allowing for some preparation. However, even with advanced computer technology, hurricanes can change direction or gain strength quickly. Hurricanes are a type of tropical cyclone that can lead to miles of mass destruction and high levels of morbidity and mortality (FEMA, n.d.). Annual morbidity and mortality rates due to hurricanes are hard to calculate because activity is very cyclical. During 2005, hurricane activity peaked and became the most active on record with a total of 27 storms (National Hurricane Center, 2014). Hurricanes are ranked by categories ranging from one to five, with one being the lowest and usually resulting in the least severe aftermath. The categories are determined by the strength of sustained winds, amount of damage, and storm surge height. Categories three, four, and five are considered major hurricanes and require both extensive planning and response.

Severe weather is another example of natural events that can lead to adverse circumstances requiring emergency planning and coordinated response activities. Examples of severe weather can include extreme heat, extreme cold, and excessive precipitation including ice, snow, and rain. Weather that causes extremes can cause damage to property and lead to adverse health events such as severe morbidity and mortality. Extreme heat has different definitions from different sources but is generally accepted to be an extended period of time with unusually hot weather conditions that can potentially harm human health (CDC, 2011a).

Hyperthermia is the inability of the human body to compensate when temperatures are elevated above 98.6°F. Although heat-related illness and deaths are preventable, 8,015 individuals died in the United States from extreme heat between 1999 and 2010 (CDC, 2015c). This accounts for more deaths than from hurricanes, lightning, tornadoes, floods, and earthquakes combined (CDC, 2015b). Heat-related illness occurs when the body is not able to compensate and properly cool itself through sweating. In many cases sweating alone will not compensate for the overheating. When humidity is high, it may be difficult for the sweat to evaporate rapidly, thereby preventing the body from releasing heat fast enough to maintain bodily function. When body temperatures rise quickly and the body cannot compensate physiologically to cool or lower body temperatures, the human brain can be severely damaged. This can lead to a heat stroke.

Milder effects of extreme heat include heat exhaustion, heat cramps, and heat rash. Heat exhaustion is due to exposure over several days to high temperatures and the lack of proper replacement of fluids. Signs of heat exhaustion include heavy sweating, paleness, muscle cramps, tiredness, weakness, dizziness, headache, nausea or vomiting, and fainting. Heat exhaustion can lead to a heat stroke if not treated. Individuals who engage in physical activities that result in excessive sweating can develop heat cramps, a sign of heat exhaustion. Heat cramps are caused by the body's depletion of salt and moisture from dehydration. Painful cramps can result from the lack of salt and moisture primarily in the muscles.

Those at risk for adverse health effects due to extreme heat include the elderly, young children, individuals with mental illness, and those with chronic illnesses. Other factors that make an individual at risk for illness or death related to extreme heat include individuals with obesity, fever, dehydration, heart disease, or who are taking prescription drugs or using alcohol (CDC, 2015c).

Although extreme heat can cause severe illness and death, extreme cold also can result in negative outcomes. Winter storms can lead to extreme cold, which can lead to adverse health conditions and even death. Health effects caused by extreme cold from winter weather may include hypothermia, household fires due to the misuse of alternate heating sources and candles, asphyxiation due to carbon monoxide poisoning, and motor vehicle accidents due to poor and hazardous road conditions (CDC, 2015e). One example of a health effect due to extreme cold is hypothermia, caused when the body is exposed to cold temperatures and cannot replace heat at a rate fast enough to compensate for the heat lost. Individuals exposed to extreme cold can become mentally confused, causing the individual to be unable to think clearly. Individuals in this state may not be able to find their way to a safe and warm location or be able to provide some way to warm the body either through adding clothes or starting a fire.

Health effects due to exposure to the extreme cold include hypothermia and frostbite. According to the CDC (2015e), hypothermia is defined by the core body temperature and can be classified as mild, moderate, or severe. Signs of hypothermia include shivering, confusion, memory loss, and drowsiness (see **Sidebar 11-4**). Individuals with a temperature below 95°F need immediate medical attention. Another health condition caused by extreme cold is frostbite, which is characterized

> **SIDEBAR 11-4**
>
> According to the CDC (2011b), warning signs of a heat stroke include extremely high body temperature (above 103°F); red, hot, and dry skin; rapid, strong pulse; throbbing headache; dizziness; nausea; confusion; and unconsciousness.

by the loss of feeling and color in various areas of the body. Certain areas of the body including the nose, ears, cheeks, chin, fingers, and toes are more prone to frostbite because blood circulation is limited and the areas are likely to be exposed to the elements.

Secondary Effects of Natural Disasters and Severe Weather

After natural disasters or severe weather, power lines and gas lines can be damaged. This can result in fires or electrocution. The lack of electrical power can also lead to the use of alternative heating sources that, if not used properly, can lead to carbon monoxide poisoning. Sources of carbon monoxide (CO) include small gasoline engines, stoves, generators, and gas ranges. CO also can be produced by charcoal-burning devices such as gas grills. Signs of CO poisoning include dizziness, headache, nausea, vomiting, and confusion. CO is colorless and odorless. It can cause loss of consciousness and result in death.

Foodborne illnesses may occur after a natural disaster when power outages are common and food may be spoiled due to a lack of refrigeration (Healthy Communities, 2015). Nurses may be asked to provide information to the public on food safety following a natural disaster. Water contamination can also occur after such events. When water contamination occurs local health officials may issue a "boil water" advisory and ask the community to boil water for 5 minutes or longer prior to consumption to reduce the risk of gastrointestinal infections. For those with a private or community well, disinfection may be required to kill any potential pathogens. Wells may be evaluated for contaminants such as fecal bacteria by local environmental health officials (CDC, 2009b). Reflect on strategies in **Contemporary Practice Highlight 11-1** to provide family and community support needs, supplies, and resources when electricity and/or water are not available due to a natural disaster.

A common role of the public health department, after disasters that cause excess cases of injury, is to open **tetanus** booster walk-in clinics to respond to the increase in minor but potentially dangerous skin wounds.

Role of the Nurse in Natural Disasters

The Association of Public Health Nurses (APHN) position paper (2014) on the role of public health nurses in disaster explains that the PHN's work at individual, family, community, and systems levels to promote health and prevent disease and thus bring critical expertise to each phase of the disaster cycle: preparedness (prevention, protection and mitigation), response, and recovery. The Joint Commission (n.d.) expects that hospital systems will be able to provide safe and effective patient care during an emergency, clearly defining staff roles, training those roles and responsibilities; and

KEY TERM

Tetanus: Tetanus is a potential health threat for persons who sustain wound injuries and is virtually 100 percent preventable with vaccination (CDC, 2014b).

CONTEMPORARY PRACTICE HIGHLIGHT 11-1

EMERGENCY PREPAREDNESS PLAN

Being prepared for a disaster is a higher need than most healthcare workers imagine. In 2014, Health Facilities Management and several partner organizations conducted an Emergency Management Survey including questions on procedures and policies on preparation for natural disasters. They found that 52 percent of respondents had experienced a winter storm requiring implementation of their emergency operations plan; 58 percent had had to go on emergency power in the past 5 years because of an emergency event; and 87 percent of respondents had had one or more events in the past 5 years that required implementation of the Emergency Preparedness Plan. Roughly 1,300 patients were evacuated from New York and New Jersey hospitals during Hurricane Sandy in 2012. In Flint, Michigan in 2016, the entire public water system was shown to be contaminated with lead and many children had dangerously high blood lead levels. Implications for the nursing workforce across all practice settings are significant. Personal preparedness, awareness of institutional disaster policies and procedures, and clear understanding of client support needs in a disaster scenario are key to meeting the public demand for emergency response.

Data from Health Facilities Management. (2014). Emergency management survey. Retrieved from www.hfmmagazine.com; Wang, Y. (2015, December 15). In Flint, Mich., there's so much lead in children's blood that a state of emergency is declared. *Washington Post*. Retrieved from https://www.washingtonpost.com/news/morning-mix/wp/2015/12/15/toxic-water-soaring-lead-levels-in-childrens-blood-create-state-of-emergency-in-flint-mich

sustaining staff competencies over time. These documents set the stage in support of the ways nurses play a significant role before, during, and after a natural disaster. Local health organizations such as health departments, hospitals, and clinics have prepared disaster plans for events such as hurricanes, tornadoes, and extreme temperatures. Nurses play an integral part in the planning process. Many nurses are developing contingency plans for clinical services in the event of a natural disaster so that client care can still be delivered to those in critical need. Others are working to ensure that resources such as supplies and personnel are available during a disaster and they can be obtained with ease and little forewarning. Prior to a natural disaster, nurses may assist or lead in developing, updating, testing, and disseminating emergency plans. Coordination of supplies and resources including personnel may fall under the role of the nurse and require extensive foresight.

During a natural disaster, nurses may need to assist with shelters that are established for those who do not have adequate housing. In shelters, nurses and other licensed healthcare providers may be engaged in support of vulnerable populations, assisting persons with disabilities, advocating for crucial medications and supplies, and in many ways providing care and support during a dramatic and emotional period of uncertainty. Nearly 500 Red Cross chapters across the United States are prepared to open emergency shelters within hours of a disaster (American Red Cross, 2015b).

Nurses also may be asked to assist in rescue, especially of those who may have injuries requiring immediate medical attention. The role of the nurse during such events may also include serving as a healthcare representative for community members and their families related to the event and their health. **Contemporary Practice Highlight 11-2** describes the facets of the roles of nurses in recent disasters. Consider how you would respond to a specific at-risk population with a local voluntary organization within your community in a natural disaster.

Personal Preparedness

The CDC and the American Red Cross have extensive documents to assist nurses for their personal preparedness as well as to help them prepared their communities. It is difficult for persons involved in response to dedicate their time when they are concerned that they or their families are not prepared.

Personal preparedness can also include volunteerism. There are several governmental and nongovernmental agencies that welcome volunteer nurses. The American Red Cross has had nurses involved in disaster response since its founding under the guidance of Clara Barton in 1885 (Oates, 1994). The Medical Reserve Corps was created after the events of 9/11 to create a system for engaging a broader healthcare community for response. Disaster response medical teams can be deployed across

---

CONTEMPORARY PRACTICE HIGHLIGHT 11-2

NURSES AND AT-RISK POPULATIONS

In times of disaster, at-risk populations are less likely to have resources for evacuation, extended time away from home, and/or recovery. There are over 16 million nurses around the world; nearly 4 million active in the United States. Nurses can have a substantial voice on behalf of at-risk populations in preparedness for, response to, and recovery of populations affected by disaster, whether in an institutional setting or a broader public health arena. There are many voluntary organizations active in disasters that need the critical thinking skills of nurses. Every community needs local teams trained for disaster response, including nurses. American Red Cross, Medical Reserve Corps, and other organizations listed with Voluntary Organizations Active in Disaster (VOAD) welcome nurses to be part of their service delivery.

Data from Kaiser Family Foundation. (2016). Total number of professionally active nurses. Retrieved from http://kff.org/other/state-indicator/total-registered-nurses/

BOX 11-1   HOME EMERGENCY KIT

Nurses need to be involved in public health education campaigns to ensure all homes, including their own, are equipped with a kit that is appropriate for any and all emergencies.

- Water: one gallon per person, per day (3-day supply for evacuation, 2-week supply for home)
- Food: nonperishable, easy-to-prepare items (3-day supply for evacuation, 2-week supply for home)
- Flashlight
- Battery-powered or hand-crank radio (NOAA Weather Radio, if possible)
- Extra batteries
- First aid kit
- Medications (7-day supply) and medical items

- Multipurpose tool
- Sanitation and personal hygiene items
- Copies of personal documents (medication list and pertinent medical information, proof of address, deed/lease to home, passports, birth certificates, insurance policies)
- Cell phone with chargers
- Family and emergency contact information
- Extra cash
- Emergency blanket
- Map(s) of the area

Reproduced from American Red Cross. (2015a). *Build a kit*. Retrieved from http://www.redcross.org/prepare/location/home-family/get-kit

---

the nation for surge support in critical incidents. **Box 11-1** provides information about home emergency kits.

Outbreaks and Emerging Infections

The World Health Organization (WHO, 2015a) defines a disease outbreak as the occurrence of cases of disease in excess of what would normally be expected in a defined community, geographical area, or season. An outbreak may occur in a restricted geographical area or may extend over several countries. It may last for a few days or weeks or for several years. A single case of a communicable disease long absent from a population or caused by an agent (e.g., bacterium or virus) not previously recognized in that community or area, or the emergence of a previously unknown disease, may also constitute an outbreak and should be reported and investigated. The public has become more aware of outbreak events and expects follow-up through disease investigation and identification. In the spring of 2006, the Illinois Department of Public Health noticed an increase in *Acanthamoeba* keratitis (AK), an infection of the eye. After further investigation, the CDC confirmed an increase in AK cases among soft contact lens wearers who were using a specific brand of multipurpose cleaning solution. Approximately 138 cases of AK were identified (CDC, 2007a). Another national outbreak involved contaminated Peter Pan and Great Value peanut butter. By the end of the investigation, 715 cases in 48 states of *Salmonella* had been identified. In the final analysis it was suggested that environmental contamination in the plant in Tennessee likely caused the outbreak

(Sheth et al., 2011). In recent decades there have been several viral infectious disease outbreaks with global implications: SARS in 2003, H1N1 in 2009, and Ebola in 2014 (Ratzan & Moritsugu, 2014). There are viruses that can pass between animals to humans and then can mutate to a human-to-human virulence. There have been drastic and consequential exposures, partly due to proximity of animals to people, partly due to the speed international travel allows for, and partly due to other and unknown factors. How nurses respond to, communicate about, and participate in these events is key to public information and safety. As this chapter was going to press, the Zika virus was in the news. It is spread primarily through the *Aedes* species of mosquito and can cause either no symptoms or sometimes those of fever, rash, joint pain, or conjunctivitis. Zika virus during pregnancy can cause a birth defect called microcephaly, as well as other severe fetal brain defects (CDC, 2016a).

Emerging infectious agents can also be used as a human-made terrorism event. Certain agents may have the potential to be mass produced and disseminated to a large population of individuals within a geographical region. These cause diseases that have not been seen in humans or that occur in a new geographical location. With ease in production and mass dissemination comes the risk for high levels of morbidity and mortality.

In many localities, epidemiologists employed at local or state health departments will conduct outbreak investigations to identify the cause of the outbreak. Although outbreaks are common, there is always a need to conduct an investigation. Primarily, outbreak investigations are conducted to identify the etiology or cause of the outbreak. Other reasons for conducting outbreak investigations include gaining knowledge about a specific disease or disease-causing agent (pathogen), providing information to the general public, and evaluating intervention or prevention activities. By gaining knowledge on pathogens or diseases caused by pathogens, future outbreaks can be avoided and current outbreaks may be better controlled to prevent further transmission. In conducting outbreak investigations, interventions and prevention activities can be evaluated, such as hospital protocols to prevent the spread of hospital-acquired infections. Investigations have also provided information to the public to reduce anxiety and to increase adherence with certain behaviors such as obtaining influenza shots or practicing proper hand hygiene. Conducting outbreak investigations have also proven to be beneficial to policymakers in the development of laws such as the requirement to vaccinate all children prior to entering school.

Role of the Nurse in Outbreaks and Role of Personal Protective Equipment

During significant outbreaks, nurses and other healthcare providers typically provide information to the general public by communicating through the media. By alerting the media about an outbreak, other cases or individuals at risk for being a possible case can be identified and provided assistance. Working with the media and the local community and having consistent messaging, can be beneficial in reducing

SIDEBAR 11-5
Epidemiologists are public health scientists who work as disease detectives in conducting investigations and studies to find the etiology or cause of an outbreak.

anxiety among the general public. The CDC (2015d) maintains a Health Alert Network (HAN), which is their primary method of sharing cleared information about urgent public health incidents with public information officers; federal, state, territorial, and local public health practitioners; clinicians; and public health laboratories (see **Sidebar 11-5**).

Personal protective equipment (PPE) is a standard resource in hospitals and less common in routine public health practice. Emerging infections, such as Ebola, biological exposures such as anthrax, and chemical exposure protection or decontamination post exposure all have specific types of recommended levels of personal protection. Whether it involves simple gloves and a mask or full head and body cover with respirator, knowledge of appropriate PPE is a crucial component of disaster planning and response, messaging to the public, and self-care (CDC, 2013b). The National Institute for Occupational Safety and Health (NIOSH) and CDC both have extensive websites to educate workers about protective safety.

Disasters Caused by Humans

Humans have sought to inflict harm on others for millennia. One of the earliest reports of bioterrorism was in the Sixth Century, BC when Assyrians poisoned enemy wells with rye ergot, a fungus that causes convulsions if ingested. Modern times have brought the concepts of weapons of mass destruction and terrorism into daily experiences across the globe.

Some events, such as the random shooter, garner large media attention and cause significant community impact (Cross & Pruitt, 2013). Human-made disasters can take other forms, such as chemical spills or massive transportation accidents.

In this section we look briefly at chemical, biological, radiation, and nuclear (CBRN) events and resources nurses should become familiar with in order to respond in these circumstances.

Biological and Chemical Agent Overview

Biological and chemical events can be both intentional and unintentional. Intentional events are usually identified as terrorist attacks and can be domestic or international. The purpose of an intentional release of a biological or chemical agent is to cause harm to the general public and disruption to daily life activities that could harm the overall economy. Unintentional events are accidents that can result in the release of a biological or chemical agent.

Biological agents have been a component of terrorist attacks since the beginning of recorded history. Terrorist attacks can be covert or overt events. Another historical example was during the 14th century when Tartars catapulted plague-contaminated cadavers into a nearby city on the Black Sea. Although the attack was successful, it also caused a continuation of the Black Death in Europe (Phillips, 2005). During the **incubation period** many biologic sources have the additional challenge that an individual can be asymptomatic and yet still communicable. This could lead to extensive secondary spread. Modes of transmission of the biological agent are contact, or person-to-person, droplet or airborne (Occupational Safety and Health Administration, n.d.).

> **KEY TERM**
> **Incubation period:** The time that lapses between when the host receives the agent and when the host presents with symptoms.

The CDC has five focus areas for dealing with a biological or chemical event. The five focus areas identified by the CDC are (a) preparedness and prevention; (b) detection and surveillance; (c) diagnosis and agent identification; (d) response; and (e) communication (CDC, 2000).

Healthcare providers may be called upon to assist in one or more of these five areas.

Bioterrorism Events

A biological agent is a living organism and can involve bacteria, viruses, or parasites. There are three distinct classes of biological agents, labeled Categories A, B, and C. They vary based on the ease of mass production and the health effects if released into a population.

Category A is characterized by agents that are easy to produce and disseminate and may have a direct mode of transmission (i.e., person to person). Category A agents of concern include variola major (smallpox), *Bacillus anthracis* (anthrax), *Yersinia pestis* (plague), *Clostridium botulinum* toxin (botulism), *Francisella tularensis* (tularemia), filoviruses including Ebola hemorrhagic fever and Marburg hemorrhagic fever, and arena viruses that include Lassa (Lassa fever) and Junin (Argentine hemorrhagic fever) (CDC, 2001a).

An example of a Category A **bioterrorism** event (see **Sidebar 11-6**) occurred less than a month after the events of September 11 when a man was admitted to a local hospital in South Florida with fever and altered mental status. The 63-year-old male was given antibiotic therapy but died 3 days later. An autopsy later revealed inhalation anthrax (CDC, 2001b). During a 2-month period, 22 cases of anthrax were identified. Five of the 22 identified cases resulted in death (CDC, 2001c). Evaluating previous bioterrorism events such as this example can assist those who must develop and implement appropriate response plans in the future. In particular, it is important to understand how the events were initially detected and the process involved in reporting them. Clues to a possible biological or chemical terrorist attack include the presence of an unusual disease case such as anthrax, an unusual increase in a disease, or an unusual pattern of death.

> **KEY TERM**
> **Bioterrorism:** The use of a biological agent to intentionally produce disease in a susceptible population.

> **SIDEBAR 11-6**
> Sources for Category A, B, C diseases/pathogens include:
> http://www.niaid.nih.gov
> https://emergency.cdc.gov/bioterrorism
> http://www.cdc.gov
> http://www.jhsph.edu

After the anthrax event of 2011, the U.S. Army Medical Research Institute of Infectious Diseases (USAMRIID) evaluated numerous biological agents to predict whether they could be used in a bioterrorist attack. In 2002, the Office of Public Health Preparedness and Response was created through the CDC. One of many funded strategies was to create a national and structural system for delivery of emergency medications for mass populations, such as anthrax prophylaxis, influenza vaccine, and others, called the SNS, or the Strategic National Stockpile (FDA, 2002). The medications and supplies in the SNS are cached in specific regions and should arrive within 12 hours of a disaster; however, localities should be prepared to use their own resources for the initial 24 to 72 hours. Hospitals and clinics may need to purchase some supplies and have them available in the event of a disaster. An all-hazards disaster plan should be in place and annual drills or tabletop exercises should be conducted to assess the feasibility of the plan.

Category B agents (see Sidebar 11-6) are relatively easy to produce and disseminate; however, not as easy as those in Category A. Although Category B agents can cause illness and death, they are far less deadly than the agents in Category A. The majority of Category B agents are transmitted indirectly. This means they are not transmitted person-to-person (direct transmission) but rather require a **vector** or vehicle. A vector is a living organism that transmits an agent to a host, such as a human. For example, the flea is a vector for typhus fever and the tick is the vector for Rocky Mountain spotted fever. A vehicle is a nonliving object that may be contaminated with an agent and can then transmit it to a host via ingestion. For example, when contaminated with a strain of salmonella, egg salad can cause salmonellosis in a host (i.e., a human).

> **KEY TERM**
>
> **Vector:** A living organism that transmits an infective agent (such as a bacteria or virus) to a host, such as a human.

For the purposes of this chapter, the focus is on Category A agents because they pose the greatest threat to public health.

Smallpox

Smallpox is a disease caused by the variola virus that has two distinct forms—variola minor and variola major (see **Sidebar 11-7**). Variola minor is less severe than variola major, with a lower fatality rate. Variola major is the most common and severe form of variola and can be easily spread from person to person. Nearly 30 percent of people infected with variola major lead to death. Symptoms of smallpox include a rash with raised bumps and high fever (CDC, 2007b).

Although the World Health Organization (2015b) declared that smallpox was eradicated in 1977 after the last known case was identified in Somalia, it may still be a plausible threat due to its high death rate and person-to-person transmission. Because smallpox is spread from person to person, should there be an outbreak, the main role of public health professionals and healthcare providers will be to contain the outbreak as much as possible through

> **SIDEBAR 11-7**
>
> Although some experts have discussed using antivirals to treat smallpox cases, only prevention through vaccination has proven to be successful in the control and elimination of smallpox.

the early identification and isolation of cases and the quarantine of individuals who may have been contaminated but are not showing signs and symptoms of disease.

Anthrax

Anthrax, a bacterial disease caused by *Bacillus anthracis*, comes in three forms: cutaneous, inhalation, and gastrointestinal. Although all three forms of anthrax can be treated with antibiotics, the gastrointestinal and inhalation forms can cause severe illness and death. Cutaneous anthrax begins with a painless skin lesion that may progress to a black eschar. Those with cutaneous anthrax may experience symptoms such as a fever and malaise. Death from cutaneous anthrax is rare if treated with an antibiotic, but as many as 20 percent of those who are not treated may die. Inhalational anthrax, however, has a higher fatality rate even with prompt initiation of antibiotics. In the bioterrorism-related anthrax cases that occurred in 2001, 45 percent of those diagnosed with inhalation anthrax died. Individuals with inhalation anthrax present with viral-like respiratory illness, and it should be included in the differential diagnosis of those presenting with unexplained upper respiratory illness and symptoms such as fever and muscle aches. Gastrointestinal anthrax may occur after consuming raw or undercooked meat that has been contaminated with anthrax. Symptoms include severe abdominal pain, fever, nausea, anorexia, and bloody diarrhea. The death rate due to gastrointestinal anthrax is reported to be around 25 to 60 percent (CDC, 2009a).

Although anthrax is not spread person to person, it can be spread through handling animal products that have been infected with the bacteria or from eating undercooked meat that has been infected. Treatment recommendations for adults with anthrax include antibiotic therapy.

Botulism

Botulism is a paralyzing disease of the muscles caused by toxin released from the bacterium *Clostridium botulinum* (see **Sidebar 11-8**). On average, 110 cases are reported annually within the United States. Botulism cannot be spread person to person, but left untreated, it has a high fatality rate. As there is antitoxin in only three states (Alaska, California, and at the CDC in Atlanta), nearly all cases of botulinum poisoning are reported.

An average of 145 cases are reported each year, of which 15 percent are foodborne and are due to the improper preparation and storage of home-canned foods. Of these cases, 65 percent are infant botulism (see **Sidebar 11-9**), primarily caused by feeding infants honey and 20 percent are wound, most of which are caused by black–tar heroin injection, especially in California (CDC, 2016b) Classic symptoms of botulism include drooping eyelids, difficulty in swallowing, dry mouth, abdominal pain,

SIDEBAR 11-8
Botulism comes in three forms: foodborne botulism, infant botulism, and wound botulism.

SIDEBAR 11-9
Infant botulism is the most common form of botulism, comprising between 60 and 75 percent of the cases each year.

nausea, vomiting, and diarrhea. Infants may be lethargic, feed poorly, and have a weak cry and poor muscle tone.

Botulism differs from many of the other bioterrorism agents because the bacteria form a toxin. This toxin causes respiratory paralysis and therefore is a concern because most persons will require mechanical ventilation. Many community-level hospitals have only a few ventilators and therefore would not be able to treat a large number of clients with botulism (Branson, Johannigman, Daughtery, & Rubinson, 2008).

Plague

Plague, caused by the bacterium *Yersinia pestis*, has three forms: pneumonic, bubonic, and septicemic. The pneumonic plague form infects the lungs and can be spread person to person via respiratory droplets. Symptoms of pneumonic plague mimic respiratory influenza and include fever, headache, shortness of breath, chest pain, and cough (CDC, 2004). Bubonic plague, the most common form of plague, is transmitted by fleas and cannot be spread person to person. Clients with bubonic plague will present with symptoms that include enlarged and tender lymph nodes, fever, headache, and overall bodily weakness. Septicemic plague cannot be spread person to person and occurs when the *Yersinia pestis* bacteria multiply in the person's blood throughout the body. This bacteremia can be a secondary effect from either pneumonic or bubonic plague or it can occur alone. Symptoms include fever, chills, and shock. Rapid treatment with an antibiotic must occur within 24 to 48 hours to reduce the risk of death (**see Sidebar 11-10**). In recent decades an average of seven people per year develop plague. There has not been a case of person-to-person infection in the United States since 1924 (National Institute of Allergy and Infectious Disease [NIAID], 2015).

> **SIDEBAR 11-10**
> Antibiotics recently licensed to prevent or treat pneumonic plague and septicemia plague include Ciprofloxacin, levofloxacin, and moxifloxacin (NIAID, 2015).

Tularemia

The incidence of tularemia in the United States is low, with approximately 100 to 200 cases reported annually. Tularemia is caused by the bacteria *Francisella tularensis* and occurs naturally within the United States. Outbreaks in Europe, in Kosovo, Spain, and Scandinavia, have sustained interest in this disease (Sjöstedt, 2007). It is often referred to as "rabbit fever" because it can be found in mammals such as infected rabbits, muskrats, prairie dogs, and even domestic cats (CDC, 2015f). Tularemia is highly infectious and can be manufactured and disseminated as an airborne weapon. Although tularemia can be manufactured as a biological weapon, it cannot be transmitted via person-to-person contact. It can be spread through the bite of a tick that carries the agent, handling of infected animal carcasses, consumption of contaminated food, or inhalation of aerosolized particles. Signs and symptoms of tularemia depend on the type of exposure or how the bacteria enter the body.

Treatment for tularemia includes antimicrobial therapy, with streptomycin, genta-micin, doxycycline, or ciprofloxacin (CDC, 2015f).

The Role of the Nurse in Bioterrorism Events

It is important for nurses to make keen observations and use deductive reasoning in evaluating clients who may have been exposed to a biological agent. Schools of nursing across the country have begun to address workforce development and nurse preparedness through curriculum enhancement (Veenema, 2006). Nurses should be on alert for, and know the resources available, to support identification of individuals who present with unusual symptoms that lack a clear diagnosis.

During an outbreak nurses need to evaluate and **triage** clients based on symptoms and severity. In large outbreaks, clients must be triaged based on the severity of symptoms. In many cases, the nurse may be the first professional to come in contact with an exposed client. Early identification and treatment could reduce the overall morbidity and mortality that result from the pandemic. In significant mass-casualty disasters, field triage might reverse the order of "worst is first" to a decision to help those most likely to survive first and leave those with poor signs of life for last. In modern times, there is more discussion on strategies to support the best ways to identify the right patient for early transport when there are massive numbers of persons with injuries. This includes uses of Respiratory, Pulse and Motor (RPM) effort assessment (Sacco et al., 2005). In addition to assessment and triage, nurses may be asked to report findings to local authorities including the public health department and provide follow-up on potential cases or contacts of confirmed cases. Samples for laboratory testing may also need to be collected and submitted with rigorous follow-up of the results with the public health department. Nurses have an opportunity to educate, inform, and mobilize communities to develop safe public health policies and programs. As a public health or school nurse, how would you advocate for improved policies and set priorities in state and city bud-gets to improve environmental conditions for children with asthma, as discussed in **Contemporary Practice Highlight 11-3**?

Nurses play an important role in planning and preparing for bioterrorism events. In many health departments, hospitals, and healthcare centers, nurses are serving as leaders in developing multilevel and multidisciplinary plans for a bioterrorism event (see **Sidebar 11-11**). In this leadership role, nurses are writ-ing protocols, coordinating personnel, and providing training opportunities for staff. Nurses also engage in drills to assess preparedness and resource needs during such events.

> **KEY TERM**
>
> **Triage:** A French word meaning *to sort*. During a disaster, it is the process of deciding who is to be treated first, who can wait, and whose life cannot be saved (Beach, 2010).

> **SIDEBAR 11-11**
>
> When a biological exposure is suspected, the nurse must conduct an immediate assessment and interview of clients and their family members that includes health history questions on environmental and occupational exposures.

CONTEMPORARY PRACTICE HIGHLIGHT 11-3

CLIMATE CHANGE

Climate change has an impact on health, including events due to an increase in disaster events. These events can and will continue to affect work for nurses. Extreme heat events can increase heat-related illness and death; Air pollution affects the prevalence and exacerbations of asthma and other respiratory conditions; Changes in vector ecology, such as changing geographic patterns of such diseases as dengue fever, malaria, Lyme disease, West Nile virus, and others will affect public health and the acute care practice environment; severe weather can have an impact on injuries, fatalities, and mental health. The public health challenges of the effects of climate change are evident, yet state and local governments are always in a struggle to balance budgets and set priorities.

Data from Centers for Disease Control and Prevention. (2016c). *Climate change and health effects wheel.* Retrieved from http://www.cdc.gov/climateandhealth/effects/; Polivka, B., Chaudry, R., & MacCrawford, J. (2012). Public health nurses' knowledge and attitudes regarding climate change. *Environmental Health Perspectives, 120*(3), 321–325. doi: 10.1289/ehp.1104025

Chemical Emergencies

Chemical agents can be either manufactured or derived from natural sources such as vegetation. At this point in time, a **chemical emergency** seems inevitable regardless of the intent. In January 2014 in West Virginia, an estimated 10,000 gallons of 4-Methylcyclohexanemethanol—an industrial chemical—spilled into the Elk River. Elk River is upstream from Charleston's municipal water intake—a water supply serving 300,000 people. A "Do Not Use" order was subsequently released by the governor because of the uncertainty over the chemicals in the water (CDC, 2014d). Although, in the final analysis, most persons who presented with symptoms related to an exposure by this chemical (nausea, vomiting, diarrhea, skin rash, itching, headache, sore throat, and cough) were treated and released without long-term consequences, the potential impact on public health for this region and downstream communities demonstrates the scope for "unseen" risks inherent in our society.

Chemical emergencies, like biological emergencies, can be either intentional or unintentional, both with potentially disastrous outcomes. An example of another unintentional chemical emergency occurred in 2005, when two freight trains collided in Graniteville, South Carolina. The collision caused the release of nearly 11,500 gallons of chlorine gas, which resulted in 9 casualties and 529 persons with injuries needing immediate medical care. The incident prompted public health officials to study the effects of chlorine gas related to health outcomes (CDC, 2005).

KEY TERM

Chemical emergency: The release of some hazardous chemical agent either unintentionally, such as through an accidental industrial release, or intentionally, as in a terrorist attack.

An example of an intentional chemical emergency involved the contamination of ground hamburger. In January 2003, 1,700 pounds of ground beef were recalled after 36 individuals complained of becoming ill or having family members who became ill after ingesting the product. Laboratory analysis revealed that nearly 100 people were ill after consuming ground beef. The tests verified that the beef had been contaminated with nicotine. Based on an extensive investigation it was discovered that the contamination did not occur in the processing plant but at a single grocery store. Upon further study, investigators found that the poisoning was caused by one individual who had contaminated nearly 200 pounds of ground beef with an insecticide containing nicotine as the main ingredient (CDC, 2003). In 2013, the Food and Drug Administration (FDA, 2013) released a tool to help prevent intentional food contamination. Whether intentional or unintentional, chemical emergencies are plausible and can lead to extensive public health consequences.

Chemical agents that could be used in a terrorist attack or could be released accidentally and lead to serious public health outcomes are categorized by either the type of chemical or by the effects the chemical has on the human body. According to the CDC (2013a), the 13 categories are the following:

- Biotoxins
- Blister agents/vesicants
- Blood agents
- Caustics (acids)
- Choking/lung/pulmonary agents
- Incapacitating agents
- Long-lasting anticoagulants
- Metals
- Nerve agents
- Organic solvents
- Riot control agents/tear gas
- Toxic alcohols
- Vomiting agents

The Role of the Nurse in Chemical Events

The role of the nurse in chemical events mirrors his or her role in bioterrorism events. Nurses can play a significant role in the early identification of a chemical agent and the assessment, triage, and treatment of affected individuals.

Radiation

Radiation, a ubiquitous form of energy, can come from either human-made sources such as medical devices or natural sources such as the sun. The release of radioactive material can result

KEY TERM

Radiation: A ubiquitous form of energy that can come from either human-made sources such as medical devices or natural sources such as the sun.

in radioactive contamination and radiation exposure. Radioactive contamination is defined as radioactive particles that are on or in an object or a living organism such as humans. For example, radioactive material can be on clothing, objects, and the skin. Internal contamination can occur when the individual inhales or ingests radioactive material. Radioactive exposure is defined as the penetration of the body by radioactive material given off in the form of particles or waves.

Adverse health effects have been documented, however, from exposure to large doses of radiation for a short period of time or from prolonged exposure to low doses (Agency for Toxic Substances and Disease Registry [ATSDR], 1999). Radiation events can include accidents or intentional release due to a terrorist attack. Although rare, in the past 50 years there have been approximately 10 different events where radiation was released that resulted in the contamination of either small groups with high exposure levels or low exposure among a large population of people.

Approximately 237 employees and rescue workers suffered effects related to the accidental release of radiation in April 1986 from a nuclear reactor located in Chernobyl, Ukraine (formerly the Soviet Union). Thirty workers died due to conditions related to radiation exposure and nearly 15,000 people living within the community suffered health conditions. There was a high incidence of thyroid cancer in young children (Demidchik, Drozd, & Biko, 2009). Over the years since this event, an increase in thyroid cancer; neurological damage; respiratory, gastrointestinal, and hemopoietic diseases; and conditions related to the exposure have been documented in individuals exposed to the radiation. The ATSDR (1999) maintains a site on individual risks for exposure.

In 2011, after an earthquake stimulated tsunami, the Fukushima Daiichi nuclear power plant was breached. There were no serious radiation-induced injuries to onsite workers; however 150,000 people were evacuated from a 12-mile zone around the plant because of radiation fears (WHO, 2013).

Radiation exposure can also be intentional. In fall 2006, United Kingdom officials began an investigation related to the death of Alexander Litvinenko, a former Russian spy contaminated with polonium-210 (Po-210). Traces of radioactive material were also found at a London sushi bar where Litvinenko was presumably poisoned. His poisoning stimulated deeper discussion about preparedness for and management of toxic chemicals (McFee, 2009). With the concern of an intentional radiation event comes the worldwide concern over dirty bombs. A dirty bomb is composed of a mixture of explosives and radioactive material that can be released when the bomb explodes. Dirty bombs are often mistaken for atomic bombs such as those used in the attacks on Hiroshima and Nagasaki in World War II. Atomic bombs are much more powerful and cause the release of large amounts of radioactive material that can spread for miles. The detonation of a dirty bomb would not cause extensive or widespread release of radioactive material. Injuries related to the explosion from a dirty bomb are the primary concern.

One effect of radiation exposure is acute radiation syndrome (ARS), also known as radiation toxicity or radiation sickness (CDC, 2014c). ARS is a characteristic result of radiation exposure where the dose is high and exposure is of short duration to the entire body. ARS has extensive physiological effects on the human body and can affect the central nervous system, cardiovascular system, and gastrointestinal system and destroy bone marrow.

ARS is identified by four clinical stages: prodromal, latent, manifest illness, and recovery or death. The prodromal stage involves symptoms such as nausea, vomiting, anorexia, and diarrhea. Those exposed can also experience confusion and loss of consciousness. The symptoms can occur within a few minutes of exposure or can occur days after the event and go on for hours, days, or weeks depending on the dosage. In the latent phase, exposed individuals may look healthy; however, destruction of bone marrow is common. In the manifest illness stage, symptoms include anorexia, fever, and malaise. In this stage, death due to infection and possible hemorrhage is likely, depending on the amount radiation exposure. In the final stage, individuals exposed to low doses of radiation for a short period of time usually recover. Death is common, however, for those who were exposed to higher levels of radiation or to low levels for an extended period of time (CDC, 2014c).

The Role of the Nurse in Radiation Events

The role of nurses and other healthcare providers during a radiological event is multifaceted. Although transfer of radioactive material from a contaminated client is rare, healthcare providers should evaluate any possible self-contamination prior to treating the client (see **Sidebar 11-12**). After the possibility of self-contamination has been eliminated, the nurse should remove the client's clothing by cutting and rolling the clothing away from the face. Once the clothes have been removed they should be placed in a double bag and closed and labeled as hazardous material. The next step is for the nurse to cleanse possible contaminated body areas with saline water. If facial contamination has occurred, eyes, nose, and mouth need to be flushed. Wounds may need to be covered with a waterproof dressing. Clients who are able to stand may be able to be decontaminated in a showering facility (CDC, 2014c). Some situations require triage of clients to prioritize those who need immediate treatment.

> **SIDEBAR 11-12**
>
> Health effects of radiation exposure vary depending on the dose and the length of exposure. Health effects can vary from mild to severe and can take days, months, or years to develop. Some studies, for example, have shown that radiation may increase the risk for cancer later in life (CDC, 2014c).

During most radiological events that require medical attention, nurses may be involved in supportive care, surveillance, treatment of primary burns, secondary infections, pain management, and follow-up for mental health support. Immediately after the event, the airway should be secured, and the client should be monitored closely for respiratory and circulatory status, blood pressure, blood gases, and other physiological markers. Clients need to be followed or closely monitored after the initial evaluation. Nurses' role may also include client education on the treatment being provided or on mechanisms to prevent secondary effects such as an infection.

Summary

The role of the nurse during emergency-related events is multifaceted. Nurses should have a role in planning and training within their organizations. In response, nurses may be required to triage patients based on symptoms, provide first-aid assistance, support an evacuation shelter, administer medications, and provide needed psychological assistance among other things. Given the risk of catastrophic disasters, nurses should consider preparing themselves beyond their workplace structure to work in austere conditions, such as through courses like Wilderness First Aid (American Academy of Orthopaedic Surgeons, 2015). This kind of training prepares one for handling medical emergencies when help is hours or even days away, a reality of catastrophic disaster situations.

Biological, chemical, and radiological events have occurred throughout history and still pose a serious threat today. Natural disasters such as hurricanes, tornadoes, and severe weather have resulted in the need for better emergency planning and preparation. The overall goal of disaster preparedness activities, the NIMS, and ICS is to provide awareness and an infrastructure for local, state, and federal agencies to prepare their communities and provide assistance before, during, and after an emergency to improve health and safety outcomes. Nurse activities in disaster preparedness are aligned to protect the public's health through a reduction in morbidity and mortality.

In most states, epidemiologists are employed to conduct outbreak investigations; however, at the local level nurses play a significant role in conducting investigations, communicating with the public, providing direct care, conducting surveillance, and interpreting early data trends. In addition to outbreak investigations, nurses follow up on isolated cases of a particular communicable disease such as tuberculosis, hepatitis, or HIV, as required by the state. Nurses assist with obtaining laboratory specimens for investigative interpretation of results. Local, state, and federal health agencies conduct regular surveillance on a number of reportable or notifiable diseases. Nurses may also be in charge of tracking diseases within a specific area or community and reporting those numbers to the state health department, which in turns reports regularly to the CDC.

In conclusion, nurses play key roles in disaster preparedness, planning, and response for a wide range of events including biological, chemical, and radiologic emergencies as well as natural disasters and outbreaks. Nurses must collaborate with other public healthcare professionals at the local, state, and federal levels to protect the safety and health of the nation and decrease morbidity and mortality during emergencies.

Reflective Practice Questions

1. Name three specific natural disasters that may cause the need for emergency planning and response activities.
2. Identify three Category A agents that may be used in a bioterrorism event.
3. What is the disaster plan at the agency where you practice? Would the personnel and supply resources sustain the community for the initial 24 hours of a disaster? How are nurses mobilized in the disaster plan? What changes would you suggest in the disaster plan?
4. You are working with families with infants and young children in hurricane-prone Florida on a public health education project. You need to create a meal plan with suggested emergency food sources that would sustain the family for 5 days without electricity. What meals would you plan and what dry foods should the family have stored for emergencies?
5. Who would you engage as partners in order to prepare a disaster preparedness and response plan for tornadoes in a trailer park for low-income families?
6. List some secondary events that may be involved with natural disasters.
7. Describe a potential role of a nurse in an incident using the ICS framework.

References

Abrams, L. G., & Pacific Northwest Annual Conference Disaster Response Team. (2009). *Master plan for disaster preparedness, response, and recovery.* Retrieved from https://s3.amazonaws.com/PNWUMC/Disaster+Response/pnwplan.pdf

Agency for Toxic Substances and Disease Registry. (1999). *Public health statement: Ionizing radiation.* Atlanta, GA: U.S. Department of Health and Human Services, Public Health Service. Retrieved from http://www.atsdr.cdc.gov/phs/phs.asp?id=482&tid=86

American Academy of Orthopaedic Surgeons. (2015). *Wilderness first aid: Emergency care in remote locations.* Burlington, MA: Jones and Bartlett Learning.

American Red Cross. (2015a). *Build a kit.* Retrieved from http://www.redcross.org/prepare/location/home-family/get-kit

American Red Cross. (2015b). *Red Cross shelters: FAQ.* Retrieved from https://intranet.redcross.org/content/redcross/categories/outreach/media-public/disaster-messaging/responding-to-disasters/faq-red-cross-shelters.html

Association of Public Health Nurses. (2014) *The role of the public health nurse in disaster preparedness, response and recovery: A position paper.* Retrieved from http://www.achne.org/files/public/APHN_RoleOfPHNinDisasterPRR_FINALJan14.pdf

Beach, M. (2010). *Disaster preparedness and management.* Philadelphia, PA: F.A. Davis.

Blanchard, W. (2007). *Guide to emergency management and related terms, definitions, concepts, acronyms, organizations, programs, guidance, executive orders & legislation: A tutorial on emergency management, broadly defined, past and present.* Retrieved from https://training.fema.gov/hiedu/docs/terms%20and%20definitions/terms%20and%20definitions.pdf

Branson, R., Johannigman, J., Daughtery, E., & Rubinson, L. (2008). Surge capacity mechanical ventilation. *Respiratory Care, 53*(1), 78–90.

Centers for Disease Control and Prevention. (2000). Biological and chemical terrorism: Strategic plan for preparedness and response. *Morbidity and Mortality Weekly Report, 49*(RR04);1–14.

Centers for Disease Control and Prevention. (2001a). Recognition of illness associated with the intentional release of a biologic agent. *Morbidity and Mortality Weekly Report, 50*(41):893–897.

Centers for Disease Control and Prevention. (2001b). Update: Investigation of anthrax associated with intentional exposure and interim public health guidelines. *Morbidity and Mortality Weekly Report, 50*(41), 889–893.

Centers for Disease Control and Prevention. (2001c). Update: Investigation of bioterrorism-related anthrax and interim guidelines for exposure management and antimicrobial therapy. *Morbidity and Mortality Weekly Report, 50*(42), 909–919.

Centers for Disease Control and Prevention. (2003). Nicotine poisoning after ingestion of contaminated ground beef—Michigan, 2003. *Morbidity and Mortality Weekly Report, 52*(18), 413–416.

Centers for Disease Control and Prevention. (2004). *Facts about pneumonic plague.* Retrieved from http://emergency.cdc.gov/agent/plague/factsheet.asp

Centers for Disease Control and Prevention. (2005). Public health consequences from hazardous substances acutely released during rail transit—South Carolina, 2005; selected states, 1999–2004. *Morbidity and Mortality Weekly Report, 54*(3), 64–67.

Centers for Disease Control and Prevention. (2007a). Acanthamoeba keratitis multiple states, 2005–2007. *Morbidity and Mortality Weekly Report, 56*(21), 532–534.

Centers for Disease Control and Prevention. (2007b). *Smallpox disease overview.* Retrieved from http://emergency.cdc.gov/agent/smallpox/overview/disease-facts.asp

Centers for Disease Control and Prevention. (2009a). *Anthrax.* Retrieved from http://www.cdc.gov/nczved/divisions/dfbmd/diseases/anthrax/technical.html

Centers for Disease Control and Prevention. (2009b). *Public water systems FAQ.* Retrieved from http://www.cdc.gov/healthywater/drinking/public/faq.html

Centers for Disease Control and Prevention. (2011a). *Climate change and extreme heat events.* Retrieved from http://www.cdc.gov/climateandhealth/pubs/ClimateChangeand ExtremeHeatEvents.pdf

Centers for Disease Control and Prevention. (2011b). *Warning signs and symptoms of heat-related illness.* Retrieved from https://www.cdc.gov/extremeheat/warning.html

Centers for Disease Control and Prevention. (2012). Tornado-related fatalities—Five states, southeastern United States, April 25–28, 2011. *Morbidity and Mortality Weekly Report, 61*(28), 529–533.

Centers for Disease Control and Prevention. (2013a). *Chemical emergencies overview.* Retrieved from https://emergency.cdc.gov/chemical/overview.asp

Centers for Disease Control and Prevention. (2013b). *Emergency response resources: Workplace safety and health topics.* Retrieved from http://www.cdc.gov/niosh/topics/emres/ppe.html

Centers for Disease Control and Prevention. (2014a). *After a tornado.* Retrieved https://www.cdc.gov/disasters/tornadoes/after.html

Centers for Disease Control and Prevention. (2014b). *Emergency wound management for healthcare professionals.* Retrieved from http://www.cdc.gov/disasters/emergwoundhcp.html

Centers for Disease Control and Prevention. (2014c). *Possible health effects of radiation exposure and contamination.* Retrieved from http://emergency.cdc.gov/radiation/healtheffects.asp

Centers for Disease Control and Prevention. (2014d). *2014 West Virginia chemical release.* Retrieved from https://emergency.cdc.gov/chemical/MCHM/westvirginia2014/

Centers for Disease Control and Prevention. (2015a). *Disaster training and response.* Retrieved from http://www.cdc.gov/nceh/hsb/disaster/training.htm

Centers for Disease Control and Prevention. (2015b). *Extreme heat prevention guide.* Retrieved from http://www.cdc.gov/nceh/hsb/disaster/training.htm

Centers for Disease Control and Prevention. (2015c). *Frequently asked questions about extreme heat.* Retrieved from http://www.cdc.gov/disasters/extremeheat/faq.html

Centers for Disease Control and Prevention. (2015d). *Health Alert Network.* Retrieved from http://emergency.cdc.gov/HAN/index.asp

Centers for Disease Control and Prevention. (2015e). *Hypothermia.* Retrieved from http://www.cdc.gov/disasters/winter/index.html

Centers for Disease Control and Prevention. (2015f). *Transmission of tularemia.* Retrieved from http://www.cdc.gov/tularemia/transmission

Centers for Disease Control and Prevention. (2016a). *About Zika.* Retrieved from http://www.cdc.gov/zika/about/index.html

Centers for Disease Control and Prevention. (2016b). *Botulism.* Retrieved from http://www.cdc.gov/botulism

Centers for Disease Control and Prevention. (2016c). *Climate change and health effects wheel.* Retrieved from http://www.cdc.gov/climateandhealth/effects/

Central United States Earthquake Consortium. (2015). *New Madrid Seismic Zone.* Retrieved from www.cusec.org

Cross, B., & Pruitt, S. (2013). Dark knights rising: The Aurora Theater and Newtown massacres and shareholder wealth. *Journal of Criminal Justice, 41*(6). doi: 10.1016/j.jcrimjus.2013.09.002

Demidchick, Y., Drozd, V., & Biko, J. (2009). Thyroid cancer in infants and adolescents after Chernobyl. *Minerva Endocrinologica.* Retrieved from https://www.researchgate.net/profile/Yuri_Demidchik/publication/

Dictionary.com (n.d.). Disaster [Def. 1]. In *Dictionary.com.* Retrieved from http://www.dictionary.com/browse/disaster?s=t

Federal Emergency Management Agency. (2004). *Position paper: NIMS and the Incident Command System.* Retrieved from http://www.fema.gov/txt/nims/nims_ics_position_paper.txt

Federal Emergency Management Agency. (2011). *Tornado outbreak of 2011 in Alabama, Georgia, Mississippi, Tennessee, and Missouri: EF scale summary.* Retrieved from http://www.fema.gov/media-library-data/20130726-1827-25045-7585/tornado_mat_app_e_508.pdf

Federal Emergency Management Agency. (2015). National Incident Management System. Retrieved from http://www.fema.gov/national-incident-management-system

Federal Emergency Management Agency. (n.d.). *Hurricane.* Retrieved from http://m.fema.gov/hurricane

Federal Emergency Management Agency, & Emergency Management Institute. (2008). Incident Command System training: ICS review material. Retrieved from http://www.training.fema.gov/emiweb/is/icsresource/assets/reviewmaterials.pdf

Field, C., Barros, V., Stocker, T., & Dahe, Q. (2012). *Managing the risks of extreme events and disasters to advance climate change adaptation.* New York, NY: Cambridge University Press.

Food and Drug Administration. (2002). Title I–*National preparedness for bioterrorism and other public health emergencies.* Retrieved from http://www.fda.gov/RegulatoryInformation/Legislation/ucm155733.htm

Food and Drug Administration. (2013). *FDA releases new tool to help prevent intentional food contamination* [Press release]. Retrieved from http://www.fda.gov/NewsEvents/Newsroom/PressAnnouncements/ucm352093.htm

Goldfinger, C., Nelson, C. H., Morey, A. E., Johnson, J. R., Patton, J., Karabanov, E., . . .Vallier, T. (2012). *Turbidite event history—Methods and implications for Holocene paleoseismicity of the Cascadia subduction zone.* U.S. Geological Survey Professional Paper 1661–F, 170.

Health Facilities Management. (2014). Emergency management survey. Retrieved from www.hfmmagazine.com

Healthy Communities. (2015). *Food safety tips in power loss.* Retrieved from http://www.healthcommunities.com/food-safety/keep-foods-safe-lose-power.shtml

International Council of Nurses. (2006). *Position statement: Nurses and disaster preparedness.* Geneva, Switzerland: International Council of Nurses.

Jones, J. (2006). Mother nature's disasters and their health effects: A literature review. *Nursing Forum, 41*, 78–87. doi: 10.1111/j.1744-6198.2006.00041.

Kaiser Family Foundation. (2016). Total number of professionally active nurses. Retrieved from http://kff.org/other/state-indicator/total-registered-nurses/

McFee, R. (2009). Death by Polonium-210: Lessons learned from the murder of former Soviet spy Alexander Litvinenko. *Seminars in Diagnostic Pathology, 26*(1), 61–67. doi: 10.1053/j.semdp.2008.12.003

National Hurricane Center. (2014). *Tropical cyclone climatology.* National Oceanic and Atmospheric Administration. Retrieved from http://www.nhc.noaa.gov/climo/

National Hurricane Center, & National Oceanic and Atmospheric Administration. (n.d.). Saffir-Simpson Hurricane Wind Scale. Retrieved from http://www.nhc.noaa.gov/aboutsshws.php

National Institute of Allergy and Infectious Disease. (2015). *Plague.* Retrieved from http://www.niaid.nih.gov/topics/plague/Pages/Default.aspx

National Oceanic and Atmospheric Administration. (2011). *The historic tornados of April, 2011.* Silver Spring, MD: U.S. Department of Commerce. Retrieved from http://www.nws.noaa.gov/om/assessments/pdfs/historic_tornadoes.pdf

National Oceanic and Atmospheric Administration. (2016). 2016 Severe Weather Awareness Campaign kickoff March 6–12. Retrieved from http://www.srh.noaa.gov/sjt/?n=svrwx_awareness

National Severe Storms Laboratory. (2015). *Severe weather 101: Tornado basics.* Retrieved from http://www.nssl.noaa.gov/education/svrwx101/tornadoes/

Oates, S. B. (1994). *A woman of valor: Clara Barton and the Civil War.* New York: Free Press.

Occupational Safety and Health Administration. (n.d.) *Infectious disease.* Retrieved from https://www.osha.gov/SLTC/healthcarefacilities/infectious_diseases.html#additional_agents

Office of Disaster Preparedness and Management. (2013). *Levels 1 to 3.* Government of the Republic of Trinidad and Tobago. Retrieved from http://www.odpm.gov.tt/node/66

Phillips, M. B. (2005). Bioterrorism: A brief history. *Northeast Florida Medicine, 56*(1), 32–35.

Polivka, B., Chaudry, R., & MacCrawford, J. (2012). Public health nurses' knowledge and attitudes regarding climate change. *Environmental Health Perspectives, 120*(3), 321–325. doi: 10.1289/ehp.1104025

Ratzan, S., & Moritsugu, K. (2014). Ebola crisis—Communication chaos we can avoid. *Journal of Health Communication: International Perspectives, 19*(11), 1213–1215. doi: 10.1080/10810730.2014.977680

Sacco, W., Navin, M., Fiedler,, K., Waddell, R., Long, W., & Buckman, R. (2005). Precise formulation and evidence-based application of resource-constrained triage. *Journal for the Society of Academic Emergency Medicine, 12*(8), 759–770.

Sheth, A. N., Hoekstra, M., Patel, N., Ewald, G., Lord, C., Clarke, C. & Zink, D. (2011). A national outbreak of Salmonella serotype Tennessee infections from contaminated peanut butter: A new food vehicle for salmonellosis in the United States. *Clinical Infectious Diseases, 53*(4), 356–362. doi: 10.1093/cid/cir407

Sjöstedt, A. (2007), Tularemia: History, epidemiology, pathogen physiology, and clinical manifestations. *Annals of the New York Academy of Sciences, 1105*, 1–29. doi: 10.1196/ annals.1409.009

The Joint Commission. (n.d.). *Guidance for disaster.* Retrieved from http://www.disaster preparation.net/resources.html

United Nations International Strategy for Disaster Reduction. (2009). *Terminology for disaster risk reduction.* Retrieved from https://www.unisdr.org/we/inform/terminology

U.S. Geological Survey. (2012). Retrieved from www.usgs.gov

Veenema, T. G. (2006). Expanding educational opportunities in disaster response and emergency preparedness for nurses. *Nursing Education Perspectives, 27*(2), 93–99.

Wang, Y. (2015, December 15). In Flint, Mich., there's so much lead in children's blood that a state of emergency is declared. *Washington Post.* Retrieved from https://www .washingtonpost.com/news/morning-mix/wp/2015/12/15/toxic-water-soaring-lead -levels-in-childrens-blood-create-state-of-emergency-in-flint-mich/

World Health Organization. (2013). *Health risk assessment from the nuclear accident after the 2011 Great East Japan earthquake and tsunami, based on a preliminary dose estimation.* Geneva, Switzerland: Author. Retrieved from http://apps.who.int/iris/bitstream/10665/78373/1 /WHO_HSE_PHE_2013.1_eng.pdf?ua=1

World Health Organization. (2015a). *Disease outbreaks.* Retrieved from http://www.who .int/topics/disease_outbreaks/en/

World Health Organization. (2015b). *Smallpox.* Retrieved from http://www.who.int/csr /disease/smallpox/en/

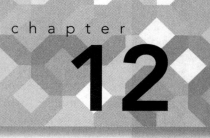

The Healthy Nurse: Finding the Balance

Jo-Ann Stankus, Paula Clutter, and Peggy Mancuso

LEARNING OUTCOMES

After reading this chapter you will be able to:

- Define health as the concept relates to the individual nurse.
- Describe the biopsychosocial model of health.
- Discuss the health implications of nutrition, sleep, activity, smoking cessation, and psychosocial well-being as they relate to the individual nurse within the nursing community.
- Discuss psychological stress, fatigue, addiction, and workplace safety issues that occur in the nursing workplace environment.
- Discuss challenges and solutions to improved health of the nursing workforce.

Introduction

Historically, medical textbooks focused on health and illness as opposite states. These two entities were portrayed as two opposing ends of a continuum within the spectrum of life and death was the ultimate marker for disease. Medical education was constructed around the biomedical model or the physiological and pathological causes of disease. Throughout this time, however, nursing education emphasized that professional nurses do more than care for those who face illness and disease. Nurses focus on families as participants in the healthcare team and promote the health of entire communities. As Florence Nightingale noted in 1859, "Surgery removes the bullet out of the limb, which is an obstruction to cure, but nature heals the wound. So it is with medicine; the function of an organ becomes obstructed; medicine, so far as we know, assists nature to remove the obstruction, but does nothing more. And what nursing has to do in either case, is to put the patient in the best condition for nature to act upon him." Nightingale realized that "nature" and "health" were irretrievably interrelated and could not be separated. The further question would be how to *know* health; what does health *look like*? In 1948 the World Health Organization defined health as "a state of complete physical, mental and social well-being and not merely the absence of disease or infirmity" (p. 100). In today's world, how do nurses attain and maintain health while they continue to promote health in those individuals in their care?

From birth to death, the concepts of care and compassion are interwoven into the many courses of the nursing curriculum. Current nursing coursework emphasizes health promotion, prevention of disease, and interventions to treat and rehabilitate patients, their families, and their communities. Nevertheless, in most nursing classrooms, the concepts of health, wellness, and illness are discussed and applied to patients and their families, with little focus on the health of the individual nurse. The insight that a healthy nurse has the ability to provide optimum care to others, and this ability is compromised if that nurse is overly fatigued or ill, is often overlooked. Advice about stress relief may be provided to nursing students, perhaps with added information about effective study habits. Nurses who work in hospitals must attend safety lectures and are required to receive a yearly flu vaccine. Nevertheless, nurses as primary caregivers often do not allow themselves enough time for self-health behaviors because they are focused on caring for others.

Sartorius (2006) noted, "Today, three types of definition of health seem to be possible and are used. The first is that health is the absence of any disease or impairment. The second is that health is a state that allows the individual to cope adequately with all demands of daily life (also implying the absence of disease and impairment). The third definition states that health is a state of balance, an equilibrium that an individual has established within himself and between himself and his social and physical environment" (p. 1). The third definition is the one that applies to nurses today as the nurse must balance "healthy altruism" with the potential for harm to the self, or "compassion fatigue." The American Nurses Association (ANA) defines a **healthy nurse** "as one who actively focuses on creating and maintaining a *balance and synergy* of physical, intellectual, emotional, social, spiritual, personal, and professional well-being. Healthy nurses live life to the fullest capacity, across the wellness/illness continuum, as they become stronger role models, advocates, and educators, personally, for

KEY TERM

Healthy nurse: The creating and maintaining of a balance and synergy of physical, intellectual, emotional, social, spiritual, personal, and professional well-being (ANA, n.d., para. 1).

their families, their communities and work environments, and ultimately for their patients" (ANA, n.d., para. 1).

The ANA in conjunction with Pfizer conducted a survey of nurses and nursing students about being a healthy nurse. The Health Risk Appraisal (HRA) was originally administered during 2013 and 2014, and ANA continues to solicit survey participants. The preliminary results of this survey allow nurses to get a glimpse at what health issues are faced by nurses and ways to improve their lives to be a health example for the patients under their care. Preliminary findings of the survey are indicated in **Box 12-1**.

Nursing is an occupation that requires a healthy mind, body, and spirit to render compassionate and safe care. Through experience, education, and training, nurses can learn healthy adaptation strategies. Ideally, nurses model health as they support healthy behaviors in their patients. If nurses are not "healthy" in mind, body, or spirit, how does their "illness" manifest itself in the ability to care for others? What happens to a nurse who is no longer able to render high-quality care to others due to illness, compassion fatigue, burnout, or occupational stress? What happens to

---

BOX 12–1   HEALTH RISK APPRAISAL FINDINGS

- The nurse respondents (82 percent) perceived that workplace stress was the highest ranked risk factor.
- The nurse respondents were concerned about the risk of injury from lifting and repositioning patients or equipment.
- Bullying and incivility in the workplace are prevalent (43 percent), as are physical assaults by patients or their family members.
- Many participants (more than 50 percent) reported heavy workloads that often necessitate working outside scheduled work hours to complete tasks, such as arriving early to work and/or staying late.
- The majority of participants are above their ideal weight range (average body mass index [BMI] was 28, which is in the "overweight" category) for their height.
- A significant personal safety risk identified is distracted driving, such as talking on the phone while driving (60 percent), eating while driving (53 percent), and texting while driving (16 percent).
- Participants reported being diagnosed by their healthcare provider with lower back pain (34 percent).
- About 20 percent eat five or more servings of fruits or vegetables per day, and 35 percent eat three or more servings of whole grains daily.
- On the positive side, most participants said they had access to worksite wellness and health promotion programs. A very low percentage said they smoke cigarettes, and 94 percent do not smoke cigarettes at all. Of those who do smoke, 56 percent are actively trying to quit.

Data from American Nurses Association. (2015b). *Health Risk Appraisal (HRA). Preliminary findings October 2013–October 2014. Executive summary.* Silver Spring, MD: Author. Retrieved from http://nursingworld.org /HRA-Executive-Summary

the newly graduated nurse who is trying to adapt to the caregiver role during the first employment year? How do the nursing students react to the constant stressors and challenges that they face in nursing school? How do nurses stay healthy? The purpose of this chapter is to focus on health issues for nursing professionals to maintain their own health.

The Biopsychosocial Health Perspective

In 1946, a young physician named George Engel conducted an unorthodox experiment on a 1-year-old girl named Baby Monica (Engel, 1977). Baby Monica was born with esophageal atresia, and she had a temporary gastrostomy tube placed while she was waiting for surgical repair of the defect. Dr. Engel and a colleague played "friendly doctor" and "somber doctor" as they interacted with the little girl. The outcome measure for this psychological experiment was the amount of Baby Monica's gastric secretion volume. When the "friendly doctor" entered the room, gastric secretions flowed abundantly. When Dr. Engel, "the somber doctor," entered the room, Baby Monica's gastric secretions stopped. This simple experiment provided evidence that the mind and the emotions that accompany human interactions produced measurable physiological changes in the body. The mind and the body

KEY TERM

Biopsychosocial model of health: The dynamic interaction of three levels—biological, psychological, and social aspects of health—that affect an individual's well-being.

were not separate. In 1977, Dr. Engel published his findings in the journal *Science,* and the **biopsychosocial model of health** became the new paradigm, thus providing new dimensions to the prevailing biomedical world view. Dr. Engel proposed that the biopsychosocial aspects of an individual represented different systems, with each system being encompassed by and influencing other systems, beginning from the very atoms within each human and culminating with the biosphere of the planet.

In 1980, Engel noted, "How physicians approach patients and the problems they present is very much influenced by the conceptual models in relationship to which their knowledge and experience are organized" (p. 535). Even so, nursing philosophies and theories help guide a nurse's thinking and practice, a practice that is based on evidence collected over time and founded on holism. Holistic human health focuses on the entire human being—including the biopsychosocial and spiritual interrelationships among individuals, families, and communities. Optimal health is achieved through balance and synchrony of these intertwined states of being. The philosophical perspectives of Florence Nightingale, Virginia Henderson, and Jean Watson teach about how the environment can positively or negatively affect health. The nursing care models of Dorothea Orem, Imogene King, and Sister Calista Roy focused on enabling individuals to care for themselves within the context of their environment, their relationships with others, and their capabilities to adapt to change. Spirituality was incorporated into the model of nursing care through the work of Henderson and Watson, and many

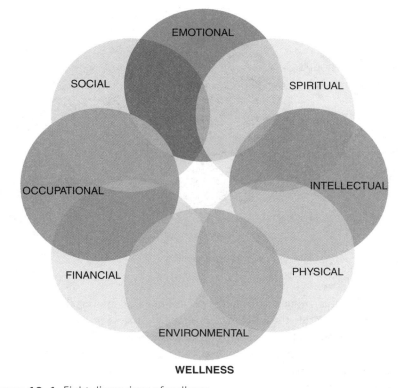

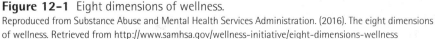

WELLNESS

Figure 12-1 Eight dimensions of wellness.
Reproduced from Substance Abuse and Mental Health Services Administration. (2016). The eight dimensions of wellness. Retrieved from http://www.samhsa.gov/wellness-initiative/eight-dimensions-wellness

epidemiological studies support the proposition that the longest lived populations are those who affirm a spiritual purpose in life (Buettner, 2009; Perry-Black, 2014; Poulain et al., 2004).

The biopsychosocial-spiritual model of health is most commonly illustrated as overlapping circles, such as the eight dimensions of wellness presented in **Figure 12-1**.

Inherent within this conceptualization of the physical, psychological, social, and spiritual aspects of health is the proposition that each area influences the other parts of the model. All four aspects of health function are interdependent. Balance and synchronicity are implied assumptions of the model. An imbalance in any of the four areas will affect the other three, thus affecting their whole being. As a nurse, this imbalance can emerge as the inability to render high-quality care to others. **Figure 12-2** depicts a more innovative way to view this model in that it allows movement in and out of each system, just like everyday life.

Life is not static; life is constantly changing, and these changes can force balance or imbalance at any given point in time, thus creating a dynamic state that

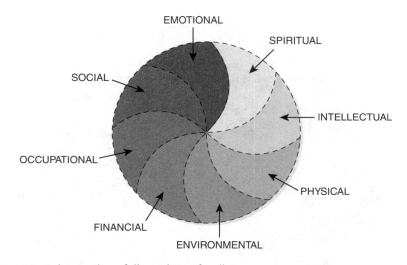

Figure 12-2 Interaction of dimensions of wellness.

affects health status. Influences from the environment or emotional changes leave biochemical trails within the individual, producing physiological changes and vice versa, with physiological changes affecting emotional, social, and spiritual aspects of health. Thinking about a stressful event may increase cortisol levels as much as experiencing the stressful event, as evidenced by posttraumatic stress disorder with both the traumatic experience and thoughts about the traumatic experience impairing health and well-being.

The manifestation of the biopsychosocial model is observed through behavior, and behaviors provide evidence of the biopsychosocial-spiritual factors that can be individually controlled or changed. Individual behaviors are vital to the creation of a healthy life. According to Dr. Jason Satterfield, "Behavior accounts for approximately 40% of premature mortality. Genetics accounts for about 30% while social factors account for about 15%. The environment accounts for only 5 percent, and health care accounts for only 10%. Together, behavior and social factors account for about 55% of premature mortality" (Satterfield, 2013, p. 26). Behaviors that affect the health of an individual nurse include choices related to nutrition, sleep, activity, and psychosocial well-being.

Health and the Individual Nurse

Nursing is the largest healthcare profession in the United States with more than 3,100,000 registered nurses (RNs; American Association of Colleges of Nursing, 2011). Nursing is a rewarding and challenging career field with opportunities to serve in a variety of specialty areas. Nurses value the capability to apply critical thinking skills through nursing interventions that alleviate suffering and improve well-being. Being part of a patient's life is an emotional and meaningful experience. A more tangible aspect of nursing as a career is the financial rewards of a nursing career. According to the May 2015 Occupational Employment and Wages data, RNs working in general medical and surgical hospitals had an average salary of $72,980 (U.S. Department of Labor, 2016). In general, RN salaries increase as nurses attain higher levels of education, engage in nursing specialty roles, assume increased job responsibilities, and advance through the nursing professional career ladders.

Although the positive aspects of nursing far outweigh the negative aspects, being a nurse is often physically and emotionally demanding. Creating and maintaining the balance and synergy of physical, intellectual, emotional, social, spiritual, personal, and professional well-being are vital skills needed by the "healthy nurse" (American Nurses Association, n.d.-a). What makes some nurses healthier than other nurses? Healthy People 2020 states personal, social, economic, and environmental factors can influence the health status of individuals and these characteristics are known as determinants of health (U.S. Department of Health and Human Services, n.d.-b).

Biological and genetic determinants of health such as age, sex, and family history of heart disease are difficult to alter. Nevertheless, a genetic tendency toward disease does not necessarily mean that a particular pathology is inevitable; and more epigenetic influences are being discovered that affect how, when, or if a particular gene is "turned on." Focusing on social and physical determinants that can affect individual behavior and health status should be addressed. Many nurses experience those positive social and physical determinants related to optimal health. These include the privilege of engaging in a career with meaningful, steady employment, good wages and benefits, and a home in a safe neighborhood, as well as generally working in safe environments. Nevertheless, negative changes in social and physical determinants of health can affect an individual's current state of health and induce negative outcomes. For example, a nurse's perception of a stressful work environment often causes that nurse to experience increased anxiety, anger, or depression, which affect that nurse's well-being and work performance.

The ANA (2015a) Code of Ethics provides a guide for professional nursing. Provision 2 of the ANA Code of Ethics states "the nurse's primary commitment is to the patient, whether an individual, family, group or community" (p. 4). An important part of nursing is providing patient-centered care. Nurses care for others but must also care for themselves by adhering to a healthy lifestyle. Provision 5 of the ANA Code of Ethics proposed that, "The nurse owes the same duties to self as to others, including the responsibility to preserve integrity and safety, to maintain competence, and to continue personal and professional growth" (p. 19). Self-care behaviors such as eating a healthy diet, getting proper physical exercise, obtaining sufficient sleep, and attending to social and spiritual needs address Provision 5 (Lachman, Swanson, & Winland-Brown, 2015).

An important nursing role is to provide patient education regarding health and wellness. Nurses should be knowledgeable about the 42 topic areas with more than 1,200 objectives in Healthy People 2020 that provides a comprehensive set of national goals and objectives for improving the health of all Americans over a 10-year period (U.S. Department of Health and Human Services, n.d.-a). Healthy People 2020 emphasizes that proper nutrition, physical activity, and a healthy body weight are essential elements of an individual's overall health and well-being. Health implications that focus on these elements can decrease an individual's risk of developing serious health problems, such as hypertension, hypercholesterolemia, obesity, diabetes, heart disease, stroke, and cancer.

Nutrition and the Nurse

The nurse provides patient education regarding maintaining a healthy diet, regular physical activity, and achieving and maintaining a healthy weight. In order to be an effective role model, the nurse must also exhibit behaviors of the healthy lifestyle, through exercise, beneficial nutrition, and maintenance of a body mass index in the normal range. Addressing a patient's obesity and discussing interventions to manage the excessive weight can be a sensitive topic for the nurse and the patient. To compound this issue, patients might not view the overweight nurse as credible if the nurse does not model self-care behaviors. As a result, patients might not be motivated to change personal health behaviors.

As noted in Box 12-1, the majority of nurse respondents to the ANA Health Risk Appraisal reported a BMI of 28, which would mean that nurses, like most U.S. residents, contribute to the nationwide obesity epidemic. Purposeful marketing of unhealthy foods and beverages, genetic or hormonal alterations of food sources, changing cultural norms, and decreased activity relate to ever-increasing prevalence of overweight and obesity in many industrialized nations (Gortmaker et al., 2011). As current demographic trends indicate, weight control is difficult for both individuals and populations. Raaijmakers, Pouwels, Berghuis, and Nienhuijs (2015) performed a systematic review of current weight loss strategies for those with a BMI of 25 or above. Effective interventions were those that included a combination of self-monitoring, counseling, communication, group support, structured nutritional plans, and individual support. Several of the studies reviewed involved web-based approaches, such as nutrition diaries (e.g., MyFitnessPal food diary—www.myfitnesspal.com) or online support groups (e.g., SparkPeople—www.SparkPeople.com). Two nonprofit nutritional guides, the Dietary Approaches to Stop Hypertension (DASH) diet and the Therapeutic Life Style (TLC) Diet, have been consistently ranked as the most beneficial approaches to general overall health, including weight loss. The commercial diet, Weight Watchers, has been ranked first at successful, long-term (1 year or more) weight loss program (Haupt, 2016). Nursing students and RNs live in a real world characterized by stress and lack of time. As such, weight management and optimal nutrition are best achieved by setting realistic goals, maintaining fitness, avoidance of weight gain, and cultivating the dieting skills of self-monitoring and stimulus control.

Smoking and the Nurse

In a 2002–2010 survey of behaviors of health professionals, licensed practical/vocational nurses were the members of the healthcare professions who reported the highest prevalence of smoking (24.9 percent), with physicians reporting the lowest prevalence of smoking at 1.95 percent (Sarna, Bialous, Nandy, Antonio, & Yang, 2014). On a positive note, RNs were the only group that reported a significant decline (11.14 percent to 7.09 percent) in smoking rates from the years 2006–2007 to 2010–2011. The Tobacco Free Nurses (n.d.) was the first national program focused on assisting nurses to quit smoking. This program provides nurses with the education and resources needed to help their patients quit smoking as well. Those nurses who successfully quit smoking become powerful role models who can share their experiences with their patients. Nurses have significant opportunities to promote and provide smoking cessation interventions and reduce tobacco use, thus addressing the goals of Healthy People 2020.

Sleep and the Nurse

Sleep is another significant aspect of health. The ANA defines healthy sleep as at least 7 hours of daily comfortable and restorative rest. Adequate sleep is vital to all humans, but sleep is especially important for nurses. In order to function effectively, nurses must obtain the many benefits associated with healthy sleep patterns. These benefits include increased energy, enhanced concentration, alertness, positive mood, increased stamina, heightened motivation, better judgment, and improved learning (American Nurses Association, 2014).

Nurses who work off-peak shifts are vulnerable to sleep deprivation. Health issues related to constant sleep deprivation include heart disease, gastrointestinal problems, diabetes, and mood disorders. Sleep deprivation could affect a nurse's ability to maintain positive interpersonal communication with patients and other healthcare professionals. More significantly, sleep deprivation is a safety issue that can have an impact on the nurse's decision-making ability and judgment, resulting in missed care, medication or treatment errors, and subsequent harm to the patient. Finally, fatigue increases the probability that a shift worker, such as a nurse, will experience a car accident related to sleep deprivation following the end of the 12-hour shift (American Nurses Association, 2014). Both the ANA and the National Sleep Foundation have determined that the following interventions promote sleep for shift workers (see **Box 12-2**).

BOX 12-2   STRATEGIES TO PROMOTE HEALTHY SLEEP

General Strategies
- Avoid nicotine.
- Keep a consistent bedtime and routine.
- Avoid alcohol and caffeine prior to bedtime.
- Engage in relaxing activities prior to bedtime such as prayer, warm bath, calming music, reading.
- Get comfortable with a supportive mattress and adequate pillows.
- Ensure your room is dark, quiet (unless you prefer soft music or white noise), and a cool but comfortable temperature.
- If you're anxiety prone, keep a pad of paper by bed to write down your worries, then let them go until morning.
- Neither starve nor stuff yourself prior to bedtime.
- Exercise earlier in the day to promote better sleep.

Strategies for Shift Workers
- Avoid long commutes and extended hours as much as possible.
- Work with others to help keep yourself alert.
- Try to be active during breaks (e.g., take a walk or exercise).
- Drink a caffeinated beverage (coffee, tea, colas) to help maintain alertness during the shift.

- Don't leave the most tedious or boring tasks to the end of your shift when you are apt to feel the drowsiest. Night shift workers are most sleepy around 4:00–5:00 a.m.
- Exchange ideas with your colleagues on ways to cope with the problems of shift work. Set up a support group at work so that you can discuss these issues and learn from each other.

Strategies for Day Sleeping
- Wear dark glasses to block out the sunlight on your way home.
- Keep to the same bedtime and wake time schedule, even on weekends.
- Eliminate noise and light from your sleep environment (use eye masks and ear plugs).
- Avoid caffeinated beverages and foods close to bedtime.
- Avoid alcohol; although it may seem to improve sleep initially, tolerance develops quickly and it will soon disturb sleep.

Data from American Nurses Association. (n.d.-b). *Healthy sleep.* Retrieved from http://www.nursingworld.org/HealthySleep; National Sleep Foundation. (n.d.). *Shift work and sleep.* Retrieved from https://sleepfoundation.org/sleep-topics /shift-work-and-sleep

Activity and the Nurse

Physical activity improves general health and fitness and decreases the risk for many chronic diseases including cardiovascular disease, diabetes, and cancers (Centers for Disease Control and Prevention, 2015). In *Physical Activity Guidelines for Americans* (U.S. Department of Health and Human Services, 2008), the Centers for Disease Control and Prevention (CDC) proposed that routine physical activity is important to an individual's health and helps to control weight, reduce the risk of heart disease, diabetes, and some cancers. In addition, routine physical activity strengthens bone and muscles, improves mental well-being, and increases the probability of living longer. The 2008 CDC guidelines for adults recommend at least 2 hours and 30 minutes (150 minutes) of moderate-intensity aerobic activity such as brisk walking every week with 2 or more days of muscle-strengthening activities that focus on the major muscle areas such as the legs, hips, back, abdomen, chest, shoulders, and arms. In general, other organizations, such as the American Heart Association, have indicated that increased levels of activity are beneficial. Albert, Butler, and Sorrell (2014) surveyed 278 hospital nurses and determined that 16 percent of nurses were inactive, 54 percent were active but did not meet guidelines for adult activity, and only 30 percent of the staff nurse respondents engaged in recommended activity levels. One strategy that has been used to promote physical activity is the use of a daily activity monitor or pedometer to measure how many steps an individual takes during the average day. Student nurses have the potential to be sedentary and less physically active due to increased time spent studying and using computers. One way to address the issue of decreased physical activity is the use of fitness monitors, which are beneficial for activity tracking as well as increasing an individual's awareness of daily physical activity.

Psychosocial Well-Being and the Nurse

Psychosocial well-being is another significant aspect of being a healthy nurse. Psychosocial well-being involves maintaining satisfactory interactions with other healthcare professionals at work, engaging in mutually beneficial relationships with family and friends, and having a sense of purpose at work. Nursing can be stressful, so effective stress management skills are essential. Workplace stress can affect the nurse's psychosocial well-being and job performance. Therapeutic communication is taught in part of the general nursing curriculum. In addition, nurses should display assertive, professional communication skills to deal effectively with stressful situations and conflict resolution.

Moral distress is a key issue that can affect the psychosocial well-being of the nurse. Moral distress occurs when the nurse knows the ethical "right action" to take but is not able to follow the course of action due to an organizational constraint. The American Association of Critical-Care Nurses (AACN, 2008) has identified personal, interpersonal, and environmental sources of moral distress. Some of the sources include disrespectful behavior, workplace violence, nurse–physician conflict, and end-of-life challenges. Nurses who experience moral distress can be stressed, anxious, and defensive with the potential to lead to burnout (see **Contemporary Practice Highlight 12-1**). Moral distress is a serious problem in nursing resulting in physical and emotional stress. Moral distress contributes to the nurse experiencing a loss of integrity and dissatisfaction with the work environment (AACN, 2008).

Improving the Health of the Nursing Workforce—Challenges and Solutions

Nurse leaders and managers realize that improving the health of the nursing workforce is an important goal, not only to promote effective patient care but to enhance the financial stability of their institutions. Employees who are experiencing

CONTEMPORARY PRACTICE HIGHLIGHT 12-1

DECREASING MORAL DISTRESS

Interventions to cope with moral distress are often not included in the nursing curriculum. Dr. Rachel Remen initiated a course for beginning medical students called "The Healer's Art" to help novice physicians become more "human" and caring. As part of the course, medical students were asked to answer three questions daily before sleeping, reflecting on the most recent happenings and proceeding toward earlier moments.

1. What surprised me today?
2. What moved me or touched me today?
3. What inspired me today?

These daily journals assisted novice practitioners to derive meaning from their educational and clinical experiences, instead of focusing entirely on skill acquisition or increasing knowledge. Identifying that meaning through journaling was found to decrease moral distress and avoid premature burnout in these students.

Data from Remen, R. N. (2013). Keeping a heart journal: It works. Retrieved from http://www.rachelremen.com /keeping-a-heart-journal/

illness cost organizations money. In this section, challenges and solutions are discussed in regard to promoting initiatives that improve the health status of nurses. Ensuring a healthy workforce is affected by both the individual behaviors nurses bring to the workforce and the context of the work environment that is shaped by organizational leadership and management. Challenges, therefore, include difficulties with assisting staff members to implement and maintain healthy behaviors as individuals, in addition to obtaining financial resources to promote health-related activities and programs.

Individual nurses and nurse leaders need to cultivate awareness of valuable health promotion resources, apply the information that promotes healthy initiatives, and disseminate knowledge obtained from these measures through professional venues. One valuable resource to improve the health of the nursing workforce is the ANA (n.d.-a) HealthyNurse™ toolkit. This toolkit provides practical tips for shift workers to help maintain a healthy diet by packing healthy meals and snacks to include fruits, vegetables, salads, low-fat meats, chicken, fish, whole-grain breads, and low fat cheese and yogurt. The toolkit tips include strategies for staying hydrated, avoiding sugar-sweetened beverages, ensuring portion control, resisting eating cookies and candy, and avoiding processed foods, which are high in sugar, fat, and salt. Furthermore, the toolkit tips suggest employers should advocate for healthier foods in the workplace, offer healthy foods in the vending machines, provide free drinking water accessible for all shifts, offer weight-loss programs and support groups, mark calorie content on cafeteria menus, and ensure healthy options at affordable prices.

The ANA HealthyNurse™ toolkit expands upon practical information to enhance sleep with a focus on maintaining a consistent bedtime and routine; avoiding nicotine, alcohol, and caffeine prior to bedtime; exercising in the daytime to enhance sleep, ensuring comfort with a supportive mattress and pillows; and engaging in relaxing activities such as prayer, relaxing music, warm bath, reading before bedtime, and journaling. If the nurse or nursing student experiences issues with anxiety, writing these down at bedtime and then letting these concerns go until morning can improve sleep.

The CDC (2015) suggested that worksite wellness programs that include a physical activity element can assist with maintaining a healthier workforce. A worksite wellness program has the potential to increase productivity and morale of the employee and reduce the employee's missed workdays. Wellness programs can also serve as marketing and recruitment tools for employees as well as a retention tool to keep high-quality and healthy employees.

The American Holistic Nurses Association (n.d.) also offers practical guidelines to manage stress. The employer should offer stress management programs and professional counseling to employees, ensure adequate staffing, have regular staff meetings incorporating discussions to communicate feelings and any issues or concerns, and maintain reasonable work schedules that enable employees to obtain adequate sleep. Individual stress relaxation exercises and biofeedback techniques can assist in managing stress. Another effective intervention to manage stress is to offer educational opportunities to improve assertive communication skills and increase the nurse's confidence when dealing with issues of conflict (see **Contemporary Practice Highlight 12-2**).

Self-care behaviors of nurses are an important aspect of being a healthy nurse. Nurses should strive to keep a balance of physical, social, psychological, and spiritual aspects of well-being to promote optimum health. Nurses have abundant resources

CONTEMPORARY PRACTICE HIGHLIGHT 12-2

TOOLKIT FOR THE WORK ENVIRONMENT

Moral distress is a key issue often ignored in the work environment. AACN's (2008) "call to action" items to address moral distress include these tactics:

1. Every nurse must recognize and identify the cause of moral distress.
2. Nurses should then state the professional duty to act on the issue.
3. Nurses must be aware of and use the internal and professional resources to address the moral distress situation.

Data from American Association of Critical-Care Nurses. (n.d.). *The 4A's to rise above moral distress.* Retrieved from http://www.aacn.org/wd/practice/docs/4as_to_rise_above_moral_distress.pdf

and a solid knowledge base of ways to promote optimum health for patients and must seek ways to apply these elements to their personal well-being. As nurses place their patients as the priority to ensure patient-centered care, nurses must also place themselves as the priority in self-care activities and be a positive role model in promoting optimum health.

The Nursing Workplace and Environment

Today's healthcare environment is dynamic and forever moving forward, which, to some, is part of the allure of nursing. The very definition of a workplace is nonstatic and can be found in many different venues, from the small rural hospital to the large urban medical center and to all the community drug stores and shops that now have their versions of miniclinics staffed by advanced practice registered nurses. Patients in the hospital are often acutely ill or have multiple chronic health conditions, and the numbers of patients and their families in the community population are growing exponentially. Giving each patient the time, compassion, and quality that is desired by the caregiver, while juggling a heavy patient workload and learning new health tecnology, is challenging. For newly graduated nurses, learning and internalizing a new role is a critical transition. Clinical situations and medical crises set the stage for difficult choices being made by nurses, which can leave them with overwhelming feelings of stress, anxiety, a lifetime of bad habits, compassion fatigue, potential workplace violence, and eventually, total burnout. According to the ANA (n.d.-c), a healthy work environment is "one that is safe, empowering, and satisfying" (para. 1). To achieve this environment, standards have been suggested by many groups representing nurses and nursing students. In a 2016 publication, the AACN listed six ways for creating and maintaining a healthy work environment: skilled communication, true collaboration, effective decision making, appropriate staffing, meaningful recognition, and authentic leadership.

Most important for the nurse, in each of these statements there is an implied collaboration that takes place between nurse and another. This collaboration takes time to foster and is developed through good communications skills with colleagues and administration. If no collaboration or unhealthy communication is part of the workplace environment, acts of incivility and bullying may take place.

Incivility, Bullying, and Workplace Violence/Workplace Safety

Nurses are considered to be compassionate, kind people; nurses are consistently voted as being the most trustworthy by the public in annual Gallup Polls. Yet in 1986 and again in 1999, Meissner asked a sentinel question that remains important today: "Nurses, are we eating our young?" This question was posed to all levels of nursing professionals—nursing students, practicing nurses, nurse educators, nurse administrators, and nurse leaders. Nurses can also face a horizontal challenge from their colleagues who may have many years of experience and sometimes show little patience for those who are new and untested. High expectations are placed on new nursing students. These expectations are self-imposed as well as inflicted on novice nurses by their supervisors and peers. Challenging situations can lead to cases of incivility and bullying in the workplace. The ANA's Code of Ethics for Nurses standard 1.5 reads in part, "The nurse creates an ethical environment and culture of civility and kindness, treating colleagues, coworkers, employees, students, and others with dignity and respect" (ANA, 2015a).

Nurses are taught to care for patients and never purposely hurt or endanger them. Sometimes what may begin as a patient's or family member's uncivil behavior escalates to verbal or physical violence. Patients and their family members are often frightened, angry, experiencing pain, tired of waiting for care, and mentally unaware of their surrounding or their actions when they come to an emergency room or are admitted to the hospital (Speroni, Fitch, Dawson, Dugan, & Atherton, 2014). This mixture of feelings combined with possible effects of medication can spark unfortunate violent occurrences, and the nurse is often the victim of this violent behavior. A study of one hospital system employing more than 5,000 nurses found "the annual workplace violence charges for the 2.1% of nurses reporting injuries were \$94,156 (\$78,924 for treatment and \$15,232 for indemnity" (Speroni et al., 2014, p. 218).

According to the CDC Workplace Violence Course for Nurses, there are four types of workplace violence: (a) Type 1 Criminal Intent, (b) Type 2 Customer/Client, (c) Type 3 Worker on Worker, and (d) Type 4 Personal Relationships (Centers for Disease Control and Prevention, n.d.; see **Box 12-3**). The type most faced by nurses in the workplace is Type II Customer/Client or Client on Worker violence.

BOX 12-3   TYPES OF WORKPLACE VIOLENCE

- Type I involves "criminal intent." In this type of workplace violence, "individuals with criminal intent have no relationship to the business or its employees."
- Type II involves a customer, client, or patient. In this type, an "individual has a relationship with the business and becomes violent while receiving services."
- Type III violence involves a "worker-on-worker" relationship and includes "employees who attack or threaten another employee."
- Type IV violence involves personal relationships. It includes "individuals who have interpersonal relationships with the intended target but no relationship to the business".

Data from Centers for Disease Control and Prevention. (n.d.). Workplace violence course for nurses. Retrieved from http://wwwn.cdc.gov/wpvhc/Course.aspx/Slide/Intro_1

In order to prevent this type of violence from occurring (or at least minimize the potential injury to the nurse, patient, and others in the area), there are key behavioral and environmental triggers that should spark the nurse's awareness that a potential violent situation may occur (CDC, n.d.). Approaches to prevent workplace violence programs include (a) organizational intervention programs, (b) education about policies related to reporting incidents, (c) strategies about ways to work with specific patient populations (e.g., those experiencing Alzheimer disease or those under the influence of drugs), (d) communication and diversity training, (e) crisis and conflict resolution, and (f) evaluation of physical environments, including the addition of panic buttons and other safety measures (ANA, 2015c; Speroni et al., 2014).

Fatigue (Physical Fatigue, Compassion Fatigue, Burnout)

Nursing requires the total commitment of the intellect, emotional intelligence, and physical capability. Caring for patients, families, and others sometimes leaves very little time for the individual nurse to engage in self-care. Many nurses experience working long shifts and extra shifts, while they engage in constant standing and lifting that places incredible strain on their bodies. Lack of sleep can exacerbate existing physical conditions or trigger new pathologies, including decreased immune functioning, gastrointestinal upset, heart disease, and poor nutritional habits (ANA, 2014). Promotion of good body mechanics, healthy eating habits, and regular sleep are key elements to maintain the health of the nursing workforce.

Physical fatigue is often coupled with sleepiness, which could lead to compassion fatigue, mental fatigue, fatal patient errors, and nurse burnout. In order to be good patient advocates, nurses must be able to be cognitively aware about what is occurring with the patients under their care (see **Box 12-4**). An extensive literature review by the ANA found, "Fatigue is linked to several types of performance deficits, including an increased risk of errors; a decline in short-term and working memory; a reduced ability to learn; a negative impact on divergent thinking, innovation, and insight; increased risk-taking behavior; and impaired mood and communication skills" (ANA, 2014, p. 2). In addition to these cognitive changes nurses with sleep deprivation and fatigue may also suffer decision regret about their clinical decisions. "Decision regret is a negative cognitive emotion that occurs when the actual outcome differs from the desired or expected outcome" (Scott, Arslanian-Engoren, & Engoren, 2014, p. 13). A study of critical-care nurses found the incident rate of decision regret is higher in nurses in critical-care units than in other units, nurses who more likely worked nights and 12-hour shifts, and nurses who did not sufficiently recover between their shifts (Scott et al., 2014).

BOX 12-4   EVIDENCE-BASED RECOMMENDATIONS

The ANA recommends the following evidence-based steps for enhancing performance and safety and patient outcomes:

- Employers should include nurse input when designing work schedules and implement a "regular and predictable schedule" that allows nurses to plan for work and personal obligations.
- Nurses should work no more than 40 hours in a 7-day period and limit work shifts to 12 hours in a 24-hour period, including on-call hours worked.
- Employers should stop using mandatory overtime as a "staffing solution."
- Employers should encourage "frequent, uninterrupted rest breaks during work shifts."
- Employers should adopt official policy that gives RNs the "right to accept or reject a work assignment" to prevent risks from fatigue. The policy should be clear that rejecting an assignment under these conditions is not patient abandonment and that RNs will not face retaliation or other negative consequences for rejecting such an assignment.
- Employers should encourage nurses to be proactive about managing their health and rest, including getting 7 to 9 hours of sleep per day; managing stress effectively; developing healthy nutrition and exercise habits; and using naps according to employer policy.

Data from American Nurses Association. (2014). *Addressing nurse fatigue to promote safety and health: Joint responsibilities of registered nurses and employers to reduce risks.* Position statement. Retrieved from https://www.michigan.gov/documents /mdch/Nurse-Fatigue-ANA-Position-Statement_475006_7.pdf

Addiction

Nursing students are always "on" and must perform at the top of their classes in order to gain entrance into a nursing school. These intense feelings of stress and anxiety do not necessarily decrease once the goal of admission to nursing school is achieved; they often increase during their time in class and clinical. Nursing students are learning a new "language," completing multiple assignments and clinical rotations, sleeping little, finding it difficult to maintain healthy eating and exercise routines, spending less time with friends and family (thus losing familiar support groups), experiencing high levels of anxiety, and some are suffering from depression (McCulloh, Nemeth, Sommers, Newman, & Amella, 2016). Some students find unhealthy ways to help cope with these feelings through the use of drugs and/or alcohol to decrease anxiety. Course content related to addictions is often taught in sociology, psychology, pharmacology, and psychiatric clinical rotations. However, little to no information is given to students about addiction issues in their personal lives or their future lives as nurse professionals. Those individuals who are practicing nursing often experience stressful events and situations. RNs must make quick decisions and implement high-stakes, lifesaving care fraught with legal liabilities for actions taken or details missed causing harm (or death) to patients. The National Council of State Boards of Nursing (2011) reported that the ANA "estimates that six to eight percent of nurses use alcohol or drugs to an extent that is sufficient to impair professional performance" (p. 1). Others estimate that nurses generally misuse drugs and alcohol at nearly the same rate (10 to 15 percent) as the rest of the population. That means that if an individual nurse works with 10 nurses, one of their coworkers may be struggling with a substance-abuse disorder (National Council of State Boards of Nursing, 2011). Nurses often turn to drugs, alcohol, and smoking as a way to relieve stress or cope with the daily events of a harsh work day. The impaired coworker may exhibit a change in personal behavior or dress or a difference in work habits (see **Box 12-5**).

A somewhat more difficult question is what to do if you think a nurse is impaired while on the job. Historically, nurses did not want to "tell" on a colleague for fear of being wrong or getting the person fired (Copp, 2009; Naegle, 2006; Puliti, 2014). According to the ANA Code of Ethics, statement 3.6, "Nurses must protect the patient, the public, and the profession from potential harm when practice appears to be impaired. The nurse's duty is to take action to protect patients and to ensure that the individual receives assistance" (ANA, 2015a, p. 13). At one point, nurses who were found impaired while at work could expect to lose their license to practice nursing. Today several options are available for those who seek assistance for their addictions. Boards of nursing in various states may offer education, probation, suspension, and peer assistance programs before revoking a license. Alternative programs for recovery from the addiction as well as peer assistance models are available in most states.

BOX 12-5 COMMON SIGNS AND SYMPTOMS OF A SUBSTANCE-ABUSING NURSE

- Increased tardiness and/or absenteeism
- Frequent unexplained absences from the nursing unit
- Work habits deteriorate
- Erratic job history
- Errors involving judgment
- Mood swings
- Medication and/or documentation errors
- Failure to do narcotics count
- Uses maximum prn dose for pain medications
- Assigned patients complain of unrelieved pain
- Sleepiness or hyperactivity

- Offers to give medications for patients assigned to other nurses
- Dishonesty
- Isolates from coworkers
- Unexplained need for money or borrowing money from coworkers
- Suspicious attitude toward others
- Change in personal grooming

Reproduced from Puliti, B. (2014). Recognizing (and reporting) substance abuse in the healthcare workplace is the duty of every nurse. *ADVANCE for Nurses.* Retrieved from http://nursing.advanceweb.com/Features/Articles/The-Impaired-Nurse.aspx

Summary

The health of the nursing workforce is undeniably associated with the present and future health of the U.S. population. This chapter has illustrated the challenges and the rewards associated with those who choose to practice in the trusted and caring profession of nursing. In order to take care of others, nurses must first and continuously take care of themselves. This self-care should be encouraged, monitored, and maintained as students enter colleges and universities and proceed to clinical nursing coursework. Lifelong health promotion strategies must be taught concurrently with course content related to caring for those who are experiencing complex acute and chronic health conditions. Student nurses need more than assistance with science, mathematics, and nursing coursework. They must also learn how to incorporate healthy personal lifestyles into their professional careers, including but not limited to effective stress management strategies. These lessons can and will be internalized and exhibited by the student nurse during the transformation to the role of a professional nurse who is responsible for the care of patients in hospital or community settings. The instance of an "unhealthy" nurse may be the first step to becoming an impaired nurse, which will be detrimental not only to the nursing workforce but to patients and their families. The healthy nurse focuses on maintaining the balance of physical, social, psychological, and spiritual aspects of well-being to promote optimum health for the nurse as well as the patient.

Reflective Practice Questions

1. Describe self-care behaviors a nurse should maintain to ensure personal health, safety, and well-being.
2. Discuss how the ANA HealthyNurse™ toolkit can be incorporated in patient education in your current work environment.
3. Identify a moral distress situation you have experienced in your work setting. Use the American Association of Critical Care Nurses (n.d.) *The 4 A's To Rise Above Moral Distress* framework to address the moral distress identified in your work environment.

References

Albert, N. M., Butler, R., & Sorrell, J. (2014). Factors related to healthy diet and physical activity in hospital-based clinical nurses. *Online Journal of Issues in Nursing, 19*(3). Retrieved from http://www.nursingworld.org/MainMenuCategories/ANAMarketplace /ANAPeriodicals/OJIN/TableofContents/Vol-19-2014/No3-Sept-2014/Healthy-Diet-and -Physical-Activity-in-Nurses.html

American Association of Critical-Care Nurses. (2008, August). *Moral distress.* Retrieved from http://www.aacn.org/WD/Practice/Docs/Moral_Distress.pdf

American Association of Critical-Care Nurses. (2016). *AACN standards for establishing and sustaining healthy work environments: A journey to excellence* (2nd ed.). Aliso Viejo, CA: Author. Retrieved from http://www.aacn.org/wd/hwe/docs/hwestandards.pdf

American Association of Critical-Care Nurses. (n.d.). *The 4A's to rise above moral distress.* Retrieved from http://www.aacn.org/wd/practice/docs/4as_to_rise_above_moral_distress.pdf

American Association of Colleges of Nursing. (2011). *Nursing fact sheet.* Retrieved from http://www.aacn.nche.edu/media-relations/fact-sheets/nursing-fact-sheet

American Holistic Nurses Association. (n.d.) *Managing stress.* Retrieved from http://www.ahna.org/Resources/Stress-Management/Managing-Stress

American Nurses Association. (2014). *Addressing nurse fatigue to promote safety and health: Joint responsibilities of registered nurses and employers to reduce risks.* Position statement. Retrieved from https://www.michigan.gov/documents/mdch/Nurse-Fatigue-ANA-Position-Statement_475006_7.pdf

American Nurses Association. (2015a). *Code of ethics for nurses with interpretive statements.* Silver Spring, MD: Author. Retrieved from http://nursingworld.org/DocumentVault/Ethics-1/Code-of-Ethics-for-Nurses.html

American Nurses Association. (2015b). *Health Risk Appraisal (HRA). Preliminary findings October 2013–October 2014. Executive summary.* Silver Spring, MD: Author. Retrieved from http://nursingworld.org/HRA-Executive-Summary

American Nurses Association. (2015c). *Incivility, bullying and workplace violence. New position statement.* Retrieved from http://nursingworld.org/MainMenuCategories/Policy-Advocacy/State/Legislative-Agenda-Reports/State-WorkplaceViolence/Incivility-Bullying-and-Workplace-Violence.html

American Nurses Association. (n.d.-a). *Healthy Nurse, Healthy Nation*™. Retrieved from http://www.nursingworld.org/healthynurse

American Nurses Association. (n.d.-b). *Healthy sleep.* Retrieved from http://www.nursingworld.org/HealthySleep

American Nurses Association. (n.d.-c). *Healthy work environment.* Retrieved from http://www.nursingworld.org/MainMenuCategories/WorkplaceSafety/Healthy-Work-Environment

Buettner, D. (2009). *The blue zones: Lessons for living longer from the people who've lived the longest.* Washington, DC: National Geographic Books.

Centers for Disease Control and Prevention. (2015). *Physical activity and health.* Retrieved from http://www.cdc.gov/physicalactivity/basics/pa-health/index.htm

Centers for Disease Control and Prevention. (n.d.). Workplace violence course for nurses. Retrieved from http://wwwn.cdc.gov/wpvhc/Course.aspx/Slide/Intro_1

Copp, M. A. (2009, April 1). Drug addiction among nurses: Confronting a quiet epidemic. Retrieved from http://www.modernmedicine.com/modern-medicine/news/modernmedicine/modern-medicine-feature-articles/drug-addiction-among-nurses-con?page=full

Engel, G. L. (1977). The clinical application of the biopsychosocial model. *American Journal of Psychiatry, 137*(5), 535–543.

Engel, G. L. (1980). The clinical application of the biopsychosocial model. *American Journal of Psychiatry, 137*(5), 535–544. doi.org/10.1176/ajp.137.5.535

Gortmaker, S. L., Swinburn, B. A., Levy, D., Carter, R., Mabry, P. L., Finegood, D. T., & Moodie, M. L. (2011). Changing the future of obesity: Science, policy, and action. *Lancet, 378,* 838–847.

Haupt, N. (2016, January 15). What is the "best diet" for you? *U.S. News and World Report.* Retrieved from http://health.usnews.com/health-news/health-wellness/articles/2016-01-05/what-is-the-best-diet-for-you

Lachman, V., Swanson, E. O., & Winland-Brown, J. (2015). The new 'code of ethics for nurses with interpretive statements' (2015): Practical clinical application. Part II. *Medsurg Nursing, 24*(5), 363–368.

McCulloh, J., Nemeth, L. S., Sommers, M., Newman, S., & Amella, E. (2016). Alcohol use, misuse, and abuse among nursing students. *Journal of Addictions Nursing, 27*(1), 12–23.

Meissner, J. E. (1999). Nurses: Are we still eating our young? *Nursing, 29*(2), 42–43.

Naegle, M. (2006, November/December). Nurses and matters of substance. *NSNA Imprint*, 58–63. Retrieved from http://nsna.org/Portals/0/Skins/NSNA/pdf/Imprint_NovDec06 _Feat_Naegle.pdf

National Council of State Boards of Nursing. (2011). *Substance use disorder in nursing: A resource manual and guidelines for alternative and disciplinary monitoring programs.* Chicago, IL: Author.

National Sleep Foundation. (n.d.). *Shift work and sleep.* Retrieved from https://sleepfoundation .org/sleep-topics/shift-work-and-sleep

Nightingale, F. (1859). *Notes on nursing: What it is and what it is not.* New York, NY: D. Appleton and Company. Retrieved from http://digital.library.upenn.edu/women /nightingale/nursing/nursing.html

Perry-Black, B. (2014). *Professional nursing concepts & challenge* (7th ed.). St. Louis, MO: Elsevier Saunders.

Poulain, M., Pes, G. M., Grasland, C., Carru, C., Ferucci, L., Baggio, G., . . . Deiana, L. (2004). Identification of a geographic area characterized by extreme longevity in the Sardinia Island: The AKEA study. *Experimental Gerontology, 39*(9), 1423–1429. doi: 10.1016 /j.exger.2004.06.016

Puliti, B. (2014). Recognizing (and reporting) substance abuse in the healthcare workplace is the duty of every nurse. *ADVANCE for Nurses.* Retrieved from http://nursing.advanceweb .com/Features/Articles/The-Impaired-Nurse.aspx

Raaijmakers, L. C., Pouwels, S., Berghuis, K. A., & Nienhuijs, S. W. (2015). Technology-based interventions in the treatment of overweight and obesity: A systematic review. *Appetite, 95*, 138–151. doi: 10.1016/j.appet.2015.07.008

Remen, R. N. (2013). Keeping a heart journal: It works. Retrieved from http://www .rachelremen.com/keeping-a-heart-journal/

Sarna, L., Bialous, S., Nandy, K., Antonio, A., & Yang, Q. (2014). Changes in smoking preva-lences among health care professionals from 2003 to 2010-2011. *Journal of the American Medical Association, 311,* 197–199. doi: 10.1001/jama.2013.284871

Sartorius, N. (2006). The meanings of health and its promotion. *Croatian Medical Journal, 47*(4), 662–664.

Satterfield, J. (2013). *Mind-body medicine: The new science of optimal health.* Chantilly, VA: The Teaching Company.

Scott, L. D., Arslanian-Engoren, C., & Engoren, M. C. (2014). Association of sleep and fatigue with decision regret among critical care nurses. *American Journal of Critical Care, 23*(1), 13–22.

Speroni, K. G., Fitch, T., Dawson, E., Dugan, L., & Atherton, M., (2014). Incidence and cost of nurse workplace violence perpetrated by hospital patients or patient visitors. *Journal of Emergency Nursing, 40*(3), 218–228.

Substance Abuse and Mental Health Services Administration. (2016). The eight dimensions of wellness. Retrieved from http://www.samhsa.gov/wellness-initiative/eight-dimensions -wellness

Tobacco Free Nurses. (n.d.). *Welcome to tobacco free nurses.* Retrieved from http://tobaccofreenurses.org/about

U.S. Department of Health and Human Services. (2008). *Physical activity guidelines for Americans.* Rockville, MD: Author. Retrieved from https://health.gov/paguidelines/guidelines/

U.S. Department of Health and Human Services, Office of Disease Prevention and Health Promotion. (n.d.-a). *Healthy People 2020.* Retrieved from https://www.healthypeople.gov/

U.S. Department of Health and Human Services, Office of Disease Prevention and Health Promotion. (n.d.-b). *Leading health indicators.* Retrieved from https://www.healthypeople.gov/2020/Leading-Health-Indicators

U.S. Department of Labor (2016, March 30). *Occupational employment and wages.* Retrieved from http://www.bls.gov/oes/

World Health Organization. (1948). Preamble to the Constitution of the World Health Organization as adopted by the International Health Conference, New York, 19–22 June, 1946; signed on 22 July 1946 by the representatives of 61 States (Official Records of the World Health Organization, no. 2, p. 100) and entered into force on 7 April 1948.

Unit III

The *Person* in Health Care

Addressing Primary Prevention and Education in Vulnerable Populations

Brian W. Higgerson

LEARNING OUTCOMES

After reading this chapter you will be able to:

- Define the term vulnerable population.
- Identify what constitutes a health disparity.
- Discuss at least three factors that contribute to health disparities.
- Understand health behaviors that are classified as primary prevention.
- Discuss how dietary practices, lack of exercise, and tobacco use may contribute to increased risk of developing major chronic diseases in the United States.
- Provide examples of how health behaviors are distributed in vulnerable populations.
- Identify three key approaches for educating and motivating clients to improve their health behaviors.
- Discuss challenges for improving health behaviors in vulnerable populations.

The editors wish to acknowledge the contributions of Diane Baer Wilson and Lisa S. Anderson to the previous edition of this chapter.

Introduction

The increased prevalence of chronic diseases in the United States has a widespread impact on individuals as well as healthcare delivery systems. A **chronic disease** is typically defined as diseases lasting more than 3 months—they are associated with decreased quality of life, increased financial burdens, and decreased life expectancy. Although chronic diseases are increasing in numbers, many of these chronic conditions are completely preventable. Recent data suggests approximately one half of all adults living in the United States have one or more chronic health conditions and one in four adults has two or more chronic diseases (Ward, Schiller, & Goodman, 2014). Heart disease, cancer, and diabetes continue to rank as the top three chronic diseases that are estimated to result in 1.2 million deaths a year (Centers for Disease Control and Prevention [CDC], 2015a). However, in learning more about the populations represented in these statistics, one might be surprised at the demographic trends. Research reveals that poor, underserved, and minority populations have higher death rates across all of these diseases. Furthermore, these individuals are also less likely to have health insurance and thus, they find it more difficult to access health care or receive high-quality health care in comparison with more affluent groups.

The purpose of this chapter is to identify **vulnerable populations** and provide a discussion on why these frequently overlooked populations are at greater risk for poor health outcomes compared to other populations. In addition, this chapter explores the role of disease prevention or risk reduction of chronic disease. Three categories of prevention are aimed at reducing health risk outcomes: primary prevention, secondary prevention, and tertiary prevention. **Primary prevention** refers to modifying health behaviors such as diet, sedentary behavior, or tobacco use to reduce one's risk of developing chronic diseases such as heart disease, stroke, cancer, and diabetes. **Secondary prevention** focuses on early detection of disease usually detected through early assessment findings or diagnostic tests or procedures, such as a prostate-specific antigen (PSA) test for prostate cancer or mammography to detect breast cancer. The goal of **tertiary prevention** is to implement strategies that will slow disease progression, limit disability from a disease, and restore individuals to their optimal level of functioning

KEY TERM

Chronic disease: A long-lasting disease that typically remains with a patient from onset to end of life and requires management of symptoms. Chronic diseases typically last longer than 3 months. Examples are cancer, cardiovascular disease, diabetes, and cerebrovascular disease. According to the U.S. Centers for Disease Control and Prevention (2015a), chronic disease is responsible for 7 out of 10 deaths in the United States.

KEY TERM

Vulnerable populations: Groups of individuals who are likely to have compromised access to health care and, therefore, are more likely to have poorer health outcomes, including higher mortality rates, compared to less vulnerable groups.

KEY TERM

Primary prevention: Actions taken to modify health behaviors such as diet, sedentary behavior, or smoking toward preventing or managing a chronic condition such as heart disease or cancer. An example is reducing one's dietary fat intake to help lower cholesterol levels and prevent one from exceeding the recommended cholesterol guidelines.

KEY TERM

Secondary prevention: Interventions focused on early detection and screening of disease, such as tuberculosis skin testing.

(Nies & McEwen, 2014). Examples of tertiary prevention strategies include cardiac rehabilitation services following a myocardial infarction or a support group for newly diagnosed diabetic clients.

The final part of this chapter details the nurse's role as an advocate for individuals within these vulnerable populations. Through education and support, nurses can play an instrumental role in encouraging vulnerable populations to participate in healthy lifestyle choices and ultimately reduce chronic conditions.

> **KEY TERM**
>
> **Tertiary prevention:** Strategies that will slow disease progression, limit disability from a disease, and restore individuals to their optimal level of functioning.

Defining Vulnerable Population

> **KEY TERM**
>
> **Poverty:** When an individual or group of individuals lacks human needs because they simply cannot afford to meet these needs.

Although a wide range of factors and income categories may be used to define **poverty**, a broad definition for poverty is when an individual or group of individuals lacks human needs because they simply cannot afford to meet these needs (Short, 2016). An unfortunate common consequence of poverty is inadequate health care or access to healthcare services. Socioeconomic status and poverty rates have more of an impact on health status and mortality rates than any specific race or culture. Over time, data have demonstrated that socioeconomic status is a strong and persistent predictor of health status. For example, adults living in poverty report higher incidence of diabetes, kidney disease, liver disease, and chronic joint pains compared to adults who were not poor. Moreover, a higher percentage of adults living in poverty reported more feelings of being hopeless, sad, or worthless compared to nonpoor adults (Blackwell, Lucas, & Clarke, 2014). A landmark study, published in 1967, examined this issue in the United States and Europe tracing back to the 17th century and reported better health and lower mortality rates were consistently associated with higher income and higher levels of education (Antonovsky, 1967). If one looks at any of several measures, the results are consistent in the relationship between socioeconomic status and mortality rates. For example, life expectancy in 2013 was 52 years in Angola, which is a very poor country, compared to 79 years in the United States, a highly developed country (World Health Organization [WHO], 2015a).

According to the U.S. Census Bureau (2014), the nation's poverty rate in 2014 was 14.8 percent, which translates to approximately 46.7 million people living in poverty. A further examination of the data reveals the disproportionate prevalence of poverty among racial groups. More African Americans (26.2 percent) and Hispanics (23.6 percent) live below the poverty line than Caucasians (10.1 percent). Likewise, according to the 2014 Census Bureau data, more African Americans (11.8 percent) and Hispanics (19.9 percent) are without medical insurance compared with Caucasians (7.6 percent).

Alarmingly, the highest percentage of group of individuals living in poverty in the United States are children under age 18 (21.1 percent), followed by adults ages 18 to 64 years (13.5 percent) and older adults over the age of 64 (10 percent; DeNavas-Walt & Proctor, 2015). Approximately 6 percent of children in the United States under the age of 19 are without health insurance (Smith & Medalia, 2015).

People with Disabilities

Vulnerable populations may include people in additional groups, such as individuals with a **disability**. Although many people with disabilities are fully functional, maintain employment, and have a high quality of life, some disabilities can make it more difficult for the individual to find employment or may limit some activities of daily living. In addition, some disabilities may place individuals at greater risk for developing comorbidities. For example, an individual with diabetes who does not control blood sugar levels is at greater risk for developing infection, having poor circulation, and developing heart disease. Thus, people with diabetes serve as another example of a potentially vulnerable population.

> **KEY TERM**
>
> **Disability:** Physical or mental impairment that substantially limits a person from completing activities of daily living.

Elderly and Young Children

Age is also a factor that can be associated with poor health outcomes. Both socioeconomic factors and physiological issues contribute to these groups being more at risk for poor health than individuals in other age groups. Elderly people are often on a fixed income and may not have health insurance to supplement governmental health plans; thus they may not be able to afford medical procedures or medications that are not covered by Medicare. Children are particularly at risk if they either are uninsured or have insufficient coverage for medical care because the lack of resources may lead to inadequate access to medical care. Children with health insurance coverage have a higher percentage of their healthcare needs met. Insured children are more likely to receive timely diagnoses of serious or chronic health conditions and thus have fewer avoidable hospitalizations (Price, Khubchandani, McKinney, & Braun, 2013).

Physiological differences also contribute to vulnerabilities. Older people, particularly those with less body mass, as well as very young children, do not tolerate extreme heat or cold temperatures. For example, these two age groups are targeted in extreme heat warnings in the summer because they are more prone to dehydration and heat stroke. Overall, however, individuals in these age categories tend to have a weaker immune response and they are often prioritized for public health initiatives such as influenza vaccination distribution, usually given in fall months.

The Interplay of Economic, Social, and Cultural Issues on Health Status

How living in poverty actually affects health and health status turns out to be a complex issue. Over the last decade, thinking has shifted from a primary focus on poverty as the prime factor related to health status to a broader focus. In reality, there is no one reason that explains why those who live in poverty are more likely to become ill, suffer from chronic conditions, and more likely to die prematurely. Many factors beyond income status are contributory to health status and chronic disease. Factors such as the state of our living environment, genetics, educational background, and our social support systems all have a considerable impact on our overall health status (WHO, 2015b). The mechanisms by which economic, social, and cultural issues are operational and affect health are not widely known, which opens research opportunities for social scientists, public health epidemiologists, as well as healthcare providers such as nurses, physicians, psychologists, and allied health professionals to explore these contextual variables. **Social determinants of health** (see **Figure 13-1**) include broad factors that can contribute to an individual's overall health status. These factors may include social-economic aspects, physical environment, and individual behaviors or characteristics (WHO, 2015b). The schema shown in Figure 13-1 depicts a widely adopted rainbow model of determinants of health, demonstrating

> **KEY TERM**
>
> **Social determinants of health:** Factors that can contribute to an individual's overall health status. These factors may include social-economic aspects, physical environment, and individual behaviors or characteristics.

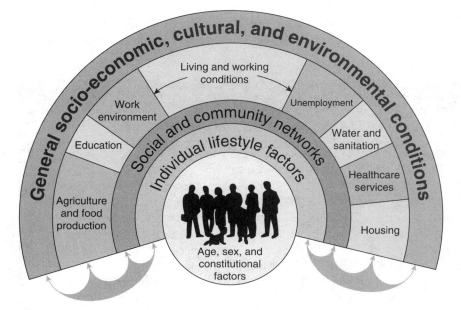

Figure 13-1 Social determinants of health.
Reproduced from Dahlgren, G., & Whitehead, M. (1991). *Policies and strategies to promote social equity in health.* Stockholm, Sweden: Institute for Futures Studies.

the layered connectivity among individual lifestyle factors and variables such as social networks and cultural-environmental influences (Dahlgren & Whitehead, 1991).

Health Disparities

Once evidence was found that overall mortality rates varied by education and socioeconomic status, more study was given to examine chronic disease rates in order to determine whether mortality rates also reflected differences across groups of individuals. **Population health** refers to the aggregation of healthcare outcomes within specified groups of individuals and the distribution of outcomes among these groups. The term **health disparities** is used to describe groups that have a disproportionate amount of disease compared to the proportion of representation in the population (see **Contemporary Practice Highlight 13-1**). When we look at the major chronic diseases we see, for example, that African American men are more likely to develop prostate cancer and have a higher mortality rate from the disease compared to Caucasian men. Moreover, African American women are approximately 9 percent more likely to die from breast cancer than Caucasian women (U.S. Cancer Statistics Working Group, 2015). Although overall deaths from cancer have declined in the United States over the past decades, from 1999–2012, the cancer death rates were higher among African American

> **KEY TERM**
>
> **Population health:** The aggregation of healthcare outcomes within specified groups of individuals and the distribution of outcomes among these groups.

> **KEY TERM**
>
> **Health disparities:** Differences in the incidence, prevalence, mortality, and burden of disease and other adverse health conditions that exist among specific population groups.

CONTEMPORARY PRACTICE HIGHLIGHT 13-1

HEALTH DISPARITIES ACROSS THE CANCER CONTINUUM OF CARE

The model shown in Figure 13-1 depicts the multifactorial aspects that may be contributory to an individual's health status. Dahlgren & Whitehead (1991) present the interrelatedness of individual factors, environmental, social, and cultural influences that together place individuals at greater risk for having a disproportionate burden of poor health care across the continuum of care and potentially suboptimal health outcomes. This model is particularly relevant for healthcare practitioners because it emphasizes the synergy created by the intersection of multiple factors. Disparities in disease outcomes may begin with differences in each of the areas of care; thus, healthcare practitioners must be diligent in completing thorough history assessments of their clients and families. By obtaining a comprehensive health history, the healthcare practitioner can develop a comprehensive understanding of the client's social determinants of health and potentially identify future risks for chronic disease.

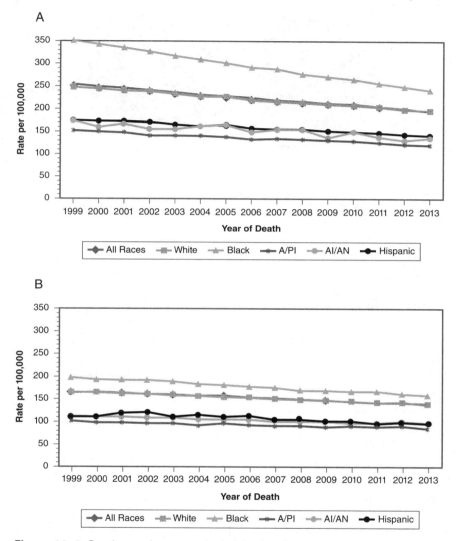

Figure 13-2 Death rates by race and ethnicity for all cancer sites combined, United States, 1999–2013. A. Male. B. Female.

Abbreviations: A/PI, Asian/Pacific Islander; AI/AN, American Indian/Alaska Native.

Reproduced from Centers for Disease Control and Prevention. (2016). *Cancer rates by race/ethnicity and sex.* Retrieved from http://www.cdc.gov/cancer/dcpc/data/race.htm

men and women compared to other ethnic/racial groups (U.S. Cancer Statistics Working Group, 2015; see **Figure 13-2**). Hypertension is also a concern among chronic diseases because of the detrimental consequences of cardiovascular disease and stroke. African Americans have the highest occurrence of hypertension and

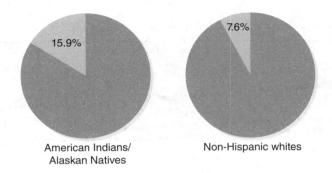

American Indians/
Alaskan Natives

Non-Hispanic whites

Figure 13–3 Rates of diagnosed diabetes.
Data from American Diabetes Association. (2016). *Statistics about diabetes.* Retrieved from http://www
.diabetes.org/diabetes-basics/statistics/

identified as a racial group most likely to develop high blood pressure at a young age (Mozaffarian et al., 2015).

Other racial and ethnic groups suffer disproportionately from chronic diseases such as diabetes. In the United States, approximately 25.8 million individuals have diabetes and an estimated 7 million of these individuals are undiagnosed (Spanakis & Golden, 2013). According to the American Diabetes Association (2016), the prevalence of diabetes is highest among American Indians/Alaskan Natives (15.9 percent) and lowest among non-Hispanic Caucasians (7.6 percent; see **Figure 13-3**).

Summary of Vulnerable Populations

Overall, there is evidence that a combination of several factors including poverty, culture, and social issues contributes to individuals being at risk for poor health outcomes including chronic disease and lower life expectancy. This section discussed minorities, people with disabilities, and very young and elderly persons as examples of groups that can be considered vulnerable for inadequate medical care and thus, more susceptible to poorer health outcomes.

Individual Health Behaviors: Primary Prevention

Evidence demonstrates a direct link between health behaviors and illness. Behaviors such as dietary practices, activity levels, use of tobacco products, or consumption of alcohol may increase our risk of developing the most prevalent chronic diseases in the United States (WHO, 2013). In fact, the top three chronic diseases in the

United States—heart disease, stroke, and cancer—are all fueled by **obesity** and by being physically inactive. In other words, if people would reduce their food intake and exercise in order to reach a body mass index (BMI) of 18–25 kg/m², many heart attacks, strokes, and cancer diagnoses would likely be averted. Research suggests that dietary intake, regular exercise, and stress reduction may contribute to lower risks or improved outcomes of chronic conditions, such as prostate cancer (Hebert et al., 2013).

In this section of the chapter we discuss the top preventable causes of death in the United States and how they are distributed in vulnerable populations (see **Contemporary Practice Highlight 13-2**). Preventable causes of death have also been quantified to show how much they contribute to the top diseases that account for the most deaths in the United States.

> **KEY TERM**
>
> **Obesity:** Having excess body fat. Obesity is clinically determined by body mass index (BMI), which is calculated by dividing a person's weight in kilograms by height in meters squared (kg/m²). A person with a BMI of 30.0 or more is defined as obese.

> **KEY TERM**
>
> **Overweight:** Having an excess of body weight that includes fat, muscle, bone, and water. Overweight is clinically determined by BMI, which is calculated by dividing a person's weight in kilometers by height in meters squared (kg/m²). A person with a BMI ranging between 25.0 and 29.9 is defined as overweight.

Obesity

Being **overweight** or obese is one of our most concerning public health issues today and the rates of obesity are increasing at alarming rates (see **Box 13-1**). The majority of Americans are overweight; more than 69 percent of the adult population has a BMI greater than 25 kg/m² (CDC, 2015b). In 2003, U.S. Surgeon General Richard Carmona, MD, MPH, said "As we look to the future and where childhood obesity will be in 20 years, it is every bit as threatening to us as is the threat of terrorism. Obesity is the threat from within" (Ornish, 2007). Dr. Carmona was responding to the fact that an obesity epidemic is a serious and costly issue in the United States, based on the significant increases in the prevalence of obesity. Rates of overweight and obesity are increasing not only in the adult population in the United States but among children as well. In 2011–2012, approximately 17 percent of children and teenagers were obese and 31 percent were either overweight or obese. Racial and ethnic inequities exist related to obesity in children. According to Ogden, Carroll, Kitt, and Flegal (2014), 22 percent of Latino children and 20 percent of African American children are estimated to be obese compared to only 14 percent of Caucasian, non-Latino children.

Causes of Obesity

Many factors contribute to becoming overweight, but being overweight results from consuming more calories than are burned each day. Eating too much and being less physically active are hallmarks of wealthy nations, where food is affordable, heavily marketed, and readily available. In addition, as wealth increases in a society,

CONTEMPORARY PRACTICE HIGHLIGHT 13-2

QUANTIFYING THE CONTRIBUTION OF UNHEALTHY LIFESTYLE BEHAVIORS IN CAUSES OF DEATH IN AMERICANS

Figure **13-4** quantifies and ranks the leading causes of death in the United States. Smoking, high blood pressure, and being overweight are the leading contributing factors to premature death. Heart attacks, stroke, cancer, and diabetes, and other physical conditions are linked to these risk factors. Health behaviors are the only known nonpharmaceutical modifiable factors for reducing risk of chronic disease. Thus, there is greater focus on these issues by the healthcare industry, food manufacturers and marketers, businesses, and organizations at all levels of our society to support individuals in disease prevention and promoting healthy lifestyles through smoking cessation, healthier diets, and more physical activity.

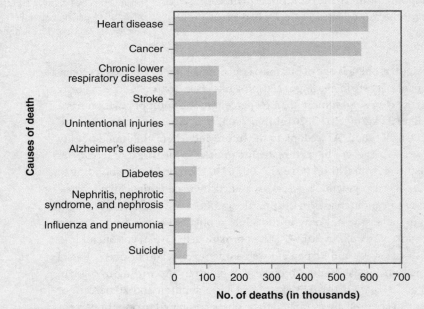

Figure 13-4 Causes of death.

Reproduced from Centers for Disease Control and Prevention. (2013). *QuickStats: Number of deaths from 10 leading causes: National Vital Statistics System, United States, 2010. Morbidity and Mortality Weekly Report, 62*(08), 155. Retrieved from http://www.cdc.gov/mmwr/preview /mmwrhtml/mm6208a8.htm

BOX 13-1 THE OBESITY EPIDEMIC

Being overweight and obesity have significantly increased among both adults and youth in the United States, and the rates continue to increase as illustrated in **Figure 13-5**. Being overweight or obese is a risk factor for diabetes, heart disease, stroke, and many types of cancer including breast cancer. Ethnic and racial inequities in weight status exist among particular groups. For example, being overweight or obese affects more than three out of every four Hispanic or African American adults. Moreover, a trending increase in obesity among children extends to adolescents in the United States. These increases prompted the U.S. government to identify an obesity epidemic to raise the public's awareness of the health consequences and suggest solutions across multiple domains such as business, health care, marketing, schools, churches, and individuals' health behavior choices. Health policy and federal funding has also increased to battle the obesity epidemic. The Healthy, Hunger-Free Kids Act of 2010 authorizes funding and establishes guidelines for school breakfast and lunch programs to improve nutritional standards for school-aged children (U.S. Department of Agriculture Food and Nutrition Service [USDA], 2014).

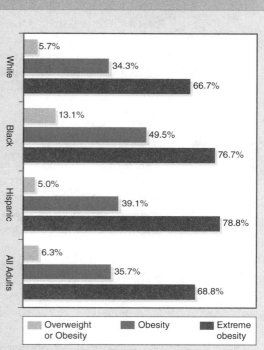

Figure 13-5 Overweight/obese adults estimated percentages by race/ethnicity.
Reproduced from National Institute of Diabetes and Digestive and Kidney Diseases. (2012). *Overweight and obesity statistics* (NIH No. 04-4158). Retrieved from http://www.niddk.nih.gov/health-information/health-statistics/Pages/overweight-obesity-statistics.aspx#b

mundane physical tasks are becoming more automated and require less physical labor; with the prospect of robotics in the future, these patterns will only increase.

Food Consumption Patterns

Changing patterns in society and the marketplace have contributed to people consuming more calories. Consumption of fast and takeaway food continues to be a prevalent pattern in the United States and is particularly widespread among children and adolescents (Jaworowska, Blackham, Davies, & Stevenson, 2013). Frequent consumption of fast-food items that are high in fat, sodium, and sugar can lead to poor dietary quality, increasing a person's risk for chronic diseases.

According to a recent Gallup poll, approximately 28 percent of Americans reported eating fast food at least once a week and 16 percent reported to consume fast food several times a week (Dugan, 2013). Fewer people cook at home, where it is easier to have control over portion sizes and the ingredients used in cooking. Eating out often translates into eating larger portions and consuming higher levels of fat and sugar. Fast food is not only convenient, it is relatively inexpensive, making it easy for working families to go to the drive-through to pick up fast food on the ride home from work.

Food Advertising

The marketing of food is a huge part of the food industry. Food advertising is so sophisticated that it targets specific gender, age, and ethnic groups. Companies place a significant focus on conducting market research so they specifically learn what appeals to various groups. Cereal manufacturers are a good example. They are very successful at marketing cereal products to kids through Saturday morning cartoons on television, so much so that these practices came under scrutiny by federal regulators. In addition to federal regulation, private groups have acted. In 2007, the Kellogg's company announced it would phase out ads targeting children under 12 as well as discontinuing the use of well-known children's characters or toys to promote products that did not meet certain nutritional guidelines (Martin, 2007). The guidelines were based on the calorie, sugar, fat, and sodium content of primarily breakfast foods. Kellogg's made its decision because of the threat of a lawsuit by two advocacy groups and private citizens who wanted to eliminate the promotion of less healthy food items to young children (Center for Science in the Public Interest, 2007).

Cola beverage companies represent another market segment that competes so heavily that they are said to have "advertising wars." They are known for state-of-the-art ad campaigns that appeal to nearly all ages but target teens and young adults. A few companies do use health to target certain groups, such as the lean microwave dinners that appeal to men and women who are health and fitness conscious or dieters with goals of losing weight.

Beverage Consumption

There have been huge shifts in the U.S. consumption patterns of beverages over the past several decades. Whereas milk used to be the top consumed beverage among youth in the United States, milk consumption has steadily decreased over the last decade and soft drinks and bottled water have significantly increased (USDA, 2011). Milk products are the highest food sources of calcium and vitamin D, providing essential nutrients for healthy bones and teeth. In earlier times, carbonated sodas were an occasional treat; however, carbonated beverages now are very popular, convenient, and inexpensive. Restaurants often provide drink refills at no charge, which add additional calories. In addition, standard serving sizes for beverages have increased substantially. In the 1960s, a small nondiet soft drink at a restaurant was generally 8 ounces and approximately 80 calories, whereas the standard now is 12 or 16 ounces resulting in consumption of 140 to 180 calories. Some convenience stores offer 24 or 36-ounce cup options; a soft drink in the latter container size contains approximately 310 calories. Consumption of soft drinks as well as sugar-sweetened drinks, such as sports and energy beverages, has particularly increased among teens and youth (Babey, Wolstein, & Goldstein, 2013).

In a 24-hour period, beverage intake can significantly contribute to higher caloric intake and more body fat contributing to a risk factor of obesity in adolescence or adulthood. Soft drink vending machines have become a controversial topic recently, especially vending machines in schools, because they offer "empty calorie" beverages—beverages that contain about 1.5 ounces of sugar and no actual nutrients. Experts observe that placing vending machines in schools sends mixed messages to students learning about health and nutrition in class during a time when obesity is at epic proportions. The average annual milk consumption by gallon decreased from 29.8 gallons in 1970 to 20.04 gallons in 2011 (USDA, 2011).

Patterns of Physical Activity

Being physically active burns more calories than sedentary behavior and thus is essential for weight control and obesity prevention. Physical activity as part of daily living has been reduced significantly in the United States. Life in schools, places of work, and communities is less physically active than in past years. Many families provide an automobile for each child of driving age. In younger children, safety may be an issue so that walking to school occurs less often as well. Television, computer, and phone use consumes many hours for school-age children and teens. Studies show that the number of hours of television watched per day is directly correlated with being overweight or obese (Twarog, Politis, Woods, Boles, & Daniel, 2015).

Policy changes in local school districts have resulted in less physical education for students in public schools; many states have used time formally designated for physical activity for adding more courses. Recent research demonstrates a positive correlation between exercise and chronic disease. Researchers found that the lack of moderate weekly physical activity was a contributing factor leading to death among individuals with cardiovascular disease, type 2 diabetes mellitus, and breast and colon cancer (Lee et al., 2012).

Obesity Consequences: Chronic Disease

There are many consequences of being overweight, including both psychological and physiological issues. Bullying, anxiety, depression, and poor academic performance are adverse outcomes associated with weight stigmatization among children (Puhl & King, 2013). Among adults, studies show that obese individuals may be discriminated against in the workplace; obese people may be less likely to be hired or have a

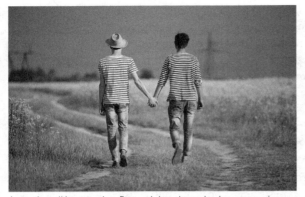

A couple walking together. Research has shown having an exercise partner increases consistency of exercise.
© Olesia Bilkei/Shutterstock

lower starting salary than nonobese individuals (O'Brien, Latner, & Hunter, 2013). Beyond these reasons, obesity is associated with early mortality and shorter life expectancy because being overweight is linked to developing chronic diseases that are the top causes of death in the United States. Although being overweight has long been tied to increased risk of developing cardiovascular disease, stroke, and diabetes, more recently published data have linked obesity to an increase in all-cause mortality risk. An analysis of the data from the Framingham Cohort Study revealed that the number of years living with obesity is directly linked to an increase of an all-cause mortality risk (Abdullah et al., 2011).

Addressing Obesity: Solutions

Losing weight can seem like such a simple thing, particularly if you are not overweight. Even healthcare providers can be judgmental in working with obese clients (Phelan et al., 2015). However, food consumption patterns are deeply rooted behaviors that are complex and are often steeped in family culture, religion, food preferences, and food availability as well as socioeconomic status. Thus, it is important to assess and understand what factors may be related to a client's weight status so that healthcare providers can effectively assist clients in improving their dietary habits and level of physical activity. The last part of this chapter deals specifically with strategies that nurses and other healthcare professionals can use to assist clients in health behavior changes when clients decide to implement healthy lifestyle choices.

Smoking and Smokeless Tobacco Control

Although cigarette smoking rates among adults have declined over the last 2 decades, approximately 16.8 percent of U.S. adults still smoke cigarettes today in spite of an increase in legislation and policies that ban smoking in restaurants, government agencies, and business offices (Jamal et al., 2015). As cigarette smoking declined, smokeless tobacco use has increased, particularly among adult men. Approximately 4 percent of adults are reported to use smokeless tobacco products, such as chewing tobacco or snuff (U.S. Department of Health and Human Services, 2014).

As early as 1930, physicians began to notice that most clients with lung cancer were smokers. It wasn't until the 1950s that definitive evidence from work by

Dr. Ernst Wynder and others established that smoking was related to significant negative health outcomes including an increased risk of developing lung cancer (Wynder, 1954). Today, we know that beyond lung cancer, smoking is also associated with increased risk of heart disease, stroke, emphysema, chronic obstructive pulmonary disease, and oral cancers. Tobacco control is estimated to prevent 8 million premature dates and increase lifespan by 20 years (Holford et al., 2014). Reducing disability, illness, and death related to tobacco use and secondhand smoke exposure is a key **Healthy People 2020** objective for primary prevention of chronic diseases in the U.S. population.

> **KEY TERM**
>
> **Healthy People 2020:** A statement of national health objectives designed to identify the most significant preventable threats to health and to establish national goals to reduce these threats in the next decade. Goals are set to help public health professionals, healthcare providers, and others work toward improving the health of citizens. Healthy People 2020 can be accessed at http://www.healthypeople.gov.

In the 1990s the government brought a lawsuit against the tobacco industry. The U.S. Tobacco Settlement was reached, whereby cigarette manufacturers were shown to be dishonest in advertising as well as in targeting children. States received funding from the settlement to help farmers transition from growing tobacco to growing other crops and support youth smoking prevention programs. Youth smoking continues to be common in high school students and, to some degree, among middle school students. This trend is of concern for a number of reasons; first and foremost, today's youth constitutes the next generation of smokers. Most adult smokers began smoking in their youth. Years of smoking can contribute to greater difficulty in quitting in adult years. Second, research by Wilson et al. (2005) demonstrated that youth who smoke are significantly more likely to have a lower intake of milk and vegetables as well as exercise less frequently than nonsmokers. These patterns were more likely in girls than boys and were evident even starting in middle school. Combining smoking with poor food intake may place youth at even higher risk of developing chronic diseases as they mature, given lower intake of protective nutrients that may offset damage from tobacco use (Wilson et al., 2005). It is important to assess smoking or tobacco use in clients when they are seen by healthcare providers for either an illness visit or a physical exam. Smoking is a very difficult habit to change and it can be easy for healthcare providers to decide that it is just too challenging to address with a client. However, it has been shown that having a healthcare provider ask patients about their smoking status and remind them of how damaging the habit is may prompt a certain percentage of clients to quit smoking, indicating that healthcare providers are perceived as powerful influencers when they articulate health promotion messages to clients. New models of delivering prevention messages are being tested for healthcare providers to ask about smoking and then refer clients to a "quit line" or online resources offered by some state health departments and organizations such as the American Cancer Society.

Client Education to Improve Health Behaviors

As already noted, health behavioral change is one of the most challenging issues that nurses and other healthcare professionals face. Behavior, such as lifestyle habits that include smoking, diet, and exercise, is learned over time, and unlike an acute condition such as an infection, cannot be changed just by taking prescription medicines. Medical knowledge has led to many advances that enable us to make organ transplants, insert heart pacemakers, and map the human genome. Yet it has been recognized that medical advances that have successfully treated acute disease are not well suited for chronic disease, which is a long-term condition that requires diligent self-management of certain health behaviors (Bandura, 2004). The complexity of health behavior has made it difficult to understand people's motivations and encourage change that will benefit those with chronic disease. For example, why is it that some people continue to smoke after a heart attack or being diagnosed with chronic lung disease? What makes it so difficult for many people to adhere to a weight-loss diet or maintain a regular exercise program?

The third section of this chapter presents health behavior change theories and tools for assessing and addressing unhealthy behaviors in clients and in various clinical and community settings.

Major Theories of Health Behaviors

There are a number of universally accepted explanations for what drives human behavior, many of which are specific to health-related behaviors. These explanations are known as models or theories and are useful in understanding why people choose to change or continue certain habits and how best to motivate them to make healthy lifestyle changes. Although there are many theories or models, some of the most commonly used health behavior theories are Social Cognitive Theory, the Health Belief Model, and the Transtheoretical Model.

Social Cognitive Theory

Social Cognitive Theory (SCT), developed by Alfred Bandura and first published in the 1970s, departed from the prevailing thought that environment was the main influence on behavior (Bandura, 1977, 1986). SCT instead is based on the idea that people's cognitive processes also influence their environment and that *reciprocal determinism,* or the constant interaction that occurs among people, their environment, and their behavior, is central to understanding behavior. The ideas of self-efficacy, the belief in one's ability to change a behavior successfully, along with self-control, the ability to maintain a change in behavior, are central to SCT. Thus, clients who firmly believe they can reduce sodium intake in their diet is more likely to succeed in meeting this goal than clients who have low confidence in their ability to adhere to new dietary guidelines.

Health Belief Model

The Health Belief Model (HBM) is one of the oldest models of health behavior and has been widely used to explain the adoption of several different health behaviors (Becker, 1974; Rosenstock, 1966). Based on the impact of personal beliefs on actions related to health, the HBM contains four main components: perceived susceptibility, perceived severity, perceived threat, and perceived benefits of action weighed against perceived barriers to action. According to the HBM (see **Figure 13-6**), clients will not consider a health-related behavioral change without first perceiving (a) that they are susceptible to a disease, (b) that the disease would have severe effects on them personally, and (c) that based on the perceived susceptibility and perceived severity, the disease is believed to be a threat. Perceiving a threat creates motivation to make changes to avoid that threat; however, final action is influenced by (d) perceived benefits of the action weighed against (e) perceived barriers to successfully taking that action.

For example, a fair-skinned woman who believes she is more susceptible to skin cancer and that the disease would affect her severely perceives sun exposure to be a threat. Her final decision to take preventive action would be based on whether she believes she can overcome the barriers to taking action (e.g., the inconvenience of wearing a hat in the sun and applying sunscreen) to realize

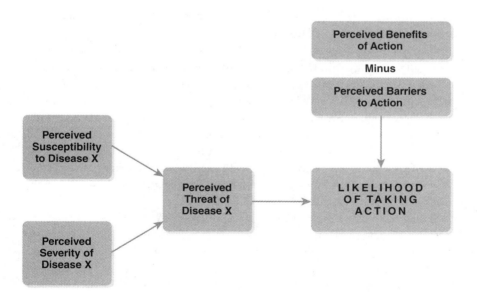

Figure 13–6 Health Belief Model.
Reproduced from Kaplan, R. M., Sallis, J. F., & Patterson, T. L. (1993). *Health and human behavior.* New York, NY: McGraw-Hill. Courtesy of James F. Sallis, PhD.

the benefits (reduced risk of sunburn and skin cancer and diminished effects of sun-related aging).

Transtheoretical Model

The Transtheoretical Model, or Stages of Change Theory (Prochaska & DiClemente, 1982), is an important tool for nurses and other healthcare professionals. This model is used to assess the client's readiness for change and is based on the premise that individuals are not all ready to accept immediate changes in their eating habits, food choices, and exercise routines. Instead, change occurs in stages: precontemplation, contemplation, preparation, action, and maintenance.

It is important to note that some stages may last for months or years. For example, it is possible for someone to be in the precontemplation stage for years or in the preparation stage for several months. In addition, the stages do not always progress in clear succession; at any stage after precontemplation, a client may relapse and have to begin the process again.

The three health behavior theories just described represent some of the most well known in the field, but many more exist and refinements and new developments arise as researchers continue their work. **Box 13-2** provides information on a few other health behavior models, including some that are newer to the field.

Client Behavioral Change

Understanding and changing health behaviors are two different things. Simply informing clients about a need to change an unhealthy behavior is unlikely to succeed in eliciting positive behavioral change. Clients should be provided a comprehensive educational strategy with the tools and resources needed to change behavior. Although it is helpful to provide clients with a tailored education program that involves more than one member of the healthcare team (e.g., nurses, physicians, dietitians, psychologists) and uses a collaborative approach, even brief interventions by primary care practitioners can be effective for unhealthy behaviors such as smoking (Aveyard, Begh, Parsons, & West, 2012). Research demonstrates that client engagement, such as client education, equips individuals with the skills and confidence to become actively engaged in their healthcare decisions and contributes to healthier outcomes, lower costs, and positive experiences (Hibbard & Greene, 2013).

Skilled nurse educators create an environment that encourages learning with trust, respect, and acceptance. Effective education actively involves clients by assessing their readiness to change, establish their own goals, and evaluate their ongoing progress in terms of these goals. Nurse educators also help clients understand the factors to provide motivation, encouragement, and ultimately sustain behavioral change. Although a variety of educational approaches exists to facilitate behavioral changes, a comprehensive model typically includes assessment, development, implementation, and evaluation.

BOX 13-2   SPOTLIGHT ON OTHER HEALTH BEHAVIOR MODELS

- *Precaution Adoption Process Model (PAPM):* Also based on stages of change, this model describes the stages people go through as they learn about a preventive behavior or activity (such as taking calcium to prevent osteoporosis), from lack of awareness through awareness and decision making to taking action (Weinstein & Sandman, 2002).

- *Human Strengths Approach:* A holistic approach to health promotion based on Leddy's Theory of Healthiness, the Human Strengths Approach focuses on the role of client strengths in maintaining health and emphasizes the importance of the nurse and client as partners, with the nurse acting as a "client resource" rather than an expert who tells the client what to do (Leddy, 2006).

- *Revised Health Promotion Model (RHPM):* This model explains the factors that influence health-promoting behaviors. Pender (1996) based this model on two other theories, Social Cognitive Theory, described in this chapter, and Expectancy-Value Theory, which is based on the concept that human behavior is rational and economical and that people will not put time and effort into working toward goals unless they value those goals and believe them to be achievable. Pender's original Health Promotion Model (HPM) was proposed as a way to integrate nursing and behavioral science viewpoints into the factors that affect health behaviors (Pender, 1996). It differed from other models in that it did not incorporate perceived fear or threat as motivating factors and thus was deemed applicable to health behaviors for which threat is not judged to be a major motivator. The RHPM, a refinement of the original HPM, is based on three major factors that influence health-promoting behaviors: (a) individual characteristics and experiences, such as prior related behavior and personal factors; (b) behavior-specific cognitions and affect (such as interpersonal influences from family, peers, situations, or perceived barriers and perceived self-efficacy); and (c) behavioral outcome (e.g., committing to a plan of action that results in behavioral change). Health-promoting behavior is the desired outcome (Pender, Murdaugh, & Parsons, 2014).

Assessing a Client

To provide clients with the skills, information, and resources they need to take steps toward making a positive health change, nurses must first assess a client's knowledge, ability, motivation, confidence, and resources for making such a change. The process should begin with a thorough assessment to formulate a comprehensive understanding of the client's current stage of change along with level of motivation to make changes. Attempting to implement an educational program without understanding client motivation can lead to failure, because unmotivated clients are much less likely to implement the suggestions and education provided by nurses. On the other hand, highly motivated clients who are ready to take action will likely need less formal education and assistance in the process. Examples of questions that can be used to assess motivation are:

- Have you ever thought about making changes in your [insert behavior; e.g., exercise habits]?
- What would you like to change about your [insert behavior] now?
- What concerns do you have about changing your [insert behavior] now?
- What has prevented you from making these changes in the past?

Assessment also involves understanding the client's knowledge and level of comprehension of the diagnosis and disease, treatment, and behaviors that the client can adopt to improve his or her health. Through this assessment process, the nurse can measure the scope of a client's knowledge and identify appropriate strategies to tailor educational interventions to meet the client's needs. Given the wide access to knowledge through the Internet and technological resources, many clients today may be more familiar with their condition than were clients 20 years ago and may require less intensive education. Other clients will have little or no knowledge of their condition and will need more information and resources. The varying range of client knowledge and technological skills makes this a crucial area to include in assessment.

Assessment should also include factors that may influence the client's ability to succeed in actualizing change that go beyond health status and motivation. It is important for healthcare professionals to realize that a client's behaviors are influenced by the interaction of physical environment, social and family networks, and the availability of resources. These factors are especially important when working with vulnerable populations. Therefore, assessment should address issues such as client literacy level, socioeconomic status, and physical and psychological stressors in home and work environments that may have a negative effect on client ability to change. Consideration of these factors can assist nurses in developing tailored plans that will be the most helpful to the client. For example, a client with low literacy levels may require simple instruction or the inclusion of a fully literate family member or close friend to help with the **health behavior change**; or a client who lives alone or is unlikely to be supported by family members may benefit from referral to a group education setting to provide social support. A client who works long hours on the job and relies frequently on restaurant food for meals may need guidance on healthy, yet convenient food choices.

> **KEY TERM**
>
> **Health behavior change:** A persistent and lasting change in a person's actions. Overweight/obesity, lack of physical activity, and dietary habits are the top three behaviors that health educators seek to change.

Creating and Implementing the Plan

Nurses can play an instrumental role in collaborating with their clients to develop and implement a behavioral change plan with a nurse–client mutual partnership. A client-driven educational approach helps to create an environment that allows clients to express their feelings, questions, and concerns and facilitates mutual goals with the nurse. Client perceptions are often more favorable when clients believe they are informed and involved in their treatment decisions, which in turn, empowers clients (Nygårdh, Malm, Wikby, & Ahlström, 2012).

Nurse educators should aim to provide information, correct misconceptions, address feelings about the recommended change, provide support, and motivate the client to foster change. Nurses may be able to validate the client's feelings about recommended changes by using language such as, "I know it's hard to . . .", "It must be difficult to . . .", or "I'd like to help you with . . .". In developing and discussing the plan, nurses should also show optimism about the chances for success to motivate the client ("I really think you'll be able to . . ." or "You seem confident in taking the necessary steps to achieve your goal of . . ."). The plan should also include follow-up appointment schedules to discuss progress and evaluate achievement of client goals. Follow-up appointments show clients that their behavioral change is important, that the nurse educator wants to spend time helping them monitor their progress, and that any obstacles encountered will be tackled together with the nurse educator.

Goal-setting is a critical part of client-centered education. Goals are most effectively created by clients with the assistance of a healthcare professional, after examining areas that need change. Clients may be encouraged to focus on only a few goals at one time and they may be more or less challenging depending on the client's confidence to achieve them. Goals should be clearly defined and include specific time frames. Clients may need "cues" from the nurse or healthcare professional to identify potential challenges and barriers that could threaten their ability to achieve their goals. The nurse educator can use feedback, reflection, summary, and problem-solving skills to encourage clients to consider ways to cope with anticipated difficulties. This process will help clients be more prepared and self-assured. Clients who have confidence to handle different situations and obstacles are more likely to achieve their goals.

Evaluating, Reassessing, and Revising

Maintaining any behavior change is often difficult. Follow-up appointments enable the nurse educator to evaluate and monitor progress, determining if the plan is appropriate. Useful questions include, "What part of the plan was most helpful?" and "What part of the plan did not work?" Such inquiries can help the nurse educator and client improve the plan, refining future goals.

Throughout the entire process, the nurse can use open-ended assessment questions that enable him or her to tailor the helping relationship to the needs of the client. Reflective statements such as, "Tell me more about…", "I hear you saying…", and summary statements are helpful to clarify and summarize what the client shares.

The Educational Environment

Nurses encounter clients in hospitals, offices, community clinics, other outpatient settings, and home settings. Client education can be provided through one-on-one instruction, or nurse educators may become involved in classroom settings through venues such as a hospital's community education program or a community outreach center. The nurse educator should be aware of the unique characteristics of each setting and how the environment can enhance educational efforts. In addition, it is important for the nurse educator to communicate with other members of the healthcare team who are working with the client (e.g., dietitians, health educators, advanced practice nurses, physicians) to ensure a coordinated and collaborative approach toward behavioral change.

Hospital Setting

The clinical setting can offer key opportunities to initiate or reinforce a client's educational plan, given the opportunities for follow-up visits with the client. Nurses can begin counseling during hospitalization, with follow-up visits scheduled to continue through the course of outpatient treatment or therapy. Recent studies show that many clients view diet and exercise education postsurgery as an opportune time to start practicing better habits—a "teachable moment" (Rock & Demar-Wahnefried, 2002). Thus, inpatient education can be an excellent beginning to the counseling process. However, time constraints in the current healthcare model may pose challenges to extensive formal client education so brief educational interventions or take-home educational materials may be appropriate strategies.

Outpatient Setting: Individual

Changing trends in the healthcare system, leading to decreased admissions and shortened length of stay in hospitals, have propelled outpatient counseling to the forefront. Because of these trends, hospitalized clients usually are those with exacerbations of their condition or severe illnesses. Therefore, during rehospitalization or an acute episode of illness, clients may not be receptive to learning. In addition, most clients require more education and follow-up than can be provided in the inpatient setting or during discharge planning sessions. Reduced time for adequate counseling and some clients' lack of readiness to learn immediately following diagnosis support the concept that client education may best be achieved outside the hospital. This trend also underscores the need to provide printed information (e.g., brochures) for clients and additional Web resources if clients have access to and familiarity with using the Internet.

Outpatient Setting: Group

Group education settings can be an effective place to provide client education. Nurse educators may become involved in leading group education sessions as part of their hospital's community education program, or they may recommend clients to programs to supplement their education. Education in a group setting can provide clients with social support through opportunities to share with others who are trying to change health behaviors. Learning from the experiences of others, hearing how others have overcome obstacles, and providing insight from their own experiences can provide clients with the motivation and reinforcement needed to help them follow through on their plans. Being with others facing similar situations can remove feelings of isolation, helping clients feel that they are not alone in their struggle to change health behaviors (Pender, 1996).

A group education program should never be a substitute for a tailored, one-on-one approach through which nurses are able to provide clients with personal support, motivation, reassessment of goals, and evaluation on progress. However, well-developed group education programs can complement individual efforts by the nurse. In referring clients to group education programs, nurses should be familiar with the program content, know its reliability and efficacy, and assess the program logistics, such as location and time offered, with the client. It is important to follow up with the client on successive visits to determine whether the client participated or what barriers may have prevented participation.

Areas to Consider in Client Education

Multiple variables contribute to a client's ability to learn, including a client's physical condition and comfort level, length of time since and adjustment to the diagnosis, financial resources, educational level, cultural context, support system, and language barriers. The Joint Commission (2010) has specific standards for client education, including assessment of client cultural and religious beliefs, learning needs, physical or cognitive limitations, and barriers to communication. Clients differ in their educational backgrounds, intellectual abilities, and attitudes toward accepting responsibility for healthy behaviors. An assessment of these issues is important for optimal client education.

To be effective in educating clients, nurses and other healthcare professionals must demonstrate greater cultural competence. Although defined in many ways and encompassed in several terms, cultural competence basically means the ability to understand and effectively relate to people from diverse groups—in terms of gender, race, age, religious background, culture, language, educational level, and socioeconomic status. Culturally competent health providers respect cultural differences in a manner that facilitates a client's ability to make decisions (Purnell, 2014). A culturally sensitive, individualized behavior change plan can affect a client's long-term physical status, function, and quality of life. Therefore, nurses must work as collaborative partners of a healthcare team with team members, such as community educators, physical therapists, and speech therapists, to better tailor client health assessment and implement the most effective education plan during the initial diagnosis, the treatment phase, or long-term follow-up period. Given the diversity of client populations, tailored educational interventions may also require allowing for client-specific cultural norms and/or providing interpreters and non-English educational materials for non-English-speaking clients. Nurses and other healthcare professionals today are often more successful in

TABLE 13-1 COMMUNICATION TECHNIQUES

Therapeutic Communication Strategies	Non-Verbal Therapeutic Communication Strategies	Non-Therapeutic Communication Strategies
Developing an initial rapport	Facing the patient and making eye contact	Abruptly initiating the conversation before the patient is comfortable in the relationship
Maintaining the patient's rights for privacy	Using a calm voice tone, maintaining eye contact, and providing a comfortable and private environment	Discussing the patient with any other individual or family member
Clarifying by rephrasing or paraphrasing what the patient has stated	Maintaining a neutral and calm affect and keeping the room, halls, and environment quiet; listening to the patient attentively	Interrupting or changing the subject away from the patient's lead on the conversation
Providing information and explaining procedures; honestly stating when you do not know an answer	Demonstrating your willingness to be present with the patient; smiling and displaying a positive attitude with your body language	Giving false reassurance or stating information when you do not know the answer
Asking broad, open-ended questions	Sitting near the patient; maintaining your presence within their comfort zone of personal space boundaries	Assuming you know the patient's feelings
Being accepting; exploring possibilities with the patient based on their value system and cultural preferences	Using touch when appropriate; keeping eye contact with the patient and avoiding lengthy sessions on the computer when in the patient's room	Making judgmental or coercive responses; displaying anger or disagreement with the patient

communicating with clients if they communicate clearly and also reflect empathy, self-awareness, honesty, gender sensitivity, cultural awareness, and knowledge. **Table 13-1** illustrates effective communication techniques as well as ineffective communication techniques.

Gender and Culture

Gender and culture are two additional factors that may have an impact on perceptions, attitudes, and the process of learning. For example, an educator may not detect the depth of depression a man with prostate cancer is experiencing. Traditional gender stereotypes may discourage some men from showing emotion or weakness. In addition, an educator may not be familiar with cultural norms that influence dietary habits among people of certain cultures. However, a sensitive educator can recognize, understand, and feel comfortable with such differences and realize when, for example, it may be appropriate to include on the healthcare team a person who can offer informed insight of the client's cultural background and the impact that this background may have on the client's cooperation with the efforts of the healthcare team.

Language and Literacy

Spoken language and literacy levels are critical for client understanding of prescribed health regimens and efforts to change health behaviors. Clients who are nonnative speakers of English may require translators or benefit from the presence of a family member who is fluent in English. Otherwise, serious misunderstandings may occur that can affect patient care and lead to negative health outcomes. For instance, a prescription labeled "once a day" could be misinterpreted by a native speaker of Spanish with limited capability in English, because in Spanish, "once" is the number 11.

Literacy, both general and health specific, also is a critical factor in client education. Fully or partially illiterate clients may have difficulty understanding oral instructions or printed materials and are unlikely to be able to access resources available on the Internet. Patients with some chronic conditions and poor literacy skills are more likely to miss their scheduled appointments or have their prescription medications filled (Muir, Logan, & Bosworth, 2013). Clients may indicate they comprehend the educational content although they do not and are embarrassed to admit their perceived deficits to the healthcare practitioner. Nurses may identify clients at risk for low health literacy skills through informal assessment techniques. Simple oral communication strategies may promote health literacy and confidence among their clients (see **Box 13-3**). These clients require special approaches and may benefit from the help of a literate family member or friend. In addition, general health literacy is important to the success of client education efforts.

Thus, the nurse educator must be aware of a client's general literacy level and familiarity with health information before embarking on a plan for health behavior change or providing printed materials as a client resource.

Personal Resources

Many healthcare providers fail to recognize the importance of understanding the whole client in achieving successful health outcomes. This is particularly true when working with certain vulnerable populations. A client facing a large number of personal stressors in his or her life that stem from living in poverty may not have the personal resources to take on the additional challenges that a health behavior change requires. In addition, if a client's physical or social home environment is inadequate in some way, it could interfere with efforts to initiate and maintain

BOX 13-3 FOCUS ON HEALTH LITERACY

Health Literacy Informal Assessment

Adults with low health literacy report feeling a sense of shame and may hide their struggles to comprehend medical information from healthcare providers. Nurses may use informal assessment strategies to identify clients who may be at a higher risk for low health literacy. The following behaviors may indicate further assessment of health literacy skills:

- Frequently miss appointments
- Fail to complete registration forms
- Unable to name medications or explain their purpose or dosing
- Identify pills by looking at them, not reading the prescription label
- Unable to provide a coherent, sequential medical history
- Show lack of follow-through on tests or referrals
- Repeatedly use statements such as "I forgot my reading glasses," "I'll read through this when I get home," or "I'm too tired to read," when the client is asked to discuss written material

Oral Communication Strategies to Promote Health Literacy

Oral communication, particularly between providers and clients in a medical setting, is a critical medium through which health education is disseminated.

The following strategies may be used to promote health literacy:

- Create a safe and respectful environment: Greet client warmly. Make eye contact. Take the time to get to know the client and earn his or her trust.
- Use speech that is easy to understand: Slow down your speaking pace. Limit content to a few key points. Be specific and concrete, not general. Use words that are simple and familiar. Avoid complex technical jargon or acronyms.
- Keep the client engaged in the conversation: Use pictures, physical models, videos, or interactive media to aid technically complex conversations. Ask open-ended questions to facilitate discussion. Get to know what the client cares about most—family, friends, work, hobbies—and incorporate those into your health discussions.
- Confirm client understanding: Ask the individual to "teach back" the educational information. Remind the individual that many people have difficulty understanding the materials. Summarize key points.

Reproduced from Center for Healthcare Strategies , Inc. (2013). *Health literacy fact sheets*. Retrieved from http://www .chcs.org/media/CHCS_Health_Literacy_Fact_Sheets_2013.pdf

change. For example, an obese client living in a subsidized housing community who does not feel safe spending time outside is unlikely to follow advice to undertake a personal walking program. Similarly, a client advised to make dietary changes but who lacks adequate transportation to a grocery store or does not live in an area where stores offer a variety of healthy foods lacks basic resources for initiating dietary change. Finally, the social home environment is an important factor to consider when working with clients to make health behavior change. Will family members support the changes the client is trying to make? A client's efforts to make a lifestyle change are often facilitated when family members contribute to the effort, such as a spouse or significant other who simultaneously participates in a smoking cessation program or an entire family agreeing to change their eating habits or undertake a regular exercise program. Lack of support from family members can deter client efforts to enact change.

Critical to personal resources is a client's socioeconomic status. A client lacking economic or educational experience may be unlikely to initiate change or even to comply with an established health regimen. An example is a case history of an elderly African American woman, nonadherent with medications for hypertension. This client presented to her primary care provider for a chief complaint of headaches and on further examination, the client was experiencing an increased blood pressure. The client was not taking her hypertension medication. Further inquiry by the provider revealed that the client was taking her blood pressure medicine every other day versus daily as prescribed, because of the cost of the medication. As a result of this finding, the provider was able to find a lower cost alternative blood pressure medication within the same antihypertensive classification.

Summary

This chapter addressed potential healthcare challenges for individuals from populations that may be at greater risk for developing chronic diseases and the consequences commonly seen in individuals with these diseases. In addition, the chapter provided an overview of health behavior theories and described the main health behaviors that contribute to the leading causes of death in the United States today. Finally, the chapter explained how to translate behavioral change education and motivation strategies for working with individuals and groups to enhance their abilities to practice health-promoting behavior for chronic disease risk reduction.

Reflective Practice Questions

1. Discuss the difference between the terms *health disparities* and *vulnerable populations*. What are the implications for practice when a nurse is working with individuals or groups from vulnerable populations?
2. This chapter discusses the issue that causes of health disparities are "multifactorial." Explain what is meant by the term multifactorial and how the Social Determinants of Health Model may be used as an assessment tool for these factors.
3. Identify three causes of the obesity epidemic. Discuss educational strategies appropriate for school-age children participating in a healthy nutrition program.

4. Discuss an appropriate behavioral change health model for a smoking cessation program among older adults. Provide a rationale for your answer as well as the main concepts of the health model.
5. Describe three strategies that may be effective when educating clients with low health literacy skills.

References

Abdullah, A., Wolfe, R., Stoelwinder, J. S., Courten, M., Stevenson, C., Walls, H. L., & Peeters, A. (2011). The number of years lived with obesity and the risk of all-cause and cause-specific mortality. *International Journal of Epidemiology, 40*(4), 985–996. http://dx.doi.org/10.1093/ije/dyr018

American Diabetes Association. (2016). *Statistics about diabetes.* Retrieved from http://www.diabetes.org/diabetes-basics/statistics/

Antonovsky, A. (1967). Social class, life expectancy and overall mortality. *Millbank Memorial Fund Quarterly, 45,* 31–73.

Aveyard, P., Begh, R., Parsons, A., & West, R. (2012). Brief opportunistic smoking cessation interventions: A systematic review and meta-analysis to compare advice to quit and offer of assistance. *Addiction, 107*(6), 1066–1073. http://dx.doi.org/10.1111/j.1360-0443.2011.03770.x

Babey, S. H., Wolstein, J., & Goldstein, H. (2013). *Still bubbling over: California adolescents drinking more soda and other sugar-sweetened beverages.* Los Angeles, CA: UCLA Center for Health Policy and Research. Retrieved from http://healthpolicy.ucla.edu/publications/search/pages/detail.aspx?PubID=1228

Bandura, A. (1977). Self-efficacy: Toward a unifying theory of behavioral change. *Psychological Review, 84,* 191–215.

Bandura, A. (1986). *Social foundations of thought and action.* Englewood Cliffs, NJ: Prentice-Hall.

Bandura, A. (2004). Health promotion by social cognitive means. *Health Education and Behavior, 31,* 143–164.

Becker, M. H. (1974). The health belief model and sick role behavior. *Health Education Monographs, 2,* 409–419.

Blackwell, D. L., Lucas, J. W., & Clarke, T. C. (2014). Summary health statistics for U.S. adults: National Health Interview Survey 2012. *Vital Health Statistics,* (10), 260.

Centers for Disease Control and Prevention. (2013). *QuickStats: Number of deaths from 10 leading causes: National Vital Statistics System, United States, 2010. Morbidity and Mortality Weekly Report, 62*(08), 155. Retrieved from http://www.cdc.gov/mmwr/preview/mmwrhtml/mm6208a8.htm

Centers for Disease Control and Prevention. (2015a). *Chronic disease overview.* Retrieved from http://www.cdc.gov/chronicdisease/overview/index.htm

Centers for Disease Control and Prevention. (2015b). *Faststats: Obesity and overweight.* Retrieved from http://www.cdc.gov/nchs/fastats/obesity-overweight.htm

Centers for Disease Control and Prevention. (2016). *Cancer rates by race/ethnicity and sex.* Retrieved from http://www.cdc.gov/cancer/dcpc/data/race.htm

Center for Healthcare Strategies, Inc. (2013). *Health literacy fact sheets.* Retrieved from http://www.chcs.org/media/CHCS_Health_Literacy_Fact_Sheets_2013.pdf

Center for Science in the Public Interest. (2007, June 14). *Kellogg makes historic settlement agreement, adopting nutrition standards for marketing foods to children* [Press release]. Retrieved from http://www.cspinet.org/new/200706141.html

Dahlgren, G., & Whitehead, M. (1991). *Policies and strategies to promote social equity in health.* Stockholm, Sweden: Institute of Future Studies.

DeNavas-Walt, C., & Proctor, B. D. (2015). *Income and poverty in the United States: 2014* (P60-252). Washington, DC: Government Printing Office.

Dugan, A. (2013). *Fast food still major part of U.S. diet.* Retrieved from http://www.gallup.com/poll/163868/fast-food-major-part-diet.aspx

Hebert, J. R., Hurley, T. G., Harmoon, B. E., Heiney, S., Hebert, C. J., & Steck, S. E. (2013). A diet, physical activity, and stress reduction intervention in men with rising prostate-specific antigen after treatment for prostate cancer. *Cancer Epidemiology, 36*(2), e128–e136. doi:10.1016/j.canep.2011.09.008

Hibbard, J. H., & Greene, J. (2013). What the evidence shows about patient activation: Better health outcomes and care experiences; fewer data on costs. *Health Affairs, 32*(2), 207–214. http://dx.doi.org/10.1377/hlthaff.2012.1061

Holford, T. R., Meza, R., Warner, K. E., Meernik, C., Jeon, J., Moolgavkar, S. H., & Levy, D. T. (2014). Tobacco control and the reduction in smoking-related premature deaths in the United States, 1964-2012. *Journal of the American Medical Association, 311*(2), 164–171. http://dx.doi.org/10.1001/jama.2013.285112

Jamal, A., Homa, D. H., O'Conner, E., Babb, S. D., Caraballo, R. S., Singh, T., . . . King, B. A. (2015). *Current cigarette smoking among adults-United States, 2005–2014.* Retrieved from http://www.cdc.gov/mmwr/preview/mmwrhtml/mm6444a2.htm?s_cid=mm6444a2_w

Jaworowska, A., Blackham, T., Davies, I. G., & Stevenson, L. (2013). Nutritional challenges and health implications of takeaway and fast food. *Nutrition Reviews, 71*(5), 310–318. http://dx.doi.org/10.1111/nure.12031

Kaplan, R. M., Sallis, J. F., & Patterson, T. L. (1993). *Health and human behavior.* New York, NY: McGraw-Hill.

Leddy, S. K. (2006). *Health promotion: Mobilizing strengths to enhance health, wellness, and well-being.* Philadelphia, PA: F.A. Davis.

Lee, I., Shiroma, E. J., Lobelo, F., Puska, P., Blair, S. N., & Katzmarzyk, P. T. (2012). Effect of physical inactivity on major non-communicable diseases worldwide: An analysis of burden of disease and life expectancy. *Lancet, 380*(9838), 219–229. http://dx.doi.org/10.1016/S0140-6736(12)61031-9

Martin, A. (2007, June 14). Kellogg to phase out some food ads to children. *New York Times.* Retrieved from http://www.nytimes.com/2007/06/14/business/14kellogg.html

Mozaffarian, D., Benjamin, E. J., Go, A. S., Arnett, D. K., Blaha, M. J., Cushman M.. . .Turner, M. B. (2015). Heart disease and stroke statistics 2015 update: A report from the American Heart Association. *Circulation, 131*(4), e29–e322. doi: 10.1161/CIR.0000000000000152

Muir, K. W., Logan, C., & Bosworth, H. B. (2013). Health literacy and glaucoma. *Current Opinion in Ophthalmology, 24*(2), 119–124. http://dx.doi.org/10.1097/ICU.0b013e32835c8b0e

National Institute of Diabetes and Digestive and Kidney Diseases. (2012). *Overweight and obesity statistics* (NIH No. 04-4158). Retrieved from http://www.niddk.nih.gov/health-information/health-statistics/Pages/overweight-obesity-statistics.aspx#b

Nies, M. A., & McEwen, M. (2014). *Community/public health nursing: Promoting the health of populations* (6th ed.). St. Louis, MO: Elsevier Saunders.

Nygårdh, N., Malm, D., Wikby, K., & Ahlström, G. (2012). The experience of empowerment in the patient–staff encounter: The patient's perspective. *Journal of Clinical Nursing, 21,* 897–904. http://dx.doi.org/10.1111/j.1365-2702.2011.03901.x

O'Brien, K. S., Latner, J. D., & Hunter, J. A. (2013). Obesity discrimination: The role of physical appearance, personal ideology, and anti-fat prejudice. *International Journal of Obesity, 37,* 455–460. http://dx.doi.org/10.1038/ijo.2012.52

Ogden, C. L., Carroll, M. D., Kitt, B. K., & Flegal, K. M. (2014). Prevalence of obesity among adults: United States, 2011–2012. *Journal of American Medical Association, 311*(8), 806–814. http://dx.doi.org/10.1001/jama.2014.732

Ornish, D. (2007, January 24). The threat from within. *Newsweek.* Retrieved from http://www.newsweek.com/id/70227

Pender, N. J. (1996). *Health promotion in nursing practice.* Stamford, CT: Appleton & Lange.

Pender, N. J., Murdaugh, C.L., & Parsons, M.A. (2014). *Health promotion in nursing practice* (7th ed.). Upper Saddle River, NJ: Prentice Hall.

Phelan, S. M., Burgess, D. J., Yeazel, M. W., Hellerstedt, W. L., Griffin, J. M., & Van Ryn, M. (2015). Impact of weight bias and stigma on quality of care and outcomes for patients with obesity. *Obesity Reviews, 16*(4), 319–326. http://dx.doi.org/10.1111/obr.12266

Price, J. H., Khubchandani, J., McKinney, M., & Braun, R. (2013). Racial/ethnic disparities in chronic diseases of youths and access to health care in the United States. *ioMed Research International,* 2013. http://dx.doi.org/10.1155/2013/787616

Prochaska, J. O., & DiClemente, C. (1982). Transtheoretical theory: Toward a more integrative model of change. *Psychotherapy: Theory, Research, and Practice, 19*(3), 276–287.

Puhl, R. M., & King, K. M. (2013). Weight discrimination and bullying. Clinical Endocrinology and Metabolism, 27(2), 117–127. http://dx.doi.org/http://dx.doi.org/10.1016/j.beem.2012.12.002

Purnell, L. D. (2014). *Guide to culturally competent health care* (3rd ed.). Philadelphia, PA: F.A. Davis.

Rock, C., & Demark-Wahnefried, W. (2002). Nutrition and survival after the diagnosis of breast cancer: A review of the evidence. *Journal of Clinical Oncology, 20* (15), 3302–3316.

Rosenstock, I. M. (1966). Why people use health services. *Millibank Memorial Fund Quarterly, 44,* 94–127.

Short, K. S. (2016). Child poverty: Definition and measurement. *Academic Pediatrics, 16*(3), S46–S51. http://dx.doi.org/10.1016/j.acap.2015.11.005

Smith, J. C., & Medalia, C. (2015). *Health insurance coverage in the United States: 2014* (P60-253). Washington, DC: Government Printing Office.

Spanakis, E. K., & Golden, S. H. (2013). Race/ethnic difference in diabetes and diabetic complications. *Current Diabetes Reports, 13*(6), 814–823. http://dx.doi.org/10.1007/s11892-013-0421-9

The Joint Commission. (2010). *Advancing effective communication, cultural competence, and patient-*and *family-centered care: A roadmap for hospitals.* Retrieved from http://www.jointcommission.org/assets/1/6/ARoadmapforHospitalsfinalversion727.pdf

Twarog, J. P., Politis, M. D., Woods, E. L., Boles, M. K., & Daniel, L. M. (2015). Daily television viewing time and associated risk of obesity among U.S. preschool aged children: An analysis of NHANES 2009–2012. *Obesity Research & Clinical Practice, 9*(6), 636–638. http://dx.doi.org/10.1016/j.orcp.2015.09.004

U.S. Cancer Statistics Working Group. (2015). *United States cancer statistics: 1999–2012 incidence and mortality web-based report.* Atlanta, GA: Department of Health and Human Services, Centers for Department of Health and Human Services, Centers for Disease Control and Prevention, and National Cancer Institute.

U.S. Census Bureau. (2014). *Poverty data.* Retrieved from https://www.census.gov/hhes/www/poverty/data/

U.S. Department of Agriculture. (2011). *Dairy market statistics.* Retrieved from http://www.ams.usda.gov/sites/default/files/media/Dairy%20Market%20Statistics%202011.pdf

U.S. Department of Agriculture Food and Nutrition Service. (2014). *School meals: Healthy-Hunger Free Kids Act.* Retrieved from http://www.fns.usda.gov/school-meals/healthy-hunger-free-kids-act

U.S. Department of Health and Human Services. (2014). *The health consequences of smoking—50 years of progress: A report of the Surgeon General, 2014.* Atlanta, GA: U.S. Department of

Health and Human Services, Centers for Disease Control and Prevention, National Center for Chronic Disease Prevention and Health Promotion, Office on Smoking and Health.

U.S. Department of Health and Human Services, Office of Disease Prevention and Health Promotion. (n.d.). *Healthy People 2020*. Retrieved from https://www.healthypeople.gov

Ward, B. W., Schiller, J. S., & Goodman, R. A. (2014). Multiple chronic conditions among US adults: A 2012 update. *Preventing Chronic Disease, 11*(E62). doi: 10.5888/pcd11.130389

Weinstein, N. D., & Sandman, P. M. (2002). The precaution adoption process model. In K. Glanz, B. K. Rimer, & F. M. Lewis (Eds.), *Health behavior and health education: Theory, research, and practice* (3rd ed., pp. 121–143). San Francisco, CA: Jossey-Bass.

Wilson, D. B., Smith, B., Speizer, I., Bean, M., Mitchell, K., Uguy, L. S., . . . Fries, E. A. (2005). Differences in food intake and exercise by smoking status in adolescents. *Preventive Medicine, 40*(6), 872–879.

World Health Organization. (2013). *A global brief on hypertension: Silent killer, global public health crisis*. Retrieved from http://www.thehealthwell.info/node/466541

World Health Organization. (2015a). *Global health observatory data repository: Life expectancy data by country*. Retrieved from http://apps.who.int/gho/data/node.main.688?lang=en

World Health Organization. (2015b). *Health impact assessment*. Retrieved from http://www.who.int/hia/evidence/doh/en/

Wynder, E. (1954). The place of tobacco in the etiology of lung cancer. *Connecticut Medicine, 18*(4), 321–330.

chapter 14

Cultural Diversity and Care

G. Elaine Patterson

LEARNING OUTCOMES

After reading this chapter you will be able to:

- Compare common value orientations associated with cultures.
- Analyze components of cultural diversity.
- Describe the components and principles of cultural competence.
- Describe the influence of technology on cultural development and communication systems.
- Discuss cultural influences on beliefs and systems related to health and illness.
- Discuss the role of culture in interactions with clients.
- Address the development of cultural competence in nursing students.
- Identify appropriate patterns, challenges, and needs of clients in the cultural domain.

Introduction

An awareness of and accommodation to the cultural aspects of health and illness behaviors enables nurses to promote health by skillfully blending professional knowledge with knowledge of the individual's or group's beliefs. People

The editors wish to acknowledge the contributions of Joan C. Engebretson and Judith A. Headley to the previous edition of this chapter.

present with practices and beliefs from their country of origin
or with practices arrived at by acculturation processes where
cultures are adapting each other's attributes, creating variations
of the original. No matter how acculturation occurs, healthcare
workers are responsible for delivering competent quality care
to an increasingly diverse population. **Culturally competent
health care** is the delivery of health care with skill, knowledge,
and sensitivity to cultural factors. This chapter identifies the
components of cultural competence and describes the principles of cultural competence, as well as strategies that foster the development of cultural competence.

Cultural Diversity and Practices

Culture is the combination of ideas, customs, skills, arts, and
other capabilities of a people or group, although as a whole, it is
more complex than any one of these elements. Culture, which is
learned from birth through language acquisition and socialization, is the process by which an individual adapts to the group's
organized way of life. This process also provides for the transmission of culture from
one generation to another. Members of the cultural group share cultural beliefs and
patterns of behavior that create a group identity, which has a powerful influence on
behavior, usually on a subconscious level. Culture is largely tacit, meaning it is not
generally expressed or discussed at a conscious level. Most culturally derived actions
are based on implicit cues rather than written or spoken sets of rules.

Although many of the underlying beliefs and value systems of a culture are stable,
all cultures are inherently dynamic and changing; therefore, it is difficult to generalize
from one situation or time to another. Cultural practices are continually adapting
to the environment, historical context, technology, and availability of resources. As
a result, the context in which people live influences, and is influenced by, cultural
practice. Anthropology (the study of cultures) and nursing are both based on a holistic perspective. Culture has a significant impact on health and illness behaviors, as
well as patterns of response. It directly influences health behaviors such as diet and
exercise. Cultural beliefs and practices also affect the types of health problems that
are attended to and the actions taken to deal with them. Activities taken to promote,
maintain, or restore health are all performed in a cultural context. Therefore, an
understanding of the client's perceptions and the context in which he or she lives
are necessary for optimal client care.

Culture also determines much of the relationship and type of communication
between a client and a healthcare provider. Given that the United States is a culturally diverse nation, nurses and other healthcare providers encounter individuals and
groups whose habits of health maintenance, reactions to illness or disease, and use

of healthcare services may differ from their own. According to the 2013 U.S. census, diverse groups that comprise the U.S. population include African American (13.8 percent), Asian American (6 percent), Pacific Islanders and Native Hawaiians (0.4 percent), and Hispanics (17.1 percent). European Americans make up 76.2 percent of the U.S. population but that number is declining. It is predicted that by the year 2020 "no racial group will comprise a majority" (Thomas, 2014, p. 7492).

Cultural Competency

With increasing diversity in the population, and the recognition that health disparities exist across ethnic groups, healthcare regulatory agencies recommend that cultural competence become a goal in the provision of health care. There is no single definition of cultural competence. However it is generally accepted that culturally competent care respects diversity in the population, acknowledging factors that can affect health and delivery of health care. These factors include race, sex, culture, age, behaviors, and communication styles. Therefore, cultural competence is measured by how well a patient's needs are met regardless of the patient's race, gender, ethnicity, sexual orientation, religion, and language (Kyeyune, 2015).

The Office of Minority Health (U.S. Department of Health and Human Services, 2016) has developed standards and recommendations that apply to the institutional level as well as to the individual provider. Institutions are mandated to provide cultural and linguistically appropriate services in health and health care. These standards are known as the national CLAS standards.

The National Center for Cultural Competency (NCCC), an established resource and publication site located at George Washington University, has as its mission to "increase the capacity of health care and mental health care programs to design, implement and evaluate culturally and linguistically competent service delivery systems to address growing diversity, persistent disparities, and to promote health and mental health equality" (NCCC, n.d., para. 1). The NCCC uses a conceptual framework developed by Cross, Baron, Dennis, and Isaacs (1989) that describes a continuum from cultural destructiveness to cultural competency. Professionals seek to counter cultural destructiveness, the lowest level of the continuum, through laws such as the Civil Rights Act of 1964 (Title VI), which mandates that healthcare providers do not discriminate according to **race**, **ethnicity**, or creed. The ethic of nonmaleficence, or "do no harm," also addresses this basic level.

The second level of the continuum, cultural incapacity, refers to unintentional practices that may be harmful to patients through ignorance, insensitive attitudes, or improper allocation of resources. Cultural blindness, the third level, is exemplified

> **KEY TERM**
>
> **Race:** A social classification that denotes a biologic or genetically transmitted set of distinguishable physical characteristics.

> **KEY TERM**
>
> **Ethnicity:** Designation of a population subgroup sharing a common social and cultural heritage.

by treating all patients alike without accommodating cultural differences. Providing translators, developing health education aimed at specific cultural groups, and creating programs that address diverse groups' access to care are good examples of cultural precompetence, which is level four. Cultural competence, level five, is best described as an ongoing learning process for the provider who can integrate cultural knowledge into individualized patient-centered care. This eventually leads to the highest level of the continuum, cultural proficiency. This framework reminds us that cultural competence is a developmental process that evolves over an extended period. Both individuals and organizations are at various levels of awareness, knowledge, and skills along the cultural competence continuum (Cross et al., 1989). Practicing in a culturally competent manner also incorporates the three aspects of evidence-based practice: best evidence from valid and clinically relevant research, the provider's clinical expertise, and the patient's values and unique preferences (Sackett et al., 2000).

Culturally competent health care must be provided within the context of a client's cultural background, beliefs, and values related to health and illness to attain optimal client outcomes. Healthcare providers have to be knowledgeable of their own cultural awareness before initiating care. According to a survey conducted by the National Council of State Boards of Nursing (NCSBN) and The Forum of State Nursing Workforce Centers, nurses from minority backgrounds represent 19 percent of the registered nurse (RN) workforce. Considering racial/ethnic backgrounds, the RN population is composed of White/Caucasian (83 percent), African American (6 percent), Asian (6 percent), Hispanic (3 percent), American Indian/Alaskan Native (1 percent), Native Hawaiian/Pacific Islander (1 percent), and other nurses (1 percent) (NCSBN, 2013). In addition to Leininger's classic work on cultural diversity, and the work of the Transcultural Nursing Society, there is a body of literature addressing the need for cultural sensitivity (Hicks, 2012); biases and ethnocentrism (Dunagan, Kimble, Gunby, & Andrews, 2014); and several others regarding nurses' role and responsibility in providing culturally sensitive care.

Most educational approaches to addressing cultural competence have focused on knowledge, attitudes, and skills. Knowledge has often focused on facts and characteristics about specific cultures. This "cookbook" approach has been criticized as leading to **stereotyping**. The approach of cultural sensitivity training attempts to address attitudes. What seems to be more valuable is for providers to learn a set of skills that enable them to provide high-quality patient care to everyone. A literature review of cultural competence and the clinical encounter (Betancourt, Corbett, & Bondaryk, 2014) concluded that healthcare providers develop the skills for a patient-centered approach that does the following: (a) assesses core cross-cultural issues, (b) explores the meaning of the illness to the patient, (c) determines the social context in which the patient lives, and (d) engages in a negotiation process with the patient.

KEY TERM

Stereotyping: Consigning cultural attributes to a group of people based on assumptions, opinions, or attitudes.

Betancourt (2006) describes the culturally diverse healthcare system as one that acknowledges and incorporates the importance of culture, assessment of cross-cultural relations, vigilance toward the dynamics that result from cultural differences, expansion of cultural knowledge, and adaptation of services to meet unique needs. Betancourt (2006) adapts five components for developing cultural sensitivity: open-mindedness, awareness of one's own cultural values, understanding of differences, knowledge, and adaptation skills, which are still being used.

1. Awareness and acceptance of cultural differences require an open-minded attitude about other worldviews. It is important to recognize that providing care based on one's own perspective may not be in the best interest of the client. Nurses who use a nonjudgmental approach in learning about a client's cultural belief system will not only gain a wealth of information, but also readily establish mutual trust in their nurse–client relationships.

2. An awareness of one's own biases and attitudes is a step toward overcoming them. Recognition of personal cultural attitudes requires conscious effort; most people are unaware of their cultural beliefs because their beliefs are so integrated into their perception of the world. It is important to note that value awareness does not mean that one tries to eliminate values. We all need to hold values in order to live our lives. The essential aspect is to become aware of our own values, so that we can better understand the values of another.

3. It is essential to recognize basic differences among cultures without promoting the superiority of one culture over another. Often, in an effort to connect with people of other cultures, people assume that there are few differences among cultures. Although recognizing similarities may be useful for making connections, it can obscure basic differences necessary for cultural understanding. For example, a European American cannot fully understand an African American without recognizing the legacy of slavery in the African American culture.

4. One of the best ways to learn about diverse cultures is to interact with people from those cultures. However, opportunities to become immersed in another culture are not always available. An alternative is to expose oneself to culturally focused literature, films, and music, which can enhance cultural understanding.

5. Adaptation includes the ability to articulate an issue from another's perspective, as well as to recognize and reduce resistance and defensiveness. The ability to admit errors is important, because resolving errors when interacting with someone from another culture allows for the exploration of cultural issues that enhance understanding and communication. It is often better to risk a confrontation than to avoid the issue, which could result in continued misperception or lost opportunity for better cultural understanding.

Cultural Diversity and Health Disparities

The richness of the increased cultural diversity of the United States has resulted in increased disparity in health and healthcare delivery. Health disparity refers to the differences in the incidence, prevalence, mortality, and morbidity that exist among different ethnic groups. Healthcare disparity addresses the difference in treatment provided to members of different racial or ethnic groups. These disparities, according to Betancourt et al. (2014) are not only unjust and unethical but costly, by not addressing preventable and treatable conditions such as asthma, diabetes, cardiovascular diseases, cancer, and HIV/AIDS.

Health disparities are common problems among African Americans, Asian Americans, and Latinos. The incident of cancer among African Americans is 10 percent higher than among Caucasians. Other chronic health issues that occur more frequently in African Americans are asthma, diabetes, and systemic lupus erythematosus (SLE). Tuberculosis and SLE have also been found to occur more frequently in Asians, Hispanics, and Native Americans. The causes for these disparities can be linked to poor access to health care, poverty, exposure to environmental problems, low educational levels, and individual and behavioral factors (Mandal, 2014).

Healthcare delivery disparities are more often experienced by racial and ethnic minorities; lesbian, gay, and transgender individuals; women; children; people with disabilities; and those from low socioeconomic backgrounds. A study by the Agency for Healthcare Research and Quality (AHRQ, 2011) found that Blacks received worse care than Whites for 41 percent of quality measures studied (heart failure, surgery, pneumonia, and influenza). Asians received worse care for 30 percent of the measures and Hispanics received worse care for 39 percent of the measures. A study by Johnson et al. (2013) found that White children were more likely to receive pain relief in the emergency room than Black or Hispanic children. Recognizing that these ethnic and racial inequalities in the provision of pain relief exist should prompt the healthcare provider to be vigilant in making sure all children are treated fairly and appropriately. Overall, it was reported that poor people of all racial and ethnic categories received worse care for 77 percent of the measures. Suggested reasons given for such disparity in care as reported by Mandal (2014) include ineffective communication between healthcare providers and patients, discrimination on the part of the provider, and lack of preventive care and proper screening measures.

The racial and ethnic background of individuals can also affect their responses to prescribed medications. In the past 2 decades pharmacogenomics research has shown significant differences among racial and ethnic groups in the metabolism, clinical effectiveness, and side effect profile of several drugs. Doctors are now able to use the **pharmacogenomics** research

KEY TERM

Pharmacogenomics: The study of how genes affect a person's response to drugs. This relatively new field combines pharmacology (the science of drugs) and genomics (the study of genes and their functions) to develop effective, safe medications and doses that will be tailored to a person's genetic makeup.

information to select the best medication for specific groups of individuals (National Institutes of Health, 2015).

Race and Ethnicity

Ethnicity refers to values, perceptions, feelings, assumptions, and physical characteristics associated with ethnic group affiliation. Often, ethnicity refers to nationality—a group sharing a common social and cultural heritage. In contrast, race typically refers to a biologic, genetically transmitted set of distinguishable physical characteristics. In some literature, however, race has often been misused to describe differences in people that have no basis in biology or science. Demographic data are commonly gathered with no differentiation of ethnicity or definitions of race. Both skin color and country of origin have been used to classify race. For example, many natives of India (considered racially Caucasian) have darker skin than do many natives of Africa.

Race and culture have significant relationships to illness states because biologic differences can make certain groups of people vulnerable to specific diseases. For example, genetic predisposition for sickle cell disease affects people of African and Mediterranean descent; and predisposition for Tay-Sachs disease affects Ashkenazi Jews. Also, certain diseases that may be attributable to a combination of genetic predisposition and lifestyle, including nutritional patterns, are more prevalent in some groups. One example is the disproportionately high prevalence of diabetes in Native Americans and Hispanics. Some diseases are connected to lifestyle risks, such as substance abuse and human immunodeficiency virus (HIV) infection, which are related to particular social behaviors. Cultural subgroups can be attributed to multiple factors that determine values, beliefs, and behaviors. Ethnicity is the most common cultural demarcation, but intraethnic variations may be more pronounced than interethnic variations, especially in a culturally pluralistic society. Other variables that have been proposed as influencing cultural groupings are religion, socioeconomic status, geographic region, age, common beliefs, and professional orientation, such as nursing and medicine.

Factors Related to Culture

Religion is an important factor in determining the values and beliefs of a culture. Religion, an organized system of beliefs, is differentiated from spirituality, which is born out of each individual's personal experience in finding meaning and significance in life. Religious faith and the institutions derived from that faith have a powerful influence over human behavior. All religions have experiential, ritualistic, ideological, intellectual, and consequential dimensions. Religious views have historically served as a unifying force for groups of people with a set of core values and beliefs.

Socioeconomic status refers to one's social status, occupation, education, economic status, or a combination of these. Socioeconomic explanations are often discounted when determining the relationships between ethnicity or race and health status or health. It is necessary to distinguish between cultural identification and the common experience of being poor in our society. By illustration, the experience of being poor in our society is different from that of being Hispanic and also must be further distinguished from being both poor and Hispanic. The impact of socioeconomic status on both morbidity and mortality measures of specific groups is highly significant and is related to health disparities; lower socioeconomic status groups have higher morbidity and mortality rates for various diseases.

The local or regional manifestations of the larger culture bring up such distinctions as rural, urban, southern, or midwestern. For example, African Americans living in the southern region of the United States may have different beliefs and behaviors than those in the northern region, based somewhat on their heritage of slavery and exposure to the civil rights movement. The age of the individuals within a cultural group also has a profound influence on their beliefs and behaviors. Value systems are tied to historically shared events that occur in childhood; therefore, each generation develops a unique value system. For example, there is much in the popular literature about the differences among the baby boomers (people born in the late 1940s and 1950s), generation X (those born in the 1960s and 1970s), and generation Y (people born in the late 1970s and 1980s).

Common beliefs or ideologies may unite a cultural group or subculture, as well as differentiate that group from the larger culture. These value systems may be related to religion (e.g., the Amish), lifestyle (e.g., communal groups), sexual orientation (e.g., gay, lesbian, and transgender groups), or political ideologies (e.g., feminist separatist groups). Social or professional orientations also often constitute a type of cultural grouping. For example, the biomedical culture of many hospitals constitutes an unfamiliar culture for many laypeople. Healthcare professionals use unique and esoteric language, as well as rituals, roles, expectations, patterns of behavior, and symbolic communication that are often alien to the layperson.

Common Myths and Errors

Errors of stereotyping are common among those who define the world by strict categories of ethnicity or race. It is also problematic to presume that all members of another culture conform to a common pattern without regard to individual characteristics or the variety found within one cultural grouping. Stereotyping, myths, and lack of knowledge in the healthcare sector often negatively affect healthcare delivery. Some common stereotyping that negatively affect healthcare delivery include the following: all Native Americans take home remedies first before seeking medical care; in Asian cultures the theory of hot and cold, acupuncture, and other traditional treatments is widely accepted and greatly influences healthcare delivery; and Blacks/African Americans believe in no pain, no gain. Numerous efforts at negative stereotyping as reported by Reichard (2014) affect the way Latina women are viewed. Such myths include that Latina women are hypersexual and promiscuous; they oppose birth control and abortion, hence the reason they have high numbers of children; and the main reason they cross the U.S. borders is to have anchor babies. Stereotyping may be less obvious in some cases, such as a nurse manager assigning all Hispanic clients to the Mexican American nurse. Such action does not take into account the differences within the Hispanic group, presumes that all Hispanics are alike, and disregards the individual.

The heterogeneity of ethnic groups is often underestimated, and the variations within ethnic groups may be as great as or greater than those between ethnic groups. For example, the Hispanic culture includes persons of Puerto Rican, Cuban, Spanish, and South and Central American origins. These groups represent many different socioeconomic backgrounds and represent the Caucasian, Mongoloid, and Negroid racial groups. Sometimes Asians from different countries and backgrounds are grouped together and treated as generic Asians, an attitude that totally ignores the historical differences among Asians. The importance of the nurse–client relationship in the delivery of culturally sensitive health care cannot be overemphasized.

Ethnocentrism is the tendency, usually unconscious, for individuals to take for granted their own values as the only objective reality and to look at everyone else through the lens of their own cultural norms and customs. Ethnocentric views often result from a lack of knowledge of other cultures and the presumption that one's own behavior is not influenced by culture. Many people of the dominant culture falsely assume that they have no cultural practices and beliefs. This restrictive view of the world perceives people and cultures with different beliefs and behaviors as culturally inferior. An extreme and more conscious form of ethnocentrism is xenophobia, an inherent fear of cultural differences, which often leads people to bolster their security in their own values by demeaning the beliefs and traditions of others. This attitude often takes the form of prejudice or racism.

> **KEY TERM**
> **Ethnocentrism:** A worldview based to a great extent on the socialization of individuals within their own culture, to the extent that such individuals believe that all others see the world as they do.

Cultural imposition is the perception that successful cultural adaptation involves a change to the cultural views of the dominant group, regardless of an individual's cultural heritage. This posits an inherent view that the dominant culture is superior, and its values are imposed upon others.

Often disguised as equal treatment for everyone, cultural blindness ignores cultural differences as if they did not exist. This view overlooks real diversity and the importance of other perspectives. The concept of the "melting pot" assumes that, in the process of **acculturation** and assimilation, everyone takes on significant aspects of the dominant culture such that the original culture is largely lost. This assimilation or melting pot view is challenged by concepts of heritage consistency, which is the degree to which one maintains practices and beliefs that reflect one's own heritage.

> **KEY TERM**
> **Acculturation:** The process of the adaptation or accommodation of an individual immigrant or immigrant group to a new culture.

Development of Cultural Patterns and Behaviors

Anthropologists have studied the similarities between cultures related to the universal experience of being human. Their major focus has been on the variation of ways that humans organize and structure their social world. Some of the factors that contribute to the development of cultural patterns and behavior are geography and migration, gender-specific roles, value orientations and cultural beliefs, and technological development.

Geography and Migration

Social groups evolve through interaction with the climate, as well as in conjunction with the availability of food and resources. The persistence of dietary patterns reflects the types of food available in a particular region. For example, fish constitutes a large portion of the traditional diet of people from Norway and the Philippines, whereas dairy products and meats are dominant in the food patterns of Finland and Germany.

Social organization falls in line with these geographic patterns. For example, the social structure of a fishing village differs from that of a nomadic group that hunts for food and from that of a settled agrarian culture. Urbanization and industrialization are also important for the way society organizes and social roles develop. Social roles become patterned and often institutionalized into hierarchical structures that reflect social, economic, and political power. These social structures and roles greatly alter people's daily lives and the economics of providing for families.

Climate, environmental conditions, and political and economic factors are very important in migration patterns. Climate change, famine, political upheaval, and overpopulation have all been responsible for migration. For example, a large wave of Irish immigrants came to the United States in the late 1840s following a potato famine that was causing starvation, disease, and death in Ireland. In the 1980s, many immigrants came to the United States to flee political unrest in El Salvador. Many Vietnamese and Southeast Asians sought political refuge and opportunities in the United States following the Vietnam War. A large number of nurses seeking professional and economic opportunities moved to the mainland United States from the Philippines in the 1980s. Even in the 1990s and the early 21st century, a large number of immigrants have steadily come to the United States seeking economic opportunities. More recently, many people have migrated from the West African countries of Liberia and Sierra Leone, fleeing from the devastation brought on by the Ebola virus.

Cultural patterns change through the sharing of ideas, beliefs, and practices that follow trade or migration. Immigrants bring cultural patterns, values, and beliefs with them. Along with their adaptation to the new host culture, they expose the host culture to a different set of cultural beliefs and practices. Both cultures assimilate aspects of the other.

The historical context of immigration is important and varies among groups. Many African Americans arrived involuntarily and endured a lengthy history of slavery. Hispanics may be immigrants seeking economic opportunity, refugees from political upheavals, or descendants of people living in the Southwest before it became a part of the United States. The fact that many Asian immigrants find it necessary to take a job with lower status than they had in their country of origin creates cultural and economic hardships for the family.

Acculturation is an important process in the adaptation, assimilation, or accommodation of immigrant groups to a new culture. This is sometimes referred to as hybridization. This is because in the process of adapting to a new culture, immigrants integrate the new culture into their beliefs and lifestyle and yet retain heritage consistency, maintaining pride in and adhering to their parent culture. This behavior is supported by the theory of orthogonal cultural identification, which argues that in pluralistic cultural environments individuals may identify with more than one culture without sacrificing one cultural identity for another. In a dualistic cultural existence, intergenerational gaps frequently develop because the youth in a family become more quickly acculturated to the dominant society, and they may challenge the more traditional values, beliefs, and customs of their parents. This, in turn, may threaten the integrity and lines of respect in the family and roles within the family and society, particularly the role of women. Conflicts that arise from intergenerational gaps can lead to the alienation of young people and families from both the ethnic culture and the general dominant culture.

Gender Roles

All cultures develop socially sanctioned roles for each gender. Over the past century, the social role for women in the United States has undergone many changes. The role of women has expanded from its traditional focus on childbearing and child rearing to include participation in the workplace and marketplace. The feminist movement has championed this expanded role and has heightened consciousness about opportunities consistent with the American values of individualism, equality, and political freedom. Furthermore, the feminist movement has challenged the values and structures developed by elite, masculine power, such as competition, strong focus on objectives and goals, the harnessing and control of nature, principle-based ethics, and productive activities. Feminists have promoted cultural practices and organizations that espouse more feminine values such as teamwork, focus on social process, working in harmony with nature, relationship-based ethics, and social connections. As people from other cultures move into the United States, these differing values and expanded roles for women may challenge the traditional family roles. In some cases where women's roles take a more traditional position, a woman may need to get her husband's or father's permission prior to receiving medical care for herself or her children.

Women have played significant roles in the healing arts as well. Historically and cross-culturally, women have discovered and preserved information about healing herbs and plants. In the Middle Ages, women were often persecuted for their knowledge of plants and other healing arts, which were deemed mysterious and suspicious. As medicine became more scientific and moved into a professional and scientific status, women were disengaged from the official healing roles (Achterberg, 2013). Women were associated with nature, and men with developing technology to tame and control nature. Women's roles in the healing arts reflected this dichotomy. With the establishment of medical professions, women's roles even in midwifery—a traditional role for women—were reduced, and physicians took over the practice and moved it into hospitals. Women who worked in medical professions were often in nonphysician roles or positions of lower power and social status, such as nurses, social workers, and physical therapists.

Basic Value Orientations and Beliefs

All cultures hold certain value orientations that are central to their cultural patterns of behavior. These values can be both implicit and explicit. They influence an individual's perception of others, direct that individual's responses to others, and reflect his or her identity. These values are the basis for understanding oneself and one's social relationships, political and economic structures, and direct and motivated behavior. These values are generally quite stable and do not change quickly. The classic work of Kluckhohn (1976) on cultures and their value orientation is still being used as a basis for research in providing insight into the core assumptions of other cultures.

In western culture and in particular the United States, these value orientations are reflected in a strong emphasis on individualism, mastery over nature, future-focused time orientation, and an action orientation to being. This can be seen in health care when the provider sees the individual who is the patient and often ignores the impact on the family. Our mastery over nature is illustrated in our efforts to understand and cure disease and control health issues. Future orientation is reflected in our goal orientation and an emphasis on the effect our actions may have on the future. Both healthcare providers and patients expect some type of action or treatment from the clinical encounter. This reflects the shared value of an action-oriented culture. The healthcare system both influences and is influenced by the general cultural orientations. Cultural conflicts may occur when we fail to recognize that our patients hold differing value orientations.

Worldviews and cosmologies essential to Judeo-Christian-Islamic beliefs differ from those of other world religions. Three dominant cosmology assumptions foundational to Judeo-Christian-Islamic beliefs are monotheism, transcendence, and dualism (Fisher, 2011). Monotheism, the belief in one god or creator who is separate from humans, contrasts with the beliefs common in many agrarian societies, whose members believe in polytheism (i.e., multiple gods with different attributes) or pantheism (i.e., the locus of the sacred in all living things). The western view of transcendence, or relating to God as separate from humans and knowing God through prayer, supplication, and rituals, can be contrasted with the eastern view of immanence, or finding God by looking inward and doing other spiritual exercises to discover the sacred. Finally, western dualism, separation of material from nonmaterial aspects of being, is in contrast to monism, or the essential unity found in both the pantheistic and eastern belief systems. Many "new age" perspectives are exploring these issues in the context of different cultural beliefs. **Contemporary Practice Highlight 14-1** provides Leininger's three modes of intervention.

CONTEMPORARY PRACTICE HIGHLIGHT 14-1

LEININGER'S THREE MODES OF INTERVENTION

In the 1970s, Madeleine Leininger began discussions on the importance of culturally competent health care, creating the discipline of transcultural nursing. Leever (2011) explored the moral foundation of cultural competence suggesting an organizational approach that emphasizes overall organizational preparedness (p. 560). Leininger (2001) identified three modes of intervention involving clinical decision making that focus on cultural practices:

1. *Cultural preservation and maintenance* refers to professional actions that retain relevant care values to support aspects of the client's culture that positively influence his or her health care.

2. *Cultural accommodation and negotiation* refers to professional actions to bridge the gap between the client's culture and biomedicine for beneficial health outcomes, by recognizing the cultural relevance of a practice and integrating it into the treatment plan, even though the cultural practice has no scientific basis.

3. *Cultural repatterning and restructuring* refers to professional actions that assist the client in making changes in, but not discarding, practices that may be harmful to his or her well-being.

You are caring for a Japanese woman with Stage II breast cancer who was admitted for a partial mastectomy. During the admission assessment, she shares with you that she knows she has cancer because she had a termination (abortion) of a pregnancy and she did not disclose this to her spouse. She also reports she is uncertain if she will take chemotherapy as recommended. She is considering performing tai chi daily instead of taking chemotherapy. Using Leininger's three modes of interventions, how would you focus your care for this client?

Technology and Culture

In contemporary western culture, as well as in much of the world, technology is widely expanding. The development of technology influences values, religion, politics, and the arts and sciences. Medical technology in particular has progressed in its development of intricate instruments that allow for more complex procedures, such as computer-based imaging, microsurgery, gene mapping, targeted therapies, and pharmacogenomics. The development of these technologies poses new ethical and cultural questions related to the human and social impact this technology may have. Often the use of these technologies challenges existing cultural values. Once the technology is available for use, it often becomes the fuel for ethical debates related to such issues as allocation of resources, fetal tissue transplantation and right to life, and genetic testing and right to privacy. Technology influences the way the world communicates and affects the type of information shared and who has access to this information. Diverse populations who may have fewer technological resources may be at a disadvantage to receiving information that will assist in improving health status as well as education in general.

Traditionally, knowledge was passed on by oral means in stories, parables, and poetry. Essential knowledge (i.e., cultural wisdom associated with oral tradition) was preserved through memory, often aided by rhythm and rhyme. Many cultures today have their roots in oral traditions. With the advent of written communication, the world became a different culture based on the type of knowledge that was conveyed and developed. Printed materials recorded information with detail, precision, and accuracy in a way that oral speech could not. The ability to read this information also facilitated discussions and formation of complex thoughts. Thus, scientific and factual information gained value, giving rise to the development of modern scholarship.

Today's electronic culture, dependent on telephones, radio, television, and computers to communicate information, has an enormous impact on the beliefs, values, and behaviors of contemporary society. In relation to health care, patients have access to a plethora of health-related information from multiple sources. This has presented new challenges for healthcare providers to help patients interpret information and make appropriate choices.

In the late 20th and early 21st centuries, people in the developed and industrialized world have been exposed to a number of different cultures, as a result of both immigration and electronic technology. Electronic media, allowing for fast and more universal dispersal of information, has promoted intercultural communication throughout the world as never before. Such communication has led to unprecedented exposure to different cultures, with results ranging from attempts to integrate diverse ideas to overt conflict and violence. Scientific and technologic advances, as well as global, political, social, and economic changes, have challenged existing cultural systems and increased the velocity of cultural change. With increasing cultural proliferation in the United States, nurses are challenged to self-evaluate their ability to carry out culturally competent care (see **Sidebar 14-1**).

SIDEBAR 14-1

Nurses must evaluate how healthcare goals are achieved when they deliver culturally competent care. How would you evaluate culturally competent care?

Ethnic Groups in North America

Culturally diverse groups in the United States have grown to substantial proportions of the population. In their practice, nurses are likely to encounter representatives of different cultures. General descriptions about these various ethnic groups may provide helpful orientations to the group. It is important to remember that there is much diversity within ethnicities and that in the processes of globalization and exposure to other cultures, these cultural beliefs are dynamic. Therefore, it is extremely important to avoid stereotyping. Reading about and engaging in discussions and activities with members of these cultural groups can help to avoid stereotypical interpretations of these groups and aid in developing cultural competency.

American Indian and Alaskan Native

According to the 2010 census, 2.9 million people, or 0.9 percent, in the United States reported to be American Indian or Alaskan Native alone (U.S. Census Bureau, 2012a). The indigenous peoples of the Americas live across the contiguous United States, Alaska, and the Aleutian Islands (Humes, Jones, & Ramirez, 2011). Only 5.6 percent of Native Americans are age 65 or older, compared to 14 percent of European Americans, indicating a shorter life expectancy. They cluster in tribal groups, with the largest concentrations located in the Pacific and western mountain regions of the United States. There is considerable variation among the tribes regarding language, beliefs, customs, health practices, and rituals. Tribes or clans constitute a social unit in which members may or may not be blood relatives, and both family and clan are powerful sources of the Native American's identity and support. Largely because of the respect for the wisdom accrued with aging, elders are typically the community leaders. Value orientations center on harmony with nature, a present-time orientation, and an integration of rituals and religion into everyday life.

Many Native Americans still adhere to folk healing practices, seeking local healers before going to a healthcare clinic. Folk healing practices may fall into the shamanic category or often be understood in a supranormal paradigm. Common health problems include diabetes, obesity, infectious disease, alcohol abuse, and diseases associated with poverty. Years of racism, dehumanization, and oppression have left a legacy in which many Native Americans may mistrust Caucasian healthcare providers.

European Americans

The largest ethnic group in North America is made up of European Americans. According to the U.S. Census Bureau (2010), those who identify themselves as White constitute the dominant culture of the U. S. and comprise approximately 75 percent of the population of the United States who describe themselves as white alone or in combination with another ethnic or race designation. Those who report their race as White alone decreased to 72% from the previous census whereas those who reported White in combination with other races grew by more than one-third of its previously reported rate in 2000 (U. S. Census, 2010). The largest emigrations from various regions in Europe occurred in the late 1700s, all through the 1800s, and into the first half of the 20th century. Many immigrants to the United States carried the European ideas of the Age of Reason, dominance over nature, and the belief in progress and technologic advancement. Their quest for freedom enhanced an abiding value of individualism. They were generally action oriented and future directed and focused on progress and productivity. Families are an important social unit among European Americans, but the value of individualism is pervasive. Although this group is diverse, the values are usually consistent with dominant values of the culture. Therefore, members of this group may not be as aware of the role that culture plays in their lives as the members of other cultural groups.

African Americans

The 2010 census estimated the number of African Americans in the United States who identified as African American alone to be 38.9 million, or 13 percent of the population (U.S. Census Bureau, 2011a). This is anticipated to increase to 61.8 million by 2060 (U.S. Census Bureau, 2012d). One-third of this population was under the age of 18 in 2000. This group is very heterogeneous and varies in economic status, religion, education, and regional background. Many African Americans are descendants of slaves who were brought to the United States; others are recent immigrants from Africa and the Caribbean islands. Within the social structure of slavery, families were dispersed and individuals were not allowed to read. Thus, a tradition of strong matriarchal family units with a rich oral tradition developed. Social organization centers on the family, kinship bonds, and the church or mosque. Some of the health disparities among African Americans may be related to the disproportional rate of poverty. Many African Americans have absorbed much of the dominant culture, but some adhere to ancestral beliefs of illness as disharmony with nature and supranormal healing rituals or folk healing. The history of slavery and the Tuskegee atrocities have made some African Americans mistrustful of receiving professional health care or participating in clinical research studies.

Asian Americans

Asian Americans who identified as Asian alone constituted 4.8% of the total U. S. population, or approximately 14.7 million people according to the 2010 census (U.S. Census Bureau, 2012b). Asian Americans are expected to represent 8 percent of the population by 2060 (U.S. Census Bureau, 2012d). Approximately two-thirds reside in the western part of the United States. This group is composed of immigrants and refugees from the Pacific Rim countries, such as China, Japan, Korea, Thailand, Laos, Vietnam, Cambodia, and the Philippines. People from Pakistan and India are often included in this group as well. There is wide diversity in language, customs, and beliefs in this group. Traditional Asian families tend to be patriarchal, revere their elders, and value achievement and honor. Certain infectious diseases, such as tuberculosis and hepatitis, are common among Asian Americans, depending on the country from which they emigrated. Stress-related diseases and suicides are high, as many do not seek mental health care because of an associated stigma and a threat to honor. Asians' traditional health practices of ten are oriented around the balance paradigm in which health is equated with balance and the unimpeded flow of energy, or "chi." Traditional healing includes the use of herbal preparations, and many families practice traditional dermabrasion procedures such as coining, pinching, or rubbing.

Pacific Islanders and Native Hawaiians

The Native Hawaiian and other Pacific Islander (NHPI) population constitutes 0.2 percent of the U.S. population in the 2010 census (U.S. Census Bureau, 2012c). Native Hawaiians are the largest subgroup (58 percent), although the majority of this group reported one or more other races as well. Nearly three fourths of this population lives in the west, with over half living in California and Hawaii.

There is great diversity in beliefs and customs. As an aggregate group, NHPIs are socioeconomically disadvantaged and underserved in terms of access to social and health services. Pacific Islanders have high rates of health-related risk behaviors, such as smoking, heavy alcohol consumption, and high fat and caloric intake, which leads to obesity. Native Hawaiians have the second highest overall cancer incidence rate and the highest age-adjusted cancer mortality rate compared to other ethnic groups, with high rates of breast, colorectal, prostate, lung, and stomach cancers (Intercultural Cancer Council, n.d.). Native Hawaiians are 2.5 times more likely to have diabetes than White residents of Hawaii of similar age. Other common illnesses among NHPIs are asthma, hypertension, and hypercholesterolemia (Hawaii Department of Health, 2015).

Hispanic or Latino Americans

According to the 2010 census report, the Hispanic population in the United States was 50.5 million in 2010, accounting for 16 percent of the U.S. population (U.S. Census Bureau, 2011b). It is projected that the Hispanic population in the United States will be approximately 128.8 million by 2060 (U.S. Census Bureau, 2012d). The majority of these immigrants come from Mexico (63 percent), with others from Puerto Rico (9.2 percent), Cuba (3.5 percent), and Central and South America (24 percent; U.S. Census Bureau, 2011b). This is the fastest growing group in the

United States. Although the Spanish language is a common factor, there is much diversity in dialects and cultural practices. This group is composed of indigenous peoples of the Americas, Spanish and other European settlers, and some African-Caribbean groups. Predominant religions are Catholicism and Pentecostalism. The family and extended family are important, and the family unit is traditionally patriarchal. Many believe that illness may be punishment for sins or the result of witchcraft or *brujería*, meaning the "evil eye." Traditional health beliefs regarding hot and cold remedies for various maladies reflect humeral balance beliefs. Healing also incorporates many spiritual elements, such as worship of saints and use of talismans. **Contemporary Practice Highlight 14-2** provides a brief case study on personal value system.

Impact of Culture on Health Care

Concepts of health and healing are rooted in culture. The concept of disease generally refers to the diagnostic label or categorization of a disorder that medicine treats, whereas the concept of illness incorporates the personal, social, and cultural aspects of the experience. Cultural practices influence an individual's behavior to promote, maintain, and restore health, and how, when, and whom they seek for help or treatment. Cultural beliefs, values, and practices are also extremely important in birth and death.

Nursing Applications

Six phenomena evidenced in all cultural groups have variations that are relevant to the provision of culturally competent nursing assessment and care and are outlined

---

CONTEMPORARY PRACTICE HIGHLIGHT 14-2

PERSONAL VALUE SYSTEM

You are working in a prenatal clinic and caring for a Korean 17-year-old who is 8 months pregnant. The family is very ashamed of their daughter and the teen's father is insisting that the girl give the baby up for adoption. The pregnant teen says she wants to keep the baby but she does not want to offend her father. Respond to the following points as you consider a culturally competent plan of care for this teen and her family.

1. Clarify your own values, beliefs, and ideas related to your heritage.
2. Identify barriers in your own life to acceptance of cultural diversity.
3. Explore activities that will increase your awareness and acceptance of this teen and her family.
4. What resources or referrals would be helpful for this teen and her family regarding the tension over the pregnancy and decisions regarding the infant?

here (Giger & Davidhizar, 2016). It is useful to understand these variations in clinical practice.

1. *Communication:* There are cultural variations in the expression of feelings, use of touch, body contact, gestures, and verbal and nonverbal communication. Language shapes experiences and influences perceptions and actions. Warmth and humor are two communication factors that are interpreted differently through various cultures. For example, many Asians may not overtly express their emotions, because they may fear "losing face."

2. *Personal space:* Spatial behavior refers to the comfort level related to personal space, meaning the area that surrounds a person's body. Spatial territoriality is the need to have and to control personal space. Cultures vary in the level of proximity to others that is acceptable. For example, western culture has three zones: the intimate zone (less than 18 in.), the personal zone (18 in. to 3 ft), and the social zone (3–6 ft). Cultural background also influences aspects of objects within space, such as orderliness, cleanliness, and structural boundaries of furniture and architecture.

3. *Time:* Cultures vary in their orientation toward time, both social time and clock time. Social time refers to patterns and orientations related to the ordering of social life, whereas clock time represents an objective, ordered approach of viewing time in a linear fashion that infers causality. Some cultures orient around cyclic approaches that attach time to natural events that repeat, such as seasons or migration patterns. For example, in mystical thought, magic or ritual may negate the temporal order of causality and reverse a bad event. All cultures contain the three orientations of future, present, and past, with one being dominant.

4. *Social organization:* Families, religious groups, kinship groups, workplace groups, and special interest groups are social organizations. Families vary in structure, dynamics, roles, and organizational patterns. Kinship structures and the relative geographic location of family members have cultural implications. Religious organizations provide not only social connections but also a context in which to understand one's relationship to the world, the cosmos, and the meaning in life.

5. *Environmental control:* Different cultures have different perceptions of the ability of an individual to control nature, the environment, and personal relationships. The locus of control may be external (i.e., an event contingent on luck or fate), internal (i.e., an event contingent on one's own behavior or characteristic), or outside (i.e., an event in harmony with nature, as in some Asian cultures). In folk medicine, for example, events are perceived as natural and unnatural. Natural events have to do with the world as God intended and the laws of nature. Unnatural events upset the harmony of nature and are outside the world of nature.

6. *Biologic variations:* In a pluralistic culture, it is important to determine those factors that are strictly biologic (i.e., genetic) and those that are ethnic adaptations related to living in a particular environment (e.g., availability of certain types of food) or in certain social conditions (e.g., socioeconomic status, lifestyle). Biologic factors to be considered are body size and structure, including variations in teeth, facial features, and skin color; variations in metabolism and enzyme production that result in drug reactions, interactions, and sensitivities; and susceptibility to disease (e.g., hypertension, diabetes, sickle cell anemia). Nutritional issues, including food preferences, habits, and patterns, as well as deficiencies such as lactose intolerance, all have medical implications.

This information is a helpful guide to thinking about cultural variations. However, no amount of factual knowledge about cultural variation can replace careful individual assessment, because there is more intracultural variation than intercultural variation.

Developing Cultural Competence in Students

Today's nursing classroom represents a diverse group of students from a variety of countries, cultural backgrounds, and life experiences. The diversity may be in the form of age, gender, ethnicity, race, sexual orientation, gender identity, religious beliefs, political orientation, abilities, and originality of thought. Educators are encouraged to respect and embrace this diversity and to devise ways to ensure that the classroom is a welcoming place where all can learn. Bednarz, Schim, and Doorenbos (2010) suggest that educators "identify issues that complicate teaching (perils), analyze barriers for themselves and their students (pitfalls), and select new strategies for working with nontraditional students (pearls)" (p. 253). It is also important that educators design learning experiences that create an environment in which students can assess their own cultural biases, respect the diversity of their peers, and acquire a knowledge base that will foster the development of cultural competence.

In 2014, Dunagan et al. identified biases and ethnocentrism as a major hurdle to cultural competent care. They agreed that nursing students' cultural competence improves when the curriculum provides appropriate cultural content. Pavlakis and Leondiou (2014) suggested that having cultural knowledge alone will not solve the problem of cultural competence, because there may be barriers that hinder the development of cultural relationships. These barriers may include language difficulties, perceived impolite behaviors such as making eye contact, role of the primary decision makers in the family, and issues of personal space and body contact. However, they believe that appropriate instruction in the classroom regarding these barriers can prepare the student to work effectively within a particular culture.

Educators can also prepare students to be culturally competent in the clinical setting by including in the curriculum simulation case studies, role playing activities, creating service and volunteer opportunities in underserved areas, and leading cultural immersion experiences (Mareno & Hart, 2014; Ume-Nwagbo, 2012). Some common examples of classroom behaviors that are motivated by culture can be found in the student–teacher relationship. The cultural background of students can influence how they perceive the authority of the teacher and how comfortable they are in interacting with faculty and asking questions or admitting that they do not understand the teacher.

Summary

Members of minority or varied cultural groups may distrust and fear the western biomedical healthcare system, of which nurses are a part. The element of trust is essential to the formation of a therapeutic nurse–client relationship, so clients need to know that nurses are receptive and nonjudgmental regarding their differences. Nurses must approach cultural competence through knowledge of self and knowledge of other cultures. To develop the ability to interact with clients appropriately, nurses should clarify their personal values, recognize the healthcare system as a culture, learn about the specific culture of each client, interact and intervene in a culturally consistent manner, and elicit feedback regularly from the client and family. Skills such as listening, explaining, acknowledging, recommending, and negotiating facilitate a nonjudgmental perspective toward the client's cultural beliefs. Nurses and clients should validate their perceptions and discuss similarities and differences in their perceptions to formulate health-related goals and interventions.

Cultural competency is a dynamic, challenging process faced by all healthcare providers, regardless of their cultural background or association. The process of sharing information in a straightforward manner demystifies other cultures and, for example, makes it possible for the nurse and client to find common ground and understand the context of differences. The nurse and patient conjointly develop an approach to address the identified concerns and the agreed-upon goals. The patient discusses his or her assets, barriers, and priorities, and the nurse shares expert knowledge and may suggest other resources. Knowledge and acceptance of the client's right to alternative solutions and modalities could be incorporated into the plan of care. Nurses should make every effort to acquire appropriate foods, people, artifacts, and so on, as well as to secure space and time for such practices. Nursing practice should always convey a message of respect to the client and their cultural practices and belief system.

Reflective Practice Questions

1. How do you feel when caring for clients whose cultural backgrounds differ from your own?
2. What are your values and beliefs regarding health and illness in relation to care of the elderly?
3. What are your biases and attitudes toward immigrant clients with various cultural backgrounds?
4. How do you feel when you observe inequities towards a minority colleague or peer?
5. What steps would you take to establish a relationship with a patient who has a different cultural background than yours?
6. How would you react if you perceive your client's values and decision-making abilities are contrary to your own ethical beliefs?

References

Achterberg, J. (2013). *Woman as healer.* (reprint). Boston, MA: Shambhala.

Agency for Healthcare Research and Quality (AHRQ). (2011). *National healthcare disparities report.* Retrieved from http://archive.ahrq.gov/research/findings/nhqrdr/nhdr11/index.html

Bednarz, H., Schim, S., & Doorenbos, A. (2010). Cultural diversity in nursing education: Perils, pitfalls, and pearls. *Journal of Nursing Education, 49*(5), 253–260. doi: 10.3928/01484834-20100115-02

Betancourt, J. R., Corbett, J., & Bondaryk, M. (2014). Addressing disparities and achieving equity: Cultural competence, ethics and health care transformation. *Chest Journal, 145*(1), 143–148.

Betancourt, J. R. (2006). Cultural competency: Providing quality care to diverse populations. *The Consultant Pharmacist, 21*(12), 988–995.

Cross, T. L., Baron, B. J., Dennis, K.W., & Isaacs, M. R.(1989). *Towards a culturally competent system of care: Vol. I. A monograph on effective services for minority children who are severely emotionally disturbed.* Washington, DC: Georgetown University, Child Development Center.

Dunagan, P. B, Kimble, L. P., Gunby, S., & Andrews, M. (2014). Attitudes of prejudice as a predictor of cultural competence among baccalaureate nursing students. *Journal of Nursing Education, 53*(6), 320–328. doi: http://dx.doi.org/10.3928/01484834-20140521-13

Fisher, J. (2011). The Four Domains Model: Connecting spirituality, health, and wellness. *Religions, 2,* 17–28. Retrieved from http://www.mdpi.com/2077-1444/2/1/17/pdf

Giger, J., & Davidhizar, R. (2016). *Transcultural nursing: Assessment and intervention* (7th ed.). St. Louis, MO: Mosby.

Hawaii Department of Health. (n.d.) *2015 summary of reported cases of notifiable diseases by county, state of Hawai`i.* Retrieved from health.hawaii.gov/docd/files/2016/05/2015-SUMMARY_NOTIFIABLE-DISEASES-BY-COUNTY-STATE-OF-HAWAII.pdf

Hicks, D. (2012). Cultural competence and the Hispanic population. *Medsurg Nursing, 21*(5), 314–315.

Humes, K. R., Jones, N. A., & Ramirez, R. R. (2011). *Overview of race and Hispanic origin: 2010.* Washington, DC: U.S. Census Bureau. Retrieved from http://www.census.gov/prod/cen2010/briefs/c2010br-02.pdf

Intercultural Cancer Council. (n.d.). *Native Hawaiians/Pacific Islanders and cancer.* Retrieved from http://nebula.wsimg.com/b21ee0fa0250ae9672cd3352a1fd16d7?AccessKeyId=4ECD43F4A65F6DBF7F21&disposition=0&alloworigin=1

Johnson, T., Weaver, M., Borrero, S., Davis, E., Myaskovsky, L., Zuckerbraun, N., & Kraemer, K. (2013). Association of race and ethnicity with management of abdominal pain in the emergency department. *Pediatrics, 132*(4), e851–e858. doi: 10.1542/peds.2012-3127

Kluckhohn, F. R. (1976). Dominant and variant value orientations. In P. J. Brink (Ed.), *Transcultural nursing: A book of readings* (pp. 63–81). Englewood Cliffs, NJ: Prentice Hall.

Kyeyune, C. (2015). Cultural competence in health care. In *NAAAS Conference Proceedings* (pp. 256–265). Scarborough, ME: National Association of African American Studies. Retrieved from http://search.proquest.com/docview/1692917915?accountid=13420

Leever, M. G. (2011). Cultural competence: Reflections on patient autonomy and patient good. *Nursing Ethics, 18*(4), 560–570. doi: 10.1177/0969733011405936

Leininger, M. (2001). *Culture care diversity and universality: A theory of nursing.* Sudbury, MA: Jones and Bartlett.

Mandal, A. (2014) What are health disparities? Retrieved from http://www.news-medical.net/health/What-are-Health-Disparities.aspx

Mareno, N., & Hart, P. L. (2014). Cultural competency among nurses with undergraduate and graduate degrees: Implications for nursing education. *Nursing Education Perspectives, 35*(2), 83–88.

National Center for Cultural Competence. (n.d.). Welcome. Retrieved from http://nccc.georgetown.edu

National Council of State Boards of Nursing. (2013). The 2013 National Nursing Workforce Survey of Registered Nurses. *Journal of Nursing Regulation, 4*(2), S3–S65.

National Institutes of Health. (2015). Pharmacogenomics fact sheet. Retrieved from https://www.nigms.nih.gov/education/pages/factsheet-pharmacogenomics.aspx

Pavlakis, A., & Leondiou, L., (2014). Multicultural nursing education in a multicultural society. *International Journal of Caring Sciences, 7*(1), 32–37.

Reichard, R. (2014). 7 lies we have to stop telling about Latina women in America. Retrieved from http://mic.com/articles/90195/7-lies-we-have-to-stop-telling-about-latina-women-in-america

Sackett, D. L., Straus, S. E., Richardson, W. S., Rosenberg, S., & Haynes, R. B. (2000). *Evidence-based medicine: How to practice and teach EBM. EBM* (2nd ed.) New York, NY: Churchill Livingstone.

Thomas, B. (2014). Health and health care disparities: The effect of social and environmental factors on individual and population health. *International Journal of Environmental Research and Public Health, 11*(7), 7492–7507.

Ume-Nwagbo, P. (2012). Implications of nursing faculties' cultural competence. *Journal of Nursing Education, 51*(5), 262–268. doi: http://dx.doi.org/10.3928/01484834-20120323-01

U.S. Census Bureau. (2010). 2010 census. Retrieved from http://www.census.gov/2010census/

U.S. Census Bureau. (2011a). The Black population: 2010. Retrieved from http://www.census.gov/prod/cen2010/briefs/c2010br-06.pdf

U.S. Census Bureau. (2011b). The Hispanic population: 2010. Retrieved from http://www.census.gov/prod/cen2010/briefs/c2010br-06.pdf

U.S. Census Bureau. (2012a). The American Indian and Alaska native population: 2010. Retrieved from http://www.census.gov/prod/cen2010/briefs/c2010br-10.pdf

U.S. Census Bureau. (2012b). The Asian population: 2010. Retrieved from https://www .census.gov/prod/cen2010/briefs/c2010br-11.pdf

U.S. Census Bureau. (2012c). The Native Hawaiian and other Pacific Islander population: 2010. Retrieved from http://www.census.gov/prod/cen2010/briefs/c2010br-12.pdf

U.S. Census Bureau. (2012d). U.S. Census Bureau projections show a slower growing, older, more diverse nation a half century from now. Retrieved from https://www.census.gov /newsroom/releases/archives/population/cb12-243.html

U.S. Department of Health and Human Services. Office of Minority Health. (2016). Cultural and linguistic competency. Retrieved from http://minorityhealth.hhs.gov/omh/browse .aspx?lvl=1&lvlid=6

Ethical Decision Making and Moral Choices: A Foundation for Nursing Practice

Phyllis Ann Solari-Twadell

LEARNING OUTCOMES

After reading this chapter you will be able to:

- Discuss the significance of the nurses' ability to reflect on ethical dimensions of nursing practice.
- Recognize the American Nurses Association (ANA) *Code of Ethics for Nurses* as the basis for nursing's contract with society.
- Understand how the patient bill of rights and advanced directives are related to nursing's professional code of ethics.
- Discuss the role, function, and underlying goals of ethics committees.
- Explain various ethical conflicts and the impact of personal values on these issues.

The editors wish to acknowledge the contributions of Kevin Valadares to the previous edition of this chapter.

Nursing's Contract with Society

The profession of nursing exists due to a contract that the profession has with the society that it serves. Fundamental to that contract are ethical decisions and behaviors on the part of those who are members of the profession. The purpose of this chapter is to provide a discourse on the **ethical** dimensions of nursing practice, including the **code of ethics** for nurses, the nurse and **moral** decision making, the patient bill of rights, advance directives, ethical principles and directives in nursing, and **organizational ethics**.

Code of Ethics

Most professions, whether its members function within healthcare settings or not, have a code of ethics. This code illustrates the standards and behaviors as a form of instructions for its members and expectations for its constituents. Basic to the nursing profession's contract with society are long-standing values and ethics. These values and ethics are the heart of the code of ethics that constitutes nursing as a profession; the code acts as a general guide primarily to the members of the profession but also informs other professional groups and society as a whole. Society, through laws and licensure, grants the nursing profession authority over certain functions that allow the profession to autonomously manage issues pertinent to the profession. "At the same time it (the profession) needs to meet the demands of the public it serves" (Kangasniemi, Pakkanen, & Korhonen, 2015, p. 1745).

"Vulnerability, as a concept related to nurses and nursing practice, illustrates actual and potential susceptibilities to making an error, breaching or failing to meet a standard, and proneness to being reported to a nurse regulatory authority" (Pugh, 2011, p. 21). The nursing profession, aware of maintaining "public trust," is expected to maintain "quality," ethical, and safe environments for care and healing of "all" members of society. Society expects that care provided by the nursing profession will be delivered with excellence, in a socially just manner, caring for "all in need regardless of their culture, socioeconomic status or beliefs" (ANA, 2010, p. 5).

What is today the ANA's *Code of Ethics for Nurses* was first created by Lystra Gretter, principal of the Farrand Training School for Nurses in Detroit in 1893. This first code was in the form of a pledge that was patterned after the physician-driven Hippocratic oath. However, because Gretter identified Florence Nightingale as having the highest ideals of nursing, the first version of this early code was called "the Florence Nightingale Pledge." This pledge has remained a part of many nursing ceremonies even after the ANA published the first official society code of ethics in 1950.

From its inception, the code of ethics for the profession of nursing has regularly been revised (1956, 1960, 1968, 1976, 1985, 2001, 2015). These revisions have kept this document relevant in a healthcare environment that is not only complex but constantly changing. No matter what the revision, there is always a focus on social justice, prevention, and addressing the causes of disease, illness, and trauma that are the source of challenging patient and client well-being. In addition, the dignity of each person, providing nursing care that is high quality and in alignment with nursing standards upholding just treatment of the nurse is always mandated for inclusion (ANA, 2015).

The International Code of Ethics for Nurses, first adopted in 1953, was most recently revised in 2012. This code provides the ethics standard for nurses worldwide. This international code for the profession of nursing also is reviewed regularly and revised in order that nursing professionals worldwide have clarity regarding respect for human rights, including the right to life, to dignity, and to be treated with respect. The intention of this code is that nurses internationally have guidance in choices that they make daily in their nursing practice. This code is intended to support nurses worldwide in saying "no" to participating in patient care that is in conflict with caring and healing.

The Nurse as the Steward of Ethical Care

Nurses often develop strong relationships with the patients they care for over time. These relationships invite the nurse to be privy to the most intimate meaningful details of a person's life. Through these relationships nurses come to understand the beliefs and values that are most important to those they care for, becoming stewards "watching over" and protecting the well-being of another from a whole-person perspective. Often the nurses' personal beliefs and values that have been formed over a lifetime continue to be shaped by the depth of these relationships with patients. Fostering a reflective nursing practice engenders a mindfulness that creates space and time to enhance the process of paying attention on purpose and without judgment. The intentional focus on mindfulness in patient care encourages personal authenticity in all relationships, both with colleagues and patients (Sherwood & Horton-Deutsch, 2012). Through this reflective practice nurses can develop an innate sense of when ethical patient care is being challenged.

Nurses, on the other hand, often find themselves in patient care situations where they are compelled to make ethical decisions that are not consistent with their professional and personal values (Radzuin, 2011, p. 39). These patient-related situations can produce *moral distress*. Moral distress is a "specific psychological response to morally challenging situations" (Fourie, 2015, p. 92). Jameton (1984) discusses moral distress as occurring in three different forms: *moral uncertainty*, which presents when one is unsure whether an ethical dilemma exists; *moral dilemma*, when two or more ethical principles or values are in conflict; and *moral distress*, when there is an identified ethical dilemma and the morally right thing to do is known, but restraints make it impossible to go forward with what is believed to be the right action. Circumstances that can provoke moral distress for nurses include "end of life care, incompetence of providers, lack of communication, witnessing unnecessary suffering, leadership style and ethical climate of unit or the institution" (O'Connell, 2015, p. 33).

"Religion has played, and will continue to play, a significant role in the lives of nurses and hence in the profession of nursing. Religion can have numerous benefits for individuals including social support, a sense of significance and answers in life that, while common to the human condition, are notoriously hard to answer—what is my purpose, why does suffering exist, and what comes after?" (Fowler, Reimer-Kirkham, Sawatzky, & Taylor, 2012, p. 383). Religious traditions are foundational in teaching many about living out ethical matters through integration of virtues, sacred teachings, and communication patterns (Fowler et al., 2012).

Patient Bill of Rights

Although nurses practice under the guidance of a professional code of ethics, a simultaneous set of directives exists with an understanding and respect for the rights and responsibilities of patients and their families. Nurses and healthcare organizations must practice a healthcare ethic that respects the role of patients in decision making concerning treatment and care choices. This often poses challenges, especially in acute care environments, where patients readily rely on clinicians to offer advice and advocate on their behalf regarding healthcare decisions.

The rights afforded to patients are couched in the framework of the ethical principle of respect for autonomy. This stands in opposition to the paternalistic culture of health care that was primarily seen through the physician–patient relationship (dominated by physicians) that existed until the 1980s. Paternalism was ineffective in taking into consideration the viewpoint of patients with respect to their own care. Patients, families, nurses, and other healthcare workers were encouraged to defer to physician decisions and subsequently worked around errors in judgment without directly addressing concerns. A hierarchy related to decision making in health care was the expected norm.

A consumer-driven society necessitates a more fluid patient bill of rights whereby patient autonomy is supported, even if nurses are presented with seemingly contrary clinical decisions by patients. It is then the responsibility of the nurse to work within his or her scope of practice to remain an advocate for patients with their best clinical interests in mind. The ethical principle of autonomy that supports a patient bill of rights also forms the grounding for all practices associated with advance directives.

Advance Directives

The 1990 Patient Self-Determination Act officially requires healthcare institutions to provide patients with information about their state's advance directives policies and procedures at the time of hospital admission or before various outpatient procedures. Almost all states provide for living wills, and most states have at least two statutes, one establishing a living will–type directive, the other establishing a proxy or durable power of attorney for health care. Despite the fact that the general public indicates the desire for an advance directive, only about "fifteen percent of the adult population has completed an advanced directive" (Cornelius, 2010, p. 251).

As previously noted with the patient bill of rights, advance directives are rooted in the ethical principle of autonomy. Supporting one's right to choose a course of action that determines both the quantity and quality of life forms the basis for the premise of an advance directive. Professionally, it serves as a guide for clinicians to respect and honor the autonomous decision of the patient when they are in a position to not be able to express their wishes. The role of nurses concerning the spirit and application of advance directives is one of advocacy. It is this advocacy that fortifies the patient/family–nurse relationship through participating in discussions with surrogates, providing guidance and referral to other resources as necessary, and identifying and addressing problems in the end-of-life decision-making process (see **Contemporary Practice Highlight 15-1**).

CONTEMPORARY PRACTICE HIGHLIGHT 15-1

CASE STUDY ON PATIENT ADVOCACY

Betty Caprice is a 38-year-old woman who lives at home with her parents. When she was admitted to the county hospital for treatment of a bladder infection, she weighed 85 pounds and appeared emaciated. She also had large pressure ulcers on the backs of her legs, indicating that she had not been moved in her bed for a long time.

Upon admission, it was discovered that Betty has breast cancer that had spread to her lungs, lymphatic system, and skeletal system. She is in obvious pain. Her mother filled out the admission papers for Betty, listing herself as her daughter's surrogate decision maker. Both she and Betty have been informed of the extent of the diagnosis of cancer. When she is alone (away from her mother), Betty says she is in terrible pain and pleads for pain medication. When pain medication is brought to the room, however, Betty's mother tells her daughter, "You're not in pain. You don't need pain medication, do you?" Betty inevitably replies that she does not want the pain medication. This scenario repeats itself two or three times a day. Even if pain medications are started, they are always stopped when Betty, in the presence of her mother, asks for them to be discontinued. Betty and her parents claim that their religion requires them to attempt to heal naturally and that pain medications would interfere with the natural healing process. A psychiatric consult was initiated and the psychiatrist has found that Betty is lucid, oriented to time and place, understands that she has terminal cancer, and can discuss her diagnosis, prognosis, and alternatives for care.

What are the ethical issues in Betty's care and what is your role as a nurse caregiver?

Ethical Principles and Narrative Ethics Within Nursing Practice

The principalist approach (**principalism**) to applying ethics to health care has dominated the field since the 1970s. This era began with the Belmont Report, which underscored the relevance of key ethical principles respect for autonomy, proliferation of justice, and exercising beneficence with patients (National Institutes of Health, 1974).

The primary argument of **narrative ethics** suggests that a core set of principles (commonly referred to as the Georgetown mantra—autonomy, beneficence, justice, nonmaleficence) used for ethical decision making are universal in scope and facilitate the objectivity of each clinical dilemma. Beauchamp and Childress (2012) indicate that these principles are drawn from a common morality that binds all persons independent of their situations. The four principles have been grounded in traditional ethical theories and medical codes (including all versions of the *Code of Ethics for Nurses*) throughout history (Beauchamp & Childress, 2012).

Another recent approach to understanding ethical dilemmas in health care comes from narratives. Supporters argue that the first-person narrative, or personal story, is a rich medium for qualitative data about the unique lives of individual people. The narrative is not only an important form of communication but also a means of making life, specifically the moral life. Narratives make sense through the examples put forth through interpretation of personal stories. "Narrative reasoning is somehow intrinsic to ethics of care" (Paulson, 2011, p. 40). "A narrative ethics of care generates insights and an ability to discern phenomena that other forms of ethics either lack, or would be hard pressed to incorporate" (Paulson, 2011, p. 28). With this in mind, when ethically challenging situations arise, it is not the medical chart, the proposed treatment, or even the ethical principles that should govern the care process (see **Sidebar 15-1**). "Narratives are not only therapeutic *means*, they are often *therapy itself*. Listening to the other, and demonstrating the willingness and ability to facilitate, mirror, interpret and understand the words and narratives of the other, are often in themselves therapeutic activities and a direct expression of caring. It is simply difficult to imagine caring without the carer understanding the spoken or broken narrative of the other" (Paulson, 2011, p. 40).

Nurses are in an ideal position to listen to the patient's story given the nature of the nurse–patient relationship. Once a trusting relationship is established with the patient, the stories unfold as part of the regular communication between the nurse and patient. "Active listening" (Bulechek, Butcher, McCloskey, &

Wagner, 2013, p. 149) or the "attending closely to and attaching significance to a patient's verbal and nonverbal message" along with "presence" (p. 580), which is defined as "being with another, both physically and psychologically, during times of need," are a few of the standardized nursing interventions employed by nurses. This nurse–patient relationship does not presuppose that it is always possible to understand fully another's experience. In some respects, patients will always be "the other" to nurses.

Confronting the vulnerability of patients, however, actualizes the vulnerability of the care providers. Nurses are challenged when they are confronted by a patient's suffering and appeal for help, which has implications for the nurse's ethical formation (Thorup, Rundquist, Roberts, & Delmar, 2012, p. 427).

Organizational Ethics and the Work Environment for Nurses

An ethical culture is described as one in which "employees appreciate the importance of ethics; recognize and freely discusses ethical concerns; seek guidance about ethical concerns; work to address ethical issues on a systems level; view ethics as an important component of the organization; understand what ethical practices are expected of them; feel empowered to act ethically; and view organizational decisions as ethical" (Cohen, Foglia, Kwong, Pearlman, & Fox, 2015, p. 170). Organizations where an ethical culture is transparent are noted to have "higher levels of employee productivity, less staff turnover, better levels of employee and patient safety, resources and cost savings along with higher levels of patient satisfaction" (p. 170).

One way that organizational ethics can be lived out on a regular basis in an intense patient care setting is through an ethics debriefing. Ethics debriefing sessions provide a safe and respectful forum where intensive care unit team members, for example, are able to share varying perspectives and feelings around issues and dilemmas they may be grappling with (irrespective of the source), validate and support one another, and provide a sense of solidarity and interconnectedness.

"These sessions also help caregivers to navigate through complex moral, professional and legal issues, clarify complex concepts and issues and develop a strategy to address these concerns in a timely manner" (Santiago & Abdool, 2011, p. 27).

Organizational ethics is related both to *clinical practices*, in that institutional business decisions affect patient care, and to *business practices*, in that many institutional issues are primarily business concerns involving financial matters, strategic planning, and compliance with regulatory processes (see **Sidebar 15-2**). There are three primary concerns related to the impact of organizational ethics on nurses. The first considers nurses as both professionals and employees in a healthcare setting whereas the second concerns the balance between patient-centered care and organizational

SIDEBAR 15-2

Organizational ethics is related to both clinical practices and business practices.

practices. Finally, an organizational **ethics committee** is a group that nurses can embrace to assist them in unraveling both clinical and nonclinical issues in a healthcare setting. Ethics committee membership includes major clinical services representation and other stakeholders involved in healthcare delivery. Ethics committee membership can include clinicians (physicians and nurses) from medicine, surgery, and psychiatry, social workers, chaplains, and community representatives (Pearlman, 2013),

Ethics Committees

Ethics committees have played clinically relevant roles in organizational settings since the 1960s. In 1992, The Joint Commission required that hospitals develop a means of addressing ethical concerns (Moeller et al., 2012), Ethics committees are the response to this mandate. Generally, the four functions of an ethics committee are:

1. Policy development, which includes development, review, recommendations, and implementation of policies that relate to the rights of patients and end-of-life decisions.
2. Education for doctors, nurses, staff, patients and family members, community members, and other interested parties. This education can be provided through development of written materials such as pamphlets or in more formal ways such as workshops and educational forums.
3. Case consultations, prospectively or retrospectively presented on clinical scenarios that are reviewed to address ethical dilemmas currently occurring or hypothetically developed.
4. Research may be done by some ethics committees for the purpose of assessing quality and the types of consultation services provided (Moeller et al., 2012).

Many argue that the consultative practice model is the primary purpose and most effective asset of an ethics committee. Ethics committees reject the notion of a sole clinician (usually a physician) overseeing all the nonclinical issues that arise in client care. Moreover, ethics committees emphasize that a collaborative philosophy among nurses, social workers, business professionals, consumers, and physicians is best suited to offer recommendations to the medical team, the family, and the client. The infusion of technological interventions into the fabric of client care has certainly complicated the ethical dilemmas that clinicians face. Nurses in particular, who arguably form the strongest bond with client and family, become immersed in the intersection between life-saving techniques that benefit care and those that burden the process.

One of the more recent consultative practices that ethics committees have been engaged in relates to operational conflicts that are primarily restricted to employee issues. Some organizations have created subcommittees that deal with ethical issues solely from an organizational perspective, as opposed to those involving direct patient care (see **Sidebar 15-3**). A relevant case study in a subsequent section illustrates this practice.

Significant Issues Related to Nursing and Ethics

In everyday nursing practice protecting patient's rights, informed consent to treatment procedures, surrogate decision making, and end-of-life care were highlighted as the most stressful patient care encounters for practicing nurses (Ulrich, Taylor, & Grady, 2010, p. 5).

Difficult staffing patterns, unethical practices of healthcare professionals, along with feeling fatigued, overwhelmed, and powerless were further compromising factors in managing ethical patient issues (Ulrich et al., 2010). Other compromising factors that nurses report as challenging their ability to effectively manage ethical issues are cultural competence and associated cross-linguistic patient care (Hart & Mareno, 2013).

Increasingly, nursing care includes care of those from another culture or country. Diversity of culture and the corresponding lack of knowledge of how to care for a patient from a different culture along with a lack of time and resources to assist nurses in increasing their cultural competence can compromise a nurse's ability to effectively address ethical issues such as protecting patient's rights, obtaining informed consent, surrogate decision making, and end-of-life care. In addition, prejudice and cultural bias, which are expressed through the expectation of the nurse that patients cared for should be able to speak/understand the same language and have similar beliefs and values, further compromises patient care and the ability to address ethical dilemmas effectively.

Organizational and management issues and relationships can also compromise the function of nursing services. Different values, beliefs, and motives by managers can also create ethical conflicts for nursing managers. **Case Study 15-1** provides an example of a relationship between a supervisor and manager that results in an ethical dilemma.

> **SIDEBAR 15-3**
>
> The underlying goals of ethics committees include:
> - To promote the rights of patients
> - To promote shared decision making between patients (or their surrogates if cognitively incapacitated) and their clinicians
> - To promote fair policies and procedures that maximize the likelihood of achieving good, patient-centered outcomes
> - To enhance the ethical tenor of healthcare professionals and healthcare institutions

CASE STUDY 15-1
MANAGEMENT CONFLICT

Ethical conflicts, often leading to poor teamwork and moral distress, are very challenging not only to patients and their families but to healthcare providers themselves (Pavlish, Helyer, Brown-Saltzman, Miers, & Squire, 2015, p. 248). Sarah was promoted to nurse manager because of her excellence in delivering patient care and recognized leadership ability. She was an excellent charge nurse, outstanding patient advocate, preceptor, and chair of the practice council. Sarah had been a medical-surgical nurse for over 10 years and enjoyed the variety of clients under her care. She only recently completed her bachelor of science in nursing degree and earned her certification in medical-surgical nursing.

When Sarah was in her position for less than 3 months, her immediate supervisor moved to another state because of his wife's promotion. This individual had been a mentor, confidant, and recognized leader in the organization. Sarah tried to make the best of the situation and follow the direction of her new supervisor. However, from the beginning, she found the new manager to have a very negative lens through which life and work were viewed. As an optimistic person, Sarah found this negativity counter to her basic instincts about people. Every time she tried to discuss this difference in viewpoint, her director would say she was naive and that the staff was taking advantage of her good nature. The director used several of Sarah's recent projects that appeared to be failures to justify her position. However, Sarah understood that the lack of successful outcomes on these projects were the result of staff illness and institutional reorganization. The crisis point in their working relationship was reached when the director told Sarah to terminate the employment of two staff members who were the most vocal in their dissatisfaction with the reorganization. These individuals were excellent clinical nurses, well liked by staff, and each had over 12 years of seniority in the organization. Sarah knew that the director did not like these nurses for reasons unrelated to reorganization and their performance. After her third sleepless night, Sarah came to you to ask for guidance.

What advice do you give?

Summary

Nurses and the healthcare team have a long history of establishing a relationship of trust and advocacy with clients. Nurses play a key role in functioning as a trusted source of information for clients concerning ethical decisions related to their care. The ANA Code of Ethics (2015) provides an ethical infrastructure that outlines the duties and responsibilities for nurses and expectations for the public. Further guidance regarding professional codes of ethics is provided in the patient bill of rights and the 1990 Patient Self-Determination Act. The practicing nurse must continually evaluate the congruency with organizational ethics and the patient-centered ethical directives in the work environment. The ethics committees of organizations are composed of multidisciplinary team members who serve as a model of ethical practice for the organization. The current age of technology and societal changes present complicated ethical dilemmas and require exercising moral decision making for nurses, clients, and their families, as well as healthcare organizations. The nurse's moral stance on ethical dilemmas issues is shaped by his or her personal values and beliefs, understanding and application of the Code of Ethics for Nurses and previous experience within the healthcare context.

Reflective Practice Questions

1. What are some of the values that you understand as being most important to you? What personal beliefs are associated with these values? How have these personal beliefs and values been formed and shaped by experiences and people throughout your life?
2. Your clinical assignment for the day includes caring for a Sikh patient who has particular religious beliefs and practices. How would you go about including his religious and spiritual beliefs and practices into his daily care?
3. If your beliefs as a nurse conflict with that of the organization in which you are working, what is your best course of action?
4. In the orientation program for your position as a new graduate nurse there is nothing included on the ethics committee. How would you go about researching the services of this resource in this institution?

References

American Nurses Association. (2010). *Nursing's social policy statement: The essence of the profession* (3rd ed.). Silver Spring, MD: Author.

American Nurses Association. (2015). *Code of ethics for nurses with interpretive statements.* Silver Spring, MD: Author.

Beauchamp, T. L., & Childress, J. F. (2012). *Principles of biomedical ethics* (7th ed.). New York, NY: Oxford University Press.

Bulechek, G. M., Butcher, H. K., McCloskey, J. M., & Wagner, C. (2013). *Nursing intervention classification system* (6th ed.). St. Louis, MO: Mosby.

Cohen, J. H., Foglia, M. B., Kwong, K., Pearlman, R., & Fox, E. (2015). How do healthcare employees rate the ethics of their organization? An analysis based on VA IntegratedEthics@Staff Survey data. *Journal of Healthcare Management, 60*(3), 169–184.

Cornelius, J. (2010). A literature review: Advanced directives and patients with implantable cardioverter defibrillators. *Journal of the American Academy of Nurse Practitioners, 22,* 250–255. doi: 10.1111/j1745-7599.2010.00499.x

Fourie, C. (2015). Moral distress and moral conflict in clinical ethics. *Bioethics, 29*(2), 91–97. doi: 10.1111/joon.12500

Fowler, M. D., Reimer-Kirkham, S., Sawatzky, R., & Taylor, E. J. (Eds.). (2012). *Religion, religious ethics, and nursing.* New York, NY: Springer.

Hart, P. L., & Mareno, N. (2013). Cultural challenges and barriers through the voices of nurses. *Journal of Clinical Nursing, 23,* 2223–2233. doi: 10.1111/jocn12500

Jameton, A. (1984). *Nursing practice: The ethical issues.* Englewood, Cliffs, NJ: Prentice Hall.

Kangasniemi, M., Pakkanen, P., & Korhonen, A. (2015). Professional ethics in nursing: An integrative review. *Journal of Advanced Nursing, 71*(8), 1744–1757. doi: 10.1111/jan12619

Moeller, J. R., Albanese, K. G., Garcher, K., Aultman, J. M., Radwany, S., & Frate, D. (2012). Functions and outcomes of a clinical medical ethics committee: A review of 100 consults. *HealthCare Ethics Committee Forum, 24*(2), 99–114. doi: 10.1007/s10730-011-9170-9

National Institutes of Health. (1974). *The Belmont report: Ethical principles and guidelines for the protection of human subjects of research.* Retrieved from http://www.hhs.gov/ohrp/regulations-and-policy/belmont-report/

O'Connell, C. (2015). Gender and the experience of moral distress in critical care nurses. *Nursing Ethics, 22*(1), 32–42. doi: 10.1177/0969733013513216

Paulson, J. E. (2011). A narrative ethics of care. *Health Care Analysis, 19*(1), 28–40. doi: 10.1007/s10728-010-0162-8

Pavlish, C. L., Helyer, J. H., Brown-Saltzman, K., Miers, A. G., & Squire, K. (2015). Screening situations for risk of ethical conflicts: A pilot study. *American Journal of Critical Care, 24*(3), 248–256. http://dx.doi.org/10.437/ajcc2015418

Pearlman, R. (2013). Ethics, committees, programs and consultation. *Ethics in Medicine.* Retrieved from https://depts.washington.edu/bioethx/topics/ethics.html

Pugh, S. (2011). A fine line: The role of personal and professional vulnerabilities in allegations of unprofessional conduct. *Journal of Nursing Law, 14*(6), 21–31. doi: 10.1891/1073-7472.14.1.21

Radzuin, L. C. (2011). Moral distress in certified registered nurse anesthetists: Implications for nursing practice. (201). *American Association of Nurse Anesthetists Journal, 79*(11), 39–45. doi: 10:1177/09697330114

Santiago, C., & Abdool, S. (2011). Conversations about challenging end-of life cases: Ethics debriefing in the medical surgical intensive care unit. *Dynamics, 2*(4), 26–30. doi: 10:1136/bmj.320.7244.1266

Sherwood, G. D., & Horton-Deutsch, S. (2012). *Reflective practice: Transforming education and improving outcomes.* Indianapolis, IN: Sigma Theta Tau International.

Thorup, C. B., Rundquist, E., Roberts, C., & Delmar, C. (2012). Care as a matter of courage: vulnerability, suffering and ethical formation in nursing care. *Scandinavian Journal of Caring Science, 26*, 427–435. doi: 10.1111/j1471-6712.2011.00944.x

Ulrich, C. M., Taylor, C., & Grady, C. (2010). Everyday ethics: Ethical issues and stress in nursing practice. *Journal of Advanced Nursing, 66*(11), 1–28. doi: 10.1111/j1365-2648.2010.05425x

Legal Issues in Nursing

Eileen K. Fry-Bowers

LEARNING OUTCOMES

After reading this chapter you will be able to:

- Identify and understand the four basic sources of law that govern nursing practice.
- Describe the role and function of a state's nurse practice act.
- Define "standard of care."
- List and describe the four elements of a professional malpractice claim that the plaintiff must prove in order to prevail.
- Discuss the nurse's role and responsibility in obtaining informed consent.
- Consider steps a registered nurse can take to protect him- or herself from disciplinary action and civil or criminal liability.

Introduction

Consider the following.

- There are more than 3.8 million registered nurses (RNs) (including advanced practice RNs) and over 900,000 licensed vocational or practical nurses (LVNs or LPNs) working in the field of nursing in the United States, making nursing the nation's largest healthcare profession (National Council of State Boards of Nursing [NCSBN], 2016e).

- The "nursing pipeline," which is measured by the number of persons passing the National Council Licensure Examination for Registered Nurses (NCLEX-RN), increased substantially from 2001 to 2011, with more than 142,000 new RN graduates passing the exam in 2011 as compared to 68,561 in 2001 (Health Resources and Services Administration [HRSA], 2013).
- Nurses make up the largest single component of any hospital staff, are the primary providers of hospital patient care, and deliver most of the nation's long-term care (American Association of Colleges of Nursing [AACN], 2011).

Approximately 63 percent of working RNs provide inpatient and outpatient care in hospitals. However, nurses are also employed in settings such as private practices, health maintenance organizations, public health agencies, primary care clinics, home health care, nursing homes, outpatient surgery centers, nursing-school-operated nursing centers, insurance and managed care companies, schools, mental health agencies, hospices, the military, industry, nursing education, and healthcare research (HRSA, 2013). In addition, although nurses work collaboratively with professionals in medicine and other fields, nurses also possess specific skills and may function independent of, not auxiliary to, medicine (AACN, 2011). Nursing roles range from direct patient care and case management to establishing nursing practice standards, developing quality assurance procedures, and directing complex nursing care systems and nurses are increasingly relied upon for delivery of an array of healthcare services, including primary and preventive care by advanced nurse practitioners, and services by certified nurse midwives and nurse anesthetists (Institute of Medicine [IOM], 2011).

The purpose of this chapter is to address the many legal issues that exist in nursing practice and to provide an overview of the steps that an RN can take to protect him- or herself from liability and disciplinary action. Given the evolution in scope and practice of nursing, the public expects nurses to enter practice prepared to become expert clinicians and, accordingly, holds nurses to increasingly higher levels of accountability with concomitant risk of liability. In fact, more and more nurses are being named as defendants in **professional malpractice** lawsuits (Reising, 2012). Therefore, nurses entering into practice in *any* environment must become aware of the structure and function of their state board of nursing (SBON) and how their state nursing practice act (NPA) governs and limits their professional behaviors. Nurses also must appreciate the risks associated with professional malpractice and understand how laws and regulations, such as federal or state privacy law, affect their daily practice. Moreover, nurses must appreciate the basic rights of patients and their personal professional role in safeguarding those rights. A thorough foundation in these matters, as provided by this chapter, equips nurses to understand connections among federal and state laws, institutional policies and procedures, professional codes of ethics and maintenance of boundaries, and their own professional practice (Porter, 2012).

Sources of Law

Understanding the interconnection among federal and state laws, institutional policies, codes of ethics, and professional nursing practice begins with identifying the sources of law that govern behavior and that are enforced by the courts. *Law* may be defined as "any system of regulations to govern the conduct of the people of a community, society or nation, in response to the need for regularity, consistency and justice based upon collective human experience" (Hill & Hill, 2011a, p. 1). There are four basic sources of law, all of which govern the practice of nursing: federal and state constitutional law, laws passed by the federal and state legislatures, the common law, and administrative law.

The primary source of all law in the United States is the federal Constitution. This document sets forth the powers and limitations of the federal government. The first 10 amendments to the Constitution, known as the Bill of Rights, address such familiar concepts as freedom of speech, press, and religion; the right to assembly; and the right not to be deprived of life, liberty, or property without due process of law, among others (National Archives and Records Administration, n.d.). Each state has a constitution as well, which is also a source of important rights. However, if there is any conflict between the provisions of a state constitution and the federal Constitution, federal law takes precedence; this is known as federal supremacy.

Although the Constitution does not explicitly provide for a right to privacy, the Supreme Court of the United States has nevertheless held that the Constitution does indeed offer such protection. This has profound implications for the practice of nursing because a right to privacy guides courts in deciding significant healthcare issues such as a patient's right to reproductive autonomy, right to refuse medical treatment, and right to die. See, for example, *Skinner v. State of Oklahoma* (1942); *Griswold v. Connecticut* (1965); *Eisenstadt v. Baird* (1972); *Roe v. Wade* (1973); *Planned Parenthood v. Casey* (1992); *Gonzales v. Carhart* (2007); *Jacobson v. Massachusetts* (1905); *Washington v. Harper* (1990); *Cruzan v. Director, Missouri Department of Mental Health* (1990); *Washington v. Glucksberg* (1997); and *Vacco v. Quill* (1997).

Congress and state legislatures serve as a second source of law. Laws written by state legislatures, generally effective once signed by the state's governor, and laws drafted by Congress, effective once signed by the president, are called statutes. For example, each state's NPA is a state statute that specifically defines the legal limits for the practice of nursing within that state. In addition, all states enact **civil laws** that dictate socially reasonable conduct, as well as criminal laws that protect the public from harmful behaviors.

> **KEY TERM**
> **Civil laws:** Laws that dictate behavior between parties.

The **common law,** or case law, develops as a result of judicial decisions made in settling disputes or "cases" and serves as a third and very important source of law. Courts allow for the resolution of disputes by providing a forum in which the facts can be heard and the law applied. Generally, the facts of the case are presented at a trial court and are heard by a judge or jury. In making her decision regarding any issue, a judge interprets relevant statutes, considers legislative intent, and compares the facts to similar prior cases. The decision rendered may then serve as "precedent" and establishes principles or rules that courts may adopt when deciding subsequent cases with similar issues or facts (Simon, 2010).

Lastly, after the state legislature or Congress passes a law, implementation of the law passes to administrative agencies under the state or federal executive branch, which then make rules and regulations for enforcement of the statute. As a result, these agencies have significant power akin to that of legislative bodies. In addition, they possess what are known as "quasijudicial" powers. When there is a conflict regarding application and interpretation of the regulations, the administrative agency has the power to adjudicate the dispute through an administrative law process, with final determination subject to review by a court. Courts generally give great deference to decisions made through this process. Examples of administrative boards affecting nursing practice include the Centers for Medicare and Medicaid Services in the U.S. Department of Health and Human Services, the National Labor Relations Board in the U.S. Department of Labor, the Federal Trade Commission, the Food and Drug Administration, and state boards of health, insurance, medicine, and, of course, nursing (Hall, 2014).

In addition to understanding the sources of law, nurses must distinguish between types of law, and in particular, civil law and criminal law. Civil law can be viewed as the law that dictates behavior between private parties. These disputes take the form of a "lawsuit" and a party's legal claim against another is called a "cause of action." Tort law and contract law are examples of civil law. **Tort law** establishes rules for socially reasonable conduct and imposes liability on a party, a "wrongdoer," for unreasonable conduct. In general, the conduct may be defined as intentional or unintentional, and different rules of law apply to each. Contract law governs agreements and the enforcement of those agreements between parties. Generally, civil cases are determined by the "preponderance of the evidence," meaning that it is more likely than not that one party is responsible for the harm to the other party (Simon, 2010).

Conversely, criminal law serves to protect the public from harm by punishing persons who break societal rules. Rather than a dispute between parties, the state brings the criminal action against the accused. The state must prove its case "beyond a reasonable doubt," a more rigorous standard than that required in a civil action. Thus, a person may be acquitted of criminal wrongdoing but may be held civilly liable.

Judicial System

As noted in the previous section, courts throughout the United States make law through an adjudicative process whereby the court reviews the facts of the case presented through evidence, applies appropriate statutes and precedent, and then renders a decision. Just as each state and territory of the United States has its own set of laws, each possesses a separate court system. In addition, the United States has a court system for deciding disputes involving federal law (known as federal question jurisdiction) or conflicts between citizens of different states meeting a minimum monetary standard (known as diversity jurisdiction).

The courts in each of these systems are organized in a tiered structure. At the lowest level is the trial court, which is generally responsible for discovering the facts and applying the law to a wide variety of subject matters. If a party is dissatisfied with the outcome of a case at the trial level, they may usually appeal the decision, as a matter of right, to the next level of court. This appellate court generally reviews only issues of law related to the dispute and does not revisit the facts of a matter. The appellate court may agree with the trial court's determination and affirm the decision of the lower court or it may disagree and reverse that decision; or the court may agree with some parts of the decision and disagree with other parts, and thus, affirm in part and reverse in part the trial court's decision (Liang, 2002).

If disappointed at the appellate level, the litigant may appeal to the next level of court, generally, the state's highest court (names vary) or the Supreme Court of the United States, depending upon in which system, federal or state, the dispute was adjudicated. Courts at this highest level generally have discretion whether or not to hear an appeal. If the court refuses to hear an appeal, the decision of the appellate court stands.

As noted, Congress and state legislatures delegate significant rule making and enforcement authority to administrative agencies. These agencies may also resolve disputes much in the same manner as a state or federal court, but these hearings do not require a jury, and the evidentiary rules may differ. If a party is dissatisfied with the outcome of this administrative hearing, he or she must first exhaust the administrative agency's appellate process before any appeal may be made to a court of law (Hall, 2014). In general, courts require that the appellant show that the decision of the agency was "arbitrary and capricious" for reversal of an administrative ruling.

Legal Issues in Nursing Practice

Safe and appropriate nursing practice requires more than knowledge of patient conditions and treatment modalities. Nurses must also clearly appreciate the legal issues that govern and impact their practice.

Regulation of Nursing Practice

As previously noted, each state, as well as the District of Columbia and all territories of the United States, have statutes that specifically define the legal limits for the practice of nursing within that state, and explicitly identify requirements for **licensure**; these statutes are generally referred to as **nurse practice acts (NPAs)** (Grant & Ballard, 2011; NCSBN, 2016d). These legal requirements protect the health, safety, and welfare of the general public and the integrity of the nursing profession. North Carolina passed the first NPA, called the Nurse Registration Act, in 1903. Prior to that time, nursing practice was unregulated and any person could define and practice nursing in any manner (Grant & Ballard, 2011). Although this first act failed to define nursing practice, minimal educational requirements for nursing, or required registration with the state, many states recognized the need to establish rules and regulations to govern the practice of nursing and followed suit. New York, in 1938, was the first state to pass an act mandating educational prerequisites and licensure by examination for anyone seeking to practice nursing in that state and identify themselves as an "RN" or "registered nurse" (Russell, 2012; Whelan, 2013). In 1955, the American Nurses Association (ANA) published a definition of nursing that served as the foundation for the many state practice acts to follow (since updated and refined on several occasions to reflect changes and expansion of nursing roles). By the 1970s, all states mandated licensure of professional (RN) and vocational or practical nursing (LVN or LPN) (ANA, n.d.; Russell, 2012). See **Box 16-1** for examples of title protection for RNs.

Most state NPAs explicitly provide for the creation of some form of an SBON. The structure and composition of these administrative agencies differ from state to state, as do their roles and authority. In general, however, an NPA typically:

> **KEY TERM**
>
> **Licensure:** The process by which a state or governmental agency grants permission to an individual to engage in a given profession for compensation.

> **KEY TERM**
>
> **Nurse practice acts (NPAs):** State or territorial statutes that define the legal limits for the practice of nursing within that state or territory and explicitly identify the requirements for licensure.

- Defines the authority, composition and powers of the SBON
- Defines nursing and the boundaries of the scope of nursing practice in the state
- Identifies types of licenses and titles
- States the requirements for licensure in the state
- Establishes standards for educational programs
- Protects titles
- Determines the grounds for disciplinary action, other violations and remedies (NCSBN, 2011a; Russell, 2012)

BOX 16-1   EXAMPLES OF STATUTORY TITLE PROTECTION FOR REGISTERED NURSES

Arizona

Only a person who holds a valid and current license to practice professional nursing in this state or in a party state pursuant to section 32-1668 may use the title "nurse," "registered nurse," "graduate nurse," or "professional nurse" and the abbreviation "RN."

Arizona Nurse Practice Act: Section 32-1636a

California

It is unlawful for any person or persons not licensed or certified as provided in this chapter to use the title "registered nurse," the letters "RN," or the words "graduate nurse," "trained nurse," or "nurse anesthetist."

It is unlawful for any person or persons not licensed or certified as provided in this chapter to impersonate a professional nurse or pretend to be licensed to practice professional nursing as provided in this chapter.

California Nurse Practice Act: Section 2796

Florida

Only persons who hold licenses to practice professional nursing in this state or who are performing nursing services pursuant to the exception set forth in s. 464.022(8) shall have the right to use the title "Registered Nurse" and the abbreviation "RN."

Florida Nurse Practice Act: Section 464.015 (1)

A person may not practice or advertise as, or assume the title of, registered nurse, licensed practical nurse, clinical nurse specialist, certified registered nurse anesthetist, certified nurse midwife, or advanced registered nurse practitioner or use the abbreviation "RN," "LPN," "CNS," "CRNA," "CNM," or "ARN.P" or take any other action that would lead the public to believe that person was certified as such or is performing nursing services pursuant to the exception set forth in s. 464.022(8), unless that person is licensed or certified to practice as such.

A violation of this section is a misdemeanor of the first degree, punishable as provided in s. 775.082 or s. 775.083.

Florida Nurse Practice Act: Section 464.015(9), (10)

Kansas

Title and abbreviation. Any person who holds a license to practice as a registered professional nurse in this state shall have the right to use the title "registered nurse" and the abbreviation "RN." No other person shall assume the title or use the abbreviation or any other words, letters, signs, or figures to indicate that the person is a registered professional nurse.

Nurse Practice Act Section: 65-1115(d)

(continues)

BOX 16-1   EXAMPLES OF STATUTORY TITLE PROTECTION
FOR REGISTERED NURSES (continued)

New York

Only a person licensed or otherwise authorized under this article shall practice nursing and only a person licensed under section sixty-nine hundred four shall use the title "registered professional nurse" and only a person licensed under section sixty-nine hundred five of this article shall use the title "licensed practical nurse." No person shall use the title "nurse" or any other title or abbreviation that would represent to the public that the person is authorized to practice nursing unless the person is licensed or otherwise authorized under this article.

New York Nurse Practice Act: Section 6903

Washington

It is unlawful for a person to practice or to offer to practice as a registered nurse in this state unless that person has been licensed under this chapter. A person who holds a license to practice as a registered nurse in this state may use the titles "registered nurse" and "nurse" and the abbreviation "RN." No other person may assume those titles or use the abbreviation or any other words, letters, signs, or figures to indicate that the person using them is a registered nurse.

Washington State Nurse Practice Act: Section 18.79.030

BOX 16-2   GENERAL DUTIES OF STATE BOARDS OF NURSING

Acting under the direction of the state NPA, the state boards of nursing generally:
1. Establish rules and regulations that define and govern safe nursing practice;
2. Set standard nursing educational requirements including developing curriculum requirements, establishing faculty-student ratios for clinical practice, and approving nursing educational programs;
3. Define the criteria and process for licensure, and issuing licenses to practice practical, professional, and advanced nursing;
4. Monitor licensee's compliance with state requirements and taking disciplinary action against licensees who demonstrate unsafe nursing practice or who fail to comply with licensure requirements.

Data from National Council of State Boards of Nursing. (2011a). *What you need to know about nursing licensure and boards of nursing*. Retrieved from https://www.ncsbn.org/Nursing_Licensure.pdf

---

It is through the implementation of the NPA that SBONs protect the public's health and ensure the safe practice of nursing by further defining qualifications for licensure, scope of practice, and title protection (NCSBN, 2011a, 2016b). **Box 16-2** lists the general duties of state boards of nursing.

For the majority of nursing students and practicing nurses, the most direct role that the SBON plays is that of granting licensure, or granting someone the right to use the title RN. Licensure is the process by which a state governmental agency grants permission to an individual to engage in a given profession for compensation. More specifically, licensure by a governmental entity provides assurance to the public that the applicant has attained the essential degree of competency necessary to perform a unique scope of practice (NCSBN, 2011a).

Licensure should be distinguished from certification, which is another type of credential that affords title protection and recognition of accomplishment but does not include a legal scope of practice. Generally, certification defines the process by which a nongovernmental agency, such as a nursing specialty organization, recognizes individuals who have met certain requirements. Often, state boards of nursing use such professional certification as a requirement toward granting authority for advanced practice RNs. Readers are encouraged to review the requirements of each state where they wish to practice as well as consult with professional practice specialty associations for specific information. A complete discussion of licensure requirements for advanced practice nursing can be found in Chapter 3.

All state boards of nursing as well as those of the District of Columbia and U.S. territories require candidates for nursing licensure (RN) to pass the NCLEX-RN® examination, which measures the competencies needed to perform safely and effectively as an entry-level RN (NCSBN, 2012).

Although most nursing students equate "passing boards" with licensure, it is important to note that the licensure examinations are used to *assist* the boards in making licensure decisions and that passage of the licensure examination alone *does not* guarantee licensure. Registered nursing candidates must also comply with all other requirements such as meeting background requirements or satisfactory completion of additional educational requirements. All applicants for licensure across the United States must meet the same set of Uniform Licensure Requirements (ULR). This ensures that expectations for education of a nursing student and the responsibilities of a nurse are consistent state to state (NCSBN, 2012). Notably, requirements for renewing licensure, such as continuing education requirements, still vary from state to state.

In recent years the NCSBN, the agency that administers the NCLEX-RN examination, has developed a new regulatory model for the profession of nursing, a **mutual recognition of licensure model**, also known as the **Nurse Licensure Compact (NLC)**, which allows a nurse to maintain one license in his or her state of residency and to practice and be "recognized" in another state, physically and/or electronically, subject to each state's practice law

KEY TERM

Mutual recognition of licensure model: A model that allows a nurse to have one license in his or her state of residency with the ability to practice (electronically or physically) across state lines in other states that participate in this model if there are no restrictions on his or her license and that person acknowledges that he or she is subject to each state's practice laws and rules (NCSBN, 2011a).

KEY TERM

Nurse Licensure Compact (NLC): A form of interstate compact specific to nurse licensure that provides an agreement between two or more states for the purpose of recognizing nurse licensure between and among a group of participating states. States must enter into one in order to achieve mutual recognition (NCSBN, 2011a).

and regulation. Any state wishing to enter into a mutual recognition agreement with another state or states must enact legislation consistent with NCSBN's NLC model legislation. In addition, the SBON must implement the legislation, usually over 1 year, and pay a $6,000 annual fee (NCSBN, 2016e). Importantly, adoption of the NLC legislation does not change or supersede a state's NPA or its administrative procedural rules. On May 4, 2015, the NCSBN Special Delegate Assembly adopted an enhanced NLC and a revised Advanced Practice Nurse Compact (APRN Compact). Currently, 25 states have enacted NLC legislation and another five states have legislation pending during the 2015–2016 legislative cycle (Illinois, Massachusetts, Minnesota, New York, and Oklahoma) (NCSBN, 2016e). A complete listing of the states that have entered into the NLC can be found online (NCSBN, 2016a). **Contemporary Practice Highlight 16-1** further addresses the significance of the nursing mutual recognition model.

No one person has the unequivocal right to practice nursing. A nursing **license** is a privilege granted by a SBON based upon the licensee meeting all requirements for initial licensure or renewal of licensure. A SBON can refuse initial licensure and can reprimand, suspend, or revoke the license of a nurse under specific circumstances as outlined in the state's NPA

KEY TERM

License: Permission to engage in an activity; a professional license allows the holder to engage in a specific activity for compensation.

CONTEMPORARY PRACTICE HIGHLIGHT 16-1

THE NURSING MUTUAL RECOGNITION MODEL

The evolution of professional nursing roles to include practice in eHealth or telehealth, interstate transport nursing, and mobile or travel nursing necessitates a practical strategy to meet the licensure challenges presented by the increased mobility of the nursing population. One such strategy has been the implementation of a mutual recognition of licensure model.

The nursing mutual recognition model, known as the Nurse Licensure Compact, allows a nurse to be licensed in his or her state of residence but practice in a remote state that is another member of the compact. It is the responsibility of the nurse to know and abide by the remote state's NPA and other applicable regulations, even if different from those of their home state.

An example of a common mutual recognition model is the driver's license. A person with a California driver's license may drive in Arizona but must abide by the driving laws of Arizona. Failure to do so can result in a traffic citation.

Between 1998 and 2015, 25 states enacted compact legislation and another 5 states are considering legislation during the 2015–2016 legislative cycle (Illinois, Massachusetts, Minnesota, New York, and Oklahoma). Although nearly half of the nation's states participate in the compact, there has been little formal evaluation of it, and controversy regarding the model persists. Consider the following arguments:

ARGUMENTS IN FAVOR OF NURSE LICENSURE COMPACT LEGISLATION

- The practice of eHealth, telehealth, and transport nursing requires the practice of nursing across state borders. Obtaining and maintaining multiple licenses is burdensome. Compact legislation allows nurses to avoid duplicative licensure and associated fees.
- Because licensure is dependent on the nurse's state of residence, the compact facilitates physical mobility, enabling nurses to take on travel or short-term assignments in other party states.

- The compact prevents implementation of state nurse licensure solutions that fail to provide reciprocal agreements or allow for appropriate information sharing and authority to discipline.
- Information sharing between states regarding nurses is promoted through the compact. Compact states have licensure and disciplinary information on each nurse, resulting in greater protection of the public.

ARGUMENTS AGAINST NURSE LICENSURE COMPACT LEGISLATION

- The state of practice, rather than the state of residence, should dictate licensure because the purpose of licensure is to grant a nurse authority to practice while protecting the health and safety of the citizens of the state in which the license is held.
- Inconsistencies between states in relation to licensure requirements, especially license renewal, remain, such as mandatory continuing education, criminal background checks, and disciplinary causes of action, which leads to the possibility of nurses working side by side with different requirements for practice.
- Many states rely upon licensure fees to sustain their operating expenses. Eliminating the need for duplicative licensure results in decreased revenue to the affected state.

- Because nurses working in a remote state are not required to register with that state's board of nursing, the state will not be aware of the actual number of nurses working in the state, making workforce predictions difficult.
- Variability in state NPAs, as well as civil and criminal laws, raises significant questions related to liability, enforcement, and administrative processes. Nurses may find themselves subject to multiple investigations and disciplinary proceedings arising from the same incident or be required to defend themselves against civil litigation in a state other than their home state.

Contact your SBON for its specific position statement on this issue. Contact information can be found through the NCSBN, https://www.ncsbn.org/contact-bon.htm

Data from American Nurses Association. (2015c). *Nurse Licensure Compact (NLC). ANA talking points.* Retrieved from http://www.nursingworld.org/MainMenuCategories/Policy-Advocacy/State/Legislative-Agenda-Reports/Licensure Compact/Nurse-Licensure-Compact-ANA-Talking-Points.pdf; National Council of State Boards of Nursing. (2016c). *Licensure compacts.* Retrieved from https://www.ncsbn.org/compacts.htm

(NCSBN, 2011a). Once granted, however, a nursing license represents a property interest that is protected by the U.S. Constitution and the laws and regulations of each state. Every state has a specific process for filing, investigating, and resolving complaints against nurses but, in each circumstance, a nurse has certain rights. In any licensure matter, nurses have a right to be informed of the allegations made against them, the right to present their account of the incident, and a right to fair and just legal procedures when action is taken against their license. Moreover, the nurse has the right to consult with legal counsel (*and should exercise this right*). In addition, the nurse must remember that any disciplinary hearing is, by its very nature, adversarial, because of the board's authority to take action; thus, anything said to a board investigator can be used against the nurse during subsequent proceedings (another important reason to consult legal counsel). The right to use the initials "RN" comes at significant personal cost, effort, and sacrifice, and with great responsibility. Each nurse is accountable for his or her own nursing practice. **Box 16-3** provides additional information on how to protect your RN license.

Standards of Nursing Care

In general, much like any statute, the specific content of a state's NPA is broad. These acts and other related regulations are designed to provide general guidelines for nurses, but they do not dictate how to perform procedures associated with the daily functions of a nurse. So then, what does govern how a nurse performs these activities? How do nurses know that their practice is appropriate? In general, nurses must consult the policies and procedures of their employer, which will usually explicitly detail the extent of their nursing responsibilities. An institution may restrict practice to a narrower responsibility than that authorized by the state's NPA,

---

BOX 16-3 PROTECT YOUR RN LICENSE

1. Review the nursing practice act and all associated rules and regulations of the state(s) where you practice.
2. Obtain personal professional liability insurance with a licensure defense protection benefit, which will cover legal costs in the event of disciplinary action.
3. Be familiar with the American Nurses Association Foundation of Nursing Package that includes *Code of Ethics for Nurses with Interpretive Statements* (ANA, 2015b); *Nursing: Scope and* *Standards of Practice*, 3rd Edition (2015d); and *Nursing's Social Policy Statement*, 3rd Edition (2010).
4. Join a national, state, or specialty nursing association and stay abreast of issues applicable to nursing practice by reading journals, standards, literature, and practice statements.

Data from DoNinger, M. L., & Dollinger, R. A. (2012). A new legal interpretation of duty for registered nurses. *Journal of Nursing Regulation*, 3(1), 21–25. http://dx.doi.org/10.1016/S2155-8256(15)30230-1

but it may never allow a nurse to take on greater responsibilities. But how does an institution determine its policies and procedures, and will those standards legally protect a nurse in the event of a disciplinary hearing or a lawsuit?

A **standard of care** can be defined as the degree of care, expertise, and judgment exercised by a reasonable person under the same or similar circumstances. The standard of care for a nurse then, "requires a nurse to use the level of care that a reasonably prudent nurse would provide under the same or similar circumstances" (Grant & Ballard, 2011, p. 253). This does not mean care must be optimal, or of extraordinary skill, nor does it mean that a nurse may not make an error in nursing judgment. It does require, however, that any error made be *reasonable* under the circumstances (Moffett & Moore, 2011).

> **KEY TERM**
>
> **Standard of care:** The degree of care, expertise, and judgment exercised by a reasonable person under the same or similar circumstances.

Sources of standards of care include professional nursing organizations, nursing literature such as peer-reviewed nursing journals, federal or state statutes or regulations (e.g., nurse–patient ratios for federal- or state-funded institutions, the state NPA), the Joint Commission, court decisions that may set new standards (which set precedent), professional experts (e.g., published authors, nursing professors) and even clinical practice guidelines (Moffett & Moore, 2011).

Hospitals and healthcare-related entities frequently look to these nursing standards of care when determining policies and procedures for their institutions. It is essential, however, that nurses recognize that standards of care are dynamic and change with advancements in health care (DoNinger & Dollinger, 2012). Nurses will be held accountable for standards existing at the time of any incident and not standards they may have learned in school. Thus, it is in any nurse's best interest to stay abreast of changes in practice—this includes ensuring that one's employer's policies and procedures are reflective of changed standards. *A nurse may not be protected in a legal dispute if he or she adhered to standards, albeit "hospital policy," that are outdated.*

Box 16-4 provides suggestions on how to keep your practice current as an RN. (Note: Specialists are held to the standard of other similarly situated specialists. A nurse holding advanced certification or licensure will be held to the standard required

---

BOX 16-4   KEEPING YOUR PRACTICE CURRENT

1. Join a nursing organization.
2. Subscribe to general professional and specialty nursing journals (often a benefit of membership in a nursing organization).
3. Review nursing articles available via the Internet. One source is the *NursingCenter* at http://www.nursingcenter.com, which provides access to clinical articles from 50 leading nursing journals.
4. Sign up for email alerts from nursing organizations and state boards of nursing.

of those having such additional training. For example, a Certified Registered Nurse Anesthetist [CRNA] or Pediatric Nurse Practitioner [PNP] would be held to the knowledge level of another similarly situated CRNA or PNP, rather than another RN working in the same setting.)

Civil Liability

When a nurse fails to provide a level of care that conforms to the standard of care for that particular nursing practice situation, he or she may be held legally accountable. Any injured party (plaintiff) can initiate a civil action against a "wrongdoer" (defendant) for unreasonable conduct. If the plaintiff can prove by a preponderance of the evidence that the defendant's action or inaction caused or contributed to the plaintiff's injuries, the defendant will be required to monetarily compensate the plaintiff. These civil actions are based on tort law and are usually classified according to whether the defendant's actions were intentional or unintentional. Even if a defendant's actions were unintentional, they can still be required to compensate the injured party.

Negligence

Negligence is unintentional conduct that falls below a standard of care established for the protection of others against unreasonable risk of harm (Hill & Hill, 2011b). Professional malpractice is a specific type of negligence that results when a professional person fails to perform their professional duties in a reasonable manner. Judges and juries rely on appropriate standards of care to determine the reasonableness of the professional's conduct. Standards of care, however, represent only one aspect of a malpractice claim; the plaintiff must prove several additional factors. Specifically, in a cause of action for negligence, and thus, professional malpractice, the plaintiff must prove the following four elements (see **Box 16-5**).

> **KEY TERM**
>
> **Negligence:** Unintentional conduct that falls below a standard of care established for the protection of others against unreasonable risk of harm.

BOX 16-5   FOUR ELEMENTS OF NEGLIGENCE

1. The defendant owed a duty to the plaintiff to use reasonable care;
2. The defendant failed to conform to this standard of care (known as breach of duty);
3. There is a reasonably close causal relationship between the defendant's conduct and the plaintiff's injuries (a two-part test); and

4. The plaintiff suffered actual loss or damages

Data from Schwartz, V. E., Kelly, K., & Partlett, D. (2015). *Prosser, Wade & Schwartz's torts: Cases and materials* (13th ed.). New York, NY: Foundation Press.

Duty

The first element of any malpractice claim is **duty**. In a case against a nurse, the plaintiff must prove that the nurse owed a legal duty to the plaintiff (usually the patient and, under some circumstances, the plaintiff's family) that required the nurse to deliver the appropriate standard of care. This duty generally arises with the commencement of the nurse–patient relationship—if there is such a relationship, there is a duty, on the part of the nurse, to act (or not act, as the case may be).

In the hospital setting, once nurses are assigned to care for a patient during their shift, this nurse–patient relationship commences and a duty arises. However, a duty can also be established when a nurse is "covering" a patient during a colleague's brief break or even when an unassigned patient on the nurse's unit needs assistance. In the clinic setting, a duty may arise through a simple telephone conversation between nurse and patient. Moreover, if a nurse witnesses a patient receiving inappropriate or inferior care from another nurse or other healthcare professional, including a physician, the law generally imposes a duty on that nurse to intervene on behalf of the patient. A nurse generally does not have a duty to render assistance at the scene of a car accident but, if the nurse does render assistance, the nurse must not give negligent care (Schwartz, Kelly, & Partlett, 2015). See **Contemporary Practice Highlight 16-2** for a discussion about **Good Samaritan laws** that addresses liability related to providing care in emergency situations. In summary, courts generally agree that if a patient presents for care, and care is given or should have been given, legal duty is established.

Breach of Duty

Once a plaintiff establishes that the nurse owed a duty of care to the patient, the plaintiff must show that the nurse showed a **breach of duty** by failing to perform according to the standard of care for that particular circumstance, specifically, that the defendant nurse failed to do what a reasonable and prudent nurse would have done or not done under the same or similar circumstances. Most often, this standard of care is established through expert testimony and the presentation of additional evidence such as a hospital manual of nursing policies and procedures.

Causation

The plaintiff must do much more than prove that the defendant nurse breached a duty owed to the patient; the plaintiff must demonstrate that the nurse caused the patient's **damages**. **Causation** is a difficult concept to grasp and a detailed discussion

---

KEY TERM

Duty: An obligation to act or refrain from acting.

KEY TERM

Good Samaritan laws: Laws enacted by a state that protect healthcare providers and other rescuers from liability if they render aid in an emergency, provided that they use reasonable and prudent judgment under the circumstances based on their education, training, and skill level.

KEY TERM

Breach of duty: Failure to perform according to a specific standard of care once a duty is established.

KEY TERM

Damages: Injuries incurred as a result of someone's negligence.

KEY TERM

Causation: A determination that if not for the conduct of the defendant, the plaintiff would not have been injured and that the consequences of such conduct were foreseeable.

CONTEMPORARY PRACTICE HIGHLIGHT 16-2

UNDERSTANDING GOOD SAMARITAN LAWS

Most states have "Good Samaritan" statutes that protect from liability those people, including trained healthcare workers, who stop to assist and provide care during an emergency. By providing this protection, states hope to encourage nurses, doctors, paramedics, and other citizens to help victims in an emergency.

Although stopping at the scene of an accident may be the appropriate action based upon your own morals and ethics, it is important that you understand your responsibilities under your state NPA and your state's Good Samaritan law. Although most states do not require people to give aid in such cases, two states, Minnesota and Vermont, have laws that require such assistance (known as "duty to rescue" laws).

Once you render care, you establish a nurse–patient relationship. As a result, you must deliver the same standard of care that a reasonable and prudent nurse would deliver under similar circumstances. Furthermore, you cannot leave the victim until you are able to transfer care to another competent provider of the same or greater skill level.

So how does a reasonably prudent nurse respond in such an emergency? A nurse should provide only that care that is consistent with his or her level of education, training, and expertise.

In general, in most states nurses will be protected from liability if they:

- Assess a patient's status, including level of responsiveness, airway, breathing, and circulation.
- Activate the emergency response system by calling or directing someone to call 911.
- Administer rescue breathing and/or chest compressions if indicated.
- Control bleeding.
- Administer emergency medications such as a glucagon kit or anaphylaxis kit (e.g., EpiPen).
- Use an automated external defibrillator if required.

The protections provided by Good Samaritan laws are limited to emergency situations away from the employment setting and they will not protect a nurse from liability resulting from grossly negligent action.

Of important note, victims rarely sue a person who tries to assist in an emergency. If you render assistance in an emergency, you will likely be protected if you act reasonably and give the best care possible under the circumstances. In summary, know the laws of the state in which you practice, act within acceptable standards of care, and know your limitations.

Data from Morrison, H., & Bagalio, S. (2015). Being a Good Samaritan. *Advance for Nurses*. Retrieved from http://nursing.advanceweb.com/article/being-a-good-samaritan.aspx

is beyond the scope of this chapter. Simply stated, the plaintiff must also show that the nurse's actions were (a) the "cause in fact" (known as the actual or "but for" cause) of the plaintiff's injuries and that (b) the consequences to the patient resulting from the nurse's actions were foreseeable (known as proximate cause).

Cause in fact or actual cause means that but for the conduct of the nurse, the patient would not have been injured. Note, however, that more than one person can be held legally responsible for an injury to a patient. In a lawsuit against a nurse, a patient need only show that the nurse's action or inaction contributed substantially to the patient's injury. Once the plaintiff demonstrates cause in fact, he or she must then show it was foreseeable that the patient could have been harmed by the nurse's action or inaction. For example, if a nurse administers a drug to a patient with known sedative effects and then fails to ensure that the patient's bedrails are in the upright position and the patient falls out of bed, the plaintiff may reasonably argue the nurse should have foreseen that the patient was at an increased risk of injury as a result of the medication administered and that the nurse should have taken precaution against such injury. All healthcare providers have a responsibility to foresee harm to those for whom they care and take steps to eliminate if possible, or at least mitigate, that harm.

Damages

Finally, the plaintiff must show that he or she indeed suffered injury or "damages" as a result of the nurse's negligent action. Courts award money damages in an attempt to return patients as nearly as possible to their preinjury condition or state. Even if the plaintiff demonstrates duty, breach of duty, and both components of causation, but the patient suffered no injury, there can be no monetary recovery. Money damages are classified as general, special, or punitive and are meant to compensate the patient for pain and suffering, disfigurement and disability, past and future medical expenses, past lost wages and future earning capacity, and so forth.

Respondeat Superior

Respondeat superior, Latin for "let the master answer," is a key legal doctrine, which holds that an employer is responsible for the actions of its employees that occur within the scope of the employment relationship (Schwartz, Kelly, & Partlett, 2015). Thus, although a nurse retains individual responsibility for his or her negligence, he or she shares the liability with their employer. The law recognizes that an employer should bear responsibility for the actions of its employees so as to encourage care in hiring and adequate supervision of employees. In addition, employers are usually in a better position to insure against risks and bear the monetary burden of claims. The doctrine of *respondeat superior* does not apply if nurses act outside the scope of their employment (or scope of practice), such as performing a procedure that only a physician may do in that institution. Moreover, if a hospital is held liable for the negligence of a nurse, the hospital may have the option of subsequently suing the nurse to recover the damages it paid (known as indemnification). (Note: The doctrine of *respondeat superior* does not apply to work performed by an independent contractor. A nurse hired as a private duty nurse is usually an independent contractor.)

> **KEY TERM**
>
> ***Respondeat superior***: A legal doctrine, which holds that the employer is responsible for the actions of its employees that occur within the scope of the employment relationship.

Defenses to Negligence

Once a lawsuit is filed against a nurse, the nurse can raise defenses to the malpractice claim. As noted earlier, a plaintiff must prove all of the elements of negligence in a nursing malpractice claim in order to win a monetary award of damages; thus, asserting that the plaintiff failed to prove just one of the four elements of the claim is a valid defense. Second, many states have enacted statutes of limitations that limit the time in which a plaintiff can bring a claim against a defendant. These laws and the cases they address vary from state to state, but if a plaintiff does not bring the cause of action within the time prescribed, their action is barred. Another valid defense that can limit a plaintiff's claim against a nurse is the plaintiff's own actions. The law will not reward a plaintiff who contributed to his or her own injury by failing to act in a reasonable and prudent manner. Examples of such plaintiff behavior are failure to follow instructions and failure to provide truthful information—if these actions contributed to the patient's injury, the court may reduce or even bar any damage award (Schwartz, Kelly, & Partlett, 2015).

Intentional Torts in Nursing

A nurse's legal liability to a patient can extend beyond negligence to other claims in tort law, known as the intentional torts. Unlike negligence, intentional torts are planned acts that cause harm to another, although this harm may not have been expected by the person who acted. In nursing, any willful act that violates the rights of a patient is an intentional tort. **Box 16-6** provides examples of intentional torts. Just as in a negligence/malpractice action, a nurse can be sued for money damages to compensate the patient for the harms caused (Pozgar, 2012).

Criminal Liability

As discussed, holding a license as an RN is a privilege, and with that privilege comes significant responsibility. Nurses must recognize that, in addition to civil liability, they may be subject to criminal liability for inappropriate actions taken, in addition

---

BOX 16-6　EXAMPLES OF INTENTIONAL TORTS

Assault—Attempting to or threatening to touch a person without his or her consent.
- Example—A nurse threatening to give a patient an injection if he or she does not comply with care.

Battery—Touching a person without his or her consent.
- Example—A nurse performing any treatment on a patient without the express or implied consent of the patient or his or her legal guardian.

False Imprisonment—Confining a person without his or her consent.
- Example—Unwarranted use of restraints or other restrictions, including pharmacologic, on a patient.

to the administrative disciplinary actions regarding licensure as noted above. Often intentional torts, such as those listed in Box 16-6, constitute criminal acts for which a nurse may be disciplined administratively and punished criminally. In addition, inappropriate administration and/or recording of controlled substances violate state and federal drug laws.

Decreasing Elements of Risk

Dealing with any action, whether it is a disciplinary, malpractice or other tort, or criminal action, can be professionally, financially, and psychologically devastating to a nurse. Thus, proactive risk reduction is essential. **Box 16-7** provides information about how nurses can reduce their own risk of lawsuit.

Medication errors, which include administering the incorrect medication, incorrect dose, or incorrect route, as well as improper administration, are a most common source of nursing negligence. **Box 16-8** lists common nursing actions leading to

---

BOX 16-7   REDUCE YOUR RISK OF LAWSUIT

1. Maintain knowledge of state NPA.
2. Comply with and keep current with changes in standards of care, employer's policies, and procedures.
3. Practice appropriate standard of nursing care (e.g., always adhere to "five rights" when administering medications, practice proper handwashing, adhere to state and federal privacy regulations).
4. Communicate clearly and consistently with patient, patient's family, and professional colleagues.
5. Document nursing care accurately, thoroughly, and consistently.
6. Practice adequate supervision of unlicensed personnel.

BOX 16-8   COMMON NURSING ACTIONS LEADING TO MALPRACTICE CLAIMS

In addition to medication errors, common nursing actions leading to malpractice claims include:

1. Failure to follow standards of care
2. Failure to use equipment in a responsible manner
3. Failure to assess and monitor
4. Failure to communicate
5. Failure to document
6. Failure to act as patient advocate or follow the chain of command
7. Failure to provide a safe environment
8. Failure to protect patient privacy (e.g., inappropriate use of social media)

Data from Melnik, T. (2013). Avoiding violations of patient privacy with social media. *Journal of Nursing Regulation, 3*(4), 39–46. http://dx.doi.org/10.1016/S2155-8256(15)30185-X; Reising, D. L. (2012). Making your nursing care malpractice-proof. *American Nurse Today, 7*(1), 24–28.

malpractice claims. In addition, increased use of unlicensed personnel to complete "nursing tasks" may place a nurse at risk for malpractice and/or disciplinary action for improper delegation, which is the delegation of a licensed activity, as defined by the state's nurse practice, to an unlicensed person.

Recognizing potential risk is the nurse's first step in protecting his or her license and avoiding liability. Second, the nurse should adhere to the principles outlined in Box 16-7 in the performance of his or her professional nursing role. Finally, yet most important, a nurse must *always* listen to the concerns of the patient and/or the patient's family *and respond* in a timely and effective manner.

Although a complete discussion of professional liability insurance is beyond the scope of this chapter, all nurses should carefully review their need to obtain such insurance. Factors to consider include the nurse's employment situation and potential risk of lawsuits (e.g., Does the nurse work in a high-risk environment such as labor and delivery?) and personal financial situation (e.g., Could the nurse afford legal representation in the event of a lawsuit or disciplinary action?).

Legal Issues in the Nurse–Patient Relationship

A nurse's duty to his or her patient supersedes all other nursing activities. The prior discussion regarding professional liability makes clear that patients have a right to receive care of a certain standard and quality. In addition, as noted at the beginning of this chapter, the Supreme Court has carved out additional patient rights. Moreover, subsequent statutes, such as the Patient Self-Determination Act (PSDA), passed as part of the Omnibus Budget Reconciliation Act of 1990, effective December 1, 1991; the Health Insurance Portability and Accountability Act (HIPAA), enacted by the U.S. Congress in 1996; and a Patient's Bill of Rights, contained in the Patient Protection and Affordable Care Act (ACA) of 2010 have provided patients with the legal means to gain control over their health care, including access to care, treatment, decision making, and security of health-related information.

The PSDA applies to all healthcare institutions receiving Medicaid funds and requires them to provide individuals receiving medical care written information about their rights under state law to make decisions about medical care, including the right to accept or refuse medical or surgical treatment. Institutions must also provide individuals with information about their right to formulate advance directives such as living wills and durable powers of attorney for health care (42 U.S.C. §§ 1395cc (a)(1) et. seq.). Patients must be made aware of their right to make decisions about these issues upon admission (in the case of hospitals or skilled nursing facilities), enrollment (in the case of health maintenance organizations), on first receipt of care (in the case of hospices), or before the patient comes under an agency's care (in the case of home health personal care agencies) (American Nurses Association, 2012).

Title II of HIPAA contains the Privacy Rule, effective in 2003, and establishes regulations for the use and disclosure of protected health information, including information about the health status, provision of health care, or payment for health care that can be linked to a person, and any part of a person's medical record (45 C.F.R. 164.501).

Prominent health-related agencies and organizations have promulgated various versions of a Patients' Bill of Rights to guide healthcare professionals and institutions in their policies of care regarding patients. Finally, after nearly a decade of unsuccessful attempts by Congress to pass formal legislation known as the Patients' Bill of Rights, many of the protections included in this legislation became part of the Patient Protection and Affordable Care Act of 2010. These rules prohibit exclusions for preexisting conditions, lifetime health insurance coverage limits, restriction of annual coverage limits and limit rescissions. In addition, the provisions guarantee direct access to certain types of providers and access to out-of-network emergency care (Jost, 2010).

All of these documents and statements stem from a common belief in the patient's right to **self-determination**. Moreover, they serve to address the public's growing mistrust of the healthcare industry, concerns over medical error, and perceptions of a preference for profits over patients. Nurses must familiarize themselves with these statements, and in particular, the American Nurses Association's *Code of Ethics for Nurses with Interpretive Statements*, which holds that nurses have moral and professional obligations to recognize the inherent rights of patients (ANA, 2015b).

> **KEY TERM**
>
> **Self-determination:** The right of every individual to control his or her own person free from interference from others.

There is a great and longstanding regard for the principle of respect for autonomy and self-determination in modern Western society, as evidenced by the following quotes from well-known legal cases:

> No right is held more sacred, or is more carefully guarded, by the common law, than the right of every individual to the possession and control of his own person, free from all restraint or interference of others, unless by clear and unquestionable authority of law. (*Union Pacific R. Co. v. Botsford*, 141 U.S. 250 [1891])
>
> Every human being of adult years and sound mind has a right to determine what shall be done with his own body; and a surgeon who performs an operation without his patient's consent commits assault, for which he is liable in damages. (*Schloendorff v. Society of New York Hospital*, 105 N.W. 92 [1914])

These basic beliefs guide the behavior of healthcare providers in regard to a patient's right to information and right to refuse treatment.

Informed Consent

A patient's right to autonomy and self-determination is most relevant to the issue of **consent**. Under modern rules, any healthcare provider has a duty to inform a patient of all relevant facts regarding a treatment or procedure prior to his or her consent to it. Although physicians, advanced practice nurses, and physician's assistants are often responsible for obtaining informed consent prior to performing procedures, the bedside nurse is also responsible for explaining all nursing procedures to the patient prior to performing them. In such cases, and under most circumstances, a patient's physical acquiescence to bedside care generally constitutes consent.

What constitutes informed consent varies according to jurisdiction, but courts apply one of three standards (Rock & Hoebeke, 2014):

Physician-based standard: Under this standard, a physician (or nurse practitioner or physician's assistant) has a duty to disclose any information that a reasonable physician in the same or similar circumstances would disclose to the patient for consent purposes.

Patient-based standard: Under this standard, a physician (or nurse practitioner or physician's assistant) must disclose any information that a reasonable patient would consider material (affect the patient's decision) in making a decision regarding his or her treatment or care.

Hybrid standard: This standard incorporates both of the above standards and generally requires that disclosure of information meet the physician-based standard and must be sufficient to provide a reasonable person with a general understanding of the procedure or course of treatment.

Regardless of standard, obtaining an informed consent generally requires that the care provider performing the treatment or procedure discuss the following information with the patient (Guido, 2013; Rock & Hoebeke, 2014):

- Patient diagnosis
- Nature and purpose of proposed course of therapy or procedure
- Expected outcomes from therapy or procedure
- Expected benefits from therapy or procedure
- Name of person performing or responsible for therapy or procedure
- Complications, risks, and side effects of therapy or procedure
- Reasonable alternatives
- Possible prognosis if therapy or procedure is not done

However, simply providing this information to a patient does not mean that the care provider obtained the informed consent of the patient. Information is but one of three elements necessary for meeting the legal requirements of an informed consent. In order for a patient's consent to a treatment or procedure to be valid, the consent must be *voluntary* and the patient must be *competent* to give his or her consent (Rock & Hoebeke, 2014).

For a consent to be voluntary, the patient must not be coerced or under any influence, including that of medication that may alter thought processes, such as a narcotic or sedative agent. Voluntary consent can be expressed verbally, such as stating "yes," or in writing, such as by signature on a consent form. Such affirmation is known as express consent. Consent can also be implied by a patient's actions, such as complying with examination; this constitutes implied consent. Silence, however, cannot be construed as consent if a reasonable person would speak before receiving treatment.

Only a competent patient can give informed consent. Most adults (minors will be discussed next) who can understand relevant information concerning their medical care, demonstrate sufficient understanding of the salient issues, and communicate their choice regarding their care are deemed to be competent. Generally, a nurse is in a very good position to assess the competency of a patient due to frequent interactions with that patient throughout a given nursing shift. Often, it is the nurse who initially detects defects in the patient's attention span, memory, or basic understanding of the situation, each of which can interfere with his or her ability to give informed consent. Any concern regarding patient competence should be immediately shared with the patient's physician or care provider performing the treatment or procedure.

It is the responsibility of the person performing the medical treatment or surgical procedure to obtain informed consent. The care provider performing the treatment or procedure should never delegate obtaining informed consent to the bedside nurse. In other words, that care provider, physician, nurse practitioner, or physician's assistant must be the one to provide the patient with the necessary information to obtain consent, such as the complications, risks, or side effects of the therapy or procedure, as discussed earlier. A nurse may be called upon to witness the consent, which means that the nurse observed the patient signing the consent form, thus giving consent to undergo the procedure. Witnessing a consent is not the same thing as obtaining consent. A nurse may also answer a patient's questions as they pertain to relevant nursing care, but must refer questions regarding medical care to the physician. Documentation of questions asked and information provided is essential. Finally, each nurse must be knowledgeable about consent policies and procedures at his or her institution, as well as be familiar with specific state requirements or issues unique to his or her area of practice (e.g., emergency department, labor and delivery, school-based clinic, etc.; see **Box 16-9**).

BOX 16-9   YOUR NURSING RESPONSIBILITY IN INFORMED CONSENT

The nurse's primary role in the informed consent process is as *patient advocate*:

- Determine your patient's level of understanding and approval of the procedure to be done or care to be given.
- Identify any patient fears and/or misconceptions and notify care provider.
- Provide information regarding nursing care associated with the procedure or treatment.
- Contact the appropriate care provider if you doubt the patient's understanding of the procedure or treatment or his or her decision-making ability.
- Document questions asked and information provided.
- Notify your supervisor or follow institution policy if you continue to believe your patient's consent is not voluntary or competent.

The nurse's secondary role in the informed consent process is to act as *witness*:

- Witness that the patient is giving consent voluntarily.
- Witness that the patient is lucid and competent to give consent.
- Witness that the signature on the consent form is, in fact, that of the patient (legal guardian or healthcare proxy agent).

Finally, ensure that the process and signed document conforms to your facility's informed consent policy.

Data from Guido, G. W. (2013). *Legal and ethical issues in nursing* (6th ed.). Upper Saddle River, NJ: Prentice Hall; Rock, M. J., & Hoebeke, R. (2014). Informed consent: Whose duty to inform? *Medsurg Nursing, 23*(3), 189–194.

Special Concerns with Informed Consent

In some circumstances, the usual rules regarding obtaining consent do not apply. Conversely, at other times, additional safeguards are warranted. Nurses working with vulnerable populations, such as minors or the elderly, and those who work in emergency department settings, must know when deviation from the usual rules is required. They must implement the appropriate informed consent rules when necessary. See **Case Study 16-1**.

Minors and Informed Consent

In general, minors, individuals under the age of 18, are incapable of providing a valid legal consent, and a parent or court-appointed guardian must provide consent for medical or surgical treatment of the minor. Several statutory exceptions exist. Many states allow minors to consent to treatment for sexually transmitted diseases, including human immunodeficiency virus (HIV); care for the prevention or treatment of pregnancy (including contraception and, in a decreasing minority of states, abortion); treatment for physical abuse; and treatment or counseling for substance abuse. In addition, a minor who can demonstrate to a court that they possess the maturity to choose or reject a particular healthcare treatment despite their chronological age may be judged to be a "mature minor" and capable of consenting to treatment (Rozovsky, 2015). An emancipated minor is one who is financially

CASE STUDY 16-1
CONSENT

Mrs. Johnson is a 93-year-old woman with a history of congestive heart failure and chronic renal insufficiency. Her present medications include inderal, lisinopril, digoxin, lasix, warfarin, and a multivitamin. She has been a widow for approximately 40 years. She has 3 living children, 9 grandchildren, and 10 great-grandchildren, most of whom she sees regularly. She lives independently in a "seniors" apartment complex, and, until recently, has participated in many of the complex's activities, including working in the community commissary several mornings a week. She uses a walker in public but manages to move about her apartment unaided. She requires assistance when grocery shopping. Her family members accompany her to medical appointments.

Several days ago, she fell following a trip to the grocery store. She was transported by emergency medical services to the local emergency department. She was diagnosed with left femoral neck fracture with displacement of the femoral head. The orthopedic surgeon has recommended hip replacement surgery. Her family is in support of this procedure.

You are the bedside nurse caring for Mrs. Johnson. In fact, you have cared for Mrs. Johnson for the past 2 days. You have found her to be quiet and cooperative and have noted none of the cantankerous behavior that her family states is characteristic of her. It is 7:30 am, you have received report from the off-going nurse, and have begun your assessment. You note that Mrs. Johnson seems a bit delayed in her responses to your questions. No other changes are noted.

At 7:45 am Dr. Bones, the orthopedic surgeon, enters the patient's room to discuss her upcoming surgery and obtain surgical consent. You remain at the bedside listening to Dr. Bones' comprehensive explanation of the procedure. Throughout his explanation, Mrs. Johnson looks at him and nods her head approvingly. Dr. Bones finally asks Mrs. Johnson if she has any questions, to which she replies, "No, sir." Dr. Bones turns to you and states that he will complete the informed consent paperwork and asks you to have Mrs. Johnson sign it.

Shortly thereafter, you bring the consent form to Mrs. Johnson and ask her to sign it. She looks at you and states, "Now Mary, I told you I cannot sign that permission slip. You didn't finish your chores. Now go," and she waves you away. Mary is not your name. Mary is the name of Mrs. Johnson's daughter.

What are the implications of Mrs. Johnson's response? Did Dr. Bones obtain an informed consent from Mrs. Johnson? What should you do?

---

independent and living apart from his or her parents or guardian, is married, or who is in the U.S. military. Emancipated minors have the same legal capacity as an adult and may consent to treatment. Nurses must be aware of the statutory requirements for the treatment of minors in their respective state of licensure and practice.

Other Consent Issues

A patient who has been adjudicated by a court as mentally incompetent, is intoxicated with alcohol or drugs, is in shock, or is unconscious is not capable of consent. A judicially declared mentally incompetent patient will have a court-appointed guardian who has the legal authority to consent to treatment. It is important to note that there may be restrictions as to what the guardian may authorize. Nurses should consult their institution policies regarding questions or concerns involving the care of the mentally incompetent patient. Often, a legal or ethics consult is needed to address treatment for these patients.

In the case of an emergency, healthcare providers may act in the absence of express consent and provide care to a patient if (Rozovsky, 2015):

1. The patient is unable to give consent due to intoxication, mental incompetence, or the patient is incoherent or unconscious.
2. There is risk of serious bodily harm if treatment is delayed.
3. A reasonable person would consent to treatment under the circumstances.
4. This patient would consent to the treatment under the circumstances (or the healthcare provider has no reason to know that the person would refuse treatment, e.g., knowing that the patient is a Jehovah's Witness or Christian Scientist).

Two additional doctrines act as exceptions to informed consent: therapeutic privilege and patient waiver. Under therapeutic privilege, the physician determines that certain information may be detrimental to the patient's physical or emotional well-being and that full disclosure should not be made. Clearly, this is risky practice and requires detailed documentation of the circumstances surrounding the decision, including the information disclosed, the information withheld, and the reasons, including medical rationale, for withholding the information (Richard, Lajeunesse, & Lussier, 2010). Under patient waiver, patients may decide that they do not wish to know or discuss the various aspects of their care and simply place their care in the hands of their trusted physician. Again, detailed documentation is essential and healthcare providers must remember that the patient can revoke the waiver (Richard et al., 2010).

Failure to Obtain Consent

Failure to obtain informed consent can have significant consequences for the healthcare team. Providers can be sued for battery, the unauthorized touching of another, or more commonly, for negligence. Because obtaining informed consent is recognized as a professional standard of care, negligence is an appropriate basis for liability. If a nurse knows or should have known that informed consent was not obtained and failed to make the physician or nursing supervisor aware, the nurse may also be liable.

Right to Refuse Medical Treatment

Just as the respect for a patient's right to self-determination dictates that a care provider must obtain informed consent prior to treatments or procedures, it also recognizes that a competent patient can refuse any proposed treatments or procedures, including those that may be life-sustaining or -saving, or motivated by religious belief. As noted, the Supreme Court recognizes that individuals have a constitutionally protected interest in refusing unwanted medical treatment (*Cruzan v. Director, Missouri Department of Health*, 1990), although many legal questions remain unanswered.

The law remains unclear in cases involving incompetent, terminally ill patients, as well as the role of family members in termination of care. Cases involving refusal or termination of care in minors are complex and a detailed discussion is beyond the scope of this chapter. However, consider the following: If a parent or parents may make such a decision to refuse care for an infant or a young child, can they make that same decision for a school-age child or an adolescent child? At what point should the older child's feelings be considered? What about a cognitively impaired school-age child or adolescent or an intellectually or emotionally precocious younger child? What if the parents disagree regarding treatment with each other or with the medical staff? Should a court-appointed guardian be allowed to make this decision? What about the feelings, opinions, and beliefs of siblings, grandparents, and other close family members? And, at what point does refusal or termination of the care of a minor constitute child neglect, maltreatment, or abuse?

As with consent, refusal of treatment must be predicated upon information. If a patient refuses care, from a simple dressing change to an invasive procedure, the nurse has a legal duty to the patient to ensure that the patient has the necessary information to make an informed refusal. For example, if a patient refuses to roll over to allow a nurse to perform skin assessment, and the patient is subsequently injured, the nurse may be liable to the patient if he or she did not explain the consequences of failing to assess the patient's skin (Plawecki, Amrhein, & Zortman, 2010).

In addition, nurses must recall their legal responsibilities under the Patient Self-Determination Act (discussed earlier in the chapter) and the various patients' bill of rights in their state, at their institution, or promulgated by their nursing organization. Each of these documents serves as a standard of care to guide nurses in their interaction with patients making healthcare decisions. Institutional legal and ethical consultations are often necessary to address questions and concerns regarding refusal of treatment by a patient or his or her family. Healthcare providers should never attempt to circumvent the difficulties of dealing with patient refusal by waiting until an emergency arises and then providing the treatment in question. Proceeding with care under the guise of an emergency violates the patient's autonomy and subjects healthcare providers to legal liability. The prudent, ethical nurse refrains from imposing his or her own beliefs or value system upon a patient or a patient's family.

Privacy

On any given shift, nurses have access to some of the most personal private information about a patient and his or her family. A right to privacy is grounded in western culture and protected by the U.S. Constitution, various state constitutions, and explicit federal and state statutes (e.g., HIPAA). In addition, the ANA *Code for Nurses* prohibits disclosure of confidential patient information, as do the ethical codes of many other professional organizations. The Joint Commission mandates that institutions maintain and adhere to policies and standards to protect patient information. Nurses must remember that a right to privacy protects more than the patient's medical record; it protects them from unauthorized photographs and news stories, as well as unauthorized observation by others, even if those others are hospital personnel or healthcare students. Importantly, advances in technology including electronic health records, telehealth, computerized medical databases, and other Internet-based technologies have increased the potential for intentional and unintentional breaches of confidentiality (ANA, 2015a).

Breach of confidentiality exposes the nurse and his or her employer to lawsuits and federal and/or state legal action. In addition, the nurse can be subjected to disciplinary action by his or her SBON and will likely lose employment because breach of confidentiality can be cause for discharge. However, there are several explicit exceptions that allow disclosure of confidential information. See **Box 16-10** for examples of exceptions that may allow disclosure of confidential information.

Note that even in the circumstances outlined in Box 16-10, the disclosure of confidential information may be limited; thus, a prudent nurse will be familiar with his or her institution's confidentiality and privacy policies as well as pertinent laws and regulations affecting their area of practice (McGowan, 2012).

BOX 16-10 EXCEPTIONS THAT MAY ALLOW DISCLOSURE OF CONFIDENTIAL INFORMATION

- The patient gives verbal or written permission to release information.
- Other healthcare workers who have a legitimate reason to know information (e.g., report to charge nurse).
- Statutory or legal duty to report (e.g., communicable diseases, child abuse, gunshot wounds, etc.).
- There is a duty to warn (e.g., serious threat to an identifiable victim).

Social Media

The number of individuals using social networking sites including Facebook, Twitter, LinkedIn, YouTube, and others has grown at a remarkable rate over the last decade. Although the phenomenon of social media can be an effective means of communicating and creating professional connections in nursing, its rise also presents unique risks for nurses. Nurses must always remain aware of their professional obligations, as well as employer policies and state and federal law, when using social media and must avoid disclosing patient-related information. Notably, some SBON have specific regulations regarding a nurse's inappropriate use of social media, while others will investigate these complaints on the basis of unprofessional conduct, unethical conduct, mismanagement of patient records, breach of confidentiality, and other grounds (NCSBN, 2011b; Spector & Kappel, 2012).

Legal Issues in Nursing Practice, Policy, and Legislation

This chapter has briefly reviewed some of the ways that nursing education, professional practice, policies, laws, and regulations intersect. The healthcare industry and its various professions are highly regulated given their impact on the public. It is in the best interest of those working in healthcare-related roles, and in particular, nurses, to keep abreast of pertinent issues including legislative and community activities that will impact professional practice. In addition, as frontline patient advocates, nurses are in an optimal position and, arguably, ethically obligated to speak out about access to care, quality of patient care, adequate hospital staffing levels and safe workplaces, and the many other issues impacting the health of the public. Speaking out takes many forms, from informed voting in local, state, and federal elections to actively advocating specific reforms through letter writing to running for elected office. Chapter 17 further addresses the nurse's role in policy making and political activism.

Each nurse should become familiar with the legislative process and with their elected federal, state, and local representatives. Excellent resources regarding this process include the *Activist Tool Kit* from the American Nurses Association (2013), the *Public Policy Advocacy Toolkit* from the National League of Nursing (n.d.), and the *AACN Advocacy 101 Tool Kit* (2016) from the American Association of Critical-Care Nurses. Many other nursing and healthcare professional organizations produce similar materials providing nurses with an in-depth review of the legislative process. Most professional nursing organizations have public policy divisions that follow and advocate for legislative and policy reforms affecting nursing, health care, and public welfare and provide their membership with information regarding these efforts—another excellent reason to join.

Nurses should also consider community service as a means of advocacy. Nurses are well-respected, highly regarded, accessible members of their communities and they possess knowledge and skills to assist people and communities to make the right choices for themselves. Participating in local or regional community activities gives nurses an opportunity to influence others on a scale not available via other means. Imagine the impact a pediatric nurse has speaking at a local parent–teacher association meeting regarding bicycle helmet safety or the effect an intensive care nurse has addressing a community group about organ donation. Nurses can stimulate significant change and influence public opinion through community education and outreach.

Summary

This chapter provided an overview of the legal issues nurses confront in their professional practice. A nurse is never "just a nurse." Those who have earned the legal right to use the initials RN after their name have a legal obligation to know about the structure and function of their SBON and how their state NPA governs and limits their professional behaviors. They must recognize that their care must conform to certain standards and they must appreciate how laws and regulations, such as federal or state privacy law, affect their daily practice. Nurses must always advocate for and work to protect the basic rights of their patients.

Reflective Practice Questions

1. You are a staff nurse working on an acute care medical-surgical nursing unit. You have recently read several peer-reviewed journal articles addressing a new technique that helps reduce the risk of decubitus ulcer occurrence in your patient population. This technique has been shown to reduce the incidence of ulcer formation by a significant amount. Your unit has not implemented this technique. What are the implications of continuing to treat patients according to current hospital protocols? What is your responsibility as a unit staff nurse?

2. According to your state NPA, which of the following procedures can you delegate to an assistant who is not an RN?
   a. Assessment of a patient upon admission to an acute care unit
   b. Administration of oral medications per physician order
   c. Obtaining regularly scheduled vital signs, which include heart rate, respiratory rate, blood pressure, and temperature
   d. Assessment of a telemetry patient's electrocardiogram tracing
   e. Administration of a hydromorphone HCL intramuscular injection

   f. Performing chest compressions during resuscitation

   g. Transcribing physician's orders

   h. Administration of intravenous antibiotics

   i. Performing discharge teaching

   j. Assessing a patient following an intervention

    What if the assistant is an LVN or LPN, or emergency medical technician employed by your facility? Does your answer change? What if your practice environment is a military hospital and your assistants are corpsmen or medics?

3. You are a staff nurse working on an acute care medical-surgical nursing unit. Yesterday, you provided care for Mrs. Baker, an 85-year-old woman who recently underwent a surgical procedure. On review of your notes from the previous day, you realize that you did not document the appearance of her wound or the dressing change you performed. What is the appropriate action to take?

4. You are an RN working in your local public health clinic. A 14-year-old girl presents for treatment of a sexually transmitted infection. During your initial assessment, she confides that her boyfriend is a 19-year-old neighbor with whom she has been sexually active for the past 6 months. She is concerned that her parents will be notified that she is seeking treatment at the clinic. What is your response? What must you consider?

5. You are a staff nurse working in a very busy emergency department. After one particularly stressful shift, you post on Facebook a detailed account of your experiences that day, including your perception that the department was "short staffed," as well a disagreement with a physician colleague over the care and disposition of a 76-year-old woman admitted for care of pneumonia. You did not include the names of the physician or patient in your post, but your position as an RN at your place of employment is noted in your Facebook profile. How would your SBON characterize this act? How would your employer characterize this act? What are possible consequences, if any, of this act?

References

American Association of Colleges of Nursing. (2011). *Nursing fact sheet*. Retrieved from http://www.aacn.nche.edu/media-relations/fact-sheets/nursing-fact-sheet

American Association of Critical-Care Nurses. (2016). *AACN Advocacy 101 Tool Kit*. Retrieved from http://www.aacn.org/wd/practice/content/publicpolicy/advocacy101.pcms?menu=practice

American Nurses Association. (n.d.). *Brief historical review of nursing and the ANA*. Retrieved from http://www.nursingworld.org/FunctionalMenuCategories/AboutANA/History/BasicHistoricalReview.pdf

American Nurses Association. (2010). *Nursing's social policy statement: The essence of the profession* (3rd ed.). Silver Spring, MD: Author.

American Nurses Association. (2012). *Nursing care and do not resuscitate (DNR) and allow natural death (AND) decisions. Position statements.* Retrieved from http://www.nursingworld.org/dnrposition

American Nurses Association. (2013). *Activists tool kit.* Retrieved from http://www.rnaction.org/site/PageServer?pagename=nstat_take_action_activist_tool_kit&ct=1

American Nurses Association (2015a). *American Nurses Association position statement on privacy and confidentiality.* Retrieved from http://www.nursingworld.org/DocumentVault/Position-Statements/Ethics-and-Human-Rights/Position-Statement-Privacy-and-Confidentiality.pdf

American Nurses Association. (2015b). *Code of ethics for nurses with interpretive statements.* Silver Spring, MD: Author.

American Nurses Association. (2015c). *Nurse Licensure Compact (NLC). ANA talking points.* Retrieved from http://www.nursingworld.org/MainMenuCategories/Policy-Advocacy/State/Legislative-Agenda-Reports/LicensureCompact/Nurse-Licensure-Compact-ANA-Talking-Points.pdf

American Nurses Association. (2015d). *Nursing: Scope and standards of practice* (3rd ed.). Silver Spring, MD: Author.

Cruzan v. Director, Missouri Department of Health, 497 U.S. 261 (1990).

DoNinger, M. L, & Dollinger, R. A. (2012). A new legal interpretation of duty for registered nurses. *Journal of Nursing Regulation, 3*(1), 21–25. http://dx.doi.org/10.1016/S2155-8256(15)30230-1

Eisenstadt v. Baird, 405 U.S. 438 (1972).

Gonzales v. Carhart, 550 U.S. 124 (2007).

Grant, D. M., & Ballard, D. (2011). *Law for nurse leaders: A comprehensive reference.* New York, NY: Springer.

Griswold v. Connecticut, 381 U.S. 479 (1965).

Guido, G. W. (2013). *Legal and ethical issues in nursing* (6th ed.). Upper Saddle River, NJ: Prentice Hall.

Health Resources and Services Administration, Bureau of Health Professions, National Center for Health Workforce Analysis. (2013). *The U.S. nursing workforce: Trends in supply and education.* Washington, DC: U.S. Department of Health and Human Services. Retrieved from http://bhpr.hrsa.gov/healthworkforce/reports/nursingworkforce/nursingworkforcefullreport.pdf

Hall, D. E. (2014). *Administrative law: Bureaucracy in a democracy* (6th ed.). Upper Saddle River, NJ: Prentice Hall.

Hill, G., & Hill, K. (2011a). Law. *The people's law dictionary.* Retrieved from http://dictionary.law.com

Hill, G., & Hill, K. (2011b). Negligence. *The people's law dictionary.* Retrieved from http://dictionary.law.com

Institute of Medicine. (2011). *The future of nursing: Leading change, advancing health.* Washington, DC: National Academies Press.

Jacobson v. Massachusetts, 197 U.S. 11 (1905).

Jost, T. (2010). Implementing health reform: A patient bill of rights. [*Health Affairs* Web log comment]. Retrieved from http://healthaffairs.org/blog/2010/06/23/implementing-health-reform-a-patient-bill-of-rights/

Liang, B. A. (2002). An overview of United States law. *Hematology/Oncology Clinics of North America, 16*(6), 1315–1330.

McGowan, C. (2012). Legal issues. Patients' confidentiality. *Critical Care Nurse*, *32*(5), 61–65. http://dx.doi.org/10.4037/ccn2012135

Melnik, T. (2013). Avoiding violations of patient privacy with social media. *Journal of Nursing Regulation*, *3*(4), 39–46. http://dx.doi.org/10.1016/S2155-8256(15)30185-X

Moffett, P., & Moore, G. (2011). The standard of care: Legal history and definitions: The bad and good news. *Western Journal of Emergency Medicine*, *12*(1), 109–112.

Morrison, H., & Bagalio, S. (2015). Being a Good Samaritan. *Advance for Nurses*. Retrieved from http://nursing.advanceweb.com/article/being-a-good-samaritan.aspx

National Archives and Records Administration. (n.d.). *The charters of freedom: The bill of rights*. Retrieved from http://www.archives.gov/exhibits/charters/bill_of_rights_transcript.html

National Council of State Boards of Nursing. (2011a). *What you need to know about nursing licensure and boards of nursing*. Retrieved from https://www.ncsbn.org/Nursing_Licensure.pdf

National Council of State Boards of Nursing. (2011b). *White paper: A nurse's guide to the use of social media*. Retrieved from https://www.ncsbn.org/Social_Media.pdf

National Council of State Boards of Nursing. (2012). *The 2011 uniform licensure requirements*. Retrieved from https://www.ncsbn.org/12_ULR_table_adopted.pdf

National Council of State Boards of Nursing. (2016a). *25 Nurse Licensure Compact (NLC) states*. Retrieved from https://www.ncsbn.org/NLC_Implementation_2015.pdf

National Council of State Boards of Nursing (2016b). *About boards of nursing*. Retrieved from https://www.ncsbn.org/about-boards-of-nursing.htm

National Council of State Boards of Nursing (2016c). *Licensure compacts*. Retrieved from https://www.ncsbn.org/compacts.htm

National Council of State Boards of Nursing (2016d). *Nurse practice act, rules and regulations*. Retrieved from https://www.ncsbn.org/nurse-practice-act.htm

National Council of State Boards of Nursing (2016e). *The national nursing database*. Retrieved from https://www.ncsbn.org/national-nursing-database.htm

National League for Nursing. (n.d.). *Public policy advocacy toolkit*. Retrieved from http://www.nln.org/professional-development-programs/teaching-resources/toolkits/advocacy-teaching/toolkit-home

Planned Parenthood v. Casey, 505 U.S. 833 (1992).

Plawecki, L. H., Amrhein, D. W., & Zortman, T. (2010). Under pressure: Nursing liability and skin breakdown in older patients. *Journal of Gerontological Nursing*, *36*(2), 23–25. doi: 10.3928/00989134-20100108-03.

Porter, J. E. (2012). Nursing professional ethics, law, and boundaries. *Journal of Nursing Law*, *15*(2), 61–63(3). http://dx.doi.org/10.1891/1073-7472.15.2.61

Pozgar, G. (2012). *Legal aspects of health care administration* (11th ed.). Sudbury, MA: Jones & Bartlett Learning.

Reising, D. L. (2012). Making your nursing care malpractice-proof. *American Nurse Today*, *7*(1), 24–28.

Richard, C., Lajeunesse, Y., & Lussier, M. (2010). Therapeutic privilege: Between the ethics of lying and the practice of truth. *Journal of Medical Ethics*, *36*, 353–357. doi: 10.1136/jme.2009.033340

Rock, M. J., & Hoebeke, R. (2014). Informed consent: Whose duty to inform? *Medsurg Nursing*, *23*(3), 189–194.

Roe v. Wade, 410 U.S. 113 (1973).

Rozovsky, F. (2015). *Consent to treatment: A practical guide* (5th ed.). New York, NY: Aspen Publishers.

Russell, K. A. (2012). Nurse practice acts guide and govern nursing practice. *Journal of Nursing Regulation, 3*(3), 36–42. http://dx.doi.org/10.1016/S2155-8256(15)30197-6

Schloendorff v. Society of New York Hospital, 105 N.W. 92 (1914).

Schwartz, V. E., Kelly, K., & Partlett, D. (2015). *Prosser, Wade & Schwartz's torts: Cases and materials* (13th ed.). New York, NY: Foundation Press.

Simon, P. N. (2010). *The anatomy of a lawsuit, revised edition.* New York, NY: LexisNexis.

Skinner v. State of Oklahoma, ex. rel. Williamson, 316 U.S. 535 (1942).

Spector, N., & Kappel, D. (2012). Guidelines for using electronic and social media: The regulatory perspective. *OJIN: The Online Journal of Issues in Nursing, 17*(3). doi: 10.3912 /OJIN.Vol17No03Man01

Union Pacific R. Co. v. Botsford, 141 U.S. 250 (1891).

Vacco v. Quill, 521 U.S. 793 (1997).

Washington v. Glucksberg, 521 U.S. 702 (1997).

Washington v. Harper, 494 U.S. 210 (1990).

Whelan, J. C. (2013). "All who nurse for hire": Nursing and the mixed legacy of legislative victories. *Nursing Outlook, 61*(5), 353–359. doi: 10.1016/j.outlook.2013.07.002

Healthcare Policy and Advocacy

Joan L. Frey and Christine K. Murphy

LEARNING OUTCOMES

After reading this chapter you will be able to:

- Define politics and policy.
- Understand political activism as a valid and significant nursing action.
- Explain the components of political competence for nurses.
- Link major policy changes and publications to nursing's call to political activism.
- Discuss integration of digital information technologies into the political environment.
- Describe how to link a public policy or advocacy resource to nursing political activism.
- Discuss strategies for getting involved in the political arena.

> *The secret to getting things done is to act.*
> —Dante Alighieri, Italian poet and
> early political activist (1265–1321)

The editors wish to acknowledge the contributions of Joanne R. Warner and Sharon Kimball to the previous edition of this chapter.

Introduction

This chapter discusses the skills, perspectives, and values that comprise political competence and why political competence is needed in nursing. In addition, strategies are presented to help nurses develop their own unique expression of political awareness and activism. The development and application of skills needed for effective political action are presented along with an essential discussion as to the reasons nursing's values are intrinsic to the development of health policies and nursing practice regulations. The discussion demonstrates that how nurses choose to express political competence is less important than the fact that nurses actually become politically active.

Evolutionary Changes to Nursing's Role in Health Policy

Florence Nightingale (May 12, 1820–August 13, 1910), celebrated English social reformer and statistician known for pioneering modern nursing care, would likely be amazed to note the advances made in nursing education and the role nurses fulfill in the care of patients and families. However, after more than a century of innovation, the tenacious nursing pioneer may just as likely be amazed to note the background role that millions of nurses choose to portray in the political arena.

Never before have the opportunities been so evident or so aligned as to provide nurses with the mandate to act in influencing and changing healthcare policies and priorities. The historical context of both the passage of the Patient Protection and Affordable Care Act in 2010 and the nearly simultaneous publication of the Institute of Medicine (IOM) report, *The Future of Nursing: Leading Change, Advancing Health* (2011), have created widespread acknowledgement of the integral importance of nurses. The prominence of nursing has been easily and appropriately woven into issues of access to care and healthcare cost efficiencies. The importance of the leadership of nursing in shaping and implementing healthcare policies and healthcare provisions at all levels of society, within healthcare organizations, and throughout healthcare systems is increasingly recognized.

The Patient Protection and Affordable Care Act

The Patient Protection and Affordable Care Act (PPACA), commonly referred to as the Affordable Care Act (ACA), was passed into law with the intention to countermand increasingly alarming trends in the health of the U.S. population, including, but not limited to low health quality measures for maternal and child mortality, lack of access to affordable health insurance, and lack of access to healthcare services amid ever-rising healthcare costs.

The major provisions embodied by the ACA include (a) expansion of access to and quality of health insurance coverage; (b) payment systems reforms including equity improvements for nursing services; (c) requirements to improve healthcare system performance through coordination of care and prevention; (d) expansion of healthcare workforce capacity; and (e) improvements in the nation's public health services across federal, state, and local organizations (Mason, Gardner, Outlaw, & O'Grady, 2016; PPACA, 2010). The U.S. nursing workforce will be directly affected by provisions of the ACA because of the increased number of insured Americans with access to health care and indirectly affected because of the need to expand primary care providers, such as advanced practice registered nurses (APRNs), with expanded scope of practice and payment options (PPACA, 2010).

The Institute of Medicine Report on the Future of Nursing

The IOM report (2011), underwritten by the Robert Wood Johnson Foundation (RWJF), accepted that the ACA represented "the broadest changes to the healthcare system since the 1965 creation of Medicare and Medicaid programs" (p. 2). As the IOM report was intended to determine how the nursing profession could be engaged to support opportunities created by the PPACA, it is important to understand the report's underlying philosophy regarding nursing's potential contributions to 21st-century health care:

> What nursing brings to the future is a steadfast commitment to patient care, improved safety and quality, and better outcomes. Most of the near-term challenges identified in the health care reform legislation speak to tradi-tional and current strengths of the nursing profession in such areas as care coordination, health promotion, and quality improvement. How well nurses are trained and do their jobs is inextricably tied to every health care quality measure that has been targeted for improvement over the past few years. Thus for nursing, health care reform provides an opportunity for the profession to meet the demand for safe, high-quality, patient-centered, and equitable health care services. We believe nurses have key roles to play as team members and leaders for a reformed and better-integrated, patient-centered health care system. (IOM, 2011, pp. xi–xii)

Nursing's Opportunity and Responsibility

The four major recommendations of the 2011 IOM report now stand as clear opportunities for nursing students, nurse faculty, and all nurses in practice. In the report, the IOM recommends that nurses must be able to (a) practice to the full extent of their education and training; (b) achieve high levels of education and training through an education system that promotes seamless academic progression; (c) participate as full partners, with physicians and other healthcare professionals, to redesign healthcare systems; and (d) develop better data collection and information infrastructure for effective workforce planning and policymaking (IOM, 2011). Nursing students must learn the true nature of their role in policymaking and politics. Nursing students should be supported in the political learning process by well-informed nurse faculty who share the 21st-century vision for fully engaged professional nurses who care for patients, represent patients, teach patients, improve patient care and care systems—who embody the legal and societal responsibilities of a nurse.

As nurses, it is our professional responsibility to look around our workplaces or our communities and ask how health care can be improved. It is also our professional responsibility to act. Action will require venturing into the world of **politics** and **policy**. It will take both a personal and collective commitment to become politically competent and active.

KEY TERM

Politics: Influencing the allocation of scarce resources (Mason et al., 2016).

KEY TERM

Policy: A plan to guide action or decisions.

If the nursing profession is to demonstrate even a modicum of influence regarding the implications of health care and healthcare policy for our nation's well-being, we need only to take a glimpse into the PPACA law (2010) and IOM report (2011) to understand that health and health care are inextricably intertwined with social, economic, and political systems. Health care is political because it involves limited resources, important needs, and varied ideas on how to match resources with needs. Health is political because health care in the United States is expensive. Decisions about the allocation of resources that go to health and health care must be made. Nurses need to be those who are involved in those political decisions. Nurses need to be vocal about the policies and politics that affect their practice, their patients, and the systems in which they work. Nurses need to take seriously the true nature of their professional status and recognize the active support required by nurses to become politically astute and involved.

There are many existing and evolving legislative and regulatory issues in nursing. Workplace environments, the nursing shortage, faculty shortages, migration of nurses, patient rights, patient safety, medical error prevention, violence prevention, individual state and interstate licensure, and scope of practice are just a few examples of the critical issues facing nursing. Health care is changing rapidly. As nurses interact with patients and their families, they are often the first providers to see clearly when and how the healthcare system is failing to meet patient needs. Nurses have a choice: to continue trying to make do while feeling victimized by changes over which they feel they have no control or to take action and find opportunities to improve the healthcare system, maintain a strong profession, and bring nursing values into politics and policy formation. Political participation by nurses is imperative to our nation's health (Woodward, Smart, & Benavides-Vaello, 2015).

Advocacy as a Professional Practice Essential

Nurses, as the largest group of healthcare providers, could generate enough power to successfully reform the healthcare system based on numbers alone. According to the National Council of State Boards of Nursing (2016), there are 3.8 million registered nurses in the United States. This reality continues to offer the nursing profession a formidable power base that is largely untapped in the day-to-day world of politics and legislation (Woodward et al., 2015). However, nursing has not developed into a cohesive, powerful professional force that could be a partial counterweight to the dominance of medicine in the policy arena (Mason et al., 2016). Involvement of only a fraction of the nation's 3.8 million registered nurses in even the smallest way could become a force for change for the nursing profession and for the healthcare system and the patients it serves (Adamson, Halpern-Paul, & Curtis, 2011; Ryan & Rosenberg, 2015; Woodward et al., 2015).

Although one person can make a difference, a large group is a powerful force to contend with (Vance, 2012); **Contemporary Practice Highlight 17-1** illustrates this point.

Advocacy through political activism engages nurses in public policy dialogues and actions to improve social, health, workplace, and organizational outcomes. It is a vital concept

> **KEY TERM**
>
> **Advocacy:** A role often performed by nurses that works to promote or protect rights, values, access, interests, and equality in health care (Mason et al., 2016).

CONTEMPORARY PRACTICE HIGHLIGHT 17-1

THE INFLUENTIAL POWER OF NURSES

The potential power of nurses' voices was made evident on September 14, 2015 when thousands of nurses worldwide rose in defense of Miss Colorado's talent monologue during the Miss America pageant. Hosts on *The View*, a daytime TV show, chose to deride the monologue of a nurse wearing scrubs "costume" apparel and doctor's stethoscope. The resulting furor against *The View* resulted in hundreds of thousands of social media messages, 5 million American Nurses Association (ANA) Facebook and Twitter account contacts, and over 38 million households reached by the news media coverage. The pushback disclaimed the program hosts' insults to the nursing profession and prompted the cancellation (albeit temporary) of advertising dollars by major contributors like Johnson & Johnson. Pamela F. Cipriano, PhD, RN, NEA-BC, FAAN, and president of the American Nurses Association, shared in her *President's Perspective* (2015) that "never before has this (banding together) been so critical as we seek to achieve the 'Future of Nursing' vision—to be full partners in changing health care for the better." Cipriano went on to add, "Nurses acting together create a strong and powerful voice that speaks up for not just nurses but the welfare of our public" (p. 3).

Data from Cipriano, P. (2015). Nurses unite with pride (and stethoscopes). *American Nurse, 47*(6), 3.

for nurses to understand and an essential professional behavior in which to engage (Mason et al., 2016). The meaning of advocacy in nursing has evolved from the simple act of performing nursing functions safely within the *Code of Ethics for Nurses*, which expresses nursing's understanding of its commitment to society (ANA, 2015a).

In addition, *The Essentials for Professional Nursing Practice* (AACN, 1996, 2006, 2008, 2011) set standards for all levels of nursing education programs that include the role of the nurse as advocate. Historically, patient loyalty to the medical profession and patient advocacy efforts were closely intertwined. This scenario prevailed until the mid-1980s when nurses began to be accountable for independent decision making and, consequently, felt empowered to question or clarify physician's orders (Mason et al., 2016). Now, as a result of centuries of care, the value of nursing behaviors, skills, and knowledge are now acknowledged, joining the nurse and physician in fighting disease. Nursing advocacy in the context of today's necessary political activism requires nurses to consider forward-thinking and comprehensive advocacy as a responsibility inherent in every professional's repertoire toward true healthcare reform (Logan, Pauling, & Franzen, 2011; Stokowski et al., 2010).

KEY TERM

Political activism: Direct and collective participation in strategies toward specific societal goals; for nursing, this action is based on explicit professional values and focuses on enhancing health.

KEY TERM

Political activity: Any activity that is directed toward the success or failure of a political party, candidate for partisan political office, or partisan political group (Mason et al., 2016, p. 414).

Political activism adds a dimension to professional nursing practice that offers the reward of having more control over patient care, outcomes, and nursing practice, especially in the important areas of access, quality, and cost of care (Hall-Long, 2010). **Political activity** differs from political activism and can be defined as an activity that is partisan in nature. The difference between political activism and political activity is important to note because, although the distinction may appear to limit a person's right to freedom of speech, the clarity provides coercion protection for government employees. Political activity restrictions do apply to approximately 60,000 nurses in the United States due to their status under government employment.

For nursing to assume its rightful place among public interest groups, peers, and lawmakers, nurses must first understand how public policy processes work and how to employ political strategies to make, implement, and continue to monitor the effect of enacted public policies (Hall-Long, 2010). This basic understanding involves knowing *who* can **influence** health and social policies, *where* nurses' influence can be applied, *what* strategies can be used to influence policy, *when* to act, and, overall, *why* it is important for nurses to advocate for public policy improvements related to health care (Mason et al., 2016).

KEY TERM

Influence: Affect the actions or opinions of others (Vance, 2012)

Defining Politics and Policy

Mason et al. (2016) define politics as the "use of relationships and power to gain ascendency among competing stakeholders to influence policy and the allocation of scarce resources" (p. 10). In AACN's *From Patient Advocacy to Political Activism: AACN's Guide to Understanding Healthcare Policy and Politics* (2010) the publication's stated goal is to "help nursing students, faculty, chairs, directors, and deans better understand the policy process, the issues facing nursing education, and how to participate in effective advocacy" (p. 2). The premise would be to heighten nurses' understanding and actively engage nursing professionals with the political processes and policies that shape their workplace to deliver better patient care. Politics also refers to the methods and tactics used to make and apply policy.

A policy is a plan to guide decisions and actions. The term may apply to a government, a private sector organization, a group, or an individual. Examples of policies include presidential executive orders, corporate privacy policies, or workplace policies and procedures. Mason et al. (2016) differentiate among public policy, social policy, health policy, institutional policy, and organizational policy. **Public policy** is defined as policy formed by governmental bodies (e.g., legislation passed by Congress) and the regulations written from that policy. **Social policy** refers to policy decisions that promote the welfare of the public. **Health policy** identifies decisions made to promote the health of individual citizens. **Institutional policies** govern workplaces (i.e., what the institution's goals are and how it will operate). **Organizational policies** are positions taken by organizations. Each type of policy can affect nurses and their practice.

Health policy is a version of public policy that pertains to health or influences the pursuit of health. It can be defined, therefore, as authoritative decisions regarding health or the pursuit of health made in the legislative, executive, or judicial branches of government that are intended to direct or influence the actions, behaviors, or decision of others (Longest, 2016). Public health–related policies come from local, state, or federal legislation; regulations; and/or court rulings that govern the provision of healthcare services. In addition to public policies, there are institutional or business policies related to health care. These policies are developed in the private sector by agencies, such as hospitals or accrediting organizations (Longest, 2016; Mason, et al., 2016).

> **KEY TERM**
>
> **Public policy:** Policy formed by governmental bodies (i.e. local, state and federal legislation) and the regulations written from that policy.

> **KEY TERM**
>
> **Social policy:** Policy decisions that are made to promote the welfare of the public.

> **KEY TERM**
>
> **Health policy:** Policy decisions that are made to promote the health of individuals.

> **KEY TERM**
>
> **Institutional policies:** Policies that govern a workplace and describe an institution's goals and how it will operate.

> **KEY TERM**
>
> **Organizational policies:** Policies that articulate positions taken by an organization.

Policy may also refer to the process of making important organizational decisions, including the identification of different alternatives such as programs or spending priorities, and choosing among them on the basis of the impact they will have. In political science the policy cycle is a tool used for the analysis of the development of a policy item; it bears some similarity to elements of the nursing process: assessment, diagnosis, outcomes/planning, implementation, and evaluation. However, in the context of a health policy cycle, the steps involve (a) policy formation phase (or the "window' of opportunity"), (b) policy implementation or rulemaking, (c) policy phase to operationalize the decision(s), and (d) policy modification or feedback phase (Longest, 2016; Mason et al., 2016). A side-by-side comparison of the familiar nursing process with policymaking phases in shown in **Table 17-1**. **Case Study 17-1** provides you with an opportunity to consider a health promotion issue and apply the concepts of the policy cycle.

In order to shape policy and become involved in politics, nurses need to develop political competence. **Political competence** is composed of the skills, perspectives, and values needed for effective political involvement within nursing's professional role as described in all levels of AACN's *The Essentials* (1996, 2006, 2008, 2011). For example, Essential V: Health Care Policy, Finance, and Regulatory Environments and Essential VIII: Professionalism and Professional Values provide fundamental expectations for nurses' engagement in shaping the patient care and professional nursing environments through engagement in health policy formation and evaluation (AACN, 2008). These same perspectives regarding the professional role expectations for nurses are represented at every level in the National League for Nursing's (NLN, 2010) *Outcomes and Competencies for Graduates of Practical/Vocational, Diploma, Associate Degree, Baccalaureate, Master's, Practice Doctorate, and Research Doctorate Programs in Nursing.* The core values related to a

KEY TERM

Political competence: The skills, perspectives, and values needed for effective political involvement.

TABLE 17-1 POLICYMAKING SIMILARITIES TO NURSING PROCESS

Nursing Process	Policymaking Process
• Assessment	• Window of opportunity
• Diagnosis	• Issue exploration
• Outcome/planning	▪ Problem
• Implementation	▪ Possible solutions
• Evaluation	▪ Political issues
	• Policy rule-making
	• Operationalize policy
	• Policy modification or feedback

CASE STUDY 17-1
DEVELOPING A HEALTH PROMOTION POLICY

Connie is employed as an emergency room (ER) nurse in a large referral hospital. She graduated from her nursing program 4 years ago and enjoys the interdisciplinary team approach to high-quality care. Connie is respected as a competent caregiver and an informal leader in the ER department. However, she has never considered herself to be political.

Through Connie's experience in the ER, she is becoming increasingly aware first-hand of issues involving children's safety, specifically child abuse and neglect deaths. She acknowledges to herself that she is becoming quite passionate about making a difference in the children's lives. In the process of researching the issue, she learned that her state has one of the worst records related to child abuse and incidences of shaken-baby syndrome. In addition, she found there was no policy or procedure established at her hospital for the maternity unit of her hospital that included teaching new parents about the fragility of infants, the state data related to child abuse, or how to prevent infant injuries.

1. What is the policy issue?
2. What assessment data does she need to collect to completely understand the issue?
3. How many different ways can this issue be framed? What policy options emerge from each of the different ways to frame the issue?
4. With whom should she network? Who would be potential allies? Who would be potential challengers to policy changes?
5. What is the policymaking body that could address this issue?
6. What would the professional risks and rewards be for her if she pursued this issue?

---

nurse's professional identity, as referenced in the NLN's *Outcomes and Competencies* monograph evolve from a baseline assessment of one's personal strengths and values as a nurse and one's contributions as a member of the healthcare team through to a higher level of commitment to inquiry and the systematic investigation of nursing-related problems and dissemination of findings—all values connecting to advocacy, safe high-quality care, leadership, and promotion of positive health policy system changes (NLN, 2010). **Table 17-2** displays an adaptation of the graduate competencies for professional identity for all types of nursing programs through examples for personal reflection. Nursing students and nurse professionals are encouraged to consult the NLN publication to learn more about the originally referenced competencies.

Political competence is needed within nursing to (a) impart the importance of voting citizenship; (b) encourage participation in professional organizations; (c) create an awareness and passion for health policy issues; (d) build knowledge of the legislative, policy processes, and legislators; and (e) actively engage in the

TABLE 17-2 GRADUATE COMPETENCIES FOR PROFESSIONAL IDENTITY

Practical/ Vocational	Associate Degree/ Diploma	Baccalaureate	Master's	Practice Doctorate	Research Doctorate
How can my personal values and strengths support my professional nursing role? What are the contributions I can make as a member of the healthcare team?	As I implement my nursing role, how will my actions reflect integrity and ethical practices? How will a commitment to evidence-based practice be evident through advocacy and safe, quality care for all?	How will my daily caring actions reflect a commitment to patient advocacy? What are the leadership values and strengths that my professional role requires me to improve?	As an advanced practice nurse, let me implement my role through definitive actions that promote real healthcare policy reform. How can I advance the profession through development of myself and others to promote positive systems changes?	How will I identify ways to interpret and transform nursing research into meaningful practice outcomes? How can a diverse patient population benefit from my nurse-scholar role to impact health policy reform?	As a research-scholar, how will I personally commit to create a preferred future for the profession of nursing? Through a dedication to inquiry into nursing-patient related questions, how will I dedicate myself to the distribution of quality research results?

Data from National League for Nursing. (2010). *Outcomes and competencies for graduates of practical/vocational, diploma, associate degree, baccalaureate, master's, practice doctorate, and research doctorate programs in nursing.* New York, NY: NLN Press.

political process (Byrd et al., 2012). Nurses can influence policy. Nurses are experts. Nurses are the healthcare systems experts. Nurses are constituents. Nurses are voters. Nurses have a great understanding of the strengths and weaknesses of the healthcare system and can use this knowledge to influence politics and policy. What nurses in many instances lack is belief in their political competence (Byrd et al., 2012; Hanks, 2013).

Why Political Competence Is Needed in Nursing

Becoming and maintaining oneself as an expert nurse is a rigorous and ongoing process of acquiring knowledge, refining skills, and assimilating into a professional role. In the NLN list of graduate competencies for professional identity (see Table 17-2), evolving knowledge, skills, and levels of competence are expected as a result of education program completion. With the acquisition of competence comes the development of confidence in the nurses' role as a politically astute professional who has the potential to influence public policy changes. Mason et al. (2016) support key reasons for nurses to demonstrate political competence (see **Box 17-1**).

Increasingly, the broad nature of societal factors existing outside the healthcare system, such as psychosocial factors, political-economic conditions, cultural issues, gender roles, and the state of the environment, is understood to influence the health status of populations. Healthcare providers are challenged to use this broad understanding and intervene with societal factors that threaten or promote health (National Advisory Council on Nursing Education and Practice, 2014; U.S. Department of Health and Human Services [USDHHS], 2014). Government reports praise nursing's historical and holistic focus to providing care and also describes nursing's crucial role in the identification of and interaction between health and social problems. Specifically, nurses are intended to be a part of the diverse group of individuals and organizations that identify national health improvement priorities; increase public awareness of health determinants and opportunities for change; assist to establish measurable goals at national, state, and local levels; strengthen policies and improve practices based on evidence and knowledge; and identify critical research, evaluation, and data collection needs (USDHHS, 2014). Political competence is needed for reform and action that influence these broad issues and opportunities.

Second, an increasingly diverse U.S. population (U.S. Census Bureau, 2011) requires a culturally competent nursing workforce that effectively joins "disparate

---

BOX 17-1   WHY DO NURSES NEED POLITICAL COMPETENCE?

- Understand factors affecting the nation's health
- Apply issues of culture and power to healthcare policy development
- Advocate for quality improvement and accountability in health care
- Engage in interdisciplinary practice partnerships

- Instill nursing's voice and values in political decision making

Data from Mason, D. J., Gardner, D. B., Outlaw, F. H., & O'Grady, E. T. (2016). *Policy and politics in nursing and health care* (7th ed.). St. Louis, MO: Elsevier.

nurses together across associations and educational institutions, and with new community partners, to change policy" (Mason et al., 2016, p. 19). Political competence is required to be able to intervene within the culturally defined power dynamics in a diverse society. Nurses who can develop political competence and use power effectively can be invaluable to their communities (AACN, 2008).

Third, nurses are accountable for the design and quality improvement of the healthcare system. The most current American Association of Colleges of Nursing baccalaureate essentials (2008) underscore the need for knowledge in policy by noting that nurses' acumen should include ". . . healthcare policies, including financial and regulatory policies, directly and indirectly influence nursing practice as well as the nature and functioning of the healthcare system" (p. 3). These policies shape responses to organizational, local, national, and global issues of equity, access, affordability, and social justice in health care. Nurses, therefore, need to understand the political dynamics at play in the healthcare system and have the requisite political skills to contribute to an improved and more accountable system. Interventions at the policy level require partnerships and the skills associated with astute interdisciplinary collaboration to advance political competence in quality improvements.

Finally, without nurse activism and political involvement, nursing values and perspective would be lost in the political debate. Mason et al. (2016) notes that nursing's voice brings the values of caring, collaboration, and collectivity to policy conversations. Nurses' experiences, in fact, are powerful ways in which human stories, coupled with scientific evidence, can illustrate the needs and impetus for healthcare policy changes (Mason et al., 2016). Nursing's values are extremely important because they can point the way to prioritize or direct specific policy decisions (Kraft & Furlong, 2015).

Political competence is a requisite nursing skill for all of these reasons. Political competence prepares nurses to fulfill many aspects of their professional role including but not limited to the following from *The Essentials of Baccalaureate Education for Professional Nursing Practice* (AACN, 2008):

- Demonstrate basic knowledge of healthcare policy, finance, and regulatory environments
- Describe how health care is organized and provided, including system and patient cost factors
- Compare the benefits and limitations of major forms of reimbursement on the delivery of healthcare services
- Examine legislative and regulatory processes relevant to the provision of health care
- Describe national statues, rules, and regulations that authorize and define professional nursing practice

- Explore the impact of sociocultural, economic, legal, and political factors that influence healthcare delivery and practice
- Examine the roles and responsibilities of the regulatory agencies and their effect on patient care quality, workplace safety, and the scope of nursing and other health professionals' practice
- Discuss the implications of healthcare policy on issues of access, equity, affordability, and social justice in healthcare delivery
- Use an ethical framework to evaluate the impact of social policies on health care, especially for vulnerable populations
- Articulate, through a nursing perspective, issues concerning healthcare delivery to decision makers within healthcare organizations and other policy areas
- Participate as a nursing professional in political processes and grassroots legislative efforts to influence healthcare policy
- Advocate for consumers and the nursing profession[1]

Political skills developed through active experiences in public policy can advance nurses' personal and professional knowledge and skills to influence public policy (Byrd et al., 2012). **Contemporary Practice Highlight 17-2** demonstrates how nurses have influenced public policy by advocating for and lobbying Congress for the establishment of a national nursing research center.

How Is Political Competence Learned?

The IOM report (2011) called for a shift in nursing activism from simple lip service to actionable and visible leadership on important health and social issues. To accomplish that shift, we need to understand how nurses learn to act politically as advocates for successful health policy legislation.

During Florence Nightingale's time and for years into the 20th century, nursing was taught as a type of apprenticeship education, strictly dedicated to patient care skills (Morin, 2010). Both academic and societal expectations for nursing have evolved over the past century to catapult the profession into controversies along issues of education levels and corresponding differentiated licensure requirements (Brown, 1967; Morin, 2010, 2012, 2014; Orsolini-Hain, 2012; Scheckel, 2009). Although those issues remain primarily unresolved, the advent of nursing education in higher institutions of learning, definitions of minimum requisite competencies, degree-attainment, and licensure testing, and expectations for the professional nurse now require involvement in changes to improve healthcare policies and systems (Blegen, Goode, Park, Vaughn, & Spetz, 2013; Morin, 2014). Instead of the public,

---

[1]Reproduced from American Association of Colleges of Nursing. (2008). *The essentials of baccalaureate education for professional nursing practice.* Washington, DC: Author. Retrieved from http://www.aacn.nche.edu/education-resources/BaccEssentials08.pdf, pp. 20–21.

CONTEMPORARY PRACTICE HIGHLIGHT 17-2

CREATION OF THE NATIONAL INSTITUTE FOR NURSING RESEARCH

In *NINR: Bringing Science to Life*, the 1983 IOM report titled *Nursing and Nursing Education: Public Policies and Private Actions* recommended a federal nursing research entity as part of the mainstream scientific community, nursing leaders, and supporters in the United States began promoting the establishment of a nursing institute at the National Institutes of Health (NIH). This coordinated effort involved lobbying Congress, the Reagan Administration, and the other institutes at NIH to establish this new institute. A few members of Congress were interested in the potential that nursing research had for improving the practice of health care. However, the administration and the NIH opposed the creation of another institute at the agency. Opponents were puzzled as to why nursing would need its own institute to do research as they viewed nursing as far removed from NIH's biomedical mission and that nurse researchers could receive funding through existing institutes. Nursing leaders launched a coordinated effort to convince NIH and Congress that nursing research would improve human response to illness and assist in maintaining and enhancing health. Congress passed the Health Research Extension Act of 1985, which included a provision that created the National Center for Nursing Research, but it was vetoed by President Reagan. Nursing organizations and their members launched another campaign to override President Reagan's veto. One by one, across the country, nurses called their senators and congressional representatives urging support for the new center, explaining that nurses were represented only among a few funded researchers at other institutes who did not understand the impact of nursing interventions on health. The aggressive campaigning by nurses convinced the House of Representatives and the Senate to override the president's veto and led to the creation of the National Center for Nursing Research. A statutory revision made the center an institute in 1993 and it is now known as the National Institute for Nursing Research (NINR). Prior to the creation of the National Center for Nursing Research, the federal government spent $9.5 million on nursing research. In 2016, Congress allocated $146.485 million for nursing research at the NINR.

Data from Cantelon, P. (2010). *NINR: Bringing science to life.* Bethesda, MD: National Institute of Nursing Research. Retrieved from https://www.ninr.nih.gov/sites/www.ninr.nih.gov/files/NINR_History_Book_508.pdf

society, or politicians continuing or allowing any nostalgic view of the profession, the future of nursing can be said to reside in the constant reimagining of the nurses' role in society and the importance of nurses as political partners for change (Gillett, 2014; Morin, 2014; Turale, 2011).

A weak link in the expectation for nurses to engage as political partners for change is creating opportunities for learning about and engaging in health policy within nursing education curricula (Byrd et al., 2012; Turale, 2011). Teaching and learning in the classroom are only the first step. Immersion in real public policy issues and the creation of clinical practice that engage students to partner with clients, clinical partners, community groups, and politicians only strengthens the learning to promote real change (O'Brien-Larivée, 2011). Although additional research needs to be encouraged to document the positive outcomes for the development of "political astuteness" as a result of health policy learning experiences, participation in service learning, and real-life issues can significantly improve the knowledge, skills, and attitudes future nurses need to develop to influence public policy (Byrd et al., 2012).

The Power of Nurses and Partnerships

Politically competent nurses bring their professional credibility, values, expertise, and background to the table. Annually, nurses rank very high as trusted professionals, above others in health care, so it is nursing's responsibility and opportunity to bring the knowledge and perspective of the profession to policy and political debates (Saad, 2016). More important, politically astute nurses need to apply their professional credibility and values to partnerships, which will multiply the potential for healthcare policy improvements and can, materially, alter local, state, and national elections (Adegola, 2013).

Networking, with the intent to form strong political partnerships, is a significant behavior for politically effective nurses. One nurse has one voice; a coalition of like-minded nurses and individuals has much greater potential to communicate the desired change and achieve the intended outcome. Networking purposely links the right people and right ideas at the right time. Nurses need to understand that whether someone is an opponent or an ally might change given the political topic, so no one should be considered a perpetual enemy. Networking is the commitment of politically competent nurses to marshal their collective strength and work collaboratively and in coalition. Our individual effectiveness is made stronger through collective action, such as through professional organizations, agency coalitions, or interdisciplinary unity around a topic.

The focus of the American Association of Retired Persons' (AARP) *Future of Nursing Campaign for Action* is a prime example of nursing's ability to partner with key organizations to transform healthcare policies and systems for the benefit of consumers (Reinhard, 2012). It was the campaign's goal to partner with the Robert Wood Johnson Foundation and the AARP's huge membership to implement the IOM's report on *The Future of Nursing: Leading Change, Advancing Health* (2011). The power of these key players (RJWF and AARP) in active collaboration with major national nursing organizations, state action coalitions, and millions of consumers, created sustainable alliances to influence changes to achieve improved health for Americans. A few of the many changes already achieved through the work of these combined and focused forces include but are not limited to development of models for nursing education progression, use of Medicare funding to support graduate nursing education, support for Federal Trade Commission anticompetitive limitations for scope of practice issues, and release of a physician fee schedule to permit registered nurse practitioners to be reimbursed for pain management services (Reinhard, 2012).

With overarching goals to reduce high-risk birth rates, improve health disparities, alleviate childhood poverty, and reduce public costs, public health nurses have taken up the banner to identify the social determinants of early childbearing in order to raise public awareness and the political will to change public and healthcare policies (Smith-Battle, 2012). Similar efforts for healthcare improvements have been undertaken by specialized coalitions of nurses, private industry, and government offices to create momentum for comprehensive changes in healthcare policies, such as pressure ulcer care and reimbursement reform (Crane & Raymond, 2011) and removal of public policy barriers to improve patient care safety (Lyder & Ayello, 2012). Advocacy for vulnerable home health patients was organized into a multiyear collaborative research initiative by the Visiting Nurse Associations of America (VNAA) and its Public Policy Council, the Visiting Nurse Service of New York (VNSNY), and representative members. The research developed a process to gather data (characteristics and numbers of patients) in order to influence changes in the allocation of resources and the delivery of care (Christopher, Duhl, Rosati, & Sheehan, 2015). These are but a few of the examples whereby nurses have shown the skills to establish and cultivate meaningful and lasting relationships to effect healthcare policy changes.

Politically competent nurses take a strategic view of issues that includes the complex context as well as consideration of diverse stakeholders and their agendas. They look beyond the immediate moment in time and consider future moves and a long-range vision. Nurses often use this strategic perspective as they incorporate clinical reasoning and multiple environmental factors into decision making. Because the long-range view is often needed for social change, politically competent nurses have the ability to persevere and not define themselves by victories and defeats.

The behaviors that describe politically competent nurses are from the classic set of nursing abilities used to provide clinical care. A slight refocusing of the lens allows these behaviors to be viewed as the pursuit of policies and political decisions supporting health. Nurses should understand their political activism as caring on a grand scale and at the highest collective level.

Incorporating Policy and Politics into Daily Practice

Becoming politically involved and gaining the skills to become politically competent can seem quite daunting. But as discussed earlier in the chapter, nurses have the power to change things. Without that empowered view of their professional role, nurses can be silent and impotent workers in an evolving healthcare system that requires their valuable input.

Nurses are already skilled advocates in daily practice and can be effective in healthcare policy change. Nurses advocate during key aspects of their professional role such as with patients and their caregivers, as teachers, and as a leader (Adamson et al., 2011). These are all transferable and natural skills that can be incorporated into shaping healthcare policy. The only difference is tailoring your communication to the audience, which in politics would be legislators. Nurses must speak up, write letters, testify, advocate, and convince decision makers of what is required for the healthcare system and the nursing profession.

If nurses can successfully match their abilities to the style and requirements of the political arena, they can find the political arena a creative expression for advocacy and social change.

Nurses in Politics

Beginning with Florence Nightingale, there have been outstanding examples of individual nurses who have used their passion, perseverance, and understanding of politics and policy to change the nursing profession and improve health care and public health. Nurse activists of previous centuries, including Florence Nightingale, Lillian Wald, and Margaret Sanger, pushed for and achieved tremendous healthcare improvements in their lifetimes.

Nurses are also making changes in the policymaking arena. In the 114th Congress, congressional calendar years 2015 to 2016, there are 435 members of the United States House of Representatives and 100 members of the United States Senate. In both the House and Senate, public service/politics is the dominantly declared occupation prior to being elected to Congress. Of the 535 members, only a small handful came from the healthcare arena prior to their election. This includes 18 doctors, three dentists, nine veterinarians, three psychologists (all in the House), an optometrist (in the Senate), a pharmacist (in the House), and four nurses (all in the House) (Manning, 2015). Those four nurses include a former emergency nurse, school nurse, psychiatric nurse, and surgical nurse who have used their leadership in the U.S. Congress to advance the healthcare system and the nursing profession.

Representative Diane Black

According to her official House of Representatives website, Representative Diane Black was first elected to Congress in 2010 to represent Tennessee's 6th Congressional District. In addition to being a former emergency room nurse, Representative Black was also a small businesswoman and educator prior to her election. With more than 40 years of experience working in the healthcare field, the congresswoman understands the importance of high-quality care and the obstacles faced by patients, healthcare providers, and employers. According to her official congressional biography, her real-world experiences as a nurse uniquely position her as a credible and effective leader on healthcare policy in Congress (Black, 2015a).

Representative Black currently serves on the House Ways and Means Committee where she is a member of the Ways and Means Health Subcommittee and serves as chair of the Ways and Means Education and Family Benefits Tax Reform Working Group. She is also a member of the House Budget Committee and the House Nursing Caucus. Although the representative opposes the ACA, she believes the nation needs to replace the ACA with a more patient-centered, market-based approach in order to expand access and work to lower costs (Black, 2015b).

Representative Lois Capps

First elected in 1998 following the death of her husband, former Representative Walter Capps, Lois Capps has been an engaged and effective leader in Congress, especially on issues related to public health. Before her election to California's 24th district, Representative Capps served as a nurse and public health advocate for the Santa Barbara School District for 20 years and taught for 10 years as a part-time instructor of early childhood education at Santa Barbara City College (Capps, 2015a).

Representative Capps is a long-time supporter of efforts to support the nursing profession as well as addressing the nursing shortage. She is the cofounder of the Congressional Nursing Caucus and sponsor of the H.R. 2713, the Title VIII Nursing Workforce Reauthorization Act. As a member of the Health subcommittee of the House Ways and Means Committee, the representative has also successfully spearheaded and passed legislation specifically to detect and prevent domestic violence against women, curb underage drinking, improve mental health services, provide emergency defibrillators to local communities, bring CPR instruction to schools, and improve Medicare coverage for patients suffering from Lou Gehrig's disease (Capps 2015b). Representative Capps retired when the 114th Congress adjourned in late 2016.

Representative Renee Ellmers

According to her biography on her website, Representative Ellmers, a former surgical nurse, was first elected in 2010 to represent the 2nd district of North Carolina. Ellmers campaigned on the theme that the nation's healthcare system is broken and that it fails to meet the needs of many Americans (Ellmers, 2016a). Congresswoman Ellmers believes that free market solutions that ensure greater choice for consumers and also preserve the fundamental patient–doctor relationship must be enacted. She is also a member of the House Energy and Commerce Health subcommittee as well as chair of the Republican Women's Policy Committee. Through her work on the subcommittee, Representative Ellmers has sponsored legislation such as H.R.398, the Trafficking Awareness Training for Health Care Act of 2015, and H.R.1348, the Health Insurance Freedom Act of 2015 (Ellmers, 2016b). Representative Ellmers lost her 2016 primary election and will not be returning to Congress in 2017.

Representative Eddie Bernice Johnson

According to Congresswoman Eddie Bernice Johnson's website, she is currently serving her 12th term in Congress representing the 30th Congressional District of Texas. Congresswoman Johnson started her career as a registered nurse in 1955 and later went on to become the Chief Psychiatric Nurse at the Veterans Administration (VA) Hospital in Dallas. She is the first nurse from Texas elected to the State House, State Senate, and the United States Congress. President Carter appointed her to serve as the Regional Director of the Department of Health, Education, and Welfare (Johnson, 2016b). While she does not sit on any House Committees with jurisdiction over health issues, Congresswoman Johnson is the founder and co-chair of the Diversity and Innovation Caucus and of the House Historical Black Colleges and Universities Caucus. Since 2011, Representative Johnson has introduced the National Nurse Act, which designates the Chief Nurse Officer, an existing position in the U.S. Public Health Service, as the National Nurse for Public Health (Johnson, 2016a).

Making a Difference Through Political Activism

For professional nurses to take the lead in policymaking and directing healthcare reform initiatives, they must be knowledgeable about political activism, engage in the development of policies with legislators, and develop the advocacy skills inherent in the future role of nursing. There are multiple ways to become actively involved; examples are discussed in the following sections.

Vote

The first and strongest step you must take to impact the public policy process is to vote. If you are not yet registered, go to https://www.usa.gov/register-to-vote to register. Without your vote, nurses are not empowered to choose, support, and vote into office a candidate who can support nursing and patient-friendly healthcare legislation. Voting is your democratic right and responsibility.

Join Your Professional Nursing Organization

Another step to take is to join your professional or specialty organization. Joining a professional nursing organization is an important way to enhance individual advocacy efforts. Professional nursing organizations are great resources for ideas and venues for networking and sharing concerns. Professional nursing organizations are able to monitor legislation and offer ways for their members to learn about health policy as well as when nurses need to interact with their policymakers. These organizations are also a great resource for information from a nursing perspective related to policy issues and policy makers. See Chapter 5 for more information about professional nursing organizations.

In addition, a wealth of information can easily be found at your state nursing organization's website. You will find information about legislative bills and proposed regulations that can affect nursing practice or the health of your patients. State nursing organizations and specialty nursing organizations also list ways for nurses to get involved, or you can sign up to receive email updates and action alerts.

Some state nursing and specialty nursing organizations sponsor annual legislative days, offer policy internships or fellowships, and conduct policy workshops, all designed to give nurses the opportunity to learn more about current healthcare issues and the legislative process.

Learn about Healthcare and Nursing Issues

Obtain a copy of and become familiar with the American Nurses Association's (ANA, 2015b) *Nursing: Scope and Standards of Practice* and your state's nurse practice act. You must be knowledgeable about state and federal regulations related to your practice, including nurse licensure requirements. Your right to practice and how you practice are outlined in the nurse practice act, which is ultimately governed by the state legislature. It is also important for nurses to keep themselves updated on any changes in their board of nursing's rules, regulations, and practice acts. You can do this by reading the board's newsletters or its website. If you do not know your board's Web address, you can access it from the National Council of State Boards of Nursing website at http://www.ncsbn.org/contact-bon.htm.

There are a number of public resources available online for you to learn about the nursing and healthcare issues. These resources are perfect for learning more about what Congress and the White House are doing in the healthcare arena, learning about important legislation, as well as reviewing in depth analysis of important healthcare issues. All of these resources are vital to becoming knowledgeable about the healthcare issues that will affect how you care for patients in order to influence your legislators. Read your local newspaper, national newsmagazines, professional journals, and newsletters from organizations to which you belong. Most professional and patient advocacy groups have websites with excellent links to other websites and resources. Sign up to receive online action alerts from organizations.

Become Familiar with the Policymaking Process

Most high school government classes cover the steps involved in bringing an idea through the legislative process to become a law or regulation. Basic "Civics 101" knowledge about the U.S. Congress, federal legislation, and basic concepts of how Congress works is vital for nurses to understand these steps so they can interact with appropriate timing and actions in the policymaking process. This information will be useful to you as you work on policy issues at the federal level, but it is also transferrable to any legislative initiatives you may be working on at the state and

local levels. One recommended site to review this content is http://www.votesmart
.org. You should also become familiar with the various Congressional committees
in **Table 17-3** that have jurisdiction over the healthcare issues that impact nursing
and quality patient care.

TABLE 17-3 CONGRESSIONAL COMMITTEE JURISDICTION

Chamber	Committee	Jurisdiction
House & Senate	Appropriations Committee Labor, Health and Human Services, Education & Related Agencies (LHHS) Subcommittee	The LHHS Appropriations Subcommittee has jurisdiction over the various agencies under the Department of Education, Department of Health and Human Services, and Department of Labor as well as other related agencies such as the Medicare Payment Advisory Commission and the Social Security Administration.
House	Energy & Commerce Health Subcommittee	The Energy & Commerce Health Subcommittee has jurisdiction over public health and quarantine; hospital construction; mental health; biomedical research and development; health information technology, privacy, and cybersecurity; public health insurance (Medicare, Medicaid) and private health insurance; medical malpractice and medical malpractice insurance; the regulation of food, drugs, and cosmetics; drug abuse.
House	Ways & Means Committee Health Subcommittee	The jurisdiction of the Ways & Means Subcommittee on Health includes bills and matters that relate to programs providing payments (from any source) for health care, health delivery systems, or health research.
Senate	Finance Committee	The committee concerns itself with matters relating to taxation and other revenue as well as health programs under the Social Security Act, including Medicare, Medicaid, the Children's Health Insurance Program, Temporary Assistance to Needy Families, and other health and human services programs financed by a specific tax or trust fund; and national social security.
Senate	Health, Education, Labor, and Pensions (HELP) Committee	The HELP Committee has jurisdiction over the country's health care, education, employment, and retirement policies, including measures relating to education and training, labor, health, and public welfare.

Data from National League for Nursing. (2014). Key congressional committees. Retrieved from http://www.nln.org
/docs/default-source/advocacy-public-policy/keycongressionalcommittees.pdf?sfvrsn=2

Know Who Represents You in Congress

Every year numerous bills are introduced at all levels of the government that will affect how nurses care for patients. With only a handful of legislators with healthcare backgrounds including four nurses in Congress, legislators make decisions every day affecting nursing and health care. *You* are the expert on nursing and patient care and your legislators value your knowledge and experience. With an ever-changing healthcare system, nurses *must* interact with their legislators. Be assured that doctors, hospitals, and other special interest groups are doing just that so nurses must do so as well to influence the legislative process. Common advocacy activities include letter writing, emails, social media posts, phone calls, and in-person visits to legislators.

If you are unsure who your legislators are, you can look them up on the Internet. The legislative websites http://www.senate.gov and http://www.house.gov will inform you who represents you at the federal level. You can also find your state and local legislators through your respective state legislature and local government websites.

KEY TERM

Social media: Forms of electronic communication (such as websites for social networking and microblogging) through which users create online communities to share information, multimedia, ideas, personal messages, and other content.

You should sign up for email information and updates from your legislators' websites as this information can be helpful in finding out their positions and when they will be in their district offices.

Many legislators also have **social media** accounts such as Twitter, Facebook, YouTube, and others. Following your legislators on their various social media accounts allows you to quickly learn about their legislative priorities and to contact them through your own social media accounts.

Build Relationships and Contact Your Legislators

It is important to get to know the players. All too often people forget that relationship building with many diverse groups and individuals is the most effective way to gain information, to be invited to participate, and to build personal and organizational intellectual capital. While your legislators are in their home district make an appointment to meet with them and offer to become a resource on healthcare and nursing issues. This is a great first step to build a relationship with your legislator before you need to request something from them. Take other nurses with you to talk about nursing issues. Invite your legislators to come and spend some time at your workplace. That is the ultimate way to teach them about what you do. Then when you call to ask them to vote for or against a bill that affects health care or specifically nursing practice, they will know you are their constituent.

When dealing directly with policymakers, you must be informed. Be concise and be clear about what you want. Writing a well-crafted letter, sending emails, sending a tweet, leaving a comment on the Facebook pages of legislators, leaving a written summary of your issue with staff, and sending thank-you notes are all ways to get one's legislators to consider one as an expert in healthcare and nursing issues. Remember that professional credibility and persuasion are important political skills. They can contact you when they need information related to nursing and health care. They will welcome the expertise of a nurse and you will be able to show your cause is important to a wide range of people. Join with other nurses who share your interests and explore ways you can work together in the political process.

Become an Effective Lobbyist

Lobbying means educating and persuading. Nurses make particularly effective lobbyists in issues that relate to health. Lobbying is not a difficult task and with your experience in health care and the nursing profession you can exert more influence than you probably realize.

Knowledge Is Power

As a nurse, you have a strong advantage in discussing legislative issues that pertain to your specialty area and health care in general. In addition to your expertise, you have your legislator's ear because you are a valued member of his or her constituency. Put the relationship you have cultivated with the legislator to work. Most legislators care very much about the opinions and positions of the people they represent. However, they are not mind readers and you must inform your legislators on your opinion on healthcare issues. Call, write, email, interact on social media or visit your legislators. Tell them what action you would like them to take. Be clear, direct, and focused, and keep your message simple.

A personal visit allows you to connect names to faces. Visiting your legislator's office, either in the capital or in his or her home district, is a worthwhile effort to make. If your legislator is not available, ask to meet his or her legislative aide who often advises the legislator on health issues. Aides and other office staff serve as gatekeepers, and legislators listen to their recommendations. Treat your legislator's staff respectfully and well. They can make a huge difference in whether your concerns get presented and acted upon. Remember to keep your professional organization informed about any contacts you make. This will help them plan further lobbying efforts, building on the relationships that other members develop with their lawmakers. **Box 17-2** provides guidelines on how to effectively lobby your legislator.

Inject Social Media into Political Activism

Traditionally, constituents would need to mail a letter, pick up the phone, or schedule a meeting to contact their legislators. Once email was introduced, advocates quickly began adding this action to their arsenal of tools to contact legislators. Congressional offices now receive thousands of emails from constituents. With the rise of social media networks such as Twitter, Facebook, LinkedIn, Pinterest, Google+, and other networks, nurses have another communication tool to easily and quickly

---

BOX 17-2   HOW TO LOBBY YOUR LEGISLATOR

1. Call in advance for an appointment.
2. Be prepared.
   - Be aware of your own prejudices and biases.
   - If you are representing an organization, be well versed on their positions.
3. Know your legislator.
   - Try to understand the basis for his/her position.
   - Know his/her record on related legislation.
   - Know his/her constituency pressures.
4. Know your issue.
   - Use your own words.
   - Admit when you don't know something and get back to them.
   - Know the status of pertinent legislation.
5. Be brief and courteous.
6. Identify yourself and establish your own credentials and expertise.
7. Give them succinct, easy-to-read literature.
8. Express your appreciation for your legislator's interest and support.
9. Leave your business card or contact information.
10. Follow up with a telephone call, email, or letter within a week.

Data from League of Women Voters. (2004). *How to lobby your legislator.* Retrieved from http://www.lwvwa.org/pdfs/lobby_your_legislator.pdf

---

communicate with their legislators. Social media are affecting the dialogue between constituents and legislators in unexpected ways (Fitch & Goldschmidt, 2015). These communications hold the same weight as writing a letter, emailing, and calling a legislator's office, but the use of social media allows nurses to immediately contact their legislator and at the same time allows the legislator's office to gauge the opinions of their constituents. In a 2015 report from the Congressional Management Foundation, 80 percent of congressional staff responding to surveys noted that less than 30 posts to their office's social media platform would cause them to "pay attention" (Fitch & Goldschmidt, 2015). This is the equivalent of a large group of constituents with one policy goal showing up to a town hall meeting. The legislator would take notice of that, but social media allows constituents to engage with their legislator instantly.

Although research on the impact of social media in advocacy is relative new, it is very easy to engage with legislators in this arena as it provides instant access. Access translates to power for nurses to improve the healthcare system and the nursing profession. Congress became an early adopter of social media and every Congressional member has at least one social media account that allows them to push out information quickly. Following your legislators on their social media accounts allows you not only to be informed on what they support but also to interact with them.

Volunteer

Many political candidates maintain websites where you can volunteer to work on their campaigns. The websites often have a link that enables you to check off the activities you are willing to do. For instance, you can do as little as volunteer to place a sign in your yard or a bumper sticker on your car. You could sign up to be an Internet leader and send email messages to friends. You could host a reception and help with fund-raising activities. Coffees, luncheons, barbecues, walkathons, and kickoff events can also be used to promote a candidate. And volunteers are always needed at the campaign office to help with phone calls and paperwork.

Donate to a Cause or Political Campaign

Time, people, and money are the resources that fuel most political activities. When we cannot afford time or recruit a group of people, we can contribute money toward a cause or candidate that supports our beliefs. Our donations support media purchases, travel, salaries, and the other costs of getting work done. Financial support of any amount is valued in electoral or issue campaigns.

Run for Office

With four nurses serving in the U.S. House of Representatives, nurses make excellent elected officials. Your interpersonal and analytical skills allow you to connect with the constituency and understand complex issues. Ethical behaviors that guide nursing practice are refreshing standards in elected office. Possible roles can range from county health boards and professional organizations to state and national legislative bodies.

Summary

Political activism provides the vehicle for social change. This chapter discussed the skills, perspectives, and values that comprise political competence and why political competence is needed in nursing. Strategies were presented to help nurses develop their own unique expression of political competence. Nurses have or can develop the skills needed for effective political action supported by nursing education programs and faculty that create meaningful learning experiences. Political discussions need and benefit from nursing's values. We lose the opportunity to improve health through policy, to control our practice, and to fulfill nursing's societal obligation to make a difference when we do not fulfill this professional responsibility. How you choose to express political competence is less important than the fact that you do it.

Reflective Practice Questions

1. Who do you know who models political competence in a professional environment? Have you seen political competence modeled in nursing practice?
2. What mentor(s) can you identify to assist you to develop your own political competence? If you don't have a mentor, can you identify someone who would be willing to help you develop your political skills?
3. What public or patient care issue draws you toward political action? What is the background story that inspires you to effect change?
4. How can you promote health and improve quality of life through political activism? Do you believe you can make a difference? What steps will you take to realize your potential for making a difference?
5. Do you belong to a state or national nursing organization? If not, choose one that will help you to fulfill your professional responsibility for advocacy. If yes, identify an issue identified by your nursing organization which can benefit from your active support.
6. When you identify an issue that requires action, how you would join with others to effect change?

References

Adamson, T., Halpern-Paul, I., & Curtis, J. A. (2011). Evolving healthcare landscape: Nurses cultivating the profession of nursing, healthcare reform, and health policy advocacy. *Journal of the Dermatology Nurses' Association*, 3(6), 357–366. doi: 10.1097/JDN.0b013e318239d21c

Adegola, M. (2013). Lessons learned from politics: Translate into healthcare delivery [Editorial]. *Association for Black Nursing Faculty Journal*, 24(1), 3-4.

American Association of Colleges of Nursing. (1996). *The essentials of master's education for advanced practice nursing*. Washington, DC: Author. Retrieved from http://www.aacn .nche.edu/education-resources/MasEssentials96.pdf

American Association of Colleges of Nursing. (2006). *The essentials of doctoral education for advanced nursing practice*. Washington, DC: Author. Retrieved from www.aacn.nche .edu/publications/position/DNPEssentials.pdf

American Association of Colleges of Nursing. (2008). *The essentials of baccalaureate education for professional nursing practice*. Washington, DC: Author. Retrieved from http://www .aacn.nche.edu/education-resources/BaccEssentials08.pdf

American Association of Colleges of Nursing. (2010). *From patient advocacy to political activism: AACN's guide to understanding healthcare policy and politics*. Washington, DC: Author. Retrieved from http://www.aacn.nche.edu/government-affairs /AACNPolicyHandbook_2010.pdf

American Association of Colleges of Nursing. (2011). *The essentials of master's education in nursing*. Washington, DC: Author. Retrieved from http://www.aacn.nche.edu/education -resources/MastersEssentials11.pdf

American Nurses Association. (2015a). *Code of ethics for nurses with interpretive statements*. Silver Spring, MD: Author. Retrieved from http://nursingworld.org/MainMenuCategories /EthicsStandards/CodeofEthicsforNurses/Code-of-Ethics-For-Nurses.html

American Nurses Association. (2015b). *Nursing: Scope of standards and practice* (3rd ed.) Silver Spring, MD: Author.

Black, D. (2015a). About me: Biography. Retrieved from http://black.house.gov/about-me /full-biography

Black, D. (2015b). Legislative work: Health. Retrieved from http://black.house.gov/issue/health

Blegen, M. A., Goode, C. J., Park, S. H., Vaughn, T., & Spetz, J. (2013). Baccalaureate education in nursing and patient outcomes. *Journal of Nursing Administration, 43*, 89–94. doi: 10.1097/NNA.0b013e31827f2028.

Brown, E. L. (1967). *Nursing for the future: A report prepared for the National Nursing Council.* New York, NY: Russell Sage Foundation.

Byrd, M. E., Costello, J., Gremer, K., Schwager, J., Blanchette, L., & Malloy, T. E. (2012). Political astuteness of baccalaureate nursing students following an active learning experience in health policy. *Public Health Nursing, 29*(5), 433–443. doi: 10.1111/j.1525-1446.2012.01032.x

Cantelon, P. (2010). *NINR: Bringing science to life.* Bethesda, MD: National Institute of Nursing Research. Retrieved from https://www.ninr.nih.gov/sites/www.ninr.nih.gov /files/NINR_History_Book_508.pdf

Capps, L. (2015a). About me: Full biography. Retrieved from http://capps.house.gov /about-me/full-biography

Capps, L. (2015b). Legislative work: Health care. Retrieved from http://capps.house.gov /issue/health

Christopher, M. A., Duhl, J., Rosati, R., & Sheehan, K. (2015). Advocacy for vulnerable patients: How grassroots organizations can influence health care policy. Using case studies to make the case for home health reimbursement. *American Journal of Nursing, 115*(3), 66–69.

Cipriano, P. (2015). Nurses unite with pride (and stethoscopes). *American Nurse, 47*(6), 3.

Crane, R., & Raymond, B. (2011). Roundtable on public policy affecting patient safety [Conference proceedings]. *Journal of Patient Safety, 7*(1), 5–10. doi: 10.1097/PTS .0b013e31820c98cd

Ellmers, R. (2016a). About Renee: Biography. Retrieved from http://ellmers.house.gov /biography/

Ellmers, R. (2016b). Issues: Healthcare. Retrieved from http://ellmers.house.gov/issues /issue/?IssueID=15532

Fitch, B., & Goldschmidt, K. (2015). *#SocialCongress 2015.* Retrieved from http://www .congressfoundation.org/projects/communicating-with-congress/social- congress-2015

Gillett, K. (2014). Nostalgic constructions of nurse education in British national newspapers. *Journal of Advanced Nursing, 70*(11), 2495–2505. doi: 10.1111/jan.12443

Hall-Long, B. (2010). Nurse matters: Assuming your role in advocacy. *Home Health Nurse, 28*(5), 309–316. Retrieved from http://journals.lww.com/homehealthcarenurse online/Fulltext/2010/07000/Nurse_Matters__Assuming_Your_Role_in_Advocacy_.4 .aspx

Hanks, R. (2013). Social advocacy: A call for nursing action. *Pastoral Psychology, 62,* 163–173. doi: 10.1007/s11089-011-0404-1

Health Research Extension Act of 1985, [Public Law 99-158]. (1985).

Institute of Medicine. (1983). *Nursing and nursing education: Public policies and private actions.* Washington, DC: National Academy Press. Retrieved from https://www.nap.edu /read/1120/chapter/1

Institute of Medicine. (2011). *The future of nursing: Leading change, advancing health.* Washington DC: National Academies Press. Retrieved from www.nap.edu/catalog .php?record_id=12956

Johnson, E. B. (2016a). Issues & legislation: Health. Retrieved from http://ebjohnson.house.gov/issues/health-care

Johnson, E. B. (2016b). Meet EBJ: EBJ's bio. Retrieved from http://ebjohnson.house.gov/about/full-biography

Kraft, M., & Furlong, S. (2015). *Public policy: Politics, analysis and alternatives* (5th ed.). Washington, DC: CQ Press.

League of Women Voters. (2004). *How to lobby your legislator*. Retrieved from http://www.lwvwa.org/pdfs/lobby_your_legislator.pdf

Logan, J. E., Pauling, C. D., & Franzen, D. B. (2011). Health care policy development: A critical analysis model. *Journal of Nursing Education, 50*(1), 55–58. doi: 10.3928/01484834-20101130-02

Longest, B. B. (2016). *Health policymaking in the United States* (6th ed.). Chicago, IL: Health Administration Press.

Lyder, C., & Ayello, E. (2012). Pressure ulcer care and public policy: Exploring the past to inform the future. *Advances in Skin and Wound Care, 25*(2), 72–76.

Manning, J. (2015). *Membership of the 114th Congress: A profile*. Washington, DC: Congressional Research Service. Retrieved from https://www.fas.org/sgp/crs/misc/R43869.pdf

Mason, D. J., Gardner, D. B., Outlaw, F. H., & O'Grady, E. T. (2016). *Policy and politics in nursing and health care* (7th ed.). St. Louis, MO: Elsevier.

Morin, K. H. (2010). Florence Nightingale: The legend continues. *Imprint, 57,* 40–43.

Morin, K. H. (2012). Evolving global education standards for nurses and midwives. *American Journal of Maternal-Child Nursing, 37,* 360–364.

Morin, K. H. (2014). Nursing education: The past, present and future. *Journal of Health Specialties, 2*(4), 136–141. doi: 10.4103/1658-600x.142781

National Advisory Council on Nursing Education and Practice. (2014). *12th annual report to the Secretary of the United States Department of Health and Human Services and the Congress of the United States*. Retrieved from http://www.hrsa.gov/advisorycommittees/bhpradvisory/nacnep/Meetings/12thannualreportpublichealthnursing.pdf

National Council of State Boards of Nursing. (2016). *The National Nursing Database.* Retrieved from https://www.ncsbn.org/national-nursing-database.htm

National League for Nursing. (2010). *Outcomes and competencies for graduates of practical/vocational, diploma, associate degree, baccalaureate, master's, practice doctorate, and research doctorate programs in nursing*. New York, NY: NLN Press.

National League for Nursing. (2014). Key Congressional committees. Retrieved from http://www.nln.org/docs/default-source/advocacy-public-policy/keycongressionalcommittees.pdf?sfvrsn=2

O'Brien-Larivée, C. (2011). Service-learning experience to teach baccalaureate nursing students about health policy. *Journal of Nursing Education, 50*(6), 332–336.

Orsolini-Hain, L. (2012). The Institute of Medicine's Future of Nursing report: What are the implications for associate degree nursing education? *Teaching and Learning in Nursing, 7,* 74–77. doi: 10.3928/01484834-20110317-02

"Patient Protection and Affordable Care Act" (Public Law 111-148, 2010).

Reinhard, S. (2012). AARP: National champions of nursing for consumers. *Nursing Economics, 30*(6), 358–359.

Ryan, S., & Rosenberg, S. (2015). Nurse practitioners and political engagement: Findings from a nurse practitioner advanced practice focus group & national online survey. Paper made possible through the RWJF Executive Nurse Fellows Program. Retrieved from http://anp-foundation.org/wp-content/uploads/2015/04/Nurse_Practitioners_and_Political_Engagement_Report.pdf

Saad, L. (2016). 2015 Gallup Poll: Nursing tops job rankings for honesty, ethics 14th year in a row. *Journal of Nursing*. Retrieved from https://www.asrn.org/journal-nursing /january1-2016.html

Scheckel, M. (2009). Nursing education: Past, present and future. In G. Roux & J. Halstead (Eds.), *Issues and trends in nursing: Essential knowledge for today and tomorrow* (pp. 27–55). Burlington, MA: Jones & Bartlett Learning.

Smith-Battle, L. (2012). Moving policies upstream to mitigate the social determinants of early childbearing. *Public Health Nursing, 29*(5), 444–454. doi: 10.1111/j.15251446.2012.01017.x

Stokowksi, L. A., Sansoucie, D. A., McDonald, K. Q., Stein, J., Robinson, C., & Lovejoy, A. (2010). Advocacy: It is what we do. *Advances in Neonatal Care, 10*(2), 75–82. doi: 10.1097/ ANC.0b013e3181d50db8

Turale, S. (2011). Preparing nurses for the 21st century: Reflecting on nursing shortage's and other challenges in practice and education [Editorial]. *Nursing and Health Sciences, 13*, 229–231. doi: 10.1111/j.1442-2018.2011.00638.x

U.S. Census Bureau. (2011). *2010 census shows America's diversity.* Retrieved from http:// www.census.gov/newsroom/releases/archives/2010_census/cb11-cn125.html

U.S. Department of Health and Human Services. (2014). *About Healthy People: Introducing Healthy People 2020.* Retrieved from http://www.healthypeople.gov/2020/about/default .aspx

Vance, S. (2012). *The influence game: 50 insider tactics from the Washington, D.C. lobbying world that will get you to yes.* Hoboken, NJ: John Wiley & Sons.

Woodward, B., Smart, D., & Benavides-Vaello, S. (2015). Modifiable factors that support political participation by nurses. *Journal of Professional Nursing*, 1–8. doi: 10.1016/j. profnurs.2015.06.005.

Unit IV

Health and *Nursing* Issues

18

Rural and Urban Healthcare Issues

Darla Adams

LEARNING OUTCOMES

After reading this chapter you will be able to:

- Describe common rural and urban health and nursing practice issues.
- Discuss the impact of the environment on the health of individuals and communities.
- Identify healthcare issues that place both rural and urban residents at risk for poor health outcomes.
- Examine health professionals' challenges in improving health outcomes in both rural and urban areas.

Introduction

Many nurses will practice in rural or urban settings or care for patients who reside in rural or urban communities. Although there are similarities across all healthcare settings, unique factors affect the healthcare needs of patients depending on the environment in which they live. All nurses need to be

The editors wish to acknowledge the contributions of Nena R. Harris, Mary R. Nichols, Wanda Bonnel, Amanda Alonzo, Patricia E. Conejo, and Sylvia Heinze to the previous edition of this chapter.

familiar with issues that affect the care they provide to their patients. And those nurses who are considering practicing in either rural or urban communities need to be familiar with the issues unique to those environments.

The U.S. Census Bureau (2010) has based the most recent classifications of urban and rural cities on the 2010 census. An **urban area (UA)** is defined as one that encompasses 50,000 or more people. An **urban cluster (UC)** encompasses a community of at least 2,500 but less than 50,000 people. The U.S. Census broadly defines a **rural** community as an area not designated as urban and having less than 2,500 inhabitants.

Currently, 19 percent of the citizens in the United States are considered to be living in a rural area, and in 30 states at least 25 percent of the citizens are considered to be in rural areas. Rural hospitals make up almost half of the total number of U.S. hospitals but are much smaller than urban hospitals; most have 25 or fewer beds and are at least 35 miles away from another hospital (American Hospital Association, 2011).

> **KEY TERM**
> **Urban area (UA):** An area that encompasses 50,000 or more people.

> **KEY TERM**
> **Urban cluster (UC):** An area that encompasses at least 2,500 but less than 50,000 people.

> **KEY TERM**
> **Rural:** Any area outside of the urban classification and having less than 2,500 people.

Those living in rural communities are afforded the benefits of living in generally safer environments with greater privacy and individual space, and better air quality. Challenges exist for rural communities because although rural populations have healthcare needs similar to urban populations, there are fewer healthcare agencies and resources available to them. Additionally, there are significant and growing problems with alcohol and drug dependence in many rural settings; however, there are also fewer mental health professionals available to provide assistance. Greater geographical distances often separate patients, providers, and specialists; this makes healthcare transportation a particular challenge in the rural setting, which can affect healthcare outcomes. Lastly, the percentage of traumatic injuries is commonly higher in rural settings with poorer healthcare outcomes often related to longer EMS response time and transport distances to level one or level two trauma centers (Goodwin & Tobler, 2013).

Rural residents began to leave the rural environment around the time of the Industrial Revolution. The Industrial Revolution, beginning at the end of the 18th century, is credited with starting the process of urbanization in cities across the United States as people left rural areas and moved to cities to take advantage of the many new opportunities. The Industrial Revolution created jobs that were not available in rural towns as advancements were made in agriculture, coal mining, textiles, steam power, and transportation. Today, the vast majority of Americans are living in urban settings and it is estimated that this trend will continue.

Advantages for those living in urban settings include increased job opportunities, exposure to diverse cultures, more amenities and entertainment, and better educational opportunities. The dense physical environment of urban settings, however, is associated with challenges related to the physical and social environment and access to health and social services. Additionally, people living in poverty tend to concentrate in inner-city UAs due to the availability of more affordable, though often substandard, housing and accessibility to public transportation. Nurses play a vital role in the health of both rural and urban communities.

This chapter introduces you to some of the health issues that are common in both urban and rural communities. First, issues specific to rural environments including rural descriptions and challenges associated with rural health care are discussed. Implications for rural nursing practice round out this section. Next, a brief history and background of public health nurses as promoters of health in urban cities are provided. An overview of selected risk factors that contribute to poor health outcomes in urban environments follows. Finally, this chapter ends with an application of the nursing process in a discussion of the role of nurses in improving the health of urban residents.

Rural Healthcare Issues

Rural Descriptions

The U.S. Census Bureau (2010) broadly defines a rural community as an area not designated as urban and having less than 2,500 inhabitants. Almost 47 percent of rural hospitals have less than 25 total beds. Rural hospitals carry the burden of increased costs per case due to fewer overall patients but continued need for a full array of services (American Hospital Association, 2011).

Although rural healthcare resources may vary from county to county, overall, fewer healthcare providers and facilities for health care are available in rural areas. Rural populations are officially considered **medically underserved populations (MUPs)**, meaning they face economic, cultural, or linguistic barriers to health care. MUP designations are made based on population-specific computations that include poverty level, percentage of population over 65 years of age, infant mortality rate, and the ratio of primary care physicians per 1,000 population (Health Resources Services Administration, n.d.). A rural area that does not qualify as an MUP, but generally has limited healthcare providers, is officially called a **health professional shortage area (HPSA).** These include shortages of healthcare providers such as those who deliver primary, dental, or mental health care. Often these designations are used in the allocation of federal grant resources to help rural communities enhance access to primary health care. **Health disparities** in rural versus

> **KEY TERM**
> **Medically underserved populations (MUPs):** This designation is assigned to healthcare service areas that face economic, cultural, or linguistic barriers to health care and is based on computations specific to community poverty level, elderly population, infant mortality rate, and ratio of primary care physicians per 1,000 population (Health Resources Service Administration, n.d.).

> **KEY TERM**
> **Health professional shortage area (HPSA):** This designation identifies defined communities that have shortages of healthcare providers such as primary care, dental, or mental health care (Health Resources Service Administration, n.d.).

> **KEY TERM**
> **Health disparities:** Differences in the incidence, prevalence, mortality, and burden of disease and other adverse health conditions that exist among specific population groups.

BOX 18-1   CHARACTERISTICS AND HEALTH DISPARITIES IN RURAL SETTINGS

Although there is great variability in rural communities, the following characteristics and health disparities commonly exist in rural settings.

- Lack of health insurance coverage
- Higher incidence of poverty
- Higher incidence of hypertension and stroke
- Delayed time to cancer diagnosis
- Increased suicide rates
- Increased injury rates from motor vehicle accidents

- Higher rates of alcohol and tobacco use by teenagers
- Fewer healthcare resources including dental and mental health services

Data from National Rural Health Association. (2013). *The future of rural health. Policy brief.* Retrieved from https://www.ruralhealthweb.org/advocate/policy-documents

---

urban settings are related to a variety of factors including economic, social, and cultural differences as well as educational differences. Rural counties often have higher minority populations who work at relatively low-paid agricultural or farm jobs and experience economic disadvantages that affect the quality of living and ability to afford health care. Additionally, rural communities often lack specialty physicians including obstetricians and pediatricians. A sample of reported health disparities in rural settings is provided in **Box 18-1**.

Healthcare Roles in Rural Settings

Having a diverse and adequate supply of healthcare providers is a challenge in many rural communities. This section describes the healthcare roles most commonly found in rural settings.

Nursing

Nurses are currently in short supply in all regions of the country, but the shortage of nurses and other healthcare providers is even worse in rural areas, presenting unique challenges. In acute care hospitals, even though a shortage of nurses exists, the census of most units does not provide enough work for nursing staff to be dedicated to a certain unit and patient population; nurses are required to "float" and provide staffing where they are needed. This means that those nurses must maintain broad, generalized nursing skills and competencies, varying from those required to care for the hospital's only pediatric patient to the critically ill young adult as well as the older adult receiving palliative care.

The rural nurse must also excel in triage and decision making. In the emergency room, on any given day, the nurse may encounter and provide care to an infant with colic, an adult with pneumonia, a woman experiencing an obstetrical emergency, and a patient who has been critically injured in a motor vehicle accident, all without the benefit of a comprehensive healthcare team consisting of specialists trained to diagnose and treat the patients' emerging health crises. The nurse must be able to make immediate and potentially life-saving decisions about when to transfer a patient via air to regional healthcare centers better equipped to meet the patient's healthcare needs—a decision that has significant financial implications, as well as patient care implications.

In the rural hospital, nurses often serve as coordinators of care, linking and coordinating services and working with other care providers to minimize the patients' length of stay. The nurse communicates with physicians, case managers, social workers, pharmacists, and other facility contacts as needed. When transferring patients to other facilities, the nurse may be responsible for contacting the facility, arranging transport (via private vehicle, ambulance, or helicopter), and communicating with the physician, patient, family, and the accepting facility. At times, nurses may be required to accompany patients when they are transferred via ambulance.

Nurses are often the coordinators of care in the rural community setting itself. It is frequently the nurse's responsibility to screen for clients with health risk factors, identify problems, and help locate specific resources including both informal and formal healthcare services. Nurses work closely with patients and informal caregivers to identify care needs and consider what health or service options are available to help the patients and families obtain the needed services. Nurses working in the broader community, such as in primary care clinics, community health, or public health nurse roles are required to balance numerous, simultaneous demands. Providing and clarifying health information for rural patients on diverse issues is a significant nursing responsibility; for example, rural healthcare nurses may be expected to provide information to patients regarding available community resources such as car seat safety inspection and how to obtain discounted prescriptions or free immunizations, as well as to make referrals to other healthcare and social agencies.

Primary Care Providers

Rural primary care providers are most likely to be nurse practitioners (NPs), physician's assistants (PAs), and general practice physicians. In many states, NPs have full practice authority, meaning they can evaluate, diagnose, prescribe, and maintain medications and other treatments under the sole authority of the state boards of nursing. In 2010, comprehensive health reform called the Patient Protection and Affordable Care Act (ACA) became law. The primary goal of the ACA is to increase access to patient care, improve quality of care, and reduce healthcare costs. As more Americans acquire healthcare coverage under the ACA, it is expected that NPs will play an even larger role in providing primary care services in rural and underserved areas.

Networking with specialists, these primary care providers are typically the backbone of the rural healthcare system. Rural primary care providers face challenges similar to those in urban settings but bring unique perspectives to coping with legal, reimbursement, and regulatory issues. These issues include reimbursement issues such as those related to system costs and fewer numbers of patients; regulatory issues, which are often designed for larger provider systems and those having regulatory officers; and legal issues such as those related to "duty to treat" and transferring patients to other healthcare facilities. Rural primary care providers often have limited peer networks or even inadequate support resources in their work settings to help them deal with these issues and challenges. Graduate health professions' programs are beginning to include education on rural issues within their curricula including clinical learning opportunities in rural settings to prepare practitioners who are able to successfully function within the rural environment. Unfortunately, there are few financial incentives for rural sites to provide educational opportunities for graduate nurses. The lack of specialty physicians in rural areas often results in general practice physicians, with the assistance of NPs and PAs, providing specialty services in areas such as obstetrics and gynecology, pediatrics, general surgery, intensive care, and emergency medicine.

Emergency Care Providers

First responder emergency medical service (EMS) providers play key roles in rural care that are different from those in urban settings. In the rural setting, it is common for EMS personnel to be volunteer firefighters or other local community volunteers who receive basic required training but not advanced life support training. When emergency calls are received, agency service providers should be staffed by the appropriately designated level of care provider. If appropriate staff are not available, however, the basic technician may need to call upon the assistance of the nearest ambulance service equipped with full-time paid and adequately trained staff, thus causing a delay in patient assistance.

Community paramedicine (CP) is an emerging healthcare profession that is helping to fill the healthcare gaps often seen in rural settings. Within the structure of a CP program, paramedics and EMS professionals may be trained to provide a variety of services expanded from their traditional emergency response roles to include things such as working with the local public health department to provide community education and health promotion programs, providing postdischarge follow-up, and providing primary care to rural citizens.

Case Manager Roles and Resources

Case management is commonly considered a system of assessment, coordination, and monitoring designed to help clients connect with appropriate health and social services, both formal and informal. Formal case manager roles vary in structure, but in rural care settings the nurse is most likely to serve as an informal case manager, helping families screen for problems and identify local resources to address those problems.

Rural case managers need adequate access to supportive resources for patient and family referrals. Appropriate social services and coordinated health care are particularly critical with the limited healthcare services and providers available in rural communities. Core services that make up a formal service network and commonly provide patient and family support in larger communities are noted in **Box 18-2.** Although many states have home- and community-based service programs to assist patients, these services may be less available to rural residents.

In rural settings, nurses can assess the community for these core services, determine the gaps in services, and then consider who might fill the gaps to provide these services if they are not available. Agencies such as AARP, National Association of Area Agencies on Aging, and local health departments often provide good starting points for identifying community resources. Parish nurse programs also can make important contributions to local service continua. People often have a trusting relationship with parish nurses from their faith communities, so the parish nurses can be excellent resources for promoting health and providing support services related to chronic health problems (Catanzaro, Meador, Koenig, Kuchibhatla, & Clipp, 2007). **Contemporary Practice Highlight 18-1** demonstrates highlights of the parish nursing role.

Other Care Providers

Recruiting and retaining all levels of qualified healthcare professionals can present major challenges in rural settings. Direct care workers such as nursing assistants, support technicians, and home health aides are often in short supply in the rural setting. To help remedy this shortage, some communities use an educational ladder approach to promote recruitment for healthcare careers, providing mobility options

---

BOX 18-2   CORE HOME-BASED COMMUNITY SERVICES NEEDED FOR RURAL POPULATIONS

Transportation
Nutritional support services
Homemaker support services
Personal care services
Home health nursing services
Chore services

Data from Administration for Community Living. (2016). Administration on Aging (AoA). Supportive services and senior centers program. Retrieved from http://www.aoa.acl .gov/AoA_Programs/HCLTC/supportive_services/

CONTEMPORARY PRACTICE HIGHLIGHT 18-1

PARISH NURSING

Parish nurses work within the faith community of rural churches to:
- Educate, counsel, and advocate for health promotion
  - Advise community members on health problem referrals
  - Develop support groups for health-related concerns

Characteristics of parish nurses:
- Registered nurses experienced in hospital- or community-based settings

- Completion of basic preparation courses in parish nursing
- Embrace the four main concepts of parish nursing:
  - Spiritual formation
  - Professionalism
  - Health and wholeness as God's intent
  - Respect of culture and diversity in the community

For more information on parish nursing, see http://www.parishnurses.org

---

for healthcare workers to increase their knowledge and levels of formal healthcare training to better serve their own communities. Volunteers also play an important role in rural health care. Rural healthcare and social support volunteers may come from social, faith, and work communities.

Common Rural Health Problems and Health Disparities

Common rural health problems mirror those of larger populations and relate to the specific rural community. Although there is great variability in rural populations, in general, rural communities have a higher percentage of their population not covered by employer-provided health or prescription insurance, more poverty, higher incidences of hypertension and stroke, longer delays in cancer diagnosis, increased chronic disease complications such as diabetes, and increased injury rates from motor vehicle accidents. Heart disease, alcohol abuse, and trauma are common in rural settings (National Rural Health Association [NRHA], 2013). Challenges exist in managing common health problems because rural populations tend to be older, the economy is agriculturally driven, and economic factors affect healthcare coverage.

Rural dwellers are often self-employed and may be uninsured or underinsured for healthcare costs. For example, self-employed farmers with their money invested in land, equipment, and operational expenses such as animals and veterinary care may not budget money to buy health insurance coverage. Although perceived as "rich" by those outside of the agricultural economy, they may have limited disposable income and may need to work another job for insurance benefits or gain insurance through a spouse's employment. Other rural workers, who are not farmers but live in the rural setting, work at low-paying jobs with limited benefits (NRHA, 2013).

As noted, rural healthcare services are vastly different from those in urban settings. Those healthcare problems requiring treatment from specialists may have increased impact because of fewer healthcare resources. Specialty services are typically limited in the rural setting because the population is geographically diverse and a specialty service would have only a few clients and not be financially viable. Even patients with obstetric care needs beyond the basic pregnancy care from primary care providers may need to drive to an urban center for services. Other specialty services, such as cardiology and neurology, are often limited in rural areas. Fortunately, the use of electronic communication through telehealth technology is now allowing rural residents to access specialists without leaving their communities.

Health Promotion Issues

Data suggest that rural community residents are more likely to smoke and be obese than urban residents and also have reduced access to healthcare services. As a result, rural residents have shorter life spans than their urban counterparts (Singh & Siahpush, 2014). This suggests a need for more culturally sensitive health promotion approaches in the rural setting. Nurses in all rural settings take on broad roles in health promotion and public health. Health promotion programs that engage and work collaboratively with community members promote a focus on the health of the larger population. In rural settings there may be fewer opportunities for education about the prevention of health problems. As in UAs, some individuals would not consider certain behaviors such as smoking and heavy drinking as a health risk and would often not consider getting outside assistance. National guidelines such as Healthy People 2020 (U.S. Department of Health and Human Services [USDHHS], n.d.) provide the nurse and other care providers with direction for community health interventions. An example of a community-wide rural substance abuse program is provided in **Box 18-3**.

Rural nurses teach in diverse settings and play a very significant role in providing patient education for health promotion and disease prevention. Educational topics nurses might provide in a given setting can vary daily, from older adults' diabetic foot care to smoking cessation. Rural nurses may educate about blood pressure at a local church event, give a talk on sexually transmitted diseases at the local high school, or explain a new diagnosis of congestive heart failure to a patient at a private care clinic. In addition they provide education at health fairs sponsored by the community where they live and even at the grocery store when someone will stop them to ask for advice. Coffee shops, gas stations, or beauty shops may offer the best places for health posters and brochures.

BOX 18-3   SUBSTANCE ABUSE: RURAL MENTAL HEALTH PROGRAM EXEMPLAR IN SOUTHEAST ALASKA

Rural populations often have limited providers and resources for dealing with substance abuse, thus, a consortium approach (including use of professional staff and village provider teams and technology) was used in southeast Alaska to help provide mental health services to residents of the region. Use of indigenous village counselors ensured that the care was culturally appropriate, promoted greater longevity of the counselors, and improved employment in the depressed area. Telepsychiatry and telehealth from larger cooperative sites were used as well. Services for assessment, early intervention, education, counseling for emergency and crisis intervention, aftercare/continuing care, relapse prevention, and community development were employed.

For more information on Rural Health Promotion Programs, see http://www.ruralhealthinfo.org/community-health /health-promotion/2/program-models

---

BOX 18-4 RURAL POPULATIONS AND COMMON HEALTH CONCERNS

Agricultural workers
- Rural occupational health and safety needs

Rural teens
- Safety needs
- Limited recreational activities
- Potential problems with drinking and drugs

Diverse patients
- At-risk groups needing safety nets such as obstetrical and pediatric care services
- Rural culture and potential distrust of outsiders

Data from National Rural Health Association. (2013). *The future of rural health. Policy brief.* Retrieved from https:// www.ruralhealthweb.org/advocate/policy-documents

---

Nurses can optimize opportunities to provide healthcare education in primary care settings as well. The challenge to rural nurses is to be knowledgeable about a wide array of topics and be able to communicate with diverse populations. Rural populations and common health concerns are listed in **Box 18-4** and discussed in the following sections.

Common Health Problems for Agricultural Workers

An agriculturally driven economy lends itself to certain occupational and environmental hazards that are unique to the rural setting. Safety issues and other potential problems are pervasive for farm workers. There are no regulatory organizations such as the Occupational Safety and Health Administration (OSHA) in family farm operations. The harvest season brings a higher incidence of accidents. Farmers may work around equipment after they are tired from working a shift at another full-time job. Often teenagers work on farms or as "summer help" at local industries. These teens may not be adequately trained for these tasks, resulting in injuries or illness. Skin cancer is another common problem with farmers and field workers. Nurses have important opportunities to teach prevention of accidents and injuries and promote appropriate screening for skin cancer.

Deaths from unintentional injuries, such as motor vehicle accidents, are also higher in rural areas. According to the NRHA (2013), one third of all motor vehicle accidents occur in the rural setting, with two thirds of all deaths from motor vehicle accidents occurring on rural roads. Nurses can play a role in educating teens and employers on potential risks they may encounter as well as general safety guidelines.

Common Health Problems for Rural Teens

Teenagers are an at-risk population in general, but certain factors may put them at increased risk in the rural setting. Because of limited recreational activities in rural areas, teens are at particular risk for alcohol abuse, drug use, and other safety issues such as drunk driving or car racing. Rural nurses can address these issues with teens as part of school health promotion activities and athletic physical exams in primary care and with parents in settings such as high school orientation programs. Rural nurses may also need to work with school officials to gain population access and lead discussions on common problems such as sexually transmitted diseases.

Rural teens may have additional challenges in obtaining access to health care. For example, the rural teenager who desires birth control may not have ready transportation to the health department clinic. Privacy may also be an issue if she gets to the health department and finds that her neighbor is the nurse staffing the clinic. Further research and strategies are needed to promote positive teen health behaviors in rural communities.

Clients with Diverse Cultural Backgrounds

Different cultural backgrounds affect the communication of health information between providers and patients. Different cultural meanings and even different languages between patients and providers can lead to health treatment misunderstandings. Issues may exist when educating to promote adherence to health prescriptions, especially if patients do not have the money or other resources to manage their healthcare problems. Sometimes rural adults have a very self-sufficient mentality that may lead to suspicion of outsiders or even an antagonistic relationship with healthcare providers. The use of complementary therapy or folk remedies is common among older adults in rural settings and may be associated with this medical skepticism and the belief that they could overcome illness without medical help (Bell et al., 2013).

Seasonal migrant or farmworkers may be another at-risk population within the rural setting. The majority of farm laborers in the United States no longer are considered migrants, but are considered settled or "shuttlers," meaning they work at a single location where they also live or are shuttled across an international border to one place of employment. Only 5 percent of farm laborers are currently considered migrant farm workers who move state to state working on a variety of crops (U.S. Department of Agriculture [USDA], 2015). Approximately 50 percent of agricultural workers are not authorized to work in the United States (USDA, 2015) and therefore may not seek out health services until a major issue has developed for fear of negative consequences such as loss of employment eligibility or even deportation. Back problems and other musculoskeletal injuries, depression, sexually transmitted diseases, and acute issues such as dehydration are all common problems in migrant workers. The NRHA (2012) provides training assistance to community health nurses and other healthcare workers to ensure that high-quality healthcare services are available along the U.S.–Mexico border.

Health Literacy in the Rural Setting

Health literacy has been described as the degree to which individuals have the capacity to obtain, process, and understand basic health information and services needed to make appropriate health decisions. Higher prevalence of poor health literacy has been linked to lower levels of education and higher poverty rates, both of which are found in many rural communities (Rural Health Information Hub, 2014).

With fewer healthcare providers and resources available, health literacy issues may present even larger problems in the rural setting. Patients with low health literacy are at greater risk of misunderstanding their diagnoses, their directions for self-medication, and their self-care instructions. All these issues affect patient quality of life and add expense to the healthcare system.

The importance of the nurse assessing each patient regarding his or her specific learning needs, learning styles, and readiness to learn is noted. Although illnesses are similar, patients are not. Nurses should also address any patient misconceptions about health problems. Diverse teaching strategies including individual education, group education, and a variety of teaching methods can help meet the needs of diverse learners in rural settings. Good patient follow-up and educational reminders such as handouts with key teaching points provide opportunity for reinforcing teaching. Broad educational approaches related to chronic diseases include classes such as stress management with relaxation training and even pet therapy. Materials to enhance local agency resources can be obtained from organizations such as the Centers for Disease Control and Prevention (CDC) and national health associations for health promotion and chronic disease management. Sharing accurate information and promoting good healthcare communication are important issues that rural nurses have the potential to influence.

Care Resources and Access to Care

Rural hospitals are typically much smaller than urban ones. Hospitals in rural areas range in size from less than 25 beds to more than 100 beds. Of the approximately 1,800 rural community hospitals, 1,332 of them are designated as critical access hospitals (CAH) by the Centers for Medicare and Medicaid Services (CMS) (Rural Health Research Centers at the University of Minnesota, North Carolina-Chapel Hill, and Southern Maine, 2015). CAHs are rural hospitals with no more than 25 beds and are at least 35 miles away from another hospital. Typically, primary care providers treat patients in small community clinics or hospitals. Local churches may also be used as sites for healthcare screening and low acuity treatment.

Rural hospitals must optimize resources to be successful. Services such as pharmacy or the laboratory may be staffed for limited hours or even be absent from the setting. Nursing supervisors often take on additional roles in obtaining necessary medications and treatments for newly admitted patients. Respiratory therapy, nutritional support, and many other specialty services may be nonexistent or provided by mobile staff who visit the agency on a scheduled basis. Patients treated by these visiting specialists in both the acute care and community settings have complex medication regimes that rural nurses must manage.

The small rural hospital, in order to meet accreditation standards, must have staff trained in a variety of areas because often they need to float or cover different unit types. Even those staff who provide palliative care for hospice patients, for example, also need to have advanced cardiac life support (ACLS) training and be prepared to provide life-sustaining care in the emergency department. Although rural hospitals may also depend on agency staff to meet staffing shortfalls, agency nurses may find it difficult to meet the demands of providing both acute and chronic care for various patients along the birth-to-death continuum. Rural nurse partners can help agency nurse partners feel welcome in unique rural settings.

Lack of Local Specialty Services

To gain access to specialty health services, rural patients and families typically need to drive to large UAs that may seem strange and forbidding. Patients with cancer, for example, may have to drive over 100 miles one way to an oncology clinic. Patients with renal failure might choose not to have dialysis rather than drive to the city. In some cases people, quite literally, would choose to die rather than leave their rural comfort zone. For transportation to these distant healthcare sites, privately owned vehicles are often the only option. Family or friends often have to miss work to take loved ones to healthcare appointments because there are no buses and very limited, if any, other types of transportation.

Patients with more specialized health problems such as cancer or HIV are particularly at a disadvantage in terms of services. Although they may rely on distant communities for access to adequate health care, there are still issues concerning the lack of local community education and educational resources to promote understanding of illnesses.

Critical Access Facilities

Many hospitals in rural areas are designated **critical access facilities**. These facilities have a limited number of beds (15–25) available for admitting patients, and their services provide a type of healthcare safety net function. To gain critical access designation they must provide 24-hour emergency services and meet specified population and geographic criteria. Critical access facilities gain Medicare reimbursement for actual costs (enabling them to be financially viable [CMS, 2013]). Besides providing a healthcare safety net, critical access facilities can benefit the community in other ways as well. For example, rural hospitals are often the largest employer in a rural community and provide some of the best paying jobs (Rural Health Information Hub, 2015).

Swing Beds

In addition to receiving in-patient care in the hospital, some patients remain hospitalized under the distinction of **swing beds** for more long-term care. These patients may have been admitted to the hospital from home, but they are not well enough to return home and do not want to go to a nursing home to receive additional treatment. Many times patients in swing beds are returning to the community hospital from a metropolitan hospital following an invasive surgery such as heart bypass or a recent stroke or an extensive wound. They still require specific therapies that cannot be provided at home.

Long-Term Care Resources

Most rural settings have easier access to a long-term care nursing facility than to hospitals, and data suggest that these facilities are well used in the rural setting (National Advisory Committee on Rural Health and Human Services, 2010). Long-term care settings are different from urban facilities in that they do not typically provide extended services such as specialty units for clients with dementia, adult day care programs, or respite services for family caregivers. Additionally, resources such as home care and assisted living are often not available in rural settings. Recruitment and sometimes retention can be challenging for these facilities.

Collaboration Among Community Providers

To stay financially viable and treat the needs of a diverse rural population, rural healthcare and service agencies may best meet patient care needs via collaborative efforts. This includes local and regional collaborations with nontraditional health agencies as well as other clinical providers.

Maximizing Traditional Healthcare Resources

Statewide incentive programs are often developed to attract physicians and their families to rural areas. When there are inadequate numbers of healthcare providers, regional services provide interim medical coverage to some rural communities that contract with these programs. This can be an incentive to retired physicians and even new physicians who are seeking extra income. Some companies provide services to fly in surgeons with more experienced specialty skills to assist local surgeons.

Collaboration between rural community health centers and hospitals can be a useful approach to extending scarce resources. Sample collaborative activities include sharing electronic patient medical record systems, electronic information systems, training and technical support for clinical providers, and health promotion and disease prevention community projects. These collaborations can also include partnered health education, combined recruitment, training, human resources, and sharing case managers and service resources. Partnerships may enable agencies to make joint efforts in qualifying for and gaining grant funds and other resources. The NRHA is a national nonprofit organization that provides leadership on rural health-care issues. A summary of the NRHA's leadership activities is provided in **Box 18-5**.

Good documentation becomes particularly important when collaboration for high-quality patient care is required. Keeping multiple providers, consultants, and those transferring between rural and urban care centers informed is a key safety issue requiring clear documentation. When there are multiple team members, the benefit of using templates and checklists for communication throughout a patient's care is obvious. Electronic health records (EHRs) that provide quick access

---

BOX 18-5   NATIONAL RURAL HEALTH ASSOCIATION

Nonprofit organization that provides leadership on rural healthcare issues

Mission is to provide leadership on rural issues through advocacy, communications, education, and research

Areas of focus include NRHA Quality Initiatives, EMS agenda for the future, and sponsorship of Rural Medical Educators and NRHA Student Group

Advocates legislative and regulatory policies and positions before Congress and the White House

Members actively participate to bring about appropriate rural health policy and legislation

Volunteer membership

For more information on the National Rural Health Association, see http://www.ruralhealthweb.org

to comprehensive patient information are needed. These resources are discussed further in the technology section later in this chapter.

Maximizing Nontraditional Healthcare Resources

> **KEY TERM**
>
> **Cooperative extension offices**: Funded by the U.S. Department of Agriculture, these offices provide leadership in programming, addressing issues of concern specific to families, youth, and rural communities.

Rural partnerships might also include less traditional partners such as schools, **cooperative extension offices,** health departments, mental health centers, and senior citizen agencies. Additionally, local chapters of agencies such as the American Heart Association, American Lung Association, and American Red Cross may be available. Rural cooperative extension offices, funded by the USDA, provide leadership in programming and address issues of concern specific to families, youth, and rural communities. Affiliated groups, such as 4-H clubs, are frequently involved in health-related community service projects. Some community colleges in rural areas offer healthcare screening and education through wellness centers operated and staffed by nursing faculty and students. Collaboration among these groups, other community agencies, and local churches can provide for the more efficient use of scarce resources to improve the health of rural residents.

Maximizing Educational Opportunities and Technology for Rural Health Care

> **KEY TERM**
>
> **Area health education centers (AHECs):** Federally funded partnerships between health science center universities and local community clinical and educational resources that work together to improve education to local multidisciplinary providers and ultimately improve patient care in underserved areas.

Developing and maximizing a rural nursing workforce can be challenging. There are fewer healthcare providers in rural settings and the skills of those available need to be maximized. Especially with the rapid pace of change, rural nurses work hard to access educational resources and keep up with changing healthcare practices. Educating new professionals, orienting new nurses, and promoting staff development can all present special challenges in rural settings. **Area health education centers (AHECs)**, community colleges, and distance education partnerships can all play important roles in this effort. Technology and rural/urban partnerships are central forces in rural health care as well.

AHECs and community colleges promote health profession education in many rural states. AHECs are federally funded partnerships between health science center universities and local health agencies. AHEC partners, with particular knowledge and expertise in the interests and needs of rural students and graduates, assist rural healthcare agencies with the facilitation of rural relationships, strategic planning, and program marketing. The continuing education offered to healthcare providers in the field enhances the level of care provided, particularly in counties where few healthcare agencies and health profession schools exist, ultimately improving patient care in underserved areas.

Community colleges play a central role in nursing education in rural states. Often these schools offer the only regional access to professional clinical education such as practical nursing and associate degree nursing programs. In addition to basic healthcare educational programs, community colleges can provide a foundation for educational career ladders that partner with distant colleges and universities. Issues that affect rural community colleges include a shortage of available clinical sites, a limited range of clinical experiences, and a shortage of nursing faculty. Extensive travel may be involved for rural nursing students to obtain clinical experiences with a variety of patients.

Because advanced clinical education programs typically are not available in rural communities, technology provides a way to extend health profession education. The concepts of "growing your own" and educational career ladders often incorporate distance education strategies that provide opportunity for students unable to travel to college campuses to continue their education. Web-based transition programs such as registered nurse to bachelor of science in nursing programs allow diverse students to access advanced education from home communities. A diverse group of healthcare providers who are more likely to stay in their rural communities and potentially improve the distribution of health profession workers to underserved areas can be developed. There are several online graduate nursing programs that provide opportunities for nurses to obtain advanced degrees as primary care NPs with an emphasis on the care of rural residents.

Integrating the use of technology into health care can change the quality of practice in rural settings. Patient simulators are a good example of opportunities for technology partnerships in the rural setting. Simulators have implications for both staff development and professional education. Simulators, available in multiple forms, are tools in healthcare education that mimic patient encounters and provide practice application of theoretical concepts and skills. In particular, new high-fidelity patient simulators (HFPS) provide students and clinicians opportunities for skill practice in a safe setting. Simulators provide an opportunity to offer a diverse range of clinical experiences to students and the current nursing workforce. Rural nursing staff can demonstrate critical assessment skills, maintain practice on unusual cases, and gain continuing education without extensive travel.

Technology partnerships are particularly important in the rural setting, providing convenience in connecting with larger urban centers and specialists. **Telehealth** and **telemedicine** use telecommunications technology to deliver, manage, and coordinate care and provide rural practitioners with the opportunity to work with practitioners in urban specialty centers. Virtual health professional teams can be developed that connect rural primary care clinics with urban specialists via telemedicine. Healthcare providers can monitor patients and/or consult with rural care providers from a distance, collaboratively diagnosing

> **KEY TERM**
> **Telehealth**: Healthcare services delivered, managed, and coordinated by nurses and other healthcare providers using electronic information and telecommunications technologies.

> **KEY TERM**
> **Telemedicine**: A component of telehealth focusing on medicine's approach to deliver, manage, and coordinate care via telecommunications technologies.

patients, designing treatment plans, and monitoring patient outcomes. Real-time, two-way visual and audio connectivity between patient and provider are made possible using assistants and specially made equipment at the rural site. With appropriate resources, settings such as primary care, long-term care, hospitals, and even patient homes can be sites for telemedicine.

Furthermore, telehealth technology can allow patient assessment data such as heart and lung sounds to be transmitted electronically to specialty providers. Digital images such as x-rays or pictures of skin lesions can be transmitted. Given the appropriate technology, healthcare providers can connect with patients and families in their homes for routine check-ins and electronic reminders. Challenges associated with telehealth technology include lack of reimbursement for telehealth services, cost of technology and technical support, practice and licensure regulations, healthcare provider resistance, limited equipment and technology support, and privacy and security concerns. Technical and administrative guidelines that include requirements for confidentiality and the ethical treatment of telehealth patients, emergency backup plans, scope of services, and follow-up plans are available and should be used to assist nurses and other healthcare workers to provide safe, quality care through telehealth technology (American Telemedicine Association, 2014).

Additional technologies that assist clinicians in promoting the public's health include the Internet, smart phones or personal digital assistants (PDAs), and electronic records. Use of web-based libraries and resources of all types promote efficient access to clinical resources. The concept of fingertip knowledge is expanded as evidence-based protocols are accessed for practice.

Use of EHRs promotes safety in patient care as well as providing data for quality assurance. Electronic records provide a systematic approach to recordkeeping and easy data retrieval for patient care. Uses include not only provider documentation, but also prescribing, insurance claims processing, data exchange, and communicating information to promote efficient patient transfers. Outcomes evaluation and continuous quality improvement are facilitated with electronic records. In 2014, three out of four hospitals in the United States had adopted at least basic EHR system (Charles, Gabriel, & Searcy, 2015). **Contemporary Practice Highlight 18-2** describes a current initiative that promotes the use of technology to improve patient safety.

Evidence-Based Practice and Quality Improvement in Rural Nursing

Quality improvement projects require leadership and time resources. In the rural setting many nurses are not baccalaureate prepared and may have a limited theory or research background for quality improvement projects. Nurses who have the educational preparation, skills, and dedicated time required to direct data collection and quality assurance studies specific to the increasingly complex needs

CONTEMPORARY PRACTICE HIGHLIGHT 18-2

TECHNOLOGY

Broad attention is currently being given to the need for appropriate technology to promote safe quality care for patients. Effective electronic record systems are one approach to communicating and transferring information across healthcare systems. Although there are federal initiatives promoting technology for a connected and seamless healthcare system, implementing technology systems can challenge and burden rural health care. Nurses have a role in both making electronic record needs known within their systems and providing ideas for point-of-care approaches. Nationally, nurses are involved in the Technology Informatics Guiding Educational Reform (TIGER) initiative. The purpose of the TIGER initiative is to increase the technology capabilities of nurses and identify best practices to facilitate effective information management. One of the TIGER goals is to establish guidelines for organizations to follow as they integrate informatics into practice and academic settings.

Data from Healthcare Information and Management Systems Society. (2016). The TIGER Initiative. Retrieved from http://www.himss.org/professionaldevelopment /tiger-initiative

of diverse patients in a technology-driven, chaotic healthcare system are needed. The common rural issue of too few people to fulfill multiple roles can challenge quality improvement efforts. Although quality assurance positions are emerging in the rural hospital, with limited staff it is often the nurse manager who attempts to advance quality assurance efforts along with a myriad of other responsibilities. Nurse leaders are needed to help organizations become more quality focused with a learning community approach that addresses ongoing professional development and culture change.

The improved healthcare outcomes linked to evidence-based practice are critical for rural settings. Because time and resource barriers may present challenges to evidence-based practice, project partnering is often a necessity for rural healthcare providers. Leaders in rural nursing organizations can promote partnerships and help promote quality initiatives. For example, a nursing specialist in pressure ulcer prevention and treatment may not be available in the rural setting, but national organizations such as the National Association of Clinical Nurse Specialists can provide resources or suggest nurse consultants.

Implications for Rural Nursing Practice and Education

The rural nurse has an opportunity to create a role to match the needs of a particular rural community. Strategies such as preparing, organizing, and collaborating can help guide readiness for practice in the rural setting. **Box 18-6** highlights sample practice tips for rural nursing.

BOX 18-6 PRACTICE TIPS FOR RURAL NURSING

The following guidelines will help you prepare for nursing practice in a rural healthcare setting:

Acquire a broad, generalist nursing education and expertise.

Use a population focus in health promotion, building on available resources and working with people in their communities to promote health.

Work with primary care settings to identify educational resources and promote best practices for problems such as farm safety, child/teen safety, and coping with chronic illnesses.

Develop community-wide interventions using resources such as schools and churches and other relevant networks.

Develop an understanding of coordinator and case manager roles, gaining familiarity with local and regional resources for client support.

Emphasize the positive, work with and build on available informal and formal community networks and resources.

Promote and encourage use of collaborations and technology to promote expanded resources for health care.

Be active in national nursing organizations that provide collegial support as well as resources for practice.

Be familiar with continuous quality improvement approaches and resources for evidence-based practice.

Preparing for a rural nursing practice includes obtaining a good generalist education that prepares one to provide care to a broad range of patients. This includes being able to identify and access resources and provider networks to assist in caring for those patients with less common health problems. This also includes being knowledgeable of common challenges in addressing rural health promotion and safety issues and effectively working with people in their communities to promote health. The rural health nurse needs to understand how to consider and apply "best" nursing approaches broadly in community health systems, gaining guidance from resources such as Healthy People 2020 (USDHHS, n.d.).

Organizing for a rural nursing practice includes knowing formal and informal resources available in the community that can extend health capacity and caregiving capabilities. This includes assessing the strengths and weaknesses of these community resources. Organizing, taking leadership in community health-building efforts, and working with local volunteers can promote ongoing projects with schools, churches, and community groups. Collaborating within local and regional networks promotes partnerships for increasing quality and efficiency of services. Examples of such collaboration can include building bridges with technology between care partners, participating with national organizations on evidence-based practice committees, and helping local healthcare organizations select and participate in meaningful quality improvement projects. Being active in nursing organizations also provides collegial support as well as resources for practice; this can help build bridges for support via regional and national organizations.

> ### BOX 18-7   COMPETENCIES FOR RURAL NURSES
>
> - Maintains broad clinical and technical skills
> - Employs critical thinking and problem solving in caregiving
> - Participates as a collaborative healthcare team member
> - Uses informatics in meeting diverse patient care needs and promoting efficient healthcare systems
> - Uses good interpersonal communication and teaching/learning strategies with culturally diverse patients and families
>
> - Promotes community-wide efforts for maintaining a healthy community
> - Uses clinical best practices and pursues quality assurance efforts
>
> Data from Institute of Medicine. (2003). *Health professions education: A bridge to quality.* Washington, DC: National Academy Press. Retrieved from http://nap.edu/10681

Nurses can do a self-assessment to make sure they have the competencies needed by rural nurses. Hurme (2007) organized 25 different competencies to include the major categories of clinical and technical skills, critical thinking, interpersonal communication, and management/organizational skills. **Box 18-7** notes the competencies needed by the rural nurse.

Urban Healthcare Issues

American cities are the hub of the U.S. economy and provide opportunities for employment, entertainment, diversity, innovation and a wide array of other benefits. Cities bring people together and attract those from diverse backgrounds, lifestyles, and social settings. Americans are moving to urban settings in large numbers (see **Figure 18-1**). According to the Center for American Progress (2015) the rich economic, educational, and social opportunities that urban centers create are attracting more Americans than ever. In fact, between 2010 and 2013, over 65,000 people relocated to Los Angeles compared to only 97,000 over the entire past decade (Center for American Progress, 2015). Despite the advantages of urban living, many urban neighborhoods face daunting challenges caused by poverty, unemployment, crime, and the unavailability of affordable and good-quality housing.

Public Health Nursing in Urban Settings: A History of Prevention and Health Promotion

Public health nursing is a specialty practice aimed at improving the health outcomes for all populations by focusing on prevention and through consideration of multiple determinants of health (American Public Health Association [APHA], Public Health Nursing Section, 2013). The specialty developed largely because of advancing scientific knowledge and public disapproval of

> **KEY TERM**
>
> **Public health nursing**: The field of nursing that specializes in improving the health care of the community or individuals in the community setting.

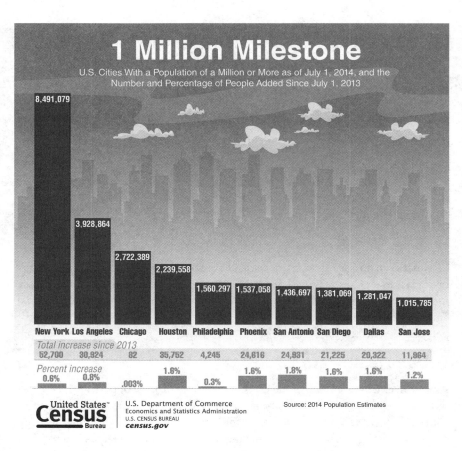

Figure 18-1 Population of the top 10 urban cities in America.
In 2000, the population per square mile for these cities were: New York City 27,012; Los Angeles 8,092; Chicago 11,892; Houston 3,501; Philadelphia 11,379; Phoenix 2,798; San Antonio 2,880; San Diego 4,020; Dallas 3,518; San Jose 5,358.

Reproduced from U.S. Census Bureau. (2015b). Ten U.S. cities now have 1 million people or more; California and Texas each have three of these places. Retrieved from http://www.census.gov/newsroom /press-releases/2015/cb15-89.html

squalid living conditions often seen within urban environments (Kulbok, Thatcher, Park, & Meszaros, 2012).

The key characteristics of public health nursing practice include "1) a focus on the health needs of an entire population, including inequities and the unique needs of subpopulations; 2) assessment of population health using a comprehensive, systematic approach; 3) attention to multiple determinants of health; 4) an emphasis on primary prevention; and 5) application of interventions at all levels—individuals, families, communities, and the systems that impact their health" (APHA, 2013, p. 2). Public health nurses have long played a role in recognizing the impact that the urban environment has had on the health of residents and addressing the health problems that often accompany urbanization. When preventing illness and promoting the health of urban residents, public health nurses must maintain a comprehensive perspective that includes all of the potential factors that may contribute to the health of the individual and population (see **Contemporary Practice Highlight 18-3**).

CONTEMPORARY PRACTICE HIGHLIGHT 18-3

HIV/AIDS

Human immunodeficiency virus (HIV) is the virus that causes acquired immune deficiency syndrome (AIDS). It is most commonly transmitted by sexual contact and use of needles that are contaminated by blood. HIV affects the immune system, attacking white blood cells and making it a challenge for infected individuals to fight off disease. AIDS is the final stage of infection and is characterized by a severely weakened immune system. In this stage of the infection, T cells are low in number and infections begin to invade the body.

HIV was first recognized in the United States in homosexual men in the early 1980s. Today, gay and bisexual men of all races are the most severely affected by HIV. Blacks/African Americans suffer the most severe burden of HIV by race. Blacks/African Americans make up only 12 percent of the U.S. population, but they accounted for 44 percent of new HIV infections in 2010 (CDC, 2014b). Although death rates have improved, HIV/AIDS remains a leading cause of death for both African American men and women; for African American women ages 35–44 years, HIV/AIDS is the number four cause of death (CDC, 2013). According to the CDC, reasons for this disparity include poverty, stigma, negative perceptions about HIV testing, increased rates of other sexually transmitted diseases, and limited HIV prevention education.

Historically, HIV has been significantly more prevalent in urban cities; rates of infection increase as city population increases. **Tables 18-1** and **18-2** illustrate the relationship between city population and HIV infections and the racial disparities for AIDS.

TABLE 18-1   PREVALENCE OF HIV INFECTION BY METROPOLITAN STATISTICAL AREA, 2013

City Population	HIV Cases per 100,000	Cumulative Number of Cases
Nonmetropolitan (< 50,000)	112.1	52,051
50,000 to 499,999	168.8	97,640
> 500,000	368.1	790,818

Data from Centers for Disease Control and Prevention. (2014a). *Diagnosis of HIV infection in the United States and dependent areas, 2014* (HIV/AIDS surveillance report, no. 26). Retrieved from http://www.cdc.gov/hiv/pdf/library/reports/surveillance/cdc-hiv-surveillance-report-us.pdf

(*continues*)

CONTEMPORARY PRACTICE HIGHLIGHT 18-3

HIV/AIDS (*continued*)

TABLE 18-2 RACIAL DISPARITIES IN HIV CASES BY POPULATION SIZE, 2012

City Population	Black/African American Residents with Diagnosed HIV Infection per 100,000	White Residents with Diagnosed HIV Infection per 100,000
Nonmetropolitan (< 50,000)	702	53
50,000 to 500,000	841	98
> 500,000	1,370	229

Data from Centers for Disease Control and Prevention, National Center for HIV/AIDS, Viral Hepatitis, STD, and TB Prevention. (2013). *HIV surveillance in urban and nonurban areas through 2013*. Retrieved from http://www.cdc.gov/hiv/pdf/2013-Urban-Nonurban-slides_508-REV-5_6-5.pdf

The Urban Environment: An Overview of Selected Risk Factors

The urban environment offers opportunities for increased job availability as well as challenges in public health issues. Risk factors that accompany urban environments are discussed including poverty, pollution, health care, and access to health care and crime and violence (see **Contemporary Practice Highlight 18-4**).

Poverty

Despite the increased opportunities for employment that exist in urban cities, poverty resulting from underemployment or unemployment continues to plague urban cities. In fact, the number of people living in concentrated poverty has nearly doubled from 7.2 million in 2000 to 13.8 million people in 2013 indicating the United States is experiencing a nationwide return of concentrated poverty including an expansion in the high-poverty ghettos and barrios (Jargowsky, 2013). **Decentralization** of urban cities has occurred as a result of the loss of employment opportunities and social capital to the suburbs leading to increased unemployment and poverty in UAs. More than one in four Black poor individuals and one in six Hispanic poor individuals lives in neighborhoods

KEY TERM

Decentralization: A process occurring in urban cities in which employment opportunities and social capital move into suburban areas. The process is suggested to be one of the causes of urban poverty.

CONTEMPORARY PRACTICE HIGHLIGHT 18-4

LEADING HEALTH INDICATORS

The CDC has identified 12 health indicators that represent areas of public health concern in the United States. These leading health indicators are:

- Access to health services
- Clinical preventive services
- Environmental quality
- Injury and violence
- Maternal, infant, and child health
- Mental health
- Nutrition, physical activity, and obesity
- Oral health
- Reproductive and sexual health

- Social determinants
- Substance abuse
- Tobacco

   Visit the websites for the National Center for Health Statistics (https://www.cdc.gov/nchs/) and Healthy People 2020 (https://www.healthypeople .gov/) for more information on these and other issues in urban cities.

Data from Centers for Disease Control and Prevention. (2011b). *Topic areas at a glance*. Retrieved from http:// www.cdc.gov/nchs/healthy_people/hp2020/hp2020 _topic_areas.htm

---

with concentrated poverty. Inner-city neighborhoods offer affordable housing and easy access to transportation attracting both immigrants and native-born poor (Jargowsky, 2013). The definition of poverty used by the U.S. Census Bureau accounts for the income of a household and number of family members living in the household. A person or family is living in poverty when they earn an income less than the set threshold. In 2014, 14.8 percent of the population (or 46.7 million people) were living in poverty in the United States (U.S. Census Bureau, 2015a). Recent reports indicate growing economic inequality, with income for those at the top of the income ladder growing considerably faster than those in the middle or bottom of the income ladder, contributing to more economic inequality (Stone, Trisi, Sherman, & Horton, 2015). **Table 18-3** provides examples of the 2015 **poverty thresholds** for families of varying types.

KEY TERM

Poverty thresholds: Income amounts set by the government that account for household size and earnings. A family whose income falls below this threshold is considered to be living in poverty.

   Growing economic inequality is especially evident in urban cities, where poverty is concentrated in inner-city neighborhoods. Concentrated poverty is described as a census tract with poverty rates of 40 percent or greater and is associated with increased crime, poorer health outcomes, failing schools, and decreased employment opportunities (Kneebone, 2014). Low-income individuals and families are less likely to have health insurance than those with greater financial means. Additionally, poor people and people of color have worse health outcomes as a result of access to care barriers and reduced quality of care. The ACA includes provisions that

TABLE 18-3 POVERTY THRESHOLDS FOR 2015 FOR VARIOUS FAMILY TYPES	
Family Type	2015 Poverty Threshold
Over 65 years old, living alone	$11,367
Over 65 years old, married couple	$14,326
Single mother with 2 children	$19,096
Single mother with 4 children	$27,853
Married couple with 2 children	$24,036
Married couple with 4 children	$31,670

Data from U.S. Census Bureau, Housing and Household Economic Statistics Division. (2015). Poverty thresholds. Retrieved from https://www.census.gov/hhes/www/poverty/methods/definitions.html

focus specifically on disparities in health care for vulnerable populations. Through the ACA, Medicaid coverage has been expanded and has increased healthcare coverage for many low-income and middle-income Americans. Unfortunately, significant restrictions to coverage still exist leaving many vulnerable individuals without healthcare coverage (Artiga, 2012). Fear of crime severely diminishes the mental and physical well-being, including cardiovascular health, of those living in economically disadvantaged neighborhoods (Browning, Cagney, & Iveniuk, 2012; Collins & Marrone, 2015), as does drug use. Nurses working with urban residents must be aware of the factors that contribute to poverty for many of its residents and its associated health-related outcomes.

The Urban Structural Environment

Substandard housing has been and continues to be a major problem in U.S. urban cities. Low-income families are disproportionately the victims of inadequate and substandard housing that exposes them to such conditions as high lead levels (see **Contemporary Practice Highlight 18-5**); poor heating or cooling; roach and rodent infestation; exposure to mold, radon gas, and other pollutants; and injuries from poor structure and inadequate upkeep (Rauh, Landrigan, & Claudio, 2008; Robert Wood Johnson Foundation Commission to Build a Healthier America, 2008). Not only does housing in urban cities affect the health status of urban residents, but the presence of food deserts also affects the health and well-being of urban residents. A food desert exists when there is lack of access to fruits, vegetables, and other healthy food choices that are also affordable (CDC, 2012). Although many factors contribute

CONTEMPORARY PRACTICE HIGHLIGHT 18-5

LEAD POISONING

Efforts at decreasing incidence of lead exposure and poisoning, mainly in children, over the last 30 years have been largely successful. A variety of organizations joined together to decrease the amount of lead poisoning that plagued urban neighborhoods. Some of these organizations included the Environmental Protection Agency, the Department of Housing and Urban Development, the Food and Drug Administration, and the Consumer Product Safety Commission. Together, the efforts of these organizations have led to the removal of lead from gasoline, paint, and toys. Furthermore, the medical community played a large role in the early screening of children and in educating parents about the dangers of lead poisoning, which include developmental, neurological, and intellectual deficits (American Academy of Pediatrics, 2005). However, more than half a million children continue to be affected each year (CDC, 2016). These children are disproportionately residents of urban neighborhoods and aging, substandard housing. Continued efforts are needed in order to continue to prevent lead poisoning, screen for exposure, and educate parents on protecting their children from the dangers of lead.

to obesity and obesity-related diseases, food deserts are particularly associated with increased risks related to obesity. Dependence on public transportation and motor vehicle transportation has contributed to increasing rates of obesity as well, due to lack of physical activity and the convenience of obtaining unhealthy meals via the drive-throughs of fast-food restaurants.

Air pollution (primarily from traffic, industry, tobacco smoke, and indoor allergens) is associated with a multitude of health conditions including respiratory disease, cardiac disease, and even death (National Institute of Environmental Health Sciences, 2016). Asthma cases in children 17 years of age or younger increased by 1.4 percent per year between 2001 and 2010 in the United States. Even worse, African American children have 1.6 times the incidence of asthma as white children (Gergen & Togias, 2015). Currently, 1 in 10 children and 1 in 12 adults have asthma (CDC, 2011a). Asthma is a complex illness that is associated with several dynamics including individual, neighborhood, and environment factors such as indoor and outdoor air quality (Keddem et al., 2015) and costs the U.S. approximately $56 billion annually (CDC, 2011a). According to the World Health Organization (2014) outdoor air pollution is estimated to result in 3.7 million premature deaths worldwide with 80 percent of these deaths caused by ischemic heart disease and strokes and 14 percent caused by chronic obstructive pulmonary disease or respiratory infections. Primary sources of air pollution for those living in urban settings include fine particles in the air from the burning of petroleum (traffic) and coal, urban smog, tobacco smoke, carbon monoxide and radon gases, allergens from cockroach and mouse droppings, mold and pollen, and building materials such as asbestos and lead (National Institute of Environmental Health Sciences, 2016). Adverse outcomes from asthma and other respiratory diseases are linked to increased use of medications, school absenteeism, hospitalizations, decreased quality of life, and death.

Tuberculosis

Tuberculosis (TB) is a respiratory illness caused by the airborne transmission of the bacteria *Mycobacterium tuberculosis*. TB spreads through the air from one person to another. Although the overall incidence of TB is falling slowly in the United States, the incidence of TB is higher in UAs primarily due to the ease of transmission among people living in crowded environments. On average, there is an increase in TB cases as the population increases; this is a reflection of a mechanism of transmission that is facilitated by increases in population. TB is particularly a threat for people infected with HIV (see **Table 18-4**).

Health Care and Access to Healthcare Services

Health care has changed dramatically in the United States over the past decade. Advances in technology, new drugs, improved medical tests and imaging, and new

TABLE 18-4 COMPARISON OF TUBERCULOSIS CASES

Cities with ≥ 1 Million Residents[+]	TB Cases per 100,000*	Cities with ≤ 600,000 Residents[+]	TB Cases per 100,000*
New York, NY	4.8	Spokane, WA	0.9
Los Angeles, CA	6.1	Portland, OR	1.5
San Francisco, CA	7.8	Augusta, GA	2.2
Houston, TX	5.9	Lancaster, PA	1.5
Washington, DC	4.5	Santa Rosa, CA	2.6

* Centers for Disease Control and Prevention, 2014

[+] Based on 2014 Census estimates

Data from Centers for Disease Control and Prevention. (2015). *Reported tuberculosis in the United States, 2014.* Atlanta, GA: U.S. Department of Health and Human Services. Retrieved from http://www.cdc.gov/tb/statistics /reports/2014/pdfs/tb-surveillance-2014-report_updated.pdf

minimally invasive procedures have changed the healthcare landscape. Evidence-based practice, including clinical practice guidelines, have improved care as healthcare providers are now being influenced to follow practice guidelines. Urban residents and communities benefit from many of these healthcare advances as well as several factors that enhance the health of urban residents. One such benefit of life in urban cities is the availability of more healthcare services for those who can access them. In general, life expectancy is longer in urban settings as compared to rural settings, and this gap in life span appears to be widening (Singh & Siahpush, 2014). The prevalence of healthcare facilities, particularly large healthcare systems, is higher in urban as compared to rural areas. Additionally, resources for assistance with basic necessities, as well as social networks centered around ethnic, cultural, religious, educational, and professional interests, are more prevalent in urban cities and may contribute to the health of urban residents.

In light of these improvements and services, many urban Americans do not have access to or cannot pay for healthcare services. Many of the country's poorest and sickest people live in poor urban inner-city neighborhoods where hospitals and healthcare providers are no longer located. Hospital expansions and relocations to areas (large urban suburbs) where a large percentage of the population is privately insured is becoming more common. Even nonprofit hospitals benefit financially when a larger percentage of their population mix has health insurance. As a result, poor communities are often left without hospitals, without primary care providers, and without healthcare services. It is has been widely accepted that as poverty increases, health decreases and that people in poor neighborhoods are less healthy than those in middle class or wealthy neighborhoods.

Barriers to health care for poor urban residents include lack of ability to pay for services, substandard housing and environmental stress, healthcare teams' lack of understanding of poverty, difficulty communicating with healthcare providers, social distance including perceived prejudice and labeling, difficult access to care, and healthcare system complexity (Loignon et al., 2015). The complexities of these existing barriers make it challenging and difficult for healthcare and social service professionals to meet the growing needs of the inner-city poor population. Clinics that serve low-income neighborhoods help fill the gaps in care as do parish nurses, community outreach centers, nonprofit organizations, and hospital-based and free clinics.

Crime and Safety

Criminal activity has long characterized urban cities and is cited by many as a reason to avoid urban cities and reside in suburban or rural areas. Fear of crime is associated with increased stress, social isolation, and anxiety, all of which reduce mental and physical well-being. Trends in criminal activity, however, indicate that violent crimes fell in the largest metropolitan areas from 1990 to 2008. Although all communities are affected by crime, poor residents living in UAs with largely minority population feel the impact disproportionately. Though crime rates are considerably higher in large cities as compared to the suburbs, the gap between these areas is declining. According to the National Center for Victims of Crime (2015), urban metropolitan areas have the highest violent crime rates compared to nonmetropolitan areas. In 2012, the rate of violent crime reported to law enforcement within UAs was 409.4 per 100,000 persons and 380.4 per 100,000 persons in cities just outside of metropolitan areas; non-metropolitan counties reported just 177.0 violent crimes per 100,000 persons. The robbery rate for metropolitan or urban cities in 2012 was 127.9 per 100,000 persons compared to a rate of 12.6 per 100,000 persons in nonmetropolitan counties (National Center for Victims of Crime, 2015). **Table 18-5** demonstrates crime type by geographical area.

Gang violence is a major source of crime in many communities in the United States. According to the Federal Bureau of Investigation (FBI) (2011) gang members are increasingly moving from UAs to suburban areas and are involved in drug trafficking, weapons trafficking, human trafficking, and other violent and nonviolent crimes. It is estimated that there are more than 1.4 million gang members in the United States today. A gang is defined as a group of individuals who come together for the purpose of identity, cohesion, and sense of belonging. Gangs are responsible for almost 50 percent of violent crimes in many districts and up to 90 percent in others (FBI, 2011). Urban gang members, when compared to rural gang members, are more concerned about their personal safety. Lack of jobs for youth, social isolation and poverty, and domestic violence in the home are factors that lead youth towards gang membership.

Gun safety is also a concern for urban residents. Members of households in urban cities are more likely to witness criminal acts such as homicide, gang activity, theft, home invasion, and selling of drugs. As a result, residents of urban cities—especially those in low-income neighborhoods—are more likely to fear victimization and possess a firearm in an effort to protect themselves and their families. Those who keep guns for protection (as opposed to hunting or other sporting hobbies) are more likely to keep the gun loaded and readily available for use in the event of threat of victimization. In 2013, 1,670 children died from a gunshot and another 9,718 were injured. The majority of these unintentional shootings occur in the home. Additionally, people who have firearm access are considered to be at twice the risk of homicide and more than three times the risk of suicide (Center for Injury Research and Prevention, 2013). Among adults, rates of intentional firearm deaths are similar in urban and rural cities. However, there is a variation in the type of firearm deaths between urban and rural cities; intentional homicides are more characteristic of urban cities, whereas suicides are more common in rural areas (Branas, Nance, Elliott, Richmond, & Schwab, 2004).

TABLE 18-5   RATE OF CRIMES PER 100,000 INHABITANTS BY POPULATION GROUP, 2014

Type of Crime	City Size > 1,000,000	City Size 500,000–999,999	City Size 250,000–499,999	Rural Areas as < 10,000
All violent crimes	658.7	874.4	717.9	282.5
All homicides	7.4	11.3	10.6	2.4
Rape	41.9	61.6	64.2	39.3
Robbery	249.2	287.8	257.2	41.3
Aggravated assault	361.3	519.8	398.6	201.7
Burglary	516.7	890.5	809.6	493.0
Motor vehicle theft	343.5	520.3	462.0	124.0

Data from Federal Bureau of Investigations. (n.d.). *2014 crime in the United States*. Retrieved from https://www.fbi .gov/about-us/cjis/ucr/crime-in-the-u.s/2014/crime-in-the-u.s.-2014/tables/table-16

The Role of the Nurse in Improving Health Outcomes in Urban Settings

The nursing process is the common link that nurses from a variety of specialties understand and use to deliver care that is patient and community centered and holistic. For public health nurses, clinical scenarios may consist of interactions with an individual person or family, a community, or policymakers. The steps of the nursing process—assessment, diagnosis, planning, implementation, and evaluation—provide the nurse with a systematic process by which the needs of urban residents are identified and actions are planned and carried out. The results of interventions are then evaluated for efficacy, sustainability, and appropriateness for the individual and community.

As a part of assessment, nurses working in urban cities must be aware of the many issues that play a role in the life of urban residents and communities. Specifically, the nurse must have an intimate knowledge of the community within which she or he works. This involves developing a knowledge base from which the nurse can make sound clinical judgments that will improve the health of individuals and the community. Assessment also includes evaluation of an individual's or community's readiness for actions aimed at improving health. Nurses make clinical judgments within the scope of nursing practice and plan for action on behalf of the individual or community. Planning for interventions can be a lengthy process as the nurse conducts ongoing assessments of patient and community needs, prioritizes appropriate interventions based on the best available evidence, and gathers resources needed for implementation of the decided interventions. Addressing the needs of the individual or family should be an interdisciplinary effort for the nurse in urban settings. Nurses must make decisions about interventions based upon whether individuals or communities have actual or potential needs, or if they are at risk for certain needs. Lastly, evaluation is an ongoing process that involves determining the attainment of the objectives identified and the success of all interventions. An improvement in health of the individual and/or community indicates success.

Summary

Rural health nursing roles require a good generalist preparation, working with the community for health promotion, being aware of resources, knowledgeably using technology tools, and having a willingness to work collaboratively with partners in care to ensure best-care practices. This includes partnerships at local, regional, and national levels. Concepts of preparing, organizing, and collaborating can guide the nurse in determining his or her readiness for practicing in rural community settings. Rural nursing provides the opportunity to practice the best of population-based care, acute care, and chronic care management skills.

Public health nurses have historically focused on the impact of environment on the health of individuals. Health and environment are very complex, interrelated issues that influence both short- and long-term health outcomes and quality of life for citizens nationally and globally. The factors that influence health include a combination of biological/genetic, psychological, emotional, lifestyle/behavioral, sociopolitical, and environmental factors; nurses must consider the role that these factors play in the health of individuals. Risk factors in the environment such as poverty can dramatically alter the health status of individuals and families. Poverty in urban cities is thought to be the result of decentralization, increased racial segregation, unemployment, and increasing economic disparities. Risk factors that play a specific role in the health of urban residents include poverty, substandard housing, air pollution, crime and violence, and access to healthcare services.

Urban cities are characterized by health-related issues that may contribute to health as well as harm health. Those suffering from poverty in urban cities encounter challenges in accessing many of the benefits of urban living, making them more vulnerable to poor health outcomes. Nursing professionals must continue to assess risk factors in the client's environment. Nurses can act as change agents and advocate for policies that improve access to care and decrease public health risk factors.

Reflective Practice Questions

1. What are your experiences working with patients from a rural setting? Urban settings? What surprises were there as you read about healthcare issues of rural patients? Urban patients?

2. What do you think are some of the similarities and differences in caring for patients in rural and urban settings? If you interviewed a patient from a rural setting and one from an urban setting with the same diagnosis, such as breast cancer, what similar concerns would you expect? What different concerns?

3. What do you see as the most important benefits of technology in rural health care? What skills would you personally need to develop in your nursing practice to effectively work in telehealth? How can you learn more about this healthcare approach?

4. Visit the NRHA's website (http://www.ruralhealthweb.org) and explore some of the links within it. If you were a nurse practicing in a rural area, what resources could you derive from this site that would help you provide better care and teaching to your patients?

5. You are working in a community health center and facilitating a support group for people with diabetes. Today, you are discussing the benefits of exercise in controlling blood glucose levels and maintaining a healthy weight. The community center is in a high-crime, low-income neighborhood with no parks, sidewalks, or exercise facilities. Group members express fear about exercising in their neighborhood. You decide to convene a group of community members in order to assess the problem in the community and come up with potential solutions. What actions would you take to conduct a full assessment of recreation barriers and resources in the community? What are some possible solutions?

References

Administration for Community Living. (2016). Administration on Aging (AoA). Supportive services and senior centers program. Retrieved from http://www.aoa.gov/AoA_programs/HCLTC/supportive_services/

American Academy of Pediatrics, Committee on Environmental Health. (2005). Lead exposure in children: Prevention, detection, and management. *Pediatrics*, *116*(4). Retrieved from http://pediatrics.aappublications.org/content/116/4/1036

American Hospital Association. (2011). *The opportunities and challenges for rural hospitals in an era of health reform. Trend watch*. Retrieved from http://www.aha.org/research/reports/tw/11apr-tw-rural.pdf

American Public Health Association, Public Health Nursing Section (2013). *The definition and practice of public health nursing: A statement of the public health nursing section*. Washington, DC: Author. Retrieved from https://www.apha.org/~/media/files/pdf/membergroups/phn/nursingdefinition.ashx

American Telemedicine Association. (2014). *Core operational guidelines for telehealth services involving provider-patient interactions*. Washington, DC: Author. Retrieved from http://www.americantelemed.org/docs/default-source/standards/core-operational-guidelines-for-telehealth-services.pdf?sfvrsn=6

Artiga, S. (2012). *Disparities in health and health care: Five key questions and answers*. Menlo Park, CA: Kaiser Family Foundation. Retrieved from http://kff.org/disparities-policy/issue-brief/disparities-in-health-and-health-care-five-key-questions-and-answers/

Bell, R. A., Grzywacz, J. G., Quandt, S.A., Neiberg, R., Lang, W., Nguyen, H., . . . Arcury, T. A. (2013). Medical skepticism and complementary therapy use among older rural African-Americans and whites. *Journal of Health Care for the Poor and Underserved, 24*(2), 777–787.

Branas, C., Nance, M., Elliott, M., Richmond, T., & Schwab, C. (2004). Urban-rural shifts in intentional firearm deaths: Different causes, same results. *American Journal of Public Health, 94*(10), 1750–1755.

Browning, C. R., Cagney, K. A., & Iveniuk, J. (2012). Neighborhood stressors and cardio-vascular health: Crime and c-reactive protein in Dallas, USA. *Social Science & Medicine, 75*(7), 1271–1279.

Catanzaro, A., Meador, K., Koenig, H., Kuchibhatla, M., & Clipp, E. (2007). Congregational health ministries: A national study of pastors' views. *Public Health Nursing, 24*(1), 6–17.

Center for American Progress. (2015). Expanding opportunities in America's urban areas. Retrieved from https://www.americanprogress.org/issues/poverty/report/2015/03/23/109460/expanding-opportunities-in-americas-urban-areas/

Centers for Disease Control and Prevention. (2011a). Asthma in the U.S.: Vital signs. Retrieved from http://www.cdc.gov/vitalsigns/asthma/

Centers for Disease Control and Prevention. (2011b). Topic areas at a glance. Retrieved from http://www.cdc.gov/nchs/healthy_people/hp2020/hp2020_topic_areas.htm

Centers for Disease Control and Prevention. (2012). A look inside food deserts. Retrieved on from http://www.cdc.gov/features/FoodDeserts/

Centers for Disease Control and Prevention. (2014a). *Diagnosis of HIV infection in the United States and dependent areas, 2014* (HIV/AIDS surveillance report, no. 26). Retrieved from http://www.cdc.gov/hiv/pdf/library/reports/surveillance/cdc-hiv-surveillance-report-us.pdf

Centers for Disease Control and Prevention. (2014b). *HIV/AIDS 101: U.S. statistics*. Retrieved from https://www.aids.gov/hiv-aids-basics/hiv-aids-101/statistics/

Centers for Disease Control and Prevention. (2015). *Reported tuberculosis in the United States, 2014*. Retrieved from http://www.cdc.gov/tb/statistics/reports/2014/pdfs/tb-surveillance-2014-report_updated.pdf

Centers for Disease Control and Prevention. (2016). *Lead*. Retrieved from http://www.cdc.gov/nceh/lead/

Centers for Disease Control and Prevention, National Center for HIV/AIDS, Viral Hepatitis, STD, and TB Prevention. (2013). *HIV surveillance report in urban and nonurban areas through 2013*. Retrieved from http://www.cdc.gov/hiv/pdf/2013-Urban-Nonurban-slides_508-REV-5_6-5.pdf

Center for Injury Research and Prevention. (2013). Gun violence: Facts and statistics. Retrieved from https://injury.research.chop.edu/violence-prevention-initiative/types-violence-involving-youth/gun-violence/gun-violence-facts-and#.Vro0tPkrIgs

Centers for Medicare & Medicaid Services. (2013). Critical access hospitals. Retrieved from https://www.cms.gov/Medicare/Provider-Enrollment-and-Certification/CertificationandComplianc/CAHs.html

Charles, D., Gabriel, M., & Searcy, T. (2015). *Adoption of electronic health record systems among U.S. non-federal acute care hospitals: 2008–2014* (ONC Data Brief no. 23). Washington, DC: Office of the National Coordinator for Health Information Technology. Retrieved from https://www.healthit.gov/sites/default/files/data-brief/2014HospitalAdoption DataBrief.pdf

Collins, R. E., & Marrone, D. F. (2015, July/September). Scared sick: Relating fear of crime to mental health in older adults. *SAGE Open*, 1–10. Retrieved from http://sgo.sagepub .com/content/spsgo/5/3/2158244015602516.full.pdf

Federal Bureau of Investigations. (n.d.). *2014 crime in the United States*. Retrieved from https://www.fbi.gov/about-us/cjis/ucr/crime-in-the-u.s/2014/crime-in-the-u.s.-2014 /tables/table-16

Federal Bureau of Investigation. (2011). 2011 National gang threat assessment: Emerging trends. Retrieved from https://www.fbi.gov/stats-services/publications/2011-national -gang-threat-assessment

Gergen, P. J., & Togias, A. (2015). Inner city asthma. *Immunology and Allergy Clinics of North America*, *35*, 101–114.

Goodwin, K., & Tobler, L. (2013). *Improving rural health: State policy options*. Washington, DC: National Conference of State Legislatures. Retrieved from http://www.ncsl.org /documents/health/RuralHealth_PolicyOptions_1113.pdf

Health Resources Services Administration. (n.d.). *Shortage designation: Health professional shortage areas and medically underserved areas/populations*. Retrieved from http://www. hrsa.gov/shortage/

Healthcare Information and Management Systems Society. (2016). The TIGER Initiative. Retrieved from http://www.himss.org/professionaldevelopment/tiger-initiative

Hurme, F. E. (2007). *Competencies for rural nursing practice*. (Doctoral dissertation, Louisi-ana State University, Baton Rouge, LA). Retrieved from http://etd.lsu.edu/docs/available /etd-04052007-112941/

Institute of Medicine. (2003). *Health professions education: A bridge to quality*. Washington, DC: National Academy Press. Retrieved from http://nap.edu/10681

Jargowsky, P. A. (2013). *Architecture of segregation: Civil unrest, the concentration of poverty, and public policy*. New York, NY: Century Foundation. Retrieved from apps.tcf.org /architecture-of-segregation

Keddem, S., Barg, F. K., Glanz, K., Jackson, T., Green, S., & George, M. (2015). Mapping the urban asthma experience: Using qualitative GIS to understand contextual factors affecting asthma control. *Social Science & Medicine*, *140*, 9–17.

Kneebone, E. (2014). *The growth and spread of concentrated poverty, 2000 to 2008–2012*. Washington, DC: Brookings Institution. Retrieved from http://www.brookings.edu /research/interactives/2014/concentrated-poverty#/M10420

Kulbok, P., Thatcher, E., Park, E., & Meszaros, P. (2012). Evolving public health nursing roles: Focus on community participatory health promotion and prevention. *Online Journal of Issues in Nursing*, *17*(2), 1–13.

Loignon, C., Hudon, C., Goulet, E., Boyer, S., De Laat, M., Fournier, N., . . . Bush, P. (2015). Perceived barriers to healthcare for persons living in poverty in Quebec, Canada: The EQUIhealThY project. *International Journal for Equity in Health*, *14*(4). doi: 10.1186 /s12939-015-0135-5

National Advisory Committee on Rural Health and Human Services. (2010). *The 2010 report to the secretary: Rural health and human services issue*. Retrieved from http://www.hrsa .gov/advisorycommittees/rural/2010secretaryreport.pdf

National Center for Victims of Crime. (2015). *Urban and rural crime*. Retrieved from http://victimsofcrime.org/docs/default-source/ncvrw2015/2015ncvrw_stats_urbanrural .pdf?sfvrsn=2

National Institute of Environmental Health Sciences. (2016). Air pollution. Retrieved from http://www.niehs.nih.gov/health/topics/agents/air-pollution/

National Rural Health Association. (2012). NRHA announces upcoming community health worker trainings as part of Clinton global initiative—America Commitment to Action. Retrieved from http://www.ruralhealthweb.org/index.cfm?objectid=F9C3F04C-C09F-4293-4FA4AE90832646F8&flushcache=1&showdraft=1

National Rural Health Association. (2013). *The future of rural health. Policy brief.* Retrieved from https://www.ruralhealthweb.org/advocate/policy-documents

Rauh, V. A., Landrigan, P. J., & Claudio, L. (2008). Housing and health: Intersection of poverty and environmental exposures. *Annals of the New York Academy of Sciences, 1136,* 276–288.

Robert Wood Johnson Foundation Commission to Build a Healthier America. (2008). *Housing and health* (Issue brief 2). Retrieved from http://www.commissiononhealth.org/PDF/e6244e9e-f630-4285-9ad7-16016dd7e493/Issue%20Brief%202%20Sept%2008%20-%20Housing%20and%20Health.pdf

Rural Health Information Hub. (2014). *Frequently asked questions: What are barriers to healthcare access in rural areas?* Retrieved from https://www.ruralhealthinfo.org/topics/healthcare-access#faqs

Rural Health Information Hub. (2015). *Community vitality and rural healthcare.* Retrieved from https://www.ruralhealthinfo.org/topics/community-vitality-and-rural-healthcare

Rural Health Research Centers at the Universities of Minnesota, North Carolina-Chapel Hill, and Southern Maine. (2015). Critical access hospital locations. Retrieved from http://www.flexmonitoring.org/data/critical-access-hospital-locations/

Singh, G. K., & Siahpush, M. (2014). Widening rural-urban disparities in life expectancy, U.S., 1969–2009. *American Journal of Preventive Medicine, 46*(2), e19–e29.

Stone, C., Trisi, D., Sherman, A., & Horton, E. (2015). *A guide to statistics on historical trends in income inequality.* Washington, DC: Center on Budget and Policy Priorities. Retrieved from http://www.cbpp.org/research/poverty-and-inequality/a-guide-to-statistics-on-historical-trends-in-income-inequality

U.S. Census Bureau. (2010). 2010 census urban and rural classification and urban area criteria. Retrieved from https://www.census.gov/geo/reference/ua/urban-rural-2010.html

U.S. Census Bureau. (2015a). *Income and poverty in the United States: 2014.* Retrieved from http://www.census.gov/library/publications/2015/demo/p60-252.html

U.S. Census Bureau. (2015b). Ten U.S. cities now have 1 million people or more; California and Texas each have three of these places. Retrieved from http://www.census.gov/newsroom/press-releases/2015/cb15-89.html

U.S. Census Bureau, Housing and Household Economic Statistics Division. (2015). Poverty thresholds. Retrieved from https://www.census.gov/hhes/www/poverty/methods/definitions.html

U.S. Department of Agriculture, Economic Research Service. (2015). Farm labor. Retrieved from http://www.ers.usda.gov/topics/farm-economy/farm-labor/background.aspx

U.S. Department of Health and Human Services, Office of Disease Prevention and Health Promotion. (n.d.). *Healthy People 2020.* Retrieved from https://www.healthypeople.gov

World Health Organization. (2014). Ambient (outdoor) air quality and health (Fact sheet no. 313). Retrieved from http://www.who.int/mediacentre/factsheets/fs313/en/

Nursing in the Global Health Community

Mary E. Riner and Barbara deRose

LEARNING OUTCOMES

After reading this chapter you will be able to:

- Describe the impact of globalization on health.
- Examine issues of the global burden of disease.
- Identify global health issues related to women's, children, and adolescents' health.
- Explore the impact of communicable and noncommunicable diseases globally.
- Describe the goals of the Human Resources for Health Approach to Universal Health Care Access.
- Describe issues related to global health security.
- Analyze issues related to the global nursing workforce, including ethical international recruitment of health professionals.
- Describe trends in education of the future nursing workforce.
- Examine international career and advocacy opportunities for nurses.

Introduction

In our current stage of global evolution, people are connected to each other across time and location in ever increasing ways. Internet connectivity allows us to know about and engage in political, humanitarian, and economic events in real time. People cross country borders permanently when they migrate due to personal choice or personal safety concerns or temporarily when they move for education, career, and personal travel. This connectivity calls for us to develop ethical, political, and social practices that promote civility and allow us to live peacefully in the midst of diversity. It implies engaging in global social responsibility that requires a shift from a local personal perspective to being a **global citizen**. Nurses are members of the global health community and being well prepared with knowledge of global health threats and systems allows us to participate in improving the health of people worldwide.

> **KEY TERM**
>
> **Global citizen:** Someone who identifies with being part of an emerging world community and whose actions contributed to building this community's values and practices (Global Citizen Initiative, n.d.).

The purpose of this chapter is to describe globalization and its impact on health, with a specific focus on global health issues related to the health of women, children, and adolescents. The global existence of various communicable and noncommunicable diseases is discussed, as well as the issues related to containing the spread of communicable diseases through global health security measures. The chapter also describes issues related to the global nursing workforce including the ethical implications of the international recruitment of nurses. The chapter ends with a discussion of what it means to internationalize the curriculum and explores the international career opportunities available to nurses.

Globalization

> **KEY TERM**
>
> **Globalization:** Increased interconnections among people of different countries that facilitate the exchange of goods, services, money, people, information, and ideas across national borders.

To understand issues related to nursing in the global health community, it is important to first explore the concept of globalization. **Globalization** from a multisectoral perspective refers "to the interconnectedness of countries through cross-border flows of goods, services, money, people, information, and ideas, the increasing openness of countries to such flows, and the development of international rules and institutions dealing with cross-border flows" (McMichael & Beaglehole, 2009, p. 9). This involves collaboration and cooperation as countries find effective ways to achieve mutual goals.

> **KEY TERM**
>
> **Global health:** Focuses on improving health of populations and promoting equity for all people regardless of national borders.

Global Health

Global health considers the health of populations in the global context and transcends a focus on country-level health problems that require **bilateral cooperation** to address, which is considered

> **KEY TERM**
>
> **Bilateral cooperation:** Refers to political, economic, or cultural relations between two sovereign states.

international health. In an attempt to establish a common definition of global health, the executive board of the Consortium of Universities for Global Health describes it as "the area of study, research, and practice that places a priority on improving health and achieving equity in health for all people worldwide" (Koplan et al., 2009, p. 1994). As such, "global health is about the improvement of health worldwide, the reduction of disparities, and protection of societies against global threats that disregard national borders" (Macfarlane, Jacobs, & Kaaya, 2008, p. 383). This includes threats to infectious disease outbreaks, societal threats from human-disasters including war and genocide, and threats to our environment. **Table 19-1** shows key dimensions of global health from multiple perspectives. Examples of globalization of health care include migration of nurses to other countries, mobility of people travelling abroad for health care, telehealth, and increase in private companies that provide health care to employees (World Health Organization [WHO], 2013).

Global Health, Illness, and Injury

Global Burden of Disease

The leading causes of death globally center on noncommunicable diseases, or what is often referred to as chronic disease. **Figure 19-1** shows the leading causes of death globally. The **global burden of disease (GBD)** index was developed by WHO in the early 1990s as a way to describe global health problems, identify trends, and help decision makers set priorities. It combines several health measures that identify diseases,

> **KEY TERM**
>
> **Global burden of disease (GBD):** Index that measures the loss of health from all causes of illness and deaths worldwide.

TABLE 19-1 DIMENSIONS OF GLOBAL HEALTH	
Dimension	Description
Geographical reach	Focuses on issues that directly or indirectly affect health but that can transcend national boundaries
Level of cooperation	Development and implementation of solutions often requires global cooperation
Individuals or populations	Embraces both prevention in populations and clinical care of individuals
Access to health	Health equity among nations and for all people is a major objective

Data from Koplan, J., Bond, D., Merson, M., Rodriquez, M., Sewankambo, N., & Wasserheit, J. (2009). Toward a common definition of global health. *Lancet, 373*, 1993–1995.

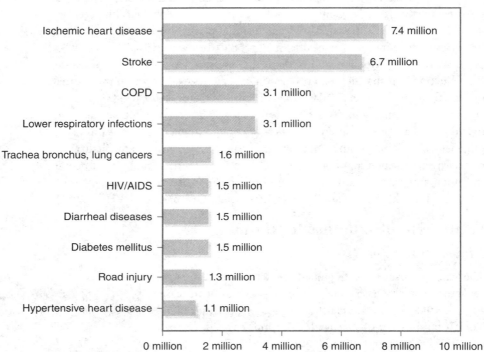

Figure 19-1 The 10 leading causes of death in the world.

Reproduced from World Health Organization. (2014c). The 10 leading causes of death in the world. Retrieved from http://www.who.int/mediacentre/factsheets/fs310/en/. Copyright 2014.

injuries, and risk factors in causing premature death, loss of health, and disability in different populations (WHO, n.d.-d). By using GBD information, countries can develop policies and budgets to guide the establishment of their health agenda.

Measure of Global Burden of Disease

An important measure of burden of disease is the **disability-adjusted life year (DALY)**. The DALY indicator assesses the burden of disease consistently across diseases, risk factors, and regions. DALYs are a measure of the years of healthy life lost due to ill health, disability, or premature death. They estimate the gap between current health status and an ideal health status, with the entire population living to an advanced age free of disease and disability. **Years of life lost (YLL)** is an estimate of the

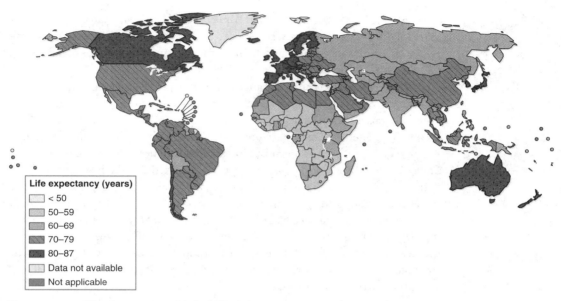

Figure 19-2 Life expectancy at birth, both sexes.

number of years a person has lost because of premature death—as a measure of
the ill health of a population (WHO, n.d.-b). These terms are used throughout the
chapter to describe the impact of various health conditions.

Life Expectancy

Life expectancy at birth varies among countries and across regions of the globe.
Understanding of the variance needs to be framed within the perspective of population development, country health priorities, and resources and current lifestyle
practices. Since 1990, life expectancy at birth has increased globally by 6 years. "A
baby born in 2012 could expect to live to 70 years on average—62 years in low-
income countries to 79 years in high-income countries (WHO, 2014a, para. 1).
Figure 19-2 shows the difference in life expectancy by country. Life expectancy
at birth is based on the death rates across all age groups in a population in a given
year—children and adolescents, adults, and the elderly.

Women's, Children's, and Adolescents' Health

Childbearing women and children are particularly vulnerable to poor health outcomes and mortality due to these stages of life. Recently the United Nations (UN)
developed work in this area and believes no woman, child, or adolescent should
face a greater risk of preventable death because of where they live or who they are

(UN, 2015). The *Global Strategy for Women's, Children's and Adolescents' Health (2016–2030)* aims to transform societies so that women, children, and adolescents everywhere can realize their rights to the highest attainable standards of health and well-being (UN, 2015).

The *Global Strategy* is universal and applies to all people (including marginalized and hard to reach), in all places (including crisis situations), and to translational issues. It focuses on safeguarding women, children, and adolescents in humanitarian and fragile settings and upholding their human rights to the highest attainable standard of health, even in the most difficult circumstances. The 2030 Vision of the *Global Strategy* is "a world in which every woman, child and adolescent in every setting realizes their rights to physical and mental health and well-being, has social and economic opportunities, and is able to participate fully in shaping prosperous and sustainable societies" (UN, 2015, p. 8). The *Global Strategy* takes a life-course approach that recognizes a person's health at each stage of life affects future health and has cumulative effects for the next generation. The *Global Strategy* adopts an integrated and multisectoral approach, recognizing that health-enhancing factors including nutrition, education, water, clean air, sanitation, hygiene, and infrastructure are essential for achieving the sustainable development goals (SDGs). It is important to note the creators of the *Global Strategy* relied on evidence-based interventions in developing their 2016–2030 recommendations.

Maternal Health

Maternal mortality is a health indicator that shows wide gaps between rich and poor, both between and within countries. "Maternal mortality is unacceptably high. About 830 women die from pregnancy- or childbirth-related complications around the world every day. By the end of 2015, roughly 303,000 women will have died during and following pregnancy and childbirth. Almost all of these deaths occurred in low-resource settings, and most could have been prevented. . . . as the healthcare solutions to prevent or manage complications are well known" (WHO, 2015c, para. 2).

All women need access to antenatal care in pregnancy, skilled care during childbirth, and care and support in the weeks after childbirth. Information collected by the WHO (2015c) reveals that "the major complications that account for nearly 75% of all maternal deaths are: severe bleeding (mostly bleeding after childbirth), infections (usually after childbirth), high blood pressure during pregnancy (pre-eclampsia and eclampsia), complications from delivery, [and] unsafe abortion" (para. 9).

Children's Health

Child morality is an important measure of health and development. Every year, approximately 6.6 million children who are under the age of 5 die (WHO, 2014a). **Figures 19-3** and **19-4** show differences in under-5 mortality rates by country in

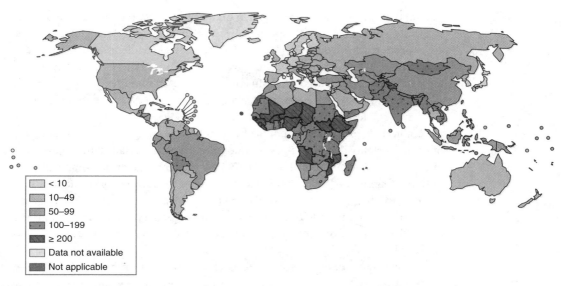

Figure 19-3 Under-5 mortality rate (probability of dying by age 5 per 1,000 live births), 1990.

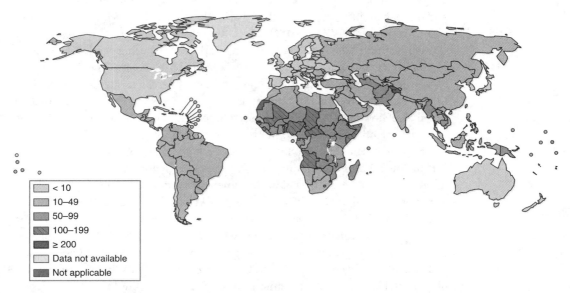

Figure 19-4 Under-5 mortality rate (probability of dying by age 5 per 1,000 live births), 2015.

1990 and 2015. Decreases since 2000 in under-5 mortality rates are accelerating in many developing countries, especially in sub-Saharan Africa. The global political collaboration achieved in 2000 by establishing the eight Millennium Development Goals (MDGs) for reducing extreme poverty and increased development assistance for health might have been a factor in faster decreases in some developing countries. Without further accelerated progress, many countries in west and central Africa will still have high levels of under-5 mortality in 2030 (Wang et al., 2014).

Remarkable financial and political efforts have been focused on the reduction of child mortality during the past few decades. Using a human rights approach to improving the welfare of children, UNICEF—the UN's agency for supporting the welfare of children—has identified key strategies for future work. The top three priorities of their *2015–2030 Agenda for #EVERYChild* are to end violence against children; put ending child poverty at the center of global poverty eradication; and renew the global efforts to end preventable newborn, child, and maternal deaths (UNICEF, 2015).

According to data compiled by WHO (2015c) on newborn outcomes, "Approximately 2.7 million newborn babies die every year and an additional 2.6 million are stillborn" (para. 10). Preterm birth is the leading killer of newborn babies worldwide. Every year, approximately 15 million babies (about 1 in 10 babies) are born preterm—born alive before 37 weeks of pregnancy (WHO, 2015f). Preterm birth complications cause more than 1 million deaths each year, and more than three quarters of these babies' lives could be saved with simple and cost-effective care (WHO, 2015f).

Bahl et al. (2012) identified key research priorities for reducing the global incidence of mortality from preterm and low-birth-weight (LBW) babies. The first category of priorities focused on health systems and policy research questions, including how to identify LBW infants born at home within 24–48 hours of birth for additional care; how to develop approaches to improve quality of care of LBW infants in health facilities; and how to improve access to hospital care for LBW infants, among others. These were followed by research priorities for improvement of the existing interventions, including how to promote early initiation of breastfeeding; improved cord care, such as chlorhexidine application; and alternative methods to Kangaroo Mother Care (KMC) to keep LBW infants warm in community settings. The highest ranked epidemiologic question suggested improving criteria for identifying LBW infants who need to be cared for in a hospital. Among the new interventions, the greatest support was shown for the development of new simple and effective interventions for providing thermal care to LBW infants, if KMC is not acceptable to the mother. **Contemporary Practice Highlight 19-1** provides an example of how advancing the educational preparation of the nursing workforce can lead to increased healthcare status of infants through the introduction of an evidence-based approach to newborn resuscitation.

INCREASING NURSING EDUCATION TO HELP BABIES BREATHE

As a very low-income country with a high rate of infant mortality, Liberia faces challenges in producing an adequate supply of well-prepared nurses and midwives. The Tubman National Institute of Medical Arts (TNIMA) at the John F. Kennedy Medical Center is the country's main educator of nurses and midwives. In order to advance the preparation of faculty, two educators received funding from the U.S. Agency for International Development (USAID) to obtain master's degrees in nursing education at Indiana University. After completing the coursework in the United States, they returned to Monrovia to complete their research study and teaching practicum. As newly certified instructors of the Helping Babies Breathe neonatal resuscitation program, they taught students, nurses, and midwives and demonstrated knowledge and skill gains among those who participated in the program.

Subsequently, in another initiative to continue building the nurse and midwife educator workforce in Liberia and ultimately decreasing the infant mortality rate, the Clinton Health Access Initiative received funding from the World Bank to enable five nursing schools to hire more faculty. This is expected to increase the number of graduates going into the nursing workforce.

Data from Bondoe, C., Wraynee, A. B., Riner, M. E., Allam, E., & Stephenson, E. (2014). Helping babies breathe: Providing an evidence-based education intervention at a tertiary referral hospital in Liberia. *Journal of Nursing Education and Practice, 4*(9), 119-127.

Adolescent Health

Based on epidemiology trend data from WHO (n.d.-b), in 2012 an estimated 1.3 million adolescents died, down from 1.5 million in 2000. The mortality rate decreased from 126 to 111 per 100,000 between 2000 and 2012. This modest decline of about 12 percent, which can be attributed to decreased AIDS mortality, continues the trend of the past 50 years. Mortality rates dropped in all regions and for all age groups except 15- to 19-year-old males in the eastern Mediterranean and the Americas regions. The leading causes of death among adolescents in 2012 were road injury, HIV, suicide, lower respiratory infections, and interpersonal violence. There are two important differences from the 2000 mortality data. HIV-related deaths have more than tripled since 2000, making it the second highest cause of mortality among adolescents. In contrast, in 2000 HIV was not even among the top 10 causes of death.

There were few significant changes in the top five causes of years lived with a disability (YLD) between 2000 and 2012, and the commonalities across regions and between high-income countries and low- and middle-income countries remain. The top five ranked causes of YLDs in 10- to 14-year-olds are unipolar depressive disorders, iron-deficiency anemia, asthma, back and neck pain, and anxiety disorders. They are similar for 15- to 19-year-olds except asthma is replaced by alcohol use disorders, the second highest cause of YLDs in 15- to 19-year-old males. These conditions are responsible for nearly 50 percent of YLDs in adolescents 10–19 years (WHO, n.d.-b).

Between 2000 and 2012 overall DALYs for adolescents decreased from 165 to 152 per 1000 population, or 8 percent, less than half of the 17 percent decline overall for all age groups. The major causes of DALYs changed little between 2000 and 2012 (WHO, n.d.-b). In 2012, depression, road injuries, iron-deficiency anemia, HIV, and intentional self-harm were the top five global causes of DALYs for adolescents. The one notable change from 2000 was that HIV ranked fourth among causes of DALYs in 2012. In 2000 it was not among the top 10. Many adolescents have health problems that require serious attention from the health sector, particularly because many conditions and behaviors that start or are reinforced during adolescence affect health across the life course.

Communicable Diseases

Communicable diseases spread from one person to another or from an animal to a person or another type of vector. The spread often happens via airborne viruses or bacteria but also through blood or other bodily fluid.

Hepatitis

Viral hepatitis is a group of infections referred to as hepatitis A, B, C, D, and E. It is a major global health challenge with nearly 400 million people living with chronic hepatitis B or C infection. It causes roughly 80 percent of liver cancers (Centers for Disease Control and Prevention [CDC], 2016b). It is responsible for more than 1 million deaths annually, mostly in low- and middle-income countries, with the highest prevalence of disease in sub-Saharan Africa and East Asia, where between 5 and 10 percent of the adult population is chronically infected.

HIV/AIDS

More than 35 million people worldwide are living with HIV (CDC, 2016a). Around 70 percent of all HIV/AIDS deaths in 2012 occurred in sub-Saharan Africa. Globally, the number of people dying from AIDS-related causes is steadily decreasing from a peak of 2.3 million deaths in 2005 to an estimated 1.6 million in 2012. With over 60 years of expertise in preventing and fighting diseases, the CDC continues to play a critical role in helping ministries of health in 60 partner countries build strong, sustainable programs that respond effectively to the HIV/AIDS epidemic. This work is supported by the U.S. President's Emergency Plan for AIDS Relief (PEPFAR). Research shows that three key prevention interventions can dramatically drive down the rate of new infections. They include antiretroviral treatment of HIV-positive persons, preventing mother-to-child transmission of HIV, and expanding voluntary medical male circumcision (CDC, 2016a).

Malaria

"In 2012, an estimated 627,000 people died of malaria—most were young children in sub-Saharan Africa" (CDC, n.d., para. 1). Within the last decade, increasing numbers of partners and resources have rapidly increased malaria control efforts. This scale-up of interventions has saved 3.3 million lives globally and cut malaria mortality by 45 percent, leading to hopes and plans for elimination and ultimately eradication. Malaria has the largest impact in Africa, where it has been extremely difficult to control (CDC, n.d.). Many reasons account for this: an efficient mosquito that transmits the infection, a high prevalence of the most deadly species of the parasite, favorable climate, weak infrastructure to address the disease, and high intervention costs that are difficult to bear in poor countries. The focus areas involved in combating malaria include public health information, science and research, prevention and control, case management, and regulating diagnostic tests and vaccines.

Tuberculosis

According to the WHO (2015b) "worldwide, 9.6 million people are estimated to have fallen ill with TB in 2014: 5.4 million men, 3.2 million women and 1.0 million children. Globally, 12% of the 9.6 million new TB cases in 2014 were HIV-positive" (p. 1). The WHO (2015b) also notes that "TB mortality has fallen 47% since 1990, with nearly all of that improvement taking place since 2000. . . In all, effective diagnosis and treatment of TB saved an estimated 43 million lives between 2000 and 2014. . . Globally, TB incidence has fallen by an average of 1.5% per year since 2000 and is now 18% lower than the level of 2000" (p. 1).

Community engagement is critical to improve the reach and sustainability of interventions related to tuberculosis (TB) and to help end TB. ENGAGE-TB—an innovative community engagement approach—was created by the WHO in 2012. Its purpose is "to better identify and treat people with TB, by involving previously unengaged nongovernmental organizations (NGOs) and other civil society organizations (SCOs). This includes a wide spectrum of community-based organizations working in primary health care, HIV, maternal and child health, education, agriculture, and livelihood initiatives" (WHO, 2015a, p. ii).

Neglected Tropical Diseases

Neglected tropical diseases (NTDs) are a diverse group of communicable diseases that prevail in tropical and subtropical conditions in 149 countries and affect more than 1 billion people, costing developing economies billions of dollars every year (CDC, 2011b). They mainly affect populations living in poverty, without adequate sanitation, and in close contact with infectious vectors and domestic animals and livestock. Some of these diseases include lymphatic filariasis, onchocerciasis, schistosomiasis, and soil-transmitted helminths such as hookworm, trachoma, and yaws. These six infections "can be controlled or even eliminated through mass administration of safe and effective medicines (mass drug administration, MDA), or other effective interventions. These diseases are known as targeted or 'tool-ready' NTDs. Along with MDA and interventions, efforts to control the vectors (e.g., mosquitoes, black flies) that transmit these diseases and improve basic water, sanitation, and hygiene are highly effective strategies against these NTDs" (CDC, 2011b, para. 1). The CDC (2011b) also notes that at the low cost of 10–50 cents per person per year, MDA-based programs are inexpensive but have an enormous benefit of helping treat or prevent several different diseases.

Noncommunicable Diseases

Chronic, noncommunicable diseases (NCDs) are the number one cause of death and disability in the world. The term NCDs refers to a group of conditions that are not mainly caused by an acute infection, result in long-term health consequences, and often create a need for long-term treatment and care. These conditions include cancers, cardiovascular disease, diabetes, and chronic lung illnesses.

All age groups and all regions of the world are affected by NCDs. NCDs are often associated with older age groups, but "evidence shows that 16 million of all deaths attributed to noncommunicable diseases (NCDs) occur before the age of 70. Of these 'premature' deaths, 82 percent occurred in low- and middle-income countries" (WHO, 2015e, para. 3). Many NCDs can be prevented by reducing common risk factors such as tobacco use, harmful alcohol use, physical inactivity, and eating unhealthy diets. Many other important conditions are also considered NCDs, including injuries and mental health disorders. The following sections identify some of the most prevalent NCDs in the world.

Cardiovascular Disease

Cardiovascular diseases are the leading causes of death in the world. "Around 3 in 10 deaths globally are caused by cardiovascular diseases. At least 80 percent of premature deaths from cardiovascular diseases could be prevented through a healthy diet, regular physical activity, and avoidance of tobacco" (WHO, 2014a, para. 4).

Mental Health

Mental disorders include depression, bipolar affective disorder, schizophrenia, and other psychoses, dementia, intellectual disabilities, and developmental disorders including autism. Depression is one of the 20 leading causes of disability world-wide, affecting around 300 million people worldwide (WHO, 2014a). Mild to moderate depression can be effectively treated with talking therapies, such as cognitive behavior therapy or psychotherapy. Antidepressants can be an effective form of treatment for moderate to severe depression but are not the first line of treatment for cases of mild depression.

Tobacco

"Tobacco kills nearly 6 million people each year. More than 5 million of those deaths are the result of direct tobacco use whereas more than 600,000 are the result of nonsmokers being exposed to secondhand smoke. Unless urgent action is taken, the annual death toll could rise to more than 8 million by 2030" (WHO, 2014a, para. 8).

Diabetes

"Almost 1 in 10 adults has diabetes. Almost 10 percent of the world's adult popu-lation has diabetes, measured by elevated fasting blood glucose ($\geq$ 126 mg/dl). People with diabetes have increased risk of heart disease and stroke. Deaths due to diabetes have been increasing since the year 2000, reaching 1.5 million deaths in 2012" (WHO, 2014a, para. 9).

Traffic Accidents

"Nearly 3,500 people die from road traffic crashes every day. Road traffic injuries are projected to rise as vehicle ownership increases due to economic growth in develop-ing countries. Strong action to improve road-use policies and enforce road-safety laws is needed to avert this rise in injuries and deaths" (WHO, 2014a, para. 10).

Disabilities

Disabilities affect people of all age groups, all demographics, and in all regions and countries. An estimated 15 percent of the world's population, or 110–190 people worldwide, experience at least one disability (WHO, 2011). Half of people with disabilities cannot afford health care and are at a higher risk of being exposed to violence (CDC, 2011a). The Convention on the Rights of Persons with Disabilities is an international agreement that will help ensure equality and participation in society of people with disabilities. To date, more than 130 countries have ratified this treaty.

A Call for Universal Healthcare Coverage

Through the Patient Protection and Affordable Care Act (PPACA) established in 2010, the United States adopted a policy strategy to increase healthcare coverage of residents in order to reduce the number of people who delay or do not receive needed treatment. This can help to address disparities in health among racial and income groups. Although the PPACA increases the number of individuals in the United States population with insurance coverage, it is not yet universal healthcare coverage, a strategy adopted by many countries and promoted by the WHO. In 2015, Margaret Chan, director-general of the WHO, described universal health coverage as "one of the most powerful social equalizers among all policy options. . .the ultimate expression of fairness" (Chan, 2015, para. 24).

The goal of universal healthcare coverage is to ensure **universal healthcare access** (WHO, 2014d). For a community or country to achieve universal healthcare coverage, several factors must be in place: a strong, efficient, well-run health system; affordable services; access to essential medicines and technologies to diagnose and treat medical problems; and a sufficient capacity of well-trained, motivated health workers (WHO, 2014d).

> **KEY TERM**
>
> **Universal healthcare access:** Has three components: physical accessibility in terms of being able to reach services, financial affordability in terms of not causing financial hardship, and acceptability to those seeking services (WHO, 2014d).

> **KEY TERM**
>
> **Health:** "A state of complete physical, mental, and social well-being, and not merely the absence of disease or infirmity, is a fundamental human right, and that the attainment of the highest possible level of health is a most important world-wide social goal whose realization requires the action of many other social and economic sectors in addition to the health sector" (WHO, 1978, p. 1).

Health for All

Universal health coverage is firmly based on the WHO constitution of 1948 that declared health a fundamental human right in the Alma-Ata Declaration. The Health for All agenda was established in the 1970s as the basis for the WHO's primary healthcare strategy to promote **health**, human dignity, and enhanced quality of life. Both the Declaration and the Health for All agenda have been widely used globally to advance a health promotion agenda.

Health Equity

Equity is paramount in the declaration. WHO defines equity as the absence of avoidable or remediable differences among groups of people, whether those groups are defined socially, economically, demographically, or geographically (WHO, n.d.-c). **Health equity** requires valuing everyone equally with focused and ongoing societal efforts to address avoidable inequalities, historical and contemporary injustices, and the elimination of health and healthcare disparities.

> **KEY TERM**
>
> **Health equity:** "The attainment of the highest level of health for all people" (U.S. Department of Health and Human Services, n.d., para. 5).

Progress in Human Rights Approach to Health

The 1978 Alma-Ata Declaration has had far-reaching influence. Recent work by the UN, the parent organization of the WHO, specifically notes how this human rights-based approach to health has been included in numerous global, regional, and national treaties and constrictions since 1978. Members of a UN System Task Team described a human rights approach to health as a progressive realization of civil, cultural, and political as well as economic and social rights as prerequisite for sustainable growth and human development of individuals, families, and societies (UN, 2012).

Sustainable Development Goals

Ensuring the availability of an appropriately prepared nursing workforce is an issue of importance within the global community, not just the nursing profession. Nurses have a key role to play in multiprofessional and interdisciplinary health teams. The work of nurses has been highlighted as one of the important factors to achieving the SDGs set for 2030 by the UN General Assembly to replace the MDGs. The eight original MDGs were an agreed-upon set of goals for improving the health and well-being of the global population that could be achieved if all countries worked together. Four of the MDGs focused specifically on health and included eradicating extreme poverty and hunger; reducing child mortality; improving maternal health; and combating HIV/AIDS, malaria, and other diseases.

By the set date of 2015, progress toward the MDGs had been made in reducing HIV, TB and malaria epidemics, child and maternal mortality, and access to safe drinking water, but still fell short of MDG targets. The SDG agenda is composed of 17 goals and has expanded to 169 targets, including an umbrella health target (SDG 3) that was built upon the unfinished business of the MDGs. The overarching message of SDG 3 is to ensure healthy lives and promote well-being at all ages. New health targets in SDG 3 address mental health, substance abuse, deaths and injuries from traffic accidents and hazardous chemicals, reproduction health, and universal health coverage. The agenda also addresses four means of implementation targets: WHO Framework Convention on Tobacco Control; research and development on vaccines and medications for communicable and NCDs; increasing health workforce in developing countries; and strengthening the capacity for early warning, risk reduction, and management of health risks (see **Box 19-1**).

Although SDG 3 is the main area for health-focused targets, many other non-health goals are considered health related and include health considerations when designing implementation strategies. In moving the agenda forward, the nursing profession will be called upon to build capacity and provide nursing research in monitoring the process, maintaining health systems, and supporting public engagement to achieve SDG goals (WHO, 2015g).

Universal Health System Components and Dimensions

Three key components comprise a universal healthcare system. They include the most basic level of care that is generally provided at a community level and involves primary care for the prevention and early intervention of health condition. Acute

BOX 19-1   ENSURE HEALTHY LIVES AND PROMOTE WELL-BEING FOR ALL AT ALL AGES—SUSTAINABLE DEVELOPMENT GOAL 3

- By 2030, reduce the global maternal mortality ratio to less than 70 per 100,000 live births.
- By 2030, end preventable deaths of newborns and children under 5 years of age, with all countries aiming to reduce neonatal mortality to at least as low as 12 per 1000 live births and under-5 mortality to at least as low as 25 per 1000 live births.
- By 2030, end the epidemics of AIDS, tuberculosis, malaria, and neglected tropical diseases and combat hepatitis, waterborne diseases, and other communicable diseases.
- By 2030, reduce by one-third premature mortality from noncommunicable diseases through prevention and treatment and promote mental health and well-being.
- Strengthen the prevention and treatment of substance abuse, including narcotic drug abuse and harmful use of alcohol.
- By 2020, halve the number of global deaths and injuries from road traffic accidents.
- By 2030, ensure universal access to sexual and reproductive healthcare services, including for family planning, information, and education and the integration of reproductive health into national strategies and programmes.
- Achieve universal health coverage, including financial risk protection, access to high-quality essential healthcare services and access to safe, effective, high-quality, and affordable essential medicines and vaccines for all.
- By 2030, substantially reduce the number of deaths and illnesses from hazardous chemicals and air, water, and soil pollution and contamination.
- Strengthen the implementation of the World Health Organization Framework Convention on Tobacco Control in all countries, as appropriate.
- Support the research and development of vaccines and medicines for the communicable and noncommunicable diseases that primarily affect developing countries, provide access to affordable essential medicines and vaccines, in accordance with the Doha Declaration on the TRIPS Agreement and Public Health, which affirms the right of developing countries to use to the full the provisions in the Agreement on Trade-Related Aspects of Intellectual Property Rights regarding flexibilities to protect public health, and, in particular, provide access to medicines for all.
- Substantially increase health financing and the recruitment, development, training, and retention of the health workforce in developing countries, especially in least-developed countries and small island developing states.
- Strengthen the capacity of all countries, in particular developing countries, for early warning, risk reduction and management of national and global health risks.

Reproduced from United Nations. (n.d.). Sustainable development goals: 17 goals to transform our world. Goal 3: Ensure healthy lives and promote well-being for all at all ages. Retrieved from http://www.un.org/sustainabledevelopment/health/. © United Nations. Reprinted with the permission of the United Nations.

care is generally provided in hospitals and specialty facilities where surgery is performed and care is managed for acute conditions. The public health level focuses on populations either with specific conditions or for geographically defined populations. Its aim is prevention and early detection.

Primary Care

As a foundation, "primary health care connects people and families with trusted health workers and supportive systems throughout their lives and provides access to services ranging from family planning and routine immunizations to treatment of illness and management of chronic conditions" (WHO, 2015d, para. 6). According to the WHO (2015d) "health systems built on strong primary health care are more resilient, efficient, and equitable" (para. 6). However, primary health care is often considered a weakness of health systems. The WHO (2015d) estimates that "more than 400 million people worldwide lack access to essential health services typically delivered through primary health care" (para. 8). Primary health care is fundamental in the prevention of epidemics, improvement of health of women and children; control of infectious diseases, and management of the rise of NCDs (WHO, 2015d).

In 2015, the Bill & Melinda Gates Foundation, World Bank Group, and the WHO partnered in an effort to assist with the improvement of primary health care around the world. The Primary Health Care Performance Initiative (PHCPI) is designed to "support countries to strengthen monitoring, tracking, and sharing of key performance indicators for primary health care" (WHO, 2015d, para. 2).

Acute Care

As the global community shifts to meet the challenge of universal health care, investing in hospitals and their performance will play a key role in success (Lewis, 2015). Reaching the expectations of universal health coverage requires renewed efforts to upgrade and strengthen hospital investments and to promote the integration of patient care across levels of care. The lack of investment and modernization of hospitals—whether in physical plant infrastructure or management systems—over the past few decades has severely impaired the potential of many expensive inpatient institutions.

Public Health

The third leg of the healthcare system stool is the public health system. Generally the responsibility of official government units, public health focuses on populations, prevention and control of illness, diseases, and injury. This work often includes early detection of outbreaks of diseases such as Ebola, early intervention in controlling spread, and reduction of harm to the population. Understanding health systems at the national and even community level is an important aspect of global health.

To be able to compare and contrast allows us to understand health systems within the context of policies, financing, distribution, service delivery, and the outcomes yielded.

Global Health Security

In a globalized world, diseases can spread rapidly across great distances via international travel and trade. A health crisis in one country can affect livelihoods and economies in many parts of the world. Such crises can result from emerging infections such as severe acute respiratory syndrome (SARS) or a new human influenza pandemic.

International Health Regulations

International health regulations have evolved in order to protect individuals and populations from widespread exposure to communicable diseases. An international legal instrument known as the International Health Regulations (IHR) is considered binding for the 196 countries across the globe who are WHO Member States. The IHR is a legal framework whose purpose is to "prevent, protect against, control and provide a public health response to the international spread of disease in ways that are commensurate with and restricted to public health risks, and which avoid unnecessary interference with international traffic and trade" (WHO, n.d.-a). The IHR calls for a multisectoral approach as most international health threats require involvement of many governmental and private community groups to cooperate, such as security, transportation, businesses, and education.

In the United States, the CDC's Global Health Security Branch (GHSB) is the agency's lead engagement office for partnerships with other U.S. government entities, multilateral institutes, and international organizations in aiding countries to achieve global health security. GHSB collaborates with the U.S. Department of State (DoS) and the U.S. Department of Defense (DoD) on global health diplomacy and biosecurity issues. It also implements CDC's strategy for Global All-Hazard Emergency Preparedness and Response and addresses concerns with international terrorism and emergency preparedness and response. Major projects within GHSB include international influenza outbreaks, biological threat reduction, and emerging pandemic threats (U.S. Department of Health and Human Services [USDHHS], n.d.). **Contemporary Practice Highlight 19-2** provides an exemplar of how nurses can engage in research in collaboration with federal agencies to address global healthcare issues.

Health Diplomacy

Global health diplomacy brings together the disciplines of public health, international affairs, management, law, and economics and focuses on negotiations that shape and manage the global policy environment for health. The relationship between

CONTEMPORARY PRACTICE HIGHLIGHT 19-2

NURSE ENGAGES IN EBOLA SURVIVOR RESEARCH

After completing her master's degree in nursing at a U.S. school of nursing, Ms. Brown, a nurse–midwife educator, returned to Liberia just in time to be faced with the Ebola virus disease (EVD) devastating the population. When the CDC established a research unit at her hospital, she signed on as the research nurse for studies on EVD, including survivor studies. One study conducted in Liberia looked at how the use of two different drugs as recommended malaria treatment for patients with suspected Ebola virus disease affected survival. They found patients who were prescribed artesunate–amodiaquine had a lower risk of death from EVD than did patients who were prescribed artemether–lumefantrine.

For more information on EVD, see Gignoux, E., Azman, A. S., de Smet, M., Azuma, P., Massaquoi, M., Job, D., . . . Ciglenecki, I. (2016). Effect of artesunate–amodiaquine on mortality related to Ebola virus disease. *New England Journal of Medicine, 374*, 23–32. doi: 10.1056/NEJMoa1504605

health, foreign policy, and trade is at the cutting edge of global health diplomacy. The goals of the WHO unit responsible for global health diplomacy include supporting the development of a more systematic and proactive approach to identify and understand key current and future changes affecting global public health and building capacity among Member States to support the necessary collective action to take advantage of opportunities and mitigate the risks for health (WHO, n.d.-a).

Nationally, advancing health diplomacy is one of the objectives of the USDHHS's Global Health Strategy, which is to "engage directly with diplomatic partners, and strengthen peer-to-peer technical, public health, and scientific relationships" (USDHHS, n.d., para. 1).

Health diplomacy efforts carried out by USDHHS can often transcend diplomatic challenges and enable the U.S. government to maintain strong and mutually beneficial ties to other countries. In cases where more traditional diplomatic relationships may be strained, USDHHS health diplomacy activities can help continue relationships with governments at a nonpolitical level or foster dialogue and develop new partnerships with academic institutions, NGOs, and civil society.

Global Nursing Workforce

The International Council of Nurses (ICN, n.d.) estimates that there may be more than 12 million nurses worldwide. According to WHO, an estimated 35 million nurse and midwives make up the greater part of the global healthcare workforce (WHO, 2009). Nurses and midwives make a substantial contribution to health delivery systems in primary, acute, and community care settings.

Definitions and Description of Practice

A common description of the practice of nursing by the ICN is provided in **Box 19-2.** It is not binding but attempts to identify common aspects of nursing found in countries around the world. The success of nursing and midwifery graduates is measured through qualification for licensure; performance assessment; delivery of safe, high-quality care; feedback from consumers, employers, and stakeholders; team collaboration; partnerships to address global health needs on a local level; and the individual's career progression and advancement (e.g., seeking advance degrees, publications, presentations, and funded research) (ICN, n.d.).

Workforce

Understanding organizational and policy workforce issues allows us to appreciate the enormous challenges faced by many countries in ensuring access to universal health coverage across different economic resources, cultures, and orientation to the design, delivery, and financing of services. In the report, *A Universal Truth: No Health Without a Workforce*, the Global Health Workforce Alliance declares that at the center of every health system are health workers with the knowledge, skills, and motivation to deliver the services (Campbell et al., 2013). Many countries are grappling with human resource health policy challenges, such as how to address shortages or surpluses and how to improve the skills, geographic distribution, and performance of health workers.

Supply, Demand, and Distribution

Understanding healthcare workforce distribution issues is important for nurse administrators. It allows for ensuring effective resource development for educating nurses around the world; monitoring their distribution within countries and across country borders; and influencing policies related to the social, political, economic, and healthcare system designs that affect nursing.

BOX 19-2   GLOBAL DEFINITION OF NURSING

Nursing encompasses autonomous and collaborative care of individuals of all ages, families, groups and communities, sick or well and in all settings. Nursing includes the promotion of health, prevention of illness, and the care of ill, disabled, and dying people. Advocacy, promotion of a safe environment, research, participation in shaping health policy and in patient and health systems management, and education are also key nursing roles (ICN, n.d.).

Estimated Global Deficit of Nurses

A Universal Truth: No Health Without a Workforce (Campbell et al., 2013) estimates a deficit of about 12.9 million skilled health professionals (midwives, nurses, and physicians) by 2035. The shortage will be most severe in the poorest countries, especially in sub-Saharan Africa, where health workers are most needed. Ensuring the availability of an appropriately prepared nursing workforce is essential to achieving health and development goals. The scarcity of nurses, and qualified health personnel overall, is one of the biggest obstacles to achieving the UN development agenda through the initial MDGs and the current SDGs.

Factors Affecting Migration

Health worker migration has been increasing worldwide over the past decades, especially from lower income countries with already fragile health systems, like those in sub-Saharan Africa. The financial crisis beginning in 2008 had worldwide impact and many countries experienced challenges to their nursing workforce. Buchan, O'May, & Dussault (2013) found that in some countries the nursing workforce was reduced while at the same time experiencing an increase in migration.

> **KEY TERM**
> **Push factors:** Those factors that make it difficult to receive a basic or advanced education in nursing or to practice in the nurse's native country.

A variety of factors influence mobility trends between countries; these can be divided into **push factors** and **pull factors**. **Box 19-3** identifies push and pull factors affecting the migration of nurses.

> **KEY TERM**
> **Pull factors:** Those factors that make migration to another country more attractive for education or practice than staying in the nurse's native country.

BOX 19-3   MAIN PUSH AND PULL FACTORS IN INTERNATIONAL NURSING MOBILITY

Push Factors
- Low pay (absolute and/or relative)
- Poor working conditions
- Lack of resources to work effectively
- Limited career opportunities
- Limited educational opportunities
- Impact of HIV/AIDS
- Unstable/dangerous work environment
- Economic instability

Pull Factors
- Higher pay (and opportunities for remittances)
- Better working conditions
- Better resourced health systems
- Career opportunities
- Provision of postbasic education
- Political stability
- Travel opportunities
- Assistance in aid work

Reproduced from Buchan, J., Parkin, T., & Sochalski, J. (2003). *International nurse mobility: Trends and policy implications.* Geneva, Switzerland: World Health Organization. Copyright 2003.

International Recruitment Practices

Beginning in the 1990s and into the 2000s, the global health community expressed concern about the likelihood of accelerated recruitment by relatively developed countries from countries with fewer resources. According to Connell and Buchan (2011) this has raised complex ethical, financial, and health questions, which have also emphasized the more complex and nuanced context of the "brain drain." Rights to health thus involve not simply a country's obligations to retain workers but also obligations in countries recruiting health workers, hence requiring considerations of transnational social justice. There are currently 57 countries considered by the WHO (2010) to be in a crisis relative to their workforce. The United States actively recruits 25.2 percent of foreign-educated nurses from these countries (Gants et al., 2012).

To address the challenge of encouraging countries and healthcare agencies to internally develop and retain an adequate workforce, the WHO Global Code of Practice on the International Recruitment of Health Personnel was developed. The code marks the first time in 30 years that WHO Member States have used the constitutional authority of the WHO to develop a code. The code establishes and promotes voluntary principles and practices for the ethical international recruitment of health personnel in a manner that strengthens each country's own health system, including effective health workforce planning, education, and retention strategies (WHO, 2010).

Nursing Education

In order to develop a common approach to educating nurses and midwives globally, WHO (2009) developed Global Standards for the Initial Education of Professional Nurses and Midwives. These standards were developed in response to the challenges resulting from the great variation of initial education around the world and a consensus that they could no longer be ignored. A survey by directors of WHO Collaborating Centres for Nursing and Midwifery found that many countries still consider initial nursing education programs at secondary school level to be sufficient, whereas some countries specify university-level education as a minimum point of entry to practice. The primary reasons for developing the standards include the increasing complexities of healthcare provision and the increasing number of health professionals at different levels and the need to ensure more equitable access to care (WHO, 2009).

The global standards for initial education provide an opportunity for countries to invest in building the capacity required to raise the standard of education of existing nursing and midwifery program to university level, thereby promoting continuous learning and ensuring professional advancement that is in line with worldwide education trends (WHO, 2009).

Faculty Needed to Educate Workforce

Although there is a great need for increased numbers of nurses and all health professionals, the ability of the global community to meet this need rests on the capacity to develop a sufficient supply of educators who are prepared for the role. Globally, health education institutions face heavy teaching loads, a shortage of educators, and competing demands for research and clinical services. In poorer countries, the major constraint is a scarcity of qualified educators to teach the next generation of professionals, without whom it would be difficult to expand the workforce (WHO, 2013). Although the shortage of prepared faculty is critical in low-income countries, it is also a barrier to admitting all qualified applicants in high-income countries.

Internationalizing the Curriculum

Increasing opportunities for students to engage in international experiences within the nursing curriculum increases their preparation as global citizens. Many schools of nursing are adopting strategies to provide students with at least one significant international experience, whether it be in the local community or through a study abroad experience. The goal of this work to internationalize the curriculum is grounded in the belief that we live in a global community and nurses need knowledge, skills, and attitudes to effectively provide health care to a diverse population, whether in their local community or abroad. In addition, students from other countries travel to receive education and schools need to be skilled in meeting their learning needs as well.

Internationalizing the curriculum involves placing learning issues within a context of other countries and trends in epidemiology, healthcare systems, and society in order to increase the global health knowledge of nursing students. Some internationalization strategies include:

- Engaging in international partnerships that provide research, learning, and service opportunities over time.
- Developing partnerships with international residents and organizations in local communities to learn about migrant and refugee populations to better serve their needs.
- Bringing visiting scholars to class and developing enrichment opportunities like lunchtime talks, cultural hours, and showing videotapes depicting international cultures are all ways to internationalize the curriculum.
- Using technology to link students across countries throughout the nursing curriculum. At one school, during predeparture sessions of a student service program between Mexico and the United States, students engaged in video self-introductions. They shared photos of a family celebration as a way to begin getting to know their Mexican counterparts (Kahn et al., 2008).
- Engaging in research and internships that provide rich opportunities for students to delve more deeply into a setting and health issue.

Nursing students often seek to include an international experience in their education programs. They see the value of shaping themselves based on firsthand experiences in other countries that allow them to expand their views of how life is lived in other cultures. The American Association of Colleges and Universities (AAC&U, n.d.) defines global learning as a critical analysis of and an engagement with complex, interdependent global systems and legacies (such as natural, physical, social, cultural, economic, and political) and their implications for people's lives and the earth's sustainability. Through global learning, students become informed, open-minded, and responsible people who are attentive to diversity across the spectrum of differences; seek to understand how their actions affect both local and global communities; and address the world's most pressing and enduring issues collaboratively and equitably (AAC&U, n.d.).

Many students seek out service-learning experiences that further their personal development and achievement of program outcomes. See **Box 19-4** for a description of how one nursing student focused her undergraduate experience in international health. Although international service learning has been a commonly accepted term, recent thought leaders have promoted a shift in thinking to global service learning, which focuses on an in-depth understanding of the country's culture, politics, and economics.

Careers and Voluntary Work in Global Nursing

Opportunities to work or volunteer abroad can be found through a wide range of organizations including governmental and humanitarian. Students at all levels of their careers choose to have a global experience that changes their perspective on the world and many times provides the launching pad for work after they complete their program. It is important to develop knowledge about the different types of organizations, their philosophy and agenda for their work, and the type of individuals

---

BOX 19-4   EXAMPLE SERVICE-LEARNING EXPERIENCE

One undergraduate student developed a passion for infants and children with malnutrition through experiences in Swaziland and Kenya. She participated in multiple curricular and cocurricular programs as an undergraduate student, including two study abroad programs to Swaziland during which she developed in-depth knowledge about child malnutrition by working in a hospital and community clinics. In her senior year she wrote a Fulbright fellowship application to support a research project with a family practice physician in Swaziland on developing effective feeding education strategies for parents. Based on this experience she is applying for graduate school to become a family nurse practitioner with a population health focus.

they are looking for and the preparation needed. This will allow you to find the best fit for your interests and skills.

Global Nursing Organizations

International nursing is of importance to multiple stakeholders around the globe. Global nursing organizations allow advancement of nursing's global agenda including efforts to address common educational preparation issues, facilitate the supply of nurses and nurse educators, and influence important policy issues. International nursing organizations advance the development of nursing in a unified manner, while allowing for individual country and culture values to be retained.

The WHO designates collaborating centers around the globe whose purpose is to provide equitable access to an adequately educated, skilled, and supported nursing and midwifery workforce to meet health needs. **Box 19-5** provides a brief overview of the mission and mandate of these collaborating centers.

The ICN is a federation of national nurses associations representing nurses in more than 128 countries. Founded in 1899, ICN is the world's first and widest-reaching international organization for healthcare professionals. Operated by nurses for nurses, ICN works to ensure high-quality nursing care for all, sound health policies globally, the advancement of nursing knowledge, and the presence worldwide of a respected nursing profession and a competent and satisfied nursing workforce. The goals of the ICN are "to bring nursing together worldwide, to advance nurses and nursing worldwide, and to influence health policy" (ICN, n.d.).

Two additional organizations that have an international focus include Sigma Theta Tau International Nursing Honor Society based in the United States and the

---

BOX 19-5   WHO COLLABORATING CENTRES FOR NURSING AND MIDWIFERY

Vision

Health for All Through Nursing and Midwifery Excellence.

Mission

To maximize the contribution of nursing and midwifery in order to advance states, member Centres, NGOs, and others interested in promoting the health of populations.

The Network will carry out advocacy and evidence based policy activities within the framework of WHA and regional resolutions and the WHO Programs of Work.

The Global Network has an elected governing body consisting of a secretariat is elected from the member collaborating Centres for a period of four years and it functions as the coordinating body of the Network.

Reproduced from World Health Organization. (n.d.-f). WHO Global Network of Collaborating Centres for Nursing and Midwifery. Retrieved from http://www.globalnetworkwhocc .com/who-we-are.html

Florence Nightingale Foundation based in the United Kingdom. These member-based nursing organizations seek to advance global scholarship.

Strategic Global Directions for Nursing and Midwifery Education

Through the efforts of multiple nursing organizations with a global focus, a common agenda has emerged that calls for unified efforts to advance nursing's development. This agenda includes midwifery, as in most countries midwifery is practiced at a level similar to nursing. On a regular basis the WHO establishes strategic directions for nursing and midwifery development that address a broad range of key issues. In the Strategic Directions for Nursing and Midwifery Development 2016–2020 draft document (WHO, 2015h), key issues include:

- Preparing for nursing's role in the Universal Health Coverage agenda by calling for education and service models that focus on providing care across the continuum of health services throughout the lifecycle for populations
- Promoting nurse and midwife models that allow practicing to the fullest scope of their education and licensure
- Ensuring high-quality education is available based on globally accepted standards for basic education
- Developing interprofessional education and practice models that facilitate collaboration
- Optimizing leadership
- Mobilizing political will to invest in building an effective nursing and midwifery workforce and governance structure

Summary

Nurses are well positioned to make a significant contribution to the health and well-being of the global population. The SDGs focus on problems that are amenable to nursing and multisectoral intervention. In order to achieve the full potential of their contributions to global population health, the nursing workforce must be effectively educated and supported at the country, state, and local levels. They must be knowledgeable about the local health problems of their communities and skilled in helping people navigate the healthcare system.

Many nursing students are engaging in study abroad experiences that move them toward global citizenship and allow them to develop their commitment to vulnerable populations globally. The ethic of health equity is fully embraced with leading health organizations around the world and sets the bar for nurses to work toward in the years to come.

Reflective Practice Questions

1. Should nurses from countries with an existing shortage of nurses be discouraged from migrating to practice nursing in another country?
2. How well have your educational experiences prepared you to practice nursing in a global society? What actions can you undertake to further increase your knowledge of global nursing workforce issues?
3. In what ways will the shift from communicable diseases to NCDs as the major causes of mortality and morbidity result in the need for a change in nursing practice?

References

American Association of Colleges & Universities. (n.d.). *Global learning value rubric*. Washington, DC: Author.

Bahl, R., Martines, J., Bhandari, N., Biloglav, Z., Edmond, K., Iyengar, S., . . . Rudan, I. (2012). Setting research priorities to reduce global mortality from preterm birth and low birth weight by 2015. *Journal of Global Health*, *2*(1), 010403. doi: 10.7189/jogh.02-010403.

Bondoe, C., Wraynee, A. B., Riner, M. E., Allam, E., & Stephenson, E. (2014). Helping babies breathe: Providing an evidence-based education intervention at a tertiary referral hospital in Liberia. *Journal of Nursing Education and Practice*, *4*(9), 119–127.

Buchan, J., O'May, F., & Dussault, G. (2013). Nursing workforce policy and the economic crisis: A global. *Journal of Nursing Scholarship*, *45*(3), 298–307.

Buchan, J., Parkin, T., & Sochalski, J. (2003). *International nurse mobility: Trends and policy implications*. Geneva, Switzerland: World Health Organization.

Campbell, J., Dussault, G., Buchan, J., Pozo-Martin, F., Guerra, M., Siyam, A., & Cometto, G. (2013). *A universal truth: No health without a workforce*. Geneva, Switzerland: Author. Retrieved from http://www.who.int/workforcealliance/knowledge/resources/hrhreport2013/en/

Centers for Disease Control and Prevention. (n.d.). *Malaria worldwide*. Retrieved from http://www.cdc.gov/malaria/malaria_worldwide/index.html

Centers for Disease Control and Prevention. (2011a). Global health programs: Global health security. Retrieved from http://www.cdc.gov/globalhealth/programs/ghs.htm

Centers for Disease Control and Prevention. (2011b). *Neglected tropical diseases*. Retrieved from http://www.cdc.gov/globalhealth/ntd/diseases/index.html

Centers for Disease Control and Prevention. (2016a). *Global HIV and tuberculosis*. Retrieved from http://www.cdc.gov/globalAIDS/default.html

Centers for Disease Control and Prevention. (2016b). *Viral hepatitis*. Retrieved from https://www.cdc.gov/hepatitis/

Chan, M. (2015). *WHO Director-General addresses ministerial meeting on universal health coverage*. Retrieved from http://www.who.int/dg/speeches/2015/singapore-uhc/en/#

Connell, J., & Buchan, J. (2011). The impossible dream? Codes of practice and the international migration of skilled health workers. *World Medical & Health Policy*, *3*(3), Article 3. doi: 10.2202/1948-4682.1175

Gants, N. R., Sherman, R., Jasper, M., Choo, C. G., Herrin-Griffith, D., & Harris, K. (2012). Global nurse leader perspectives on health systems and workforce challenges. *Journal of Nursing Management*, *20*, 433–443.

Gignoux, E., Azman, A. S., de Smet, M., Azuma, P., Massaquoi, M., Job, D., . . . Ciglenecki, I. (2016). Effect of artesunate–amodiaquine on mortality related to Ebola virus disease. *New England Journal of Medicine, 374*, 23–32. doi: 10.1056/NEJMoa1504605

Global Citizen Initiative. (n.d.). *Definition of the global citizen.* Retrieved from http://www.theglobalcitizensinitiative.org

International Council of Nurses. (n.d.). *About ICN.* Retrieved from http://www.icn.ch/abouticn.htm

Kahn, H., Stelzner, S. M., Riner, M. E., Soto-Rojas, A. E., Henkle, J., Veras-Godoy, H. A., . . . Martinez-Mier, E. A. (2008). Creating international, multidisciplinary, service-elearning experiences. In A. Dailey-Hebert, E. D. Sallee, & L. M. DiPadova (Eds.), *Service-eLearning: Educating for citizenship in a technology-rich world* (pp. 95–105). Charlotte, NC: Information Age.

Koplan, J., Bond, D., Merson, M., Rodriquez, M., Sewankambo, N., & Wasserheit, J. (2009). Toward a common definition of global health. *Lancet, 373*, 1993–1995.

Lewis, M. (2015). *Better hospitals, better health systems: The urgency of a hospital agenda.* Retrieved from http://www.cgdev.org/publication/better-hospitals-better-health-systems-urgency-hospital-agenda

Macfarlane, S. B., Jacobs, M., & Kaaya, E. E. (2008). In the name of global health: trends in academic institutions. *Journal of Public Health Policy, 29*(4), 383–401.

McMichael, A., & Beaglehole, R. (2009). The global context for public health. In R. Beaglehole & R. Bonita (Eds.), *Global public health: A new era* (2nd ed., pp. 1–22). Oxford, England: Oxford University Press.

UNICEF. (2015). *The 2030 Agenda for Sustainable Development. An Agenda for #EVERYChild 2015.* Retrieved from http://www.unicef.org/agenda2030/69525_81485.html

United Nations. (n.d.). Sustainable development goals: 17 goals to transform our world. Goal 3: Ensure healthy lives and promote well-being for all at all ages. Retrieved from http://www.un.org/sustainabledevelopment/health/

United Nations. (2012). *Health in the post-2015 UN Development* Agenda. Retrieved from http://www.un.org/millenniumgoals/pdf/Think%20Pieces/8_health.pdf

United Nations. (2015). *United Nations Global Strategy for Women's, Children's and Adolescents' Health: 2016–2030.* Retrieved from http://www.who.int/life-course/partners/global-strategy/global-strategy-2016-2030/en/

U.S. Department of Health and Human Services. (n.d.). *Global health topics: Health diplomacy.* Retrieved from http://globalhealth-stage.icfwebservices.com/global-health-topics/health-diplomacy/

U.S. Department of Health and Human Services, Office of Disease Prevention and Health Promotion. (n.d.). *Healthy People 2020: Disparities.* Retrieved from http://www.healthypeople.gov/2020/about/foundation-health-measures/Disparities

Wang, H., Liddell, C. A., Coates, M. M., Mooney, M. D., Levitz, C. E., Schumacher, A. E., . . . Murray, C. J. L. (2014). Global, regional, and national levels of neonatal, infant, and under-5 mortality during 1990–2013: A systematic analysis for the Global Burden of Disease Study 2013. *Lancet, 384*(9947), 957–979. http://doi.org/10.1016/S0140-6736(14)60497-9

World Health Organization. (1978). *Declaration of Alma-Ata.* Retrieved from http://www.who.int/publications/almaata_declaration_en.pdf

World Health Organization. (2009). *Global standards for the initial education of professional nurses and midwives.* Retrieved from http://www.who.int/hrh/nursing_midwifery/hrh_global_standards_education.pdf

World Health Organization. (2010). WHO Global Code of Practice on the International Recruitment of Health Personnel. Retrieved from http://www.who.int/hrh/migration/code/code_en.pdf?ua=1

World Health Organization. (2011). Summary: World report on disability. Retrieved from http://www.who.int/disabilities/world_report/2011/accessible_en.pdf

World Health Organization. (2013). *Transforming and scaling up health professional education and training: Policy brief on faculty development*. Retrieved from http://whoeducation guidelines.org/sites/default/files/uploads/whoeduguidelines_PolicyBrief_Faculty Development.pdf

World Health Organization. (2014a). *10 facts on the state of global health*. Retrieved from http://www.who.int/features/factfiles/global_burden/facts/en/

World Health Organization. (2014b). Life expectancy at birth, both sexes, 2012. Retrieved from http://gamapserver.who.int/mapLibrary/Files/Maps/Global_LifeExpectancy_bothsexes_2012.png

World Health Organization. (2014c). *The 10 leading causes of death in the world*. Retrieved from http://www.who.int/mediacentre/factsheets/fs310/en/

World Health Organization. (2014d). *What is universal health coverage?* Retrieved from http://www.who.int/features/qa/universal_health_coverage/en/

World Health Organization. (2015a). *Empowering communities to end TB with the ENGAGE-TB approach*. Retrieved from http://www.who.int/tb/publications/2015/engage_tb_brochure/en/

World Health Organization. (2015b). *Global Tuberculosis Report 2015*. Retrieved from http://www.who.int/tb/publications/global_report/gtbr2015_executive_summary.pdf

World Health Organization. (2015c). *Maternal mortality*. Retrieved from http://www.who.int/mediacentre/factsheets/fs348/en/

World Health Organization. (2015d). *New partnership to help countries close gaps in primary health care*. Retrieved from http://www.who.int/mediacentre/news/releases/2015/partnership-primary-health-care/en/

World Health Organization. (2015e). *Noncommunicable diseases*. Retrieved from http://www.who.int/mediacentre/factsheets/fs355/en/

World Health Organization. (2015f). *Preterm birth*. Retrieved from http://www.who.int/mediacentre/factsheets/fs363/en/

World Health Organization. (2015g). *SDG 3: Ensure healthy lives and promote wellbeing for all at all ages*. Retrieved from http://www.who.int/topics/sustainable-development-goals/targets/en/

World Health Organization. (2015h). *Strategic directions for nursing and midwifery development 2016–2020*. Retrieved from http://www.who.int/hrh/news/2015/13_11_2015_SDNM_consultation_draft_zero.pdf?ua=1

World Health Organization. (2015i). Under-five mortality rate (probability of dying by age 5 per 1000 live births), 1990. Retrieved from http://gamapserver.who.int/mapLibrary/Files/Maps/global_underfivemortality_1990.png

World Health Organization. (2015j). Under-five mortality rate (probability of dying by age 5 per 1000 live births), 2015. Retrieved from http://gamapserver.who.int/mapLibrary/Files/Maps/global_underfivemortality_2015

World Health Organization. (n.d.-a) *About the international health regulations*. Retrieved from http://www.euro.who.int/en/health-topics/emergencies/international-health-regulations/about-the-international-health-regulations

World Health Organization. (n.d.-b). *Adolescent health epidemiology*. Retrieved from http://www.who.int/maternal_child_adolescent/epidemiology/adolescence/en/

World Health Organization. (n.d.-c). *Equity*. Retrieved from http://www.who.int/healthsystems/topics/equity/en/

World Health Organization. (n.d.-d) *Global burden of disease*. Retrieved from http://www.who.int/topics/global_burden_of_disease/en/

World Health Organization. (n.d.-e). *Global health diplomacy*. Retrieved from http://www.who.int/trade/diplomacy/en/

World Health Organization. (n.d.-f). WHO Global Network of Collaborating Centres for Nursing and Midwifery. Retrieved from http://www.globalnetworkwhocc.com/who-we-are.html

Informatics, Healthcare Technology, and Nursing Practice

Josette Jones and Cathy R. Fulton

LEARNING OUTCOMES

After reading this chapter you will be able to:

- Explain the Health Information Technology for Economic and Clinical Health (HITECH) Act and its subsequent impact on health care.
- Define meaningful use.
- Describe how current technology affects health delivery systems.
- Identify ways nurses can encourage patients and their family to become more engaged in health care.
- Describe how social media can be appropriately used to share patient information and contribute to disease management.
- Explain how health information exchange (HIE) allows healthcare providers to share medical information with their own patients as well as with other providers.
- Define nursing informatics and its importance to nursing practice.
- Describe how social media provides both the potential to improve health and to cause harm.

The editors wish to acknowledge the contributions of Elizabeth M. LaRue, Susan K. Newbold, Gilan EL Saadawi, and Karen L. Courtney to the previous edition of this chapter.

Health Information Technology for Economic and Clinical Health (HITECH) Act: Promotes the adoption of electronic health records and meaningful use of health information.

Meaningful use (MU): Using health information technology to engage healthcare consumers in their care with the ultimate goal of achieving better care coordination and population and public health and also improving the quality, safety, and efficiency of health care and reducing health disparities.

Health information technology (HIT): Information technology applied to health care, making it possible for healthcare providers to better manage patient care through secure use and sharing of health information.

Patient engagement framework (PEF): A model created to guide healthcare organizations in developing and strengthening their patient engagement strategies through the use of HIT-based tools and resources (collectively known as eHealth).

Patient activation: The skills and confidence that equip patients to become actively engaged in their health care.

Nursing informatics: The specialty that integrates nursing science with computer science and multiple information management and analytical sciences to identify, define, manage, and communicate data, information, and knowledge for nursing practice.

Introduction

Since the implementation of the **Health Information Technology for Economic and Clinical Health (HITECH) Act** in 2009, many changes have occurred in healthcare delivery and the ways by which consumers and providers communicate about health. **Meaningful use (MU)**, which is based on the use of **health information technology (HIT)**, is driving healthcare practice and delivery. The **patient engagement framework (PEF)** guides how the healthcare provider, including the nurse, interacts with the consumer. The ultimate aim of this interaction is to create an environment of **patient activation**, in which the patient becomes actively engaged in participating in the management of his or her health care, recovery, and/ or well-being.

The PEF capitalizes on the use of HIT and occurs through, but is not limited to, the use of web-based applications, telehealth services, and mHealth (mobile health) applications. Such applications are also referred to as e-Health (World Health Organization, 2016). Common eHealth venues include but are not limited to (a) mHealth, which is the provision of health services and information via wireless devices such as smartphones, tablet computers, and telemonitoring devices (Doswell, Braxter, Dabbs, Nilsen, & Klem, 2013); and (b) telehealth, which is the use of electronic applications and telemetry sensors to enhance provider–patient interactions. Nurses, and especially nurse informaticists (informaticians), play an important role in fostering a culture of patient activation by taking an active leadership role in integrating these trends in nursing practice. Nurses are also crucial in contributing to the development of the policies necessary to retaining the quality of health care while reducing costs and promoting better patient outcomes when using HIT.

This chapter introduces the reader to concepts related to the use of healthcare technology in the current HCDS and its impact on nursing. The chapter also describes how this evolution in healthcare technology has led to a new domain of informatics and created a new specialty of **nursing informatics**.

Health Information Technology for Economic and Clinical Health Act

The Health Information Technology for Economic and Clinical Health Act, enacted as part of the American Recovery and Reinvestment Act of 2009, was signed into law on February 17, 2009, to promote the adoption of **electronic health records (EHRs)** and meaningful use of HIT. The underlying premise of the HITECH Act is that electronic medical records facilitate documentation of the healthcare services rendered by providers and institutions; this documentation is used to justify billing and control the escalating costs of health care. The HITECH Act was a direct response to the earlier findings of the Institute of Medicine (IOM) (Corrigan, 2005) on the myriad physical and moral harms occurring as a result of the structure and delivery of the U.S. healthcare system (Huston, 2013; Silverman, 2013).

> **KEY TERM**
>
> **Electronic health records (EHRs):** Electronic versions of a patient's medical history that is maintained by the provider over time and may include all of the key administrative clinical data relevant to that person. It automates access to information and has the potential to streamline the clinician's workflow.

The subsequent IOM 2011 *Future of Nursing* report (Altman, Butler, & Shern, 2016) reiterated that it is nurses who are being called upon to fill expanding **informatics** roles and master technological tools and information systems while collaborating and coordinating patient care in healthcare teams. Nurse leaders must think about how technology will expand and support the practice of nursing and proactively create training programs to ensure that every nurse has the competencies and skills needed to use the technology appropriately (Huston, 2013). Nurses are at the forefront to take an active role in patient engagement as stipulated in the MU objectives (HealthIT. gov, 2015). MU is defined as using HIT to engage healthcare consumers in their care with the ultimate goal of achieving better care coordination and population and public health and also improving the quality, safety, and efficiency of health care and reducing health disparities.

> **KEY TERM**
>
> **Informatics:** The study and practice of creating, storing, finding, manipulating, and sharing information.

Healthcare Delivery Systems Post HITECH Act

The evolving design of current healthcare delivery systems (HCDS) is a direct response to the concern of rising healthcare costs, disparity in access to care, and the lack of uniform quality and efficiency measures. Technology allows healthcare providers and consumers to capture and share health data from patient registration to diagnoses to post discharge, realigning the way health care can be delivered within and across settings. EHR systems are seen as important factors in the realignment of healthcare delivery, as they allow providers to share health information and create a continuum of care eliminating or at least reducing inconsistencies. In addition,

HIT has created opportunities for consumers to formally connect to their providers between visits via patient portals and/or secure messages.

HIT also includes many social media tools that have been made available for healthcare professionals and consumers including social networking platforms, forums, blogs, wikis, Twitter feeds, media sharing, virtual reality, and gaming environments (Ventola, 2014). These tools provide opportunities for professional networking and education, engaging patients in their care, providing patient education on demand, and connecting consumers with other consumers to discuss their health concerns through support groups and share useful tips on improving health. Yet, if used inappropriately, these tools carry potential risks to the consumers and providers regarding breaches of **protected health information (PHI)**, violations of personal–professional boundaries, distribution of poor quality or incorrect information, and licensing and other legal issues (Ventola, 2014). In summary, EHRs**, health information exchanges (HIEs)** of various sizes and forms; structured communication between providers, insurance companies, consumers, and government agencies; and unstructured and informal methods of sharing health information have changed the face of healthcare delivery in the United States creating opportunities and challenges for nursing.

> **KEY TERM**
>
> **Protected health information (PHI):**
> As stipulated by U.S. law, any health information about an individual's status, his/her provision of health care, or payment for health care that is created or collected by a "covered entity." Covered entities include but are not limited to providers (including nurses), insurance companies, governmental entities, and auxiliary care staff including social workers.

> **KEY TERM**
>
> **Health information exchanges (HIEs):** Electronic exchanges of health information from one healthcare professional to another to improve the continuity, quality, safety, and efficiency of healthcare delivery.

Patient Engagement and Activation

Engaging patients and families in their health is one of the pillars of the HITECH Act. MU guidelines require that all patients are provided with an electronic copy of their electronic health information (including diagnostic test results, problem list, medication lists, medication allergies, discharge summary, and procedures) upon request (HealthIT.gov, 2015). Patients must also have the ability to view their health information online and download and transmit the information to other providers or health institutions (see **Table 20-1**). For more information on the MU requirements for providers and institutions, visit the Centers for Medicare & Medicaid (CMS) website (2016b).

Patient engagement is an MU concept that stipulates having patients take a more active role (i.e., engagement) in managing their own health. When patients are engaged in their health care, it is thought that engagement may improve quality and safety of patient care, leading to improved patient outcomes, improved healthcare experience, and lower healthcare costs (Barello, Graffigna, Vegni, & Bosio, 2014). This requirement to engage patients shifts the control from the healthcare

TABLE 20-1 ELIGIBLE PROFESSIONAL OBJECTIVES AND MEASURES

1	Protect electronic protected health information created or maintained by the CEHRT through the implementation of appropriate technical capabilities.
2	Use clinical decision support to improve performance on high-priority health conditions.
3	Use computerized provider order entry for medication, laboratory, and radiology orders directly entered by any licensed healthcare professional who can enter orders into the medical record per state, local, and professional guidelines.
4	Generate and transmit permissible prescriptions electronically (eRx).
5	Health Information Exchange—The EP who transitions their patient to another setting of care or provider of care or refers their patient to another provider of care provides a summary care record for each transition of care or referral.
6	Use clinically relevant information from CEHRT to identify patient-specific education resources and provide those resources to the patient.
7	The EP who receives a patient from another setting of care or provider of care or believes an encounter is relevant performs medication reconciliation.
8	Patient electronic access—Provide patients the ability to view online, download, and transmit their health information within 4 business days of the information being available to the EP.
9	Use secure electronic messaging to communicate with patients on relevant health information.
10	Public Health Reporting—The EP is in active engagement with a public health agency to submit electronic public health data from CEHRT except where prohibited and in accordance with applicable law and practice.

Abbreviations: CEHRT, certified electronic health record technology; EP, eligible profressional.

Reproduced from Centers for Medicare & Medicaid Services. (2016a). Eligible professional objectives and measures. Retrieved from https://www.cms.gov/Regulations-and-Guidance/Legislation/EHRIncentivePrograms/Downloads/2016_EPTableOfContents.pdf

provider alone to the patient. Patient engagement starts with patient *activation*, the motivation of a patient to start engaging in healthcare decisions for the benefit of his or own health. Nurses play a central role in activating patients as they facilitate patient–provider communications and are trained to actively elicit care preferences and promote disease self-management. Healthcare practitioners are called upon to value the patient's perspectives and preferences and incorporate these into the planning and delivery of health care (Barello et al., 2014), thus creating a "*connected*

BOX 20-1   ENGAGING PATIENTS IN HEALTHCARE DECISIONS: WHAT NURSES CAN DO

- Inform, educate, and promote the importance of the patient engagement to your patients and their family members.
- Involve patients through patient advisory groups or patient advocates.
- Post information signs in health clinics and offices to encourage patients to ask questions on how they can get involved in their health care.
- Provide "how-to" tutorials (for example, YouTube tutorial) to help patients with accessing patient portals.

- Thank patients for using the health portal, demonstrating appreciation for their efforts in using the technology.
- Provide opportunities for unstructured, informal communication via social media platforms (e.g., Twitter, Facebook, Instagram, etc.), which are used to disseminate activation-related information to patients.

health" ecosystem. "Connected health" uses technology to provide access to critical personal and population health information and improve communication between healthcare providers, patients, and their families. Efforts to foster "connected health" will be successful only if the following three elements are present: (a) access to the information, (b) provider and consumer adoption, and (c) actionable information for intended receiver.

How can the nurse activate the patient and his/her family to become engaged in his/her care? **Box 20-1** provides examples of nursing actions that can be used to facilitate the development of a "connected health" ecosystem and patient engagement in health care.

Communication Platforms for Healthcare Providers and Consumers

HIT provides nurses with several means by which to engage patients and loved ones in their care. The care of patients involves many different providers, all wanting to share patient information and discuss their approaches to the patient's health and disease management. Keeping in mind the **Health Insurance Portability and Accountability Act (HIPAA)** requirement that any means of communicating PHI must be secured and confidential, it is not unexpected that over the last decade effort has been focused on developing platforms for providing secure access and sharing

KEY TERM

Health Information Portability and Accountability Act (HIPAA): A U.S. law providing privacy standards to protect patients' health records and other health information provided to health plans, doctors, hospitals, and other healthcare providers.

of health information locally or enterprisewide, and even cross-organizational. Commonly used platform types in the healthcare environment vary from secure point-to-point communication systems to Internet-based portals. Specific HIT use of informal communication platforms include patient support websites/forums (such as PatientsLikeMe, Facebook, **Figure 20-1**) as well as (to a lesser extent) clinician–patient communication platforms, also known as patient portals. Examples of these various platform types are discussed further in the next sections.

Patient Support Sites and Forums

Patient support sites and forums are very similar in nature to the use of **social media**. The most important difference between patient support sites and the use of generic social media sites is that support sites and forums are designed to cater specifically to patients (and sometimes clinicians) and are typically focused on a specific patient population and healthcare condition, such as diabetes or breast cancer, to site a few examples. The discussion forum, which is a very common feature of patient support sites,

> **KEY TERM**
>
> **Social media:** Forms of electronic communication (such as websites for social networking and microblogging) through which users create online communities to share information, multimedia, ideas, personal messages, and other content.

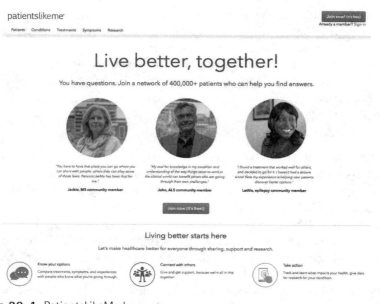

Figure 20-1 PatientsLikeMe homepage.
Courtesy of PatientsLikeMe.

allows for organized discussion of user-generated topics. Clinician involvement is not excluded from support sites and/or forums; there do exist sites and forums that use clinician feedback to patients.

Patient Portals

A **patient portal** is a HIT-based communication venue between patients and their providers, used for the sharing of patient health information. These portals are almost always Internet-based and are growing in use by clinicians and patients.

> **KEY TERM**
>
> **Patient portal:** A secure online website that gives patients convenient 24-hour access to personal health information from anywhere with an Internet connection.

Patients often wish to leave their providers and staff electronic or phone messages when a question or concern arises between visits. Patients benefit from all types of communication via secure messaging, patient portal, or personal email allowing them quicker access to vital services (such as prescription refills) and allowing after-hours communication with providers. Finally, and perhaps most important for nurses, patient portals are a part of the MU regulations and providing a means for patient engagement. Patient engagement focuses on the relationship between patients and their healthcare providers as they work together to "promote and support active patient and public involvement in health and healthcare and to strengthen their influence on healthcare decisions" (Carman et al., 2013, p. 223). Yet the term patient engagement is also used synonymously with patient activation and patient- and family-centered care. Although these concepts are related, they are not identical. Patient activation refers to an "individual's knowledge, skill, and confidence for managing his/her own health and health care," whereas engagement is defined as "actions individuals take for their health and to benefit from health care" (Carman et al., 2013, p. 223).

Social Media

Social media is defined for the purpose of this chapter as publicly available online platforms over which large numbers of users can exchange casual, conversational-type messages with each other and also post these messages for the global audience to read. Social media platforms may be based on the Internet (web or website based) or alternately be present in the form of "apps" (short for applications) for smartphone users. The most popular social media websites include Facebook and Twitter; other examples of popular social media venues include Instagram, YouTube, and Google Plus.

Because of the diversity of social media platforms there are clearly ways in which all of these exchange types can be used to influence health care. For example, an influential nursing leader can use social media to enhance healthcare delivery by posting important health messages on a global public venue such as Twitter or Facebook (global status). Private exchanges on social media have the benefit of protecting health information and can been used for patients to converse about their medical conditions, or, in some cases, even engage in synchronous as well as asynchronous messaging with an expert nurse or other healthcare provider on private pages. However, it is important for patients to understand that exchange of medical information over nonsecured platforms such as social media implies that the consumer is voluntarily disclosing PHI, and is thus losing HIPAA protection.

Multimedia-type exchanges, as seen with newer social media venues such as Tumblr, Instagram, YouTube, and others, have limited text capabilities; nonetheless, the clinician can use these venues to deliver important healthcare-related information via pictures or videos. In particular, as of this writing, one author has personally noted that Instagram is known for peer-to-peer sharing of images and descriptions of self-made healthy foods, in the hope that consumers will replicate a healthy lifestyle by trying to create these foods. Furthermore, it was also noted that YouTube is commonly used by professionals and healthcare consumers alike for videos that discuss important health topics and demonstrate physical therapies and fitness routines that can activate consumers. The nature of social media creates significant risks of violating HIPAA and state privacy regulations.

The informal nature of social networking sites such as Facebook and Twitter creates substantial potential for disclosing PHI and violating HIPAA even when patient names are not shared. A clinician, staff member, or patients and their families, unaccustomed to mass communication, might be misquoted; consumers may misunderstand the advice, intentionally or not (Landry, 2015). Healthcare employees have been terminated for tweets that violate HIPAA rules; discovered Facebook and MySpace conversations have led to insurance coverage litigation; civil complaints have been filed alleging libel/defamation of clinicians in the use of online rating sites. For this reason, a cautionary approach to social media in the healthcare context is strongly advised (Eytan et al., 2011). Therefore, it is clear that nurses must not only take some responsibility for the quality and accuracy of content posted to social media venues that they moderate but also take all possible measures (i.e., ongoing training, regular revisions of policies and procedures) to ensure that information disclosure rules (both governmental HIPAA-related and organizationally related) are not violated intentionally or unintentionally. Because of the potential for misuse of social media in healthcare situations, the American Nurses Association (n.d.) and the National Council of State Boards of Nursing (2011) have both published resources that nurses and nursing students can use to guide their practice in the appropriate use of social media in patient care. Spector and Kappel (2012) also offer guidelines for the use of electronics and social media.

Health Information Exchange

A health information exchange (HIE) may be defined as all forms of transfer of health-related information (data), structured and unstructured. As part of the HITECH Act, HIE is defined as electronic exchange of health information and interoperability between providers (hospitals and medical group practices) and independent laboratories, radiology centers, pharmacies, payers, public health departments, and other providers (Vest, 2016; Walker, Pan, Johnston, & Adler-Milstein, 2005). The value of electronically exchanging health information is the standardization of data. Once standardized, the data transferred can seamlessly integrate into the recipients' EHR, further improving patient care and avoiding duplication or unnecessary services (Office of the National Coordinator [ONC], 2016). HIEs are also the cornerstone for the patient-centered medical home (see **Contemporary Practice Highlight 20-1**), a collaborative approach to deliver primary care.

Structured Use of Health Information Exchange

The structured, formal use of HIE data can potentially facilitate provider–provider communication and benefit the quality of healthcare delivery in a number of ways. For example, healthcare delivery can be improved by:

KEY TERM

Clinical decision support system (CDSS): Software applications designed to provide clinicians and/or patients with knowledge and person-specific information, filtered or presented at appropriate times, to enhance healthcare interventions.

- Sharing patient information in a timely manner with other providers, allowing more interaction within a patient's care team; and
- Enabling a **clinical decision support systems (CDSS)**; CDSS is a concept that assists clinicians in making patient treatment decisions. CDSS, when enriched with HIE and implemented in an HIT-based format, can provide automated alerts, suggestions, and other useful information on a purely automated basis, requiring no third human party to enhance the value of the health care given.

CONTEMPORARY PRACTICE HIGHLIGHT 20-1

PATIENT-CENTERED MEDICAL HOME

The patient-centered medical home is a healthcare setting that facilitates partnerships between individual patients and their personal healthcare team (i.e., physician, nurses, therapists, pharmacist, dietitian, etc.) and when appropriate, the patient's family. Adapted from the Agency for Healthcare Research and Quality (AHRQ, 2007) definition, the medical home can be defined as "an approach based on the principles of MU to the delivery of primary care that is patient centered, comprehensive, coordinated, accessible to all and committed to quality and safety" (Patient-Centered Primary Care Collective, 2015).

There are limitations to the structured, formal use of HIE data between providers, however. The scope of use for structured HIEs in the United States is often limited to within-state care. Therefore, consumers requiring multistate care (often those individuals who live on state borders or require specialized health care from larger healthcare centers) may not see as great a benefit from structured, formalized HIE compared to those who live and are treated within the same state.

Thus, the HIE has the potential to create *silos* of nonshared patient data despite the fact that it was originally designed to essentially perform the opposite action. Nonetheless, it is important to understand that major improvements are being created in the *interoperability* of information within structured HIEs, increasingly allowing for health data exchanges across state lines. Such interoperability is also inherently dependent upon the states' intergovernmental cooperation as well as federal incentives for interstate cooperation.

Another important consideration is the fact that structured HIE is not as amenable to patient–patient and most patient–provider communications, given that these communications are almost exclusively free-text in nature. Patients, furthermore, do not widely have access to methods in which to give and receive structured healthcare information; such exchange is typically limited to portals that are designed to send formal laboratory and x-ray data to patients. However, it is possible that in the future if structure is given to currently unstructured communication, future informal/unstructured communications could be stored and exchanged via structured HIE.

Unstructured Use of Health Information Exchange

Besides a formal and governmentally regulated HIE, HIE can also take place informally through consumer-mediated HIE. A consumer-mediated exchange provides consumers/patients with access to their health information, allowing them to manage their health care online. As mentioned previously, consumers/patients in control of their own health information participate actively in their care by:

- Sharing their health information with all providers
- Identifying and correcting wrong or missing health information
- Identifying and correcting incorrect billing information
- Tracking and monitoring their own health (ONC, 2015, 2016)

Social media are typically used for this informal exchange of health information between two patients or between a patient and provider. Such informal usage of HIE can be both beneficial in improving the patient's health and problematic in causing harm to the patient or provider. Social media allows for the user to (a) find information tailored to the consumer/patient needs; (b) adapt the information to the user's preferences and learning styles; (c) provide access to information on demand, independent of time and geographical location; (d) interact with providers between healthcare visits; and (e) to share anonymously sensitive information or information that is uncomfortable to share face to face (Hull et al., 2016; Robinson, Patrick, Eng, & Gustafson, 1998; Schatz, 2015).

The growing use of social media for HIE, though, raises questions about quality, confidentiality, and security and even potential harm for consumers/patients and providers. Inaccurate and inappropriate information, poorly designed applications, and misleading claims can result in negative outcomes such as inappropriate treatment, delays in seeking medical care (Robinson, 2007; Robinson et al., 1998; Schatz, 2015), and exposure of PHI in an unsecured and potentially harmful way. Yet as Holly Potter, vice president of public relations at Kaiser Foundation Health Plan states, consumers and providers have different expectations for health information communication to date than a decade ago:

> *Social media is already integral to how people now live their lives and, increasingly, it plays an important role in how they manage their health. If we want to be relevant partners, helping our members and their families manage their health, it is our obligation to learn how to engage—safely, respectfully, and authentically.* (Holly Potter, Vice President of Public Relations at Kaiser Foundation Health Plan, as cited in Eytan et al., 2011)

Impact of Health Information Technology on Nursing

The impact of HIT on nursing practice has been significant. HIT has changed nursing practice in a number of ways. For example, nurses are required to expand their clinical knowledge base to encompass a focus on the structure and algorithm of the clinical health data, information, and knowledge used by nurses. Additionally, nurses must learn to capitalize on the use of technology to support and expand care beyond the traditional healthcare settings, i.e., community and telehealth care settings.

HIT is also serving to define nursing research programs that are related to the application of HIT to nursing practice. Current priorities for nursing research on the use of health technology are related to the development of nursing standards and terminologies, databases for clinical information, patients as users of information technology, mHealth (the practice of health care using mobile devices), and issues of data privacy and confidentiality.

The influence of HIT on nursing practice is going to continue to grow, affecting nursing education, research, and practice. To remain current and safe in an increasingly technology-dependent practice environment, nurses must commit to seeking opportunities for continuing education across the lifespan of their career.

One means by which nurses can expand their knowledge about HIT and represent nursing's perspective on issues related to the use of HIT in clinical practice is by joining professional organizations dedicated to HIT. There are a number of local, regional, national, and international organizations that provide nurses with opportunities for networking and professional development in the areas of informatics and HIT. Such organizations include the American Medical Informatics Association (AMIA), the International Medical Informatics Association (IMIA), the Healthcare Information and Management Systems Society, and the American Nursing Informatics Association.

Implications for Nursing Education

As the healthcare system continues to evolve, HIT competencies must be adjusted accordingly. Most efforts to define core HIT competencies have been adopted from those demonstrated by informatics professionals and those using HIT in their practice. The HIT core competencies address both the factual knowledge (information that one can recite or discuss) and practical skills (ability to accomplish a task) (Friedman, 2013; Valenta, Meagher, Tachinardi, & Starren, 2016). In order to streamline the integration of HIT in education, the IMIA has formulated recommendations competencies related to healthcare information technology needed by nurses and other healthcare professionals. See **Table 20-2** for examples of healthcare information technology competencies recommended for beginning nurses. It is essential for nurses practicing in today's technology-driven healthcare environment to be both computer and information literate.

> **KEY TERM**
> **Computer literacy:** Practical knowledge of hardware and software and also the different ways in which software applications can facilitate and/or support practice.

Computer literacy is defined as a practical knowledge of hardware and software and also the different ways in which software applications can facilitate and/or support practice. Information that the nurse should have to demonstrate computer literacy includes basic computer terms such as central processing unit (CPU), internal memory, bits, and bytes. A computer-literate nurse also understands that different magnetic or optical storage devices can be used for data storage and that data can be stored sequentially (i.e., tapes) or randomly (i.e., disks).

A computer-literate nurse also understands that computers and tablets also possess input devices (including keyboards, styluses, mice, scanners, and in the clinic—medical sensors), as well as output hardware (monitors, printers, speakers, etc.). Resources such as printers, scanners, storage space, applications, etc. can be shared through network systems such as a LAN (local area network) or WAN (wide area network) or be in "the cloud" (stored on a remote server and accessed via the Internet). Computer hardware always requires *software* to function. Software, also known as the *application* or simply *app*, is defined as a set of instructions written in a structured programming language and translated in binary code.

TABLE 20-2 RECOMMENDED HEALTH INFORMATION TECHNOLOGY COMPETENCIES FOR BEGINNING NURSES	
Computer Literacy	• Understanding basic computer terminology like data and database systems, hardware, software, network • Ability to use personal computers: text processing, spreadsheets, database management systems • Ability to communicate electronically including electronic data exchange with other providers, Internet use • Understanding basic concepts of sensor-based and ambient technology in health care, home care, and assisted living
Information Literacy	• Understanding of the characteristics and functionalities of information systems in health care • Responsible use of information processing tool for nursing decision making • Knowledge of health-related terminologies and standards, nomenclatures, and vocabularies for documenting and communicating nursing care • Understanding of ethical and security issues when using HIT
Nursing Practice Management	• Apply methods of project and change management • Illustrate nursing workflow when using HIT • Describe impact of HIT on the clinical workflow

Data from Hovenga, E. J. S. (2013). Health workforce competencies needed for a digital world. *Studies in Health Technology and Informatics, 193*, 141–168; Mantas, J., Ammenwerth, E., Demiris, G., Hasman, A., Haux, R., Hersh, W., . . . Wright, G.(2010). Recommendations of the International Medical Informatics Association (IMIA) on Education in Biomedical and Health Informatics (first revision). *Methods of Information in Medicine, 49*(2), 105–120.

Information literacy is the ability to define an information need, locate pertinent information, and apply the information correctly. Nurses are knowledge workers and information literacy is an important component of nursing practice. Storing and retrieving large quantities of information are facilitated by technology. Information literacy complements basic nursing skills as the information being accessed, used, and evaluated is health related and intended to support the consumer/patient in his or her care. Nursing, as an evidence-based practice, is information intensive. To positively affect disease management, nurses must be able to provide up-to-date, high-quality, patient-centered information.

Implications for Nursing Research

The research agenda related to the impact of HIT on nursing must reflect changes in context while affirming commitment to the core nursing concepts of *patient, health*, and *nursing*. Applying technology to patient care while still maintaining the "human" touch inherent in nursing care is a professional imperative. It is also important to determine how to apply the use of HIT most effectively to improve patient care outcomes. Reflective of the current challenges in nursing practice and the existing information and communication infrastructure, the recommended priorities for research focus on (a) using data, information, and knowledge to deliver and manage patient care; (b) defining and describing data and information for patient care; (c) acquiring and delivering knowledge from and for patient care; (d) investigating new technologies to create better tools for patient care; (e) applying patient care workflows in innovative practice models; (f) integrating systems for interdisciplinary care delivery; and (g) critical assessment of nursing applications of HIT (Bakken, Stone, & Larson, 2008; Moen & Mæland Knudsen, 2013).

Implications for Nursing Practice

As mentioned earlier, using technology both to improve quality of care and decrease healthcare costs is increasingly critical in the U.S. HCDS. Translating this to nursing practice means finding a means by which to provide safe, high-quality nursing care while still being efficient and cost effective. As the recent IOM report *The Future of Nursing* (2011) suggested, it is nurses who will be called upon to fill expanding roles in HIT and informatics and to master technological tools, ranging from the effective design and implementation of EHRs to the use of biometrics, genomics and genetics, healthcare robotics, and information systems. Nurses play a key role in the collaboration and coordination of patient care and are a vital link connecting patients with other healthcare providers. Nurses must proactively reflect on how emerging technologies will support and expand the practice of nursing.

Finally, nurses must increasingly ask how and why technology should be implemented. What parameters need to be put into place to determine its ethical use? Just because something can be done using technology does not mean that it should be done or is without risk (Huston, 2013). The implementation of the HIT should be based on the:

- Clinical impact of the intervention after carefully assessing the need, safety, effectiveness, and efficacy of the HIT;
- Magnitude of the clinical impact and social acceptance of the HIT intervention; and
- Clinical impact of the intervention, weighed against its risks of exposing PHI.

Nursing Informatics: What Is It?

In attempting to arrive at the truth, I have applied everywhere for information, but in scarcely an instance have I been able to obtain hospital records fit for any purposes of comparison. If they could be obtained, they would enable us to decide many other questions. . .they would show the subscribers how their money was being spent. . .what amount of good was really being done. (Nightingale, 1863, as quoted in Barnett, Jenders, & Chueh, 1993, p. 1046; Ozbolt & Saba, 2008, p. 199)

With these prophetic words (as noted by Ozbolt & Saba, 2008), Florence Nightingale planted the seeds of intertwined health sciences: health services, evidence-based practice, and nursing informatics. She called for standardized clinical records that could be analyzed to assess and improve care processes and patient outcomes. Nursing informatics thus springs from the root of modern nursing.

Nursing Informatics and the Chain of Care

Nursing is an important link in the chain of patient care as nurses are often identified as both the coordinators and providers of patient care. In order to manage both of these nursing functions, nurses need ways to capture, store, and retrieve all types of patient data, such as demographic data, assessment and diagnostic data, health insurance data, and treatment data, at the point of patient care. All these data form a basis for planning the patient care and treatment, getting feedback on the patient's progress, and suggesting actions for health promotion and disease prevention. Blum (1986) classified and defined the then-current clinical information systems according to the three types of objects that these systems processed: data, information, and knowledge. Data were defined as discrete entities that are described objectively without interpretation; information is data that are interpreted, organized, or structured; knowledge is information that is synthesized so that relationships are identified and organized (Blum, 1986). Planning the patient's care and treatment, getting feedback on the patient's progress, and suggesting actions for health promotion and disease prevention are based on the nurse's understanding of the relationships between each individual datum and by putting each datum in context. Each of these concepts/actions represents increasing complexity and requires greater application of human intellect.

History and Evolution of Nursing Informatics

Graves and Corcoran (1989) built upon Blum's (1986) definitions and included them as key components of nursing informatics practice. Graves and Corcoran defined nursing informatics (NI) practice as a "combination of computer science, informatics science, and nursing science, designed to assist in the management and processing of nursing data, information, and knowledge to support the practice of nursing and the delivery of nursing care" (p. 227). In later years, a fourth concept, wisdom, was added to the conceptual framework of nursing knowledge. R. R. Nelson (1989) and R. Nelson (2002) defined wisdom as the appropriate use of knowledge to deal with complex problems or specific human needs. "While knowledge focuses on what is known, wisdom focuses on the appropriate application of that knowledge. For example, a knowledge base may include several options for managing an anxious family, while wisdom would decide which option is most appropriate for a specific family" (American Nurses Association, 2008, p. 5).

Over the years, the definition of NI has evolved. The American Nurses Association (2008) currently defines NI as "a specialty that integrates nursing science, computer science, and information science to manage and communicate data, information, knowledge, and wisdom in nursing practice" (p. 1). The definition of nursing informatics used by the International Medical Informatics Association was updated in 2009 by the special interest group on NI to state "NI science and practice integrates nursing, its information and knowledge and their management with information and communication techniques to promote the health of people, families, and communities worldwide" (IMIA, 2009). The Health Information and Management Systems Society (2016) defines nursing informatics as "the specialty that integrates nursing science with multiple information management and analytical sciences to identify, define, manage, and communicate data, information, knowledge, and wisdom in nursing practice. NI supports nurses, consumers, patients, the interprofessional healthcare team, and other stakeholders in their decision making in all roles and settings to achieve desired outcomes. This support is accomplished through the use of information structures, information processes, and information technology" (para. 1).

Practical Uses of Informatics in Nursing

Informatics has been applied to many aspects of nursing practice including nursing management, nurse clinical practices, nursing education, and nursing research (Choi, Yang, & Lee, 2014). Darvish, Bahramnezhad, Keyhanian, & Navidhamidi (2014) stated that nurses' competencies related to informatics can be classified in three areas: (a) computer skills, including computerized searching and documenting patient demographical information and safely use of computer and networks; (b) informatics knowledge, including the basic understanding of the manual systems and computerized information systems and its impact on the providers; and (c) informatics skills, i.e., the interpretation of the flow of information within the hospital system.

In the area of nursing management, most hospital information systems are equipped with nursing management services like automation of work schedules, budgets, and quality assurance. EHR and other clinical information systems assist the clinical practices of nurses such as automation of patient records, monitoring of vital signs, and automatic billing and generation of work plans. HIT has also facilitated the transition of care from the healthcare institution to where people live (Jones & Brennan, 2002) as exemplified by gerontechnology (see **Contemporary Practice Highlight 20-2**). Nurses are also being supported by computers, networks, and distance learning programs to continue their education. Nursing research is also facilitated by various Internet resources like Medline and the adoption of standardized nursing languages.

CONTEMPORARY PRACTICE HIGHLIGHT 20-2

GERONTECHNOLOGY

The worldwide population is aging. With a growth rate higher than the population as a whole, elderly people today are one of the largest social groups. These demographic changes pose big challenges and, as a result, these challenges occupy an increasingly significant role in national and international health policies. Social policies encourage the idea of "aging in place," where older people remain in their own homes and communities, because this is considered to be the best solution in terms of the health, quality of life, and social connections of elderly people, as well as in economic terms. For this purpose, new technologies such as information and communication technologies and assistive technologies play an important role (Rodeschini, 2011). Gerontechnology is the interdisciplinary field that observes the connection between older people and technology. It uses the appropriate design and new technologies to promote independent living and autonomy in the elderly people, while strengthening the support of their networks. In other words, gerontechnology is about matching technology to make health, housing, mobility, communication, leisure, and work easier for older people. Examples of gerontechnologies can range from simple tools such as a handheld magnifier to more complex systems like remote monitoring, smart tools for medication management, and fall detector systems. Gerontechnologies can help older adults living longer and more safely at home.

Nursing Informatics: Relationships to Other Fields

As all of the aforementioned definitions of NI hint, NI is a part of a bigger trend in informatics. As the AMIA (2016a) notes, the science of informatics drives innovation that is defining future approaches to information and knowledge management in biomedical research, clinical care, and public health. All work in informatics is motivated by the need to create new solutions—often using information technology—that enhance biomedical science, the health of the populace, and the quality and safety of care that is provided to individuals when they are ill. Informatics researchers develop, introduce, and evaluate new biomedically motivated methods in areas as diverse as data mining (deriving new knowledge from large databases), natural language or text processing, cognitive science, human interface design, decision support, databases, and algorithms for analyzing large amounts of data generated in public health, clinical research, or genomics/proteomics.

The science of informatics is inherently interdisciplinary, drawing on (and contributing to) a large number of other component fields, including computer science, decision science, information science, management science, cognitive science, and organizational theory. For example, bioinformatics, public health informatics, dental informatics, and chemical informatics all include the name of the core scientific discipline. Likewise, the term "health informatics" is used to capture applied research and practice in clinical and public health informatics, and AMIA is now using the term "medical informatics" solely to refer to the branch of clinical informatics that

TABLE 20-3 ANCC INFORMATICS NURSE CERTIFICATION ELIGIBILITY CRITERIA

Criterion	Eligibility Qualifications
Licensure	• Active licensure as a registered nurse in the United States or its territory **OR** • Hold the legal equivalency of U.S. registered nurse licensure in another country
Practice	• Equivalent of 2 years of full-time practice as a registered nurse **AND** • At least 2,000 hours of practice in informatics nursing over the last 3 years **OR** • At least 1,000 hours of practice in informatics nursing over the last 3 years **plus** 12 hours of earned academic semester credit in informatics courses within a graduate nursing informatics program **OR** • Earned graduate degree from an informatics nursing program with at least 200 hours practicum (faculty-supervised) in informatics nursing
Education	• Baccalaureate-level or higher degree in nursing **OR** • Bachelor-level degree in a related discipline or field
Continuing Education	• Complete a minimum of 30 hours of continuing education related to nursing informatics in the last 3 years

Data from American Nurses Credentialing Center. (2016b). Informatics nursing certification eligibility criteria. Retrieved from http://www.nursecredentialing.org/informatics-eligibility.aspx

deals with disease diagnosis and management, with an emphasis on physicians (and therefore parallel to "dental informatics" or "nursing informatics") (AMIA, 2016b).

Certification for Informatics Nurses

A nurse can become certified as an informatics nurse by applying to sit for a certification exam through the American Nurses Credentialing Center (ANCC, 2016a) and paying the examination fee. The ANCC Informatics Nursing board certification examination is a competency-based examination that provides a valid and reliable assessment of the entry-level clinical knowledge and skills of registered nurses in the informatics specialty. The eligibility criteria for a nurse practicing in the United States is listed in **Table 20-3**.

Summary

It was recognized over a decade ago that the success of HIT implementations relies not only on IT professionals but also on physicians, nurses, and other health professionals who are the direct users of the technology (Ash & Bates, 2005). Studies have indicated that using HIT not only improves the quality of health care, but it can also have a positive impact on nurses' attitudes (Waneka & Spetz, 2010). Including informatics concepts in nursing program curricula is necessary to provide nurses with the competencies they need to effectively use HIT in their practice. Nursing informatics has emerged as a new specialty to fulfill the demand for nurses with expertise in the application HIT.

Reflective Practice Questions

1. What types of HIT are you currently using in your clinical experiences as a nursing student? What benefits to the use of HIT have you identified? What disadvantages to HIT have you experienced in the clinical setting?
2. Explain the value of the PEF for nursing practice. List three potential ways you can implement this framework in your future nursing practice.
3. You are working as a registered nurse in a clinic and a patient asks you to participate in a public Facebook site for diabetes patients and their significant others. In your future role as a nurse and healthcare provider, what precautions would you need to take in order to participate?
4. What are the possible roles of the nurse informaticist when implementing a new EHR system in a clinic?

References

Agency for Healthcare Research and Quality. (2007). Defining the patient centered medical home. Retrieved from https://www.pcmh.ahrq.gov/page/defining-pcmh

Altman, S. H., Butler, A. S., & Shern, L. (2016). *Assessing progress on the Institute of Medicine report "The Future of Nursing."* Washington, DC: National Academies Press.

American Medical Informatics Association. (2016a). Informatics core: Science of informatics. Retrieved from https://www.amia.org/about-amia/science-informatics

American Medical Informatics Association. (2016b). Nursing informatics. Retrieved from http://www.amia.org/programs/working-groups/nursing-informatics

American Nurses Credentialing Center. (2016a). Informatics nursing. Retrieved from http://nursecredentialing.org/InformaticsNursing

American Nurses Credentialing Center. (2016b). Informatics nursing certification eligibility criteria. Retrieved from http://www.nursecredentialing.org/informatics-eligibility.aspx

American Nurses Association. (n.d.). *Social networking principles toolkit.* Retrieved from http://www.nursingworld.org/socialnetworkingtoolkit.aspx

American Nurses Association. (2008). *Nursing informatics: Scope and standards of practice.* Silver Spring, MD: Author.

Ash, J. S., & Bates, D. W. (2005). Factors and forces affecting EHR system adoption: Report of a 2004 ACMI discussion. *Journal of the American Medical Informatics Association, 12*(1), 8–12.

Bakken, S., Stone, P. W., & Larson, E. L. (2008). A nursing informatics research agenda for 2008–18: Contextual influences and key components. *Nursing Outlook, 56*(5), 206–214. e203. doi: 10.1016/j.outlook.2008.06.007

Barello, S., Graffigna, G., Vegni, E., & Bosio, A. (2014). The challenges of conceptualizing patient engagement in healthcare: A lexicographic literature review. *Journal of Participatory Medicine, 6*, e9.

Barnett, O. G., Jenders, R. A., & Chueh, H. C. (1993). The computer-based clinical record: Where do we stand. *Annals of Internal Medicine, 119*(10), 1046–1048.

Blum, B. I. (1986). Clinical information systems—a review. *Western Journal of Medicine, 145*(6), 791–797.

Carman, K. L., Dardess, P., Maurer, M., Sofaer, S., Adams, K., Bechtel, C., & Sweeney, J. (2013). Patient and family engagement: A framework for understanding the elements and developing interventions and policies. *Health Affairs, 32*(2), 223–231.

Centers for Medicare & Medicaid Services. (2016a). Eligible professional objectives and measures. Retrieved from https://www.cms.gov/Regulations-and-Guidance/Legislation/EHRIncentivePrograms/Downloads/2016_EPTableOfContents.pdf

Centers for Medicare & Medicaid Services. (2016b). 2016 program requirements. Retrieved from https://www.cms.gov/Regulations-and-Guidance/Legislation/EHRIncentive Programs/2016ProgramRequirements.html

Choi, M., Yang, Y. L., & Lee, S.-M. (2014). Effectiveness of nursing management information systems: A systematic review. *Healthcare Informatics Research, 20*(4), 249–257.

Corrigan, J. M. (2005). Crossing the quality chasm. In P. P. Reid, W. D. Compton, J. H. Grossman, & G. Fanjiang (Eds.), *Building a better delivery system: A new engineering/health care partnership* (pp. 95–97). Washington, DC: National Academies Press.

Darvish, A., Bahramnezhad, F., Keyhanian, S., & Navidhamidi, M. (2014). The role of nursing informatics on promoting quality of health care and the need for appropriate education. *Global Journal of Health Science, 6*(6), 11–18.

Doswell, W., Braxter, B., Dabbs, A. D., Nilsen, W., & Klem, M. (2013). mHealth: Technology for nursing practice, education, and research. *Journal of Nursing Education and Practice, 3*(10), 99–109.

Eytan, T., Benabio, J., Golla, V., Parikh, R., Stein, S., & Garfield, S. (2011). Social media and the health system. *Permanente Journal, 15*(1), 71–74.

Friedman, C. P. (2013). What informatics is and isn't. *Journal of the American Medical Informatics Association, 20*(2), 224–226. doi: 10.1136/amiajnl-2012-001206

Graves, J. R., & Corcoran, S. (1989). The study of nursing informatics. *Image: The Journal of Nursing Scholarship, 21*(4), 227–231.

Health Information and Management Systems Society. (2016). What is nursing informatics? Retrieved from http://www.himss.org/what-nursing-informatics

HealthIT.gov. (2015). Meaningful use definition & objectives. Retrieved from https://www.healthit.gov/providers-professionals/meaningful-use-definition-objectives

Hovenga, E. J. S. (2013). Health workforce competencies needed for a digital world. *Studies in Health Technology and Informatics, 193*, 141–168.

Hull, S. J., Abril, E. P., Shah, D. V., Choi, M., Chih, M.-Y., Kim, S. C., . . . Gustafson, D. H. (2016). Self-determination theory and computer-mediated support: Modeling effects on breast cancer patient's quality-of-life. *Health Communication*, 1–10.

Huston, C. (2013). The impact of emerging technology on nursing care: Warp speed ahead. *Online Journal of Issues in Nursing, 18*(2), 1.

Institute of Medicine. (2011). *The future of nursing: Leading change, advancing health.* Washington, DC: National Academies Press.

International Medical Informatics Association. (2009). IMIA-NI: Definition of nursing informatics updated. Retrieved from https://imianews.wordpress.com/2009/08/24/imia-ni-definition-of-nursing-informatics-updated/

Jones, J. F., & Brennan, P. F. (2002). Telehealth interventions to improve clinical nursing of elders. *Annual Review of Nursing Research, 20*(1), 293–322.

Landry, K. E. (2015). Using eHealth to improve health literacy among the patient population. *Creative Nursing, 21*(1), 53–57.

Mantas, J., Ammenwerth, E., Demiris, G., Hasman, A., Haux, R., Hersh, W., . . . Wright, G. (2010). Recommendations of the International Medical Informatics Association (IMIA) on Education in Biomedical and Health Informatics (first revision). *Methods of Information in Medicine, 49*(2), 105–120.

Moen, A., & Mæland Knudsen, L. M. (2013). Nursing informatics: Decades of contribution to health informatics. *Healthcare Informatics Research, 19*(2), 86–92. doi: 10.4258/hir.2013.19.2.86

National Council of State Boards of Nursing. (2011). White paper: A nurse's guide to the use of social media. Retrieved from https://www.ncsbn.org/11_NCSBN_Nurses_Guide _social_media.pdf

Nelson, R. (2002). Major theories supporting health care informatics. In S. P. Englebardt & R. Nelson (Eds.), *Health care informatics: An interdisciplinary approach* (pp. 3–27). St. Louis, MO: Mosby.

Nelson, R. R. (1989). What is private and what is public about technology? *Science, Technology & Human Values*, *14*(3), 229–241.

Office of the National Coordinator. (2015). Patient-generated health data. Retrieved from https://www.healthit.gov/policy-researchers-implementers/patient-generated-health-data

Office of the National Coordinator. (2016). *What is HIE?* Retrieved from https://www.healthit .gov/providers-professionals/health-information-exchange/what-hie

Ozbolt, J. G., & Saba, V. K. (2008). A brief history of nursing informatics in the United States of America. *Nursing Outlook*, *56*(5), 199–205. e192.

Patient-Centered Primary Care Collective. (2015). The patient centered medical home. Retrieved from http://www.pcpcc.org/about/medical-home

Robinson, B. (2007). The ultimate health care record. *Government Health IT*, *2*, 22–24.

Robinson, T. N., Patrick, K., Eng, T. R., & Gustafson, D. (1998). An evidence-based approach to interactive health communication: A challenge to medicine in the information age. *JAMA*, *280*(14), 1264–1269.

Rodeschini, G. (2011). Gerotechnology: A new kind of care for aging? An analysis of the relationship between older people and technology. *Nursing & Health Sciences*, *13*(4), 521–528. doi: 10.1111/j.1442-2018.2011.00634.

Schatz, B. R. (2015). National surveys of population health: Big data analytics for mobile health monitors. *Big Data*, *3*(4), 219–229.

Silverman, R. D. (2013). EHRs, EMRs, and health information technology: To meaningful use and beyond. *Journal of Legal Medicine*, *34*(1), 1–6. doi: 10.1080/01947648.2013.768134

Spector, N., & Kappel, D. (2012). Guidelines for using electronic and social media: The regulatory perspective. *Online Journal of Issues in Nursing*, *17*(3), Manuscript 1. doi: 103912?OJIN.Vol17No03Man01

Valenta, A. L., Meagher, E. A., Tachinardi, U., & Starren, J. (2016). Core informatics competencies for clinical and translational scientists: What do our customers and collaborators need to know? *Journal of the American Medical Informatics Association*, *23*(4), 835–839. doi: 10.1093/jamia/ocw047

Ventola, C. L. (2014). Social media and health care professionals: Benefits, risks, and best practices. *Pharmacy and Therapeutics*, *39*(7), 491–520.

Vest, J. R. (2016). Geography of community health information organization activity in the United States: Implications for the effectiveness of health information exchange. *Health Care Management Review*. [Epub ahead of print]

Walker, J., Pan, E., Johnston, D., & Adler-Milstein, J. (2005). The value of health care information exchange and interoperability. *Health Affairs*, *24*, W5.

Waneka, R., & Spetz, J. (2010). Hospital information technology systems' impact on nurses and nursing care. *Journal of Nursing Administration*, *40*(12), 509–514.

World Health Organization. (2016). eHealth. Retrieved from http://www.who.int/topics /ehealth/en/

Understanding Genetics and Genomics Nursing Competencies

Donna Zucker

LEARNING OUTCOMES

After reading this chapter you will be able to:

- Discuss the importance of genetics and genomics to the profession of nursing.
- Identify the evolutionary history of the science of genetics and genomics.
- Describe the relevance of genetic and genomic research to the discipline of nursing practice and science.
- Describe and discuss the genetics and genomics competencies that influence nursing.
- Explore various online resources that will increase nursing competencies in genetics and genomics.

Introduction

Theories of heredity and spontaneous generation have been studied since the times of Hippocrates, Aristotle, Pythagoras, Leeuwenhoek, and Darwin. But it was not until Gregor Mendel's (1822–1884) experiments with pea plants that the rules of heredity were established and a new science of genetics emerged. Three decades after his death this work was seen to have a profound influence on several scientists whose work confirmed Mendel's experiments. Almost a century passed before scientists demonstrated that **genes** code for proteins.

> **KEY TERM**
> **Genes:** Basic physical and functional units of heredity that are made up of DNA and act as instructions to make molecules called proteins.

Of interest to scientists were the discoveries of gene disorders such as chromosomal abnormalities (e.g., Down syndrome), gene deletion disorders (e.g., Duchenne muscular dystrophy), and multifactorial disorders (e.g., diabetes and cancer). Over the past 50 years genetic scientists have given health providers detailed genetic information that aims to improve the diagnosis of diseases, can provide early detection of future genetic disease in the next generation, and create opportunities for targeted therapies and pharmaceuticals to treat certain diseases. This specialty is known as **pharmacogenomics**.

> **KEY TERM**
> **Pharmacogenomics:** The study of how genes affect a person's response to drugs. This relatively new field combines pharmacology (the science of drugs) and genomics (the study of genes and their functions) to develop effective, safe medications and doses that will be tailored to a person's genetic makeup.

This chapter discusses the rapidly changing field of genetics/genomics and its impact on nursing practice. Key terms are provided to help nurses learn the language of genetics, helping nurses to contribute to interdisciplinary teams of healthcare providers about the role genetics plays in health care. The chapter also discusses the genetics/genomics competencies for nursing practice that have been developed for today's practicing nurses enabling them to competently care for individuals and families. This chapter provides a comprehensive set of tools using the nursing process that will contribute to their growing competence in understanding genetics.

Growing Influence of Genetics and Genomics on Nursing

> **KEY TERM**
> **Human Genome Project (HGP):** An international project that mapped and sequenced the entire human genome.

The **Human Genome Project (HGP)** was initiated in 1990; and the results of the first draft of the HGP in 2001 changed the face of health and nursing care (International Human Genome Sequencing Consortium, 2001). The HGP was later completed in August 2003; this international collaboration resulted in the sequencing of the human genome and reported early data analysis with a look toward future possibilities.

The HGP sequencing has revealed many significant and new facts about the structure and function of our genetic code. Previously it was thought that the human genome consisted of 80,000 to 140,000 genes, but the total number is now estimated at around 30,000 with only about 2 percent coding for proteins and about 50 percent consisting of repeat sequences or "junk DNA" (NHGRI, n.d.). According to Dr. Francis Collins, the director of the National Institutes for Health (NIH), and former director of the National Human Genome Research Institute, all data that are generated by this project is freely accessible to the scientific community with no limits placed on its use (https://www.genome.gov/10000779). Collins suggested that the knowledge uncovered by the HGP be shared worldwide and that very high scientific standards be applied to conduct in-depth analyses of the data. The HGP was not only an opportunity for scientific exploration but it also carried a significant scientific responsibility. To date **genetics** and **genomics** science is a specialty discipline conducted by interdisciplinary team members including nurses, doctors, bench scientists, ethicists, and counselors.

> **KEY TERM**
> **Genetics:** Study of individual genes and their impact on relatively rare single gene disorders.

> **KEY TERM**
> **Genomics:** Study of all the genes in the human genome together, including their interactions with each other, the environment, and the influence of other psychosocial and cultural factors.

As with all new scientific knowledge the goals for new knowledge related to genetics are to translate innovations and findings into practice. In order to remain current with practice, nursing students are now learning genetics/genomics concepts in the curriculum, reading publications with genetics/genomics content, and applying this new knowledge to their nursing practice. Nurses should know about genetics and genomics to have a role in conducting interdisciplinary genetics research and to become informed leaders in both nursing practice and education. Nursing pioneers in genetics and genomics nursing, Jean Jenkins and Kathy Calzone (Jenkins & Calzone, 2007), were instrumental in developing nurse-specific competencies (American Nurses Association [ANA], 2008). Their work has been instrumental in setting priorities in genetics nursing research.

Relevance to Nursing Practice, Education, and Research

Being up to date in a rapidly growing field of science such as genetics or genomics requires nurses to engage in lifelong learning activities, for example, consulting the literature often, reading research studies, attending conferences, and participating in webinars. Among the milestone publications affecting nursing knowledge in the area of genetics and genomics was the report of the Human Genome Project in 2001 (NHGRI, 2001).

The Human Genome Project

The HGP is composed of a vast international consortium of researchers whose goal was the complete mapping and understanding of all the genes of human beings. We inherit two **alleles** for each gene, one from each parent. All our genes together

> **KEY TERM**
> **Alleles:** One of two or more versions of a gene. An individual inherits two for each gene, one from each parent.

are known as our **human genome**. Human **deoxyribonucleic acid (DNA)** contains all of our genes and our heredity material. Our **genotype** is our own unique collection of genes. The HGP revealed that there are about 20,500 genes and identified their locations. Essentially this provides geneticists with a "map" of the inheritable instructions for the development and functions of a human being (National Human Genome Research Institute, 2015d). The HGP is now housed as an institute at the NIH, the National Human Genome Research Institute (NHGRI). Two major outcomes of the HGP were sharing the information with people and societies worldwide, as well as an analysis of the ethical and moral implications of this new genetic information.

A recent initiative of the HGP is the Cancer Genome Atlas (http://cancergenome.nih.gov) that generated multidimensional maps of the genetic abnormalities seen in 33 different tumor types. With this information, care providers can improve cancer prevention, early detection, and treatment. This is an example of a larger effort at large-scale storage of cancer-specific clinical data. The aim is to promote sharing between researchers and clinicians for improved patient health.

Global Genetics and Genomics Community

In order for nurses to become more knowledgeable about the emerging information related to genetics and genomics, the Global Genetics and Genomics Community (G3C) was created as a way to access online case study-based information about basic genetic and genomic concepts, which were developed using the nursing process as a framework (G3C, 2015). The content is designed for entry-level nursing students, and many nurse experts contributed to the development of this information. For nursing students, the case studies are focused on ethnically diverse exemplars, family health, chronic conditions such as diabetes and cardiovascular disease, and includes direct-to-consumer information.

Genetics and Genomics Competencies for Nurses

G3C was developed to augment faculty teaching of genetics and genomics content and is based on the *Essentials of Genetic and Genomic Nursing* (ANA, 2008). First published in 2006, the purpose of these guidelines is to provide nurses with the information and education needed to demonstrate competency in providing genetic and genomic information to individuals and families in their nursing practice areas. This is not limited to newborn assessments but includes the risk for acute and chronic conditions across the lifespan and development of health-promoting activities for all citizens. In 2008 these guidelines were enhanced by the inclusion of knowledge and practice outcome indicators for each competency. These competencies are made of five domains and incorporate the entire family.

The first domain is *Professional Responsibilities*. In this domain nurses are to incorporate genetic and genomic knowledge and skills into their professional practice. In addition to working within their scope of practice, they will apply genetic and genomic science to areas of patient advocacy, education, technical skills, and having an awareness of one's own values and beliefs related to genetic and genomic science.

The second domain is *Professional Practice*. Nurses will apply and integrate genetic and genomic knowledge using the nursing process. These steps include collecting a comprehensive health and physical assessment and health history, generating a family pedigree, analyzing findings to determine a plan of care, and evaluating the client's (meant here as client and family) understandings after receiving genetic and genomic information.

The third domain is *Identification,* in which the nurse identifies ethical, societal, and legal issues related to genetic and genomic information and technologies. For example, the nurse will identify issues that may negatively influence the rights of all clients' decision making.

The fourth domain is *Referral Activities*. In this domain the nurse acts as facilitator for the client to provide referrals for specialized services. For example, the nurse would schedule a referral for genetic testing or consultation with a genetic specialist.

The fifth domain is *Provision of Education, Care, and Support*. In this domain the nurse manages the care of the client while incorporating genetic and genomic information and health promoting strategies into the encounters. This may start at the beginning of care and continue across the plan of care. The competencies also include essential knowledge elements and provide possible or suggested clinical practice indicators (ANA, 2008).

Essentials of Baccalaureate Education of Professional Nursing Practice

The *Essentials of Baccalaureate Education of Professional Nursing Practice* (American Association of Colleges of Nursing, 2008) provide a framework for baccalaureate nurse education for the 21st century. This framework provides faculty with an outline of concepts related to genetics and genomics that should be integrated into all baccalaureate nursing programs. Among the nine education essentials is a focus on health promotion and population health with an emphasis on nurses keeping abreast of the rapidly changing genetics and genomics information that influence patient health and outcomes. Several skills and competencies address the need for assessing for genetic factors that may influence health, including using a **pedigree** and standardized symbolic language for genetic risk assessment;

KEY TERM

Pedigree: A graphic illustration of a family health history using standardized symbols.

conducting a health history for possible genetic risks; becoming familiar with individual and family needs requiring genetic technology and treatments; and being alert to new and customized therapies to improve patient outcomes (ANA, 2008).

Although both of these competency frameworks form a strong foundation for genetics and genomics competencies, several other documents of note exist and inform nursing practice standards. These include the *Scope and Standards of Advanced Practice Nursing in Oncology* (Brant & Wickham, 2013) and the International Society of Nurses in Genetics's (ISONG) *Genetics and Genomics Scope and Standards of Practice* (ANA & ISONG, 2007).

Precision Medicine, Consumer Protection, and Ethics

Precision Medicine

Formally known as personalized medicine, the term **precision medicine** is used to refer to medical treatments that are individualized to patients based upon genetic, environmental, and lifestyle factors. Personalized health care may eliminate trial and error approaches to treatment, enable us to detect illnesses before they become symptomatic, and provide illness prevention strategies. President Obama dedicated $215 million dollars in 2015, to a new Precision Medicine Initiative (PMI) (NIH, n.d.-a). It calls for the voluntary participation of more than 1 million American children and adults in building a big data set, allowing scientists to amass a large amount of information to develop precise treatments and preventive therapies for specific needs in people. Some elements gathered include genetic, lifestyle, and environmental characteristics.

It is anticipated that the information gathered through this initiative will allow scientists to first and foremost develop measures of risk for a variety of diseases based on environmental exposures, genetics factors, and their interactions. Next the initiative hopes to identify the causes of individual differences in response to commonly used drugs (commonly referred to as pharmacogenomics). This initiative will also allow scientists to discover biological markers that signal increased or decreased risk of developing common diseases and develop new disease classifications and relationships. The plan will rely on the use of mobile health (mHealth) technologies to correlate persons' activity, physiological measures, and environmental exposures with health outcomes. Such mHealth tools hope to empower study participants with data and information to improve their own health through self-monitoring. Finally this initiative will create a platform to enable trials of targeted therapies (NIH, n.d.-b).

This underscores the importance of nurses expanding their competencies to genetics and genomics science, including knowledge of big data sets and their usefulness in health and wellness. To address this cutting-edge information and most up-to-date changes in this specialty, the Centers for Disease Control and Prevention (CDC) have a dedicated website with multiple resources including books, articles, and weblinks (http://www.cdc.gov/genomics/default.htm /public/features/precision_med.htm). **Contemporary Practice Highlight 21-1** further addresses the role of the nurse in serving as patient advocates in the use of precision medicine.

Biorepositories or specimen libraries now contain thousands of samples of blood, saliva, and other specimens that may contain DNA and valuable genetic information. Such repositories are very useful in families with cancer histories and other chronic conditions with the aim of preventing disease in future generations or monitoring disease treatment (Biorepositories and Biospecimen Research Branch, 2015). Nurses must have the skills and knowledge to advocate for and respond accurately to any questions clients may have regarding their biological specimens and treatment. For example, each state in the United States has its own public health regulations as to what tests are included in newborn screenings. It is usually between 3 and 8 standard tests, yet many states include up to 53 newborn screening tests (Baby's First Test, 2016). These tests screen for deficiencies in enzymes, amino acids, fatty acids, hemoglobin, endocrine, and other organic acids, as well as other inherited disorders including hearing disorders (Baby's First Test, 2015).

CONTEMPORARY PRACTICE HIGHLIGHT 21–1

PRECISION MEDICINE AND NURSING'S ROLE

Maria is pregnant and has heard that there will be genetic tests done when her baby is born. She asks you (because you are a friend and a nurse) what tests are done and what they will tell her about her baby. Maria is Hispanic and has concerns about the diabetes that is common in her family. She also asks you if you know what they do with the blood samples once the tests are completed (http://www.babysfirsttest.org).

Advocacy is nursing's primary role to ensure that moral, ethical, and legal guidelines are followed. For example, nurses can deliver accurate information, facilitate referrals for specialists, and use reflective practice to ensure professional treatment of all clients and their families. In addition, the professional nurse will understand issues that may affect patient autonomy and decision making and strive for patients to be voluntary participants in their care, without coercion or undue pressure from external forces. Finally, competent nurses can collaborate with interdisciplinary team members to address ongoing ethical issues and identify emerging conflicts.

Consumer Protection

Protecting families and communities is of central importance to the HGP. A specific entity, the **Ethical, Legal, and Social Implications (ELSI) Research Program** focuses on social, legal, and policy implications of genetic research (NHGRI, 2015a). At the onset of the HGP work it was clear that ethical and legal concerns for the protection of the public were priorities. Individual issues include individuals' rights to privacy and confidentiality of their genetic information. Equally important is the "fairness" in the use of genetic information by insurers, employers, courts, schools, adoption agencies, and the military, among others. Considerations such as the psychological impact, stigmatization, and discrimination concerns due to individuals' genetic differences also must be considered. Questions arise such as "Have individuals received adequate information and given informed consent in making decisions regarding reproductive issues?" At the societal level, education about capabilities, limitations, and social risks of clinical genetic conditions is essential for not only healthcare providers, but also for the general public and those who have genetic conditions. Some questions remain unanswered. Who will receive advanced genetic technologies? Will citizens remain up to date on environmental changes made to their food and their ability to choose nongenetically modified products?

> **KEY TERM**
>
> **Ethical, Legal, and Social Implications (ELSI) Research Program:** Fosters basic and applied research on the ethical, legal, and social implications of genetic and genomic research for individuals, families, and communities.

Laws are now in place that protect citizens from the information contained in genetic screening tests. Thirteen years after first being introduced to the legislature, the **Genetic Information Nondiscrimination Act (GINA)** was signed into law in 2008 as a protection against discrimination in the workplace and for personal insurance (NHGRI, 2015b). The bill was intended to allow Americans to take advantage of the benefits of genetic testing without fear of losing their health insurance or their jobs. Since passage of this law, health insurers are prohibited from requesting or requiring genetic information of individuals or their family members or using it for decisions regarding coverage, rates, or preexisting conditions. It also prevents employers from using genetic information in decisions regarding hiring, firing, promotion, or any other terms of employment (such as benefits). These protections extend to those who legally participate in research using genetic testing, counseling, and education (NHGRI, 2015c).

> **KEY TERM**
>
> **Genetic Information Nondiscrimination Act (GINA):** Law that prevents workplace and insurance discrimination based on genetic medical history.

There are some instances in which GINA does not apply. These include members of the military, someone who is already ill and has been diagnosed, and the use of genetic information in regard to life, long-term care, or disability insurance.

Direct-to-Consumer Products

Consumer products to determine heredity and DNA analysis, available through social media and online shopping sites, present consumers and providers with a variety of concerns and questions. In 2015 a systematic review of health science literature was completed in order to understand more about this phenomenon (Covolo, Rubinelli, Ceretti, & Gelatti, 2015). Authors found that genetic testing information provided by the companies to the consumer is not comprehensive. They concluded that the tests offered are not informative, have little predictive power, and do not measure genetic risk appropriately. Although there was no proof of negative effects on consumers the authors suggested this might be a function of very few studies examining consumer perceptions; thus more research is needed.

It is important for nurses to have an awareness of various ways consumers receive information about genetic tests and the implications these products may have on consumers' health. Genetic home testing kits such as *23 and Me* (http://23andme.com), for example, are marketed to buyers who want to know more about their heritage. Ethical issues arise concerning who or what entity is responsible for the uncertainties that may develop associated with these gene test results, as well as fear associated with new knowledge about susceptible conditions such as heart disease, diabetes, and Alzheimer's disease. Worldwide, providers are concerned about quality and oversight of these tests. Prepared with this important information, nurses can provide accurate information about these websites and products to clients and their families.

Another approach the nurse can take is to recommend consumers consult their healthcare providers for information about genetic testing. Reasonable concerns for quality oversight over genetic technologies and products have been addressed though several channels. The first is the U.S. Food and Drug Administration (USFDA) that must authorize all test kits as meeting standards of quality (http://www.fda.gov). This oversight also applies to drug labeling, ensuring all drugs complete a drug review process for safety and effectiveness (USFDA, 2015).

The second office overseeing quality is the NIH Genetic Testing Registry (GTR) that makes information about genetic tests easily accessible to healthcare providers, researchers, and others. This registry draws on the experts at the NIH and other specialists to act as consultants about the content and usefulness of the GTR. A third quality resource is the Evaluation of Genomic Applications in Practice and Prevention (http://www.egappreviews.org/about.htm). This initiative was launched by the CDC in 2004 to establish and evaluate a systematic, evidence-based process for assessing genetic tests and other applications of genomic technology in transition from research to clinical and public health practice. This is in response to the need for providers to offer safe and useful tests to their clients and families.

Theory Applicable to Genetics and Genomics

The Family Systems Genetic Illness Model

"There is a clear need for a conceptual model that describes genomic conditions in psychosocial terms and provides a guide to clinical practice and research" (Rolland & Williams, 2006, p. 37). The Family Systems Genetic Illness Model (FSGIM) was developed from an earlier model, the Family Systems–Illness (FSI) Model (Rolland, 1994). The FSGIM is tailored to address the complexities of genetic and environmental factors associated with common chronic health conditions. It is a good psychosocial framework for nursing in that it considers the type of genetic illness in relation to the individual life stage and within the context of the belief system and culture of the individual or family. See **Figure 21-1** for an illustration of the FSI model.

An important feature of using this theory for genetic and genomic disorders is that it provides a typology for looking at the onset of the genetic diagnosis, and whether it is acute or chronic and nonsymptomatic or symptomatic. Consideration of all of these phases has implications for the individual or family's treatment. Further, the theory takes into account the developmental level such as childhood, middle adulthood, and adulthood. This type of framework allows nurses to create and describe psychosocial interventions based on the onset of diagnosis and its severity, the stages in life, and whether the disorder is acute, chronic, treatable, or in some cases fatal.

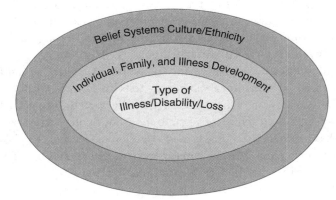

Figure 21-1   Family Systems–Illness Model.

Reproduced from Rolland, J. S. (1994). *Families, illness, and disability: An integrative treatment model.* New York, NY: Basic Books.

Nursing Process Applied to Genetics

All professional nurses use the nursing process in caring for their patients. The steps are similar for staff nurses and advanced practice nurses caring for individuals and families seeking care for genetics and genomics consultation, referral, and treatment. Specific differences are seen in the scope of practice for each level of nursing. This section focuses on the skills, attitudes, and knowledge necessary for the novice and baccalaureate prepared generalist nurse. Lea (2008) emphasized that nurses understand the ethical implications associated with genetic and genomic nursing care, including "informed decision making, informed consent and genetic testing, genetic and genomic research testing protection, maintaining privacy and confidentiality of genetic information, preventing genetic discrimination and strengthening genetic and genomic care around the world" (p. 3).

Nursing Assessment: Completing a Family History and Pedigree

Many tools are available for genetic and genomic nursing assessment. In the field of genetics and genomics, it is essential nurses know the importance of and techniques used in eliciting at least a three-generation family health history. This most often is learned by practicing with your own family, for example, by filling in a family tree or "pedigree" (NHGRI, 2015d). Among the many articles and sites addressing this skill, the NHGRI (2015d) website includes an educational module on how to create a family health history using a pedigree and a **genogram** (see **Figures 21-2** and **21-3**). Nurses can also become astute in determining an individual genetic **phenotype** based on basic assessment and history taking.

> **KEY TERM**
> **Genogram:** Includes demographic information about family members and how they are related to one another.

Consumers can also archive their family health histories using reliable websites or portals. For example, the Surgeon General's website My Family Health Portrait (U.S. Department of Health and Human Services, 2014) is an online personal electronic

> **KEY TERM**
> **Phenotype:** An individual's observable traits, such as height, eye color, and blood type.

health record that can be updated and shared by consumers as needed to assist their healthcare providers in the provision of care. This provides an opportunity for consumers to maintain a file of their own personal health record in a format that is easy to use and share with healthcare providers.

Nursing Diagnosis Related to Genetics and Genomics Health Issues

Genetics and genomics nursing has a long history mostly in the area of genetic counseling. The International Society of Nurses in Genetics, founded in 1988,

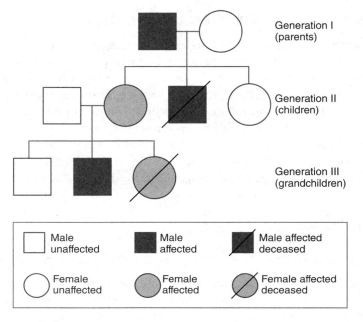

Figure 21-2 Pedigree.

Reproduced from National Human Genome Research Institute. (2010). Image gallery: Pedigree. Retrieved from https://www.genome.gov/dmd/img.cfm?node=Photos/Graphics&tid=85218. Courtesy of Darryl Leja, National Human Genome Research Institute

is a global organization dedicated to genomic health care, education, research, and scholarship. "Genetics nurses help people at risk for, or affected by diseases with a genetic component achieve and maintain health. . . .A genetics nurse is a licensed professional nurse with special education and training in genetics" (ISONG, n.d., para. 1).

Those qualified can become board certified in advanced genetic nursing by the American Nurses Credentialing Center (2015). Both nurses and midwives have to integrate genetics and genomics into family and individual assessments. Additionally, they must consider the importance of nursing interventions, referrals to specialists, and care planning based on nursing diagnoses. See **Box 21-1** for a listing of nursing diagnoses that may be appropriate for patients experiencing genetic disorders. The ANA and ISONG (2007) have also developed the Genetics/ Genomics Scope and Standards of Practice, which outlines nurse competencies based on the nursing process.

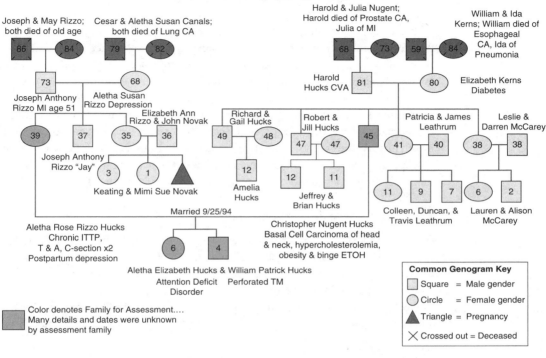

Figure 21-3 Genogram.

BOX 21-1   NURSING DIAGNOSES RELEVANT TO GENETICS DISORDERS

- Anticipatory grieving
- Anxiety
- Interrupted family processes

- Powerlessness
- Spiritual distress

Reproduced from LeMone, P., Burke, K., Dwyer, T., Levett-Jones, T., Moxham, L., Reid-Searl, K., . . . Raymond, D. (2014). *Medical-surgical nursing* (2nd Australian ed.). Melbourne, Australia: Pearson.

Nursing Role in Care Planning

Depending upon the nature of the diagnosis and specific genetic concern, genetic healthcare providers must demonstrate the leadership required to help families face stressful treatment decisions, such as surgery or chemotherapy. Participation of all interdisciplinary team members is often coordinated by the nurse and requires a plan of care including appropriate referrals to medical and surgical specialists as well as psychosocial and spiritual consultants.

It is essential for nurses to understand the essential role they play in delivering care to patients with genetic concerns. **Contemporary Practice Highlight 21-2** represents an example of an unfolding case study that has been excerpted from the Global Genetics and Genomics Community website (http://g-3-c.org/en/), most commonly referred to as G3C. The G3C website is a free access learning portal containing 15 such unfolding case studies. Using a selected unfolding case study, the learner can select various parts of a condition-specific patient encounter (e.g., health history, counseling, referral) and practice communication skills. Knowledge prompts and questions are also included along the way, located in the sidebars, directing the learner to more information on the topic.

Nursing Role in Implementation

One of the most important roles in genetic/genomic nursing is implementing the identified plan and advocating for the individual and family. One strategy is to begin by providing accurate and informative information, clarifying any areas of uncertainty, and reviewing or reinforcing information given and received. The nurse has responsibility for coordinating care, addressing health teaching and health promotion needs, and providing consultation and counseling care to the patient and family members.

Nursing Evaluation

In the evaluation phase of the nursing process, the primary goal of the nurse is to evaluate the extent to which the patient and family members understand the plan of care so that they can make informed and voluntary decisions about their care. This includes ensuring they received answers to their questions especially pertaining to legal and long-term consequences of their decisions.

CONTEMPORARY PRACTICE HIGHLIGHT 21-2

ETHICAL CASE STUDY RELATED TO GENETICS AND GENOMICS: GENETIC TESTING FOR A FAMILY WITH CYSTIC FIBROSIS HISTORY

"Lisa is a healthy 19-year-old woman who has come to the hospital to visit her 21-year-old brother, Mark, who has cystic fibrosis (CF). He has been admitted with a lung infection. She has recently learned that she is pregnant and has some questions. Lisa's brother suggested that she talk with you since he feels you have been so responsive to his questions." (G3C example, http://g-3-c.org/en/case/3/).

Summary

This chapter has provided an introduction to genetics and genomics nursing. Since the completion of the HGP and the mapping of the entire human genome, the field of genetics/genomics is rapidly evolving. Nurses are responsible for staying up to date with these rapid changes in consultation, diagnosis, and treatment of genetic/genomic disorders. Adopting nursing genetic/genomic competencies will ensure that nursing care is accurate, informed, and ethical. A variety of educational resources are available through nursing and government organizations. The nurse of the future will be an important member of an interdisciplinary team requiring specialized genetic/genomic information to predict, diagnose, and manage specific diseases.

Reflective Practice Questions

1. What type of activities can you engage in to recognize your own attitudes and values related to genetic and genomic science that may affect the way you care for patients?
2. Draw a three-generation pedigree with your own family. What did you learn in the process?
3. What is the role of the nurse in talking to a mother about her worries regarding her child's developmental milestones and the genetic tests the doctor has ordered?
4. Name three high-priority genetics/genomics competencies a new nurse should have. Why are these competencies a high priority?

References

American Association of Critical Care Nurses. (2008). *Essentials of baccalaureate education for professional nursing practice*. Washington, DC: Author. Retrieved from http://www.aacn.nche.edu/education-resources/BaccEssentials08.pdf

American Nurses Association. (2008). *Essentials of genetic and genomic competencies* (2nd ed.). Silver Spring, MD: Author. Retrieved from http://www.genome.gov/Pages/Careers/HealthProfessionalEducation/geneticscompetency.pdf

American Nurses Association & International Society of Nurses in Genetics. (2007). *Genetics and genomics nursing: Scope and standards of practice*. Silver Spring, MD: Author.

American Nurses Credentialing Center. (2015). *Advanced genetics nursing*. Retrieved from http://www.nursecredentialing.org/AdvancedGenetics

Baby's First Test. (2015). *Newborn screening, Massachusetts*. Retrieved from http://www.babysfirsttest.org/newborn-screening/states/Massachusetts

Baby's First Test. (2016). *Newborn Screening*. Retrieved from http://www.babysfirsttest.org

Biorepositories and Biospecimen Research Branch. (2015). *Mission and goals.* Retrieved from https://biospecimens.cancer.gov/about/overview.asp

Brant, J., & Wickham, R. (2013). *Statement on the scope and standards of advanced practice nursing.* Pittsburgh, PA: Oncology Nursing Society Press.

Covolo, L., Rubinelli, S., Ceretti, E., & Gelatti, U. (2015). Internet-based direct-to-consumer genetic testing: A systematic review. *Journal of Medical Internet Research, 17*(12), e279. doi: 10.2196/jmir.4378

Global Genetic Genomic Community. (2015). *About G3C.* Retrieved from http://g-3-c.org /en/about/

International Human Genome Sequencing Consortium. (2001). Initial sequencing and analysis of the human genome. *Nature, 409,* 860–921. doi: 10.1038/35057062

International Society of Nurses in Genetics. (n.d.). *What is a genetics nurse?* Retrieved from http://www.isong.org/ISONG_genetic_nurse.php

Jenkins, J., & Calzone, K. (2007). Establishing the essential nursing competencies for genetics and genomics. *Journal of Nursing Scholarship, 39*(1), 10–16.

Lea, D. H. (2008). Genetic and genomic healthcare: Ethical issues of importance to nurses. *Online Journal of Issues in Nursing, 13*(1), Manuscript 4.

LeMone, P., Burke, K., Dwyer, T., Levett-Jones, T., Moxham, L., Reid-Searl, K., . . . Raymond, D. (2014). *Medical-surgical nursing* (2nd Australian ed.). Melbourne, Australia: Pearson.

National Human Genome Research Institute. (2001). *2001: First draft of the human genome sequence released.* Retrieved from https://www.genome.gov/25520483/

National Human Genome Research Institute. (2010). Image gallery: Pedigree. Retrieved from https://www.genome.gov/dmd/img.cfm?node=Photos/Graphics&id=85218

National Human Genome Research Institute. (2015a). *ELSI Research Program.* Retrieved from http://www.genome.gov/ELSI/#al-1

National Human Genome Research Institute. (2015b). *Genetic discrimination: Legislative history of GINA.* Retrieved from http://www.genome.gov/10002077#al-4

National Human Genome Research Institute. (2015c). Genetic Information Nondiscrimination Act of 2008. Retrieved from https://www.genome.gov/10002328/

National Human Genome Research Institute. (2015d). *Your family health history.* Retrieved from https://www.genome.gov/Pages/Education/Modules/YourFamilyHealthHistory.pdf

National Institutes of Health. (n.d.-a). *About the Precision Medicine Initiative Cohort Program.* Retrieved from https://www.nih.gov/precision-medicine-initiative-cohort-program/

National Institutes of Health. (n.d.-b). *Precision Medicine Initiative Cohort Program—Frequently asked questions.* Retrieved from https://www.nih.gov/precision-medicine-initiative-cohort -program/precision-medicine-initiative-cohort-program-frequently-asked-questions

Rolland, J.S. (1994). *Families, illness and disability: An integrative treatment model.* New York, NY: Basic Books.

Rolland, J. S., & Williams, J. K. (2006). Toward a psychosocial model for the new era of genetics. In S. M. Miller, S. H. McDaniel, J. S. Rolland, & S. L. Feetham (Eds.), *Individuals, families, and the new era of genetics.* New York, NY: Norton.

U.S. Department of Health and Human Services. (2014). *My family health portrait.* Retrieved from https://familyhistory.hhs.gov/FHH/html/index.html

U.S. Food and Drug Administration. (2015). FDA's drug review process: continued. Retrieved from http://www.fda.gov/Drugs/ResourcesForYou/Consumers/ucm289601.htm

Glossary

Academic progression programs: Nursing programs that facilitate the seamless articulation or transition from one degree in nursing to another degree (e.g., LPN to RN, ASN to BSN, ASN to MSN, BSN to PhD).

Accreditation: A process by which an institution's (e.g., school of nursing's) programs, policies, and practices are reviewed by an external accrediting body to determine whether professional standards are being met.

Accreditation Commission for Education in Nursing (ACEN): This commission is an accrediting body and Title IV gatekeeper for federal funds for all types of nursing education programs.

Acculturation: The process of the adaptation or accommodation of an individual immigrant or immigrant group to a new culture.

Active failures: Errors and violations caused by acts performed by workers (e.g., nurses) closest to the sharp end of the system (e.g., patient care) that affect system safety most directly (Reason, 1997).

Adverse event: A patient safety event that resulted in harm to a patient (TJC, 2016).

Advanced beginner: Someone who has limited experience with a given situation (Benner, 1984).

Advocacy: A role often performed by nurses that works to promote or protect rights, values, access, interests, and equality in health care (Mason et al., 2016).

Agency for Healthcare Research and Quality (AHRQ): The health services research arm of the U.S. Department of Health and Human Services, complementing the biomedical research mission of its sister agency, the National Institutes of Health. It is a home to research centers that specialize in major areas of healthcare research such as quality improvement and patient safety, outcomes and effectiveness of care, clinical practice and technology assessment, and healthcare organization and delivery systems.

Alleles: One of two or more versions of a gene. An individual inherits two for each gene, one from each parent.

American Association of Colleges of Nursing (AACN): A professional organization in nursing that serves baccalaureate nursing and higher degree nursing education programs by influencing the quality of nursing education and practice through research, advocacy efforts, policy making, development of quality educational standards and indicators, and faculty development.

American Nurses Association (ANA): A professional organization for nurses that develops various standards of nursing practice and promotes change through policy development.

American Society of Superintendents of Training Schools of Nursing: A national nursing organization founded in 1893 to elevate the standards of nursing education; later became the National League for Nursing Education, and ultimately, the National League for Nursing.

Apprenticeship model: A model of nursing education that was prevalent during the first half of the 20th century, where student nurses learned nursing practice by providing service to hospitals.

Area health education centers (AHECs): Federally funded partnerships between health science center universities and local community clinical and educational resources that work together to improve education to local multidisciplinary providers and ultimately improve patient care in underserved areas.

Benchmark: Quality performance measurement data shared among healthcare providers and organizations for quality improvement and safety. The National Committee for Quality Assurance maintains benchmarking data.

Bilateral cooperation: Refers to political, economic, or cultural relations between two sovereign states.

Biopsychosocial model of health and illness: The dynamic interaction of three levels—biological, psychological, and social aspects of health—that affect an individual's well-being.

Bioterrorism: The use of a biological agent to intentionally produce disease in a susceptible population.

Blunt end: Levels of strategic and other top-level decision-making persons or groups in an organization that affect the work at the point of care delivery (the sharp end) (Reason, 1997).

Bolton Act of 1942: Legislation that created the U.S. Cadet Nurse Corps, a program subsidized by the federal government and designed to quickly prepare nurses to meet the needs of the armed forces, civilian and government hospitals, and war industries.

Breach of duty: Failure to perform according to a specific standard of care once a duty is established.

Case-control studies: Research that retrospectively compares the characteristics of one individual with certain medical conditions to another who does not have the medical condition.

Causation: A determination that if not for the conduct of the defendant, the plaintiff would not have been injured and that the consequences of such conduct were foreseeable.

Center for Medicare and Medicaid Services (CMS): A U.S. federal agency that administers Medicare, Medicaid, and the State Children's Health Insurance Program. It provides information for healthcare professionals, regional governments, and consumers in regard to how an organization meets the standards set by the agency itself.

Certification: "A process by which a nongovernmental agency or association certifies that an individual licensed to practice a profession has met certain predetermined standards specified by that profession for specialty practice" (ANA, 1979, p. 67); a designation earned by a person to ensure that he or she is qualified to perform a task or job.

Chemical emergency: The release of some hazardous chemical agent either unintentionally, such as through an accidental industrial release, or intentionally, as in a terrorist attack.

Chronic disease: A long-lasting disease that typically remains with a patient from onset to end of life and requires management of symptoms. Chronic diseases typically last longer than 3 months. Examples are cancer, cardiovascular disease, diabetes, and cerebrovascular disease. According to the U.S. Centers for Disease Control and Prevention (2015), chronic disease is responsible for 7 out of 10 deaths in the United States.

Civil laws: Laws that dictate behavior between parties.

Clinical care protocols: Clinical practice guidelines that reflect the most up-to-date practice based on evidence for reference and knowledge with the goal of having the latest scientific knowledge available to clinicians to make decisions about care. Elements include systematic literature review and the consensus of expert decision makers and consumers who consider the evidence and make recommendations.

Clinical decision support system (CDSS): Software applications designed to provide clinicians and/or patients with knowledge and person-specific information, filtered or presented at appropriate times, to enhance healthcare interventions.

Code of ethics: Standards and behaviors of a profession or organization directed towards its constituents.

Cognitive task analysis: A technique for interview data collection and analysis to describe the cognitive work and influencing factors surrounding situations that led to and resulted in decisions.

Collaboration: Working jointly with other healthcare professionals in a collegial manner. A process whereby healthcare professionals work together to improve patient/client outcomes (ANA, 2015).

Collegiality: Sharing authority and responsibility to reach a prescribed goal or outcome. Power and responsibility are shared and mutual respect and collaboration are desired (AACN, 2016).

Commission on Collegiate Nursing Education (CCNE): Affiliated with the American Association of Colleges of Nursing, this commission is an accrediting body for baccalaureate and higher degree nursing education programs.

Common law: Law that develops as a result of judicial decision; also known as case law.

Communication: "All the cognitive, affective and behavioral responses that can be used to convey a message to another person" (Watson, 1979, p. 33). Communication can be verbal, such as through one's words, how these words are expressed, the tone used in expressing these words, and their pace, clarity, timing, and relevance. Communication can also be nonverbal, where words are not used, but meanings or expressions are communicated via body language, facial expressions, and the use of touch, space, and/or sound. Communication can be varied through the aspect of one's culture as well.

Competencies: Measurable levels of knowledge, skills, and attitudes required to perform in a professional role.

Competent: Someone with 2 to 3 years of experience who is consciously aware of a given situation in its individual parts and can develop a long-range action plan (Benner, 1984).

Complex systems: Systems in which work includes both cognitive and physical demands and is characterized by dynamism, large numbers of parts and connectedness between parts, high uncertainty, and risk (Woods et al., 2010).

Computer adaptive testing (CAT): An interactive testing format used on the NCLEX-RN to adjust the type of question and level of testing difficulty based on the test taker's previous response. In the NCLEX-RN examination, the testing continues until the student either achieves a consistent level of test item difficulty that indicates a satisfactory performance level and passing of the examination, does not achieve a consistent level of testing difficulty required to indicate a satisfactory performance level and thus fails the examination, or completes all of the test items on the examination or time expires on the test.

Computer literacy: Practical knowledge of hardware and software and also the different ways in which software applications can facilitate and/or support practice.

Consent: A patient's acquiescence to care; it must be informed, voluntary, and competently made in order to be valid.

Continuing nursing education: Ongoing education that nurses take part in after they have achieved basic preparation and licensure.

Controlled trial: Research in which there is a treatment group and a group that does not receive the treatment (control group) so that comparisons can be made about the effectiveness of an intervention on a specific health issue and health outcome.

Cooperative extension offices: Funded by the U.S. Department of Agriculture, these offices provide leadership in programming, addressing issues of concern specific to families, youth, and rural communities.

Core measures: Used to measure the quality of care provided by a hospital and its providers for clients with a specific diagnosis such as heart failure, pneumonia, or acute myocardial infarction. These measures are determined by the Center for Medicare and Medicaid Services, the Joint Commission, and the American Hospital Association, and provide a basis for value-based purchasing of healthcare services.

Critical access facilities: Small rural hospitals that are the sole community hospital providers and are reimbursed by the Centers for Medicare and Medicaid Services for actual costs.

Critical thinking: A systematic process of assessing, grouping, and evaluating data to determine the best plan of action for each patient care issue.

Culturally competent health care: The ability to deliver health care with knowledge of and sensitivity to cultural factors that influence the health and illness behaviors of an individual client, family, or community.

Culture: The pattern of ideas, customs, and behaviors shared by a particular group of people or society which distinguishes them from the other.

Curriculum: The overall structure of learning experiences within nursing education programs that reflects a school of nursing's mission and philosophy, program outcomes, course of study, learning experiences, and program evaluation methods.

Damages: Injuries incurred as a result of someone's negligence.

Deaconess: Woman with some educational background who was selected by the church to provide care to the sick.

Decentralization: A process occurring in urban cities in which employment opportunities and social capital move into suburban areas. This process is suggested to be one of the causes of urban poverty.

Delegation: The transfer of the performance of a selected nursing task in a selected situation to a competent individual authority (National Council of State Boards of Nursing, 1995); the process by which a registered nurse directs another person to perform nursing skills and activities that the person would not normally carry out while still retaining accountability for those activities (National Council of State Boards of Nursing, 2016).

Descriptive studies: Research conducted in order to describe characteristics of selected variables or a certain phenomenon.

Disability: Physical or mental impairment that substantially limits a person from completing activities of daily living.

Disability-adjusted life year (DALY): Combines years of life lost due to premature mortality and years of life lost due to time lived in states of less than full health.

Disaster preparedness: A multitude of activities that are conducted before, during, and after an event that may involve extensive destruction.

Deoxyribonucleic acid (DNA): Contains the biological instructions that make each species unique. It, along with the instructions it contains, is passed from adult organisms to their offspring during reproduction.

Duty: An obligation to act or refrain from acting.

Electronic health records (EHR): Electronic versions of a patient's medical history that is maintained by the provider over time and may include all of the key administrative clinical data relevant to that person. It automates access to information and has the potential to streamline the clinician's workflow.

Ethical: Reasons for decisions about how one ought to act.

Ethical, Legal, and Social Implications (ELSI) Research Program: Fosters basic and applied research on the ethical, legal, and social implications of genetic and genomic research for individuals, families, and communities.

Ethics committee: Ideally, a multidisciplinary group of healthcare professionals and consumers charged with ethics education, policy formation, and review and consultation within an organizational setting.

Ethnicity: Designation of a population subgroup sharing a common social and cultural heritage.

Ethnocentrism: A worldview based to a great extent on the socialization of individuals within their own culture, to the extent that such individuals believe that all others see the world as they do.

Evidence-based nursing (EBN): Clinical decision making by nurses that is a combination and integration of the best research evidence; it also includes the nurse's clinical expertise and patient values and preferences about a specific type of care.

Evidence-based practice (EBP): The process of problem solving using the best research evidence in clinical decision making for patient care. It is a combination of a systematic search for and critical appraisal of the most relevant research available to answer a specific clinical question, with the clinician's own clinical expertise and patient values and preferences included (Melnyk & Fineout-Overholt, 2015).

Expert: Someone with the vast experience to intuitively assess a given situation and accurately target the problem area without being distracted by other unrelated symptoms (Benner, 1984).

Fixation: Failure to revise the assessment of a situation as new information becomes available (Woods et al., 2010).

Florence Nightingale: The founder of professional nursing in England.

Gaps: Another term for latent conditions or error-producing factors (Woods et al., 2010).

Genes: Basic physical and functional units of heredity that are made up of DNA and act as instructions to make molecules called proteins.

Genetic Information Nondiscrimination Act (GINA): Law that prevents workplace and insurance discrimination based on genetic medical history.

Genetics: Study of individual genes and their impact on relatively rare single gene disorders.

Genogram: Includes demographic information about family members and how they are related to one another.

Genomics: Study of all the genes in the human genome together, including their interactions with each other, the environment, and the influence of other psychosocial and cultural factors.

Genotype: An individual's collection of genes.

Global burden of disease (GBD): Index that measures the loss of health from all causes of illness and deaths worldwide.

Global citizen: Someone who identifies with being part of an emerging world community and whose actions contributed to building this community's values and practices (Global Citizen Initiative, n.d.).

Global health: Focuses on improving health of populations and promoting equity for all people regardless of national borders.

Globalization: Increased interconnections among people of different countries that facilitate the exchange of goods, services, money, people, information, and ideas across national borders.

Goldmark Report: Published in 1923, this report recommended that nursing education develop educational standards, schools of nursing adopt a primary focus on education and be moved to universities, and nurse educators receive advanced education.

Good Samaritan laws: Laws enacted by a state that protect healthcare providers and other rescuers from liability if they render aid in an emergency, provided that they use reasonable and prudent judgment under the circumstances based on their education, training, and skill level.

Health: "A state of complete physical, mental, and social well-being, and not merely the absence of disease or infirmity, is a fundamental human right, and that the attainment of the highest possible level of health is a most important world-wide social goal whose realization requires the action of many other social and economic sectors in addition to the health sector" (WHO, 1978, p. 1).

Health behavior change: A persistent and lasting change in a person's actions. Overweight/obesity, lack of physical activity, and dietary habits are the top three behaviors that health educators seek to change.

Health disparities: Differences in the incidence, prevalence, mortality, and burden of disease and other adverse health conditions that exist among specific population groups.

Health equity: "The attainment of the highest level of health for all people" (U.S. Department of Health and Human Services, n.d., para. 5).

Health information exchanges (HIEs): Electronic exchanges of health information from one healthcare professional to another to improve the continuity, quality, safety, and efficiency of healthcare delivery.

Health Information Portability and Accountability Act (HIPAA): A U.S. law providing privacy standards to protect patients' health records and other health information provided to health plans, doctors, hospitals, and other healthcare providers.

Health information technology (HIT): Information technology applied to health care, making it possible for healthcare providers to better manage patient care through secure use and sharing of health information.

Health Information Technology for Economic and Clinical Health (HITECH) Act: Promotes the adoption of electronic health records and meaningful use of health information.

Health literacy: An individual's capacity to obtain, process, and understand the basic health information needed to make appropriate health decisions.

Health policy: Policy decisions that are made to promote the health of individuals.

Health professional shortage area (HPSA): This designation identifies defined communities that have shortages of healthcare providers such as primary care, dental, or mental health care (Health Resources Service Administration, n.d.).

Healthy nurse: The creating and maintaining of a balance and synergy of physical, intellectual, emotional, social, spiritual, personal, and professional well-being (ANA, n.d., para. 1).

Healthy People 2020: A statement of national health objectives designed to identify the most significant preventable threats to health and to establish national goals to reduce these threats in the next decade. Goals are set to help public health professionals, healthcare providers, and others work toward improving the health of citizens. Healthy People 2020 can be accessed at http://www.healthypeople.gov.

Hindsight bias: The natural tendency for humans looking back from an accident to consistently overstate what could have been anticipated in foresight and to see only a simplified path of decision making related to the specific accident (Woods et al., 2010).

Human factors: Human factors (ergonomics) is the scientific discipline concerned with the understanding of interactions among humans and other elements of a system and the profession that applies theory, principles, data, and other methods to design in order to optimize human well-being and overall system performance (Human Factors and Ergonomics Society, 2016).

Human genome: The total gene complement, about 3 billion base pairs of DNA, contained in the human chromosomes.

Human Genome Project (HGP): An international project that mapped and sequenced the entire human genome.

Incubation period: The time that lapses between when the host receives the agent and when the host presents with symptoms.

Influence: Affect the actions or opinions of others (Vance, 2012).

Informatics: The study and practice of creating, storing, finding, manipulating, and sharing information.

Information literacy: The ability to define an information need, locate pertinent information, and apply the information correctly.

Institute of Healthcare Improvement (IHI): A not-for-profit organization seeking to improve health care around the world. IHI's work is funded primarily through fee-based program offerings and services, and also through the support of a group of foundations, companies, and individuals. It conducted the 5 Million Lives Campaign.

Institute of Medicine (IOM): Provides a vital service by working outside the framework of government to ensure scientifically informed analysis and guidance. Its mission is to serve as an adviser to the nation to improve health, and it provides unbiased, evidence-based, and authoritative information and advice concerning health and science policy to policymakers, professionals, and leaders in every sector of society and to the public at large.

Institutional policies: Policies that govern a workplace and describe an institution's goals and how it will operate.

Instruction: Teaching and learning strategies and experiences faculty and students engage in to achieve the elements of a curriculum.

Interprofessional collaborative practice: "When multiple health workers from different professional backgrounds work together with patients, families, carers [sic], and communities to deliver the highest quality of care" (WHO, 2010, p. 13).

Latent conditions: Error-producing factors like poor design, gaps in supervision, undetected system failures, lack of training, and the like arising from the decision-making levels (blunt end) of organizations that combine with active failures to result in adverse events (Reason, 1997).

Layers of defense: Organizational safeguards in place to prevent anticipated injury, damage, or failure (Reason, 1990).

Leapfrog Group: A voluntary program aimed at mobilizing employer purchasing power to alert the U.S. health industry on "leaps" in healthcare safety, quality, and customer value so they will be recognized and rewarded. Among other initiatives, Leapfrog works with its employer members to encourage transparency and easy access to healthcare information as well as providing rewards for hospitals that have a proven record of high-quality care.

License: Permission to engage in an activity; a professional license allows the holder to engage in a specific activity for compensation.

Licensure: The process by which a state or governmental agency grants permission to an individual to engage in a given profession for compensation.

Lillian Wald: A public health nurse who founded Henry Street Settlement House to provide home nursing care to the immigrant populations on the Lower East Side of New York.

Linda Richards: Purported to be the first educated nurse in the United States, a graduate of the New England Hospital for Women and Children in Boston.

Loss of situation awareness: Failure to maintain accurate tracking of the multiple processes or systems in time (Woods et al., 2010).

Magnet status: The Magnet Recognition Program, established by the American Nurses Credentialing Center in 1993, recognizes healthcare organizations that demonstrate excellence in nursing practice and adherence to national standards for the organization and delivery of nursing services.

Mary Mahoney: The first African American graduate nurse.

Meaningful use (MU): Using health information technology to engage healthcare consumers in their care with the ultimate goal of achieving better care coordination and population and public health and also improving the quality, safety, and efficiency of health care and reducing health disparities.

Medical error: Failure of a planned action to be completed as intended or the use of a wrong plan to achieve an aim (IOM, 2000).

Medically underserved populations (MUPs): This designation is assigned to healthcare service areas that face economic, cultural, or linguistic barriers to health care and is based on computations specific to community poverty level, elderly population, infant mortality rate, and ratio of primary care physicians per 1,000 population (Health Resources Service Administration, n.d.).

Membership: The state of being a member or person in a group, in this case, a professional nursing organization.

Mentor: Someone who develops a long-term relationship with a mentee, without assessment or evaluation (Huybrecht et al., 2011).

Meta-analyses: The summarizations of the results of several quantitative studies critically reviewed, synthesized, and evaluated to answer a specific clinical question about the effectiveness of an intervention across multiple studies in different settings.

Mildred Montag: Developed the concept for associate degree in nursing programs.

Mindfulness: The ability to scrutinize and refine expectations based on new information and/or contextual aspects of a situation (Langer, 1989).

Mistakes: Planning failures—"deficiencies or failures in the judgmental and/or inferential processes involved in the selection of an object or in the specification of the means to achieve it" (Reason, 1990, p. 9).

Moral: Overlaps with "ethical" but is more aligned with personal beliefs and cultural values.

Mutual recognition of licensure model: A model that allows a nurse to have one license in his or her state of residency with the ability to practice (electronically or physically) across state lines in other states that participate in this model if there are no restrictions on his or her license and that person acknowledges that he or she is subject to each state's practice laws and rules (NCSBN, 2011).

Narrative ethics: The use of stories to emphasize the importance of context, contingency, and circumstances in recognizing, evaluating, and resolving moral problems applied to health care.

National Council Licensing Examination for Registered Nurses (NCLEX-RN): This examination must be taken by all graduates of diploma, associate degree, and baccalaureate degree nursing programs prior to a license being issued. Successful completion of the examination is a requirement for practice as a registered nurse.

National Council of State Boards of Nursing (NCSBN): The nursing regulatory body given the task of providing a means to ensure that those who are licensed to practice as nurses are "safe" in terms of their knowledge base.

National Database of Nursing Quality Indicators (NDNQI): The American Nurses Association established these indicators in 1998 and has continued to update the database adding new measures over the years. Previously managed by the University of Kansas School of Nursing, NDNQI was acquired by Press Ganey in 2014. Participating organizations use the database to collect and report unit-specific data. Members receive relevant national comparative data and annual trended comparisons. Nursing-sensitive indicators reflect the structure, process, and outcomes of nursing care.

National League for Nursing Commission for Nursing Education Accreditation (NLN CNEA): Affiliated with the National League for Nursing, this commission is an accrediting body for PN/VN, Diploma, ASN/ADN, BSN, MSN and DNP nursing programs.

National League for Nursing Education (NLNE): A professional nursing organization that fostered excellence in nursing education by supporting nursing education research, engaging in policymaking and advocacy efforts related to nursing education, and promoting faculty development. It was the precursor to the National League for Nursing.

Near-miss event: Also known as "close call," "no harm," or "good catch." A patient safety event that did not cause harm as defined by the term sentinel event. (TJC, 2016).

Negligence: Unintentional conduct that falls below a standard of care established for the protection of others against unreasonable risk of harm.

Nightingale Schools: Schools of nursing developed by Florence Nightingale that promoted student nurses learning the theory and practice of nursing outside of hospital control.

Novice: Someone who has no experience with a given situation (Benner, 1984).

Nurse Licensure Compact (NLC): A form of interstate compact specific to nurse licensure that provides an agreement between two or more states for the purpose of recognizing nurse licensure between and among a group of participating states. States must enter into one in order to achieve mutual recognition (NCSBN, 2011).

Nurse practice acts (NPAs): State or territorial statutes that define the legal limits for the practice of nursing within that state or territory and explicitly identify the requirements for licensure.

Nurse training school of Women's Hospital of Philadelphia: Established in 1872, reputed to be the first permanent school of nursing in the United States.

Nurses' Associated Alumnae of the United States and Canada: Originally founded in 1896 with the intent of achieving licensure for nurses; became the American Nurses Association.

Nursing informatics: The specialty that integrates nursing science with computer science and multiple information management and analytical sciences to identify, define, manage, and communicate data, information, and knowledge for nursing practice.

Nursing specialty organization: A professional nursing organization that has a particular clinical focus.

Obesity: Having excess body fat. Obesity is clinically determined by body mass index (BMI), which is calculated by dividing a person's weight in kilograms by height in meters squared (kg/m^2). A person with a BMI of 30.0 or more is defined as obese.

Organizational ethics: Ethical analyses and actions taken by healthcare organizations.

Organizational policies: Policies that articulate positions taken by an organization.

Overweight: Having an excess of body weight that includes fat, muscle, bone, and water. Overweight is clinically determined by BMI, which is calculated by dividing a person's weight in kilometers by height in meters squared (kg/m^2). A person with a BMI ranging between 25.0 and 29.9 is defined as overweight.

Patient activation: The skills and confidence that equip patients to become actively engaged in their health care.

Patient engagement framework (PEF): A model created to guide healthcare organizations in developing and strengthening their patient engagement strategies through the use of HIT-based tools and resources (collectively known as eHealth).

Patient portal: A secure online website that gives patients convenient 24-hour access to personal health information from anywhere with an Internet connection.

Patient safety: Freedom from accidental injury (IOM, 2000).

Pay-for-performance: An important movement in healthcare insurance. Providers under this arrangement are rewarded for meeting preestablished targets for delivery of healthcare services.

Pedigree: A graphic illustration of a family health history using standardized symbols.

Performance outcomes: A predetermined set of goals that are met consistently when the same standards of care are given.

Pharmacogenomics: The study of how genes affect a person's response to drugs. This relatively new field combines pharmacology (the science of drugs) and genomics (the study of genes and their functions) to develop effective, safe medications and doses that will be tailored to a person's genetic makeup.

Phenotype: An individual's observable traits, such as height, eye color, and blood type.

Policy: A plan to guide action or decisions.

Political activism: Direct and collective participation in strategies toward specific societal goals; for nursing, this action is based on explicit professional values and focuses on enhancing health.

Political activity: Any activity that is directed toward the success or failure of a political party, candidate for partisan political office, or partisan political group (Mason et al., 2016, p. 414).

Political competence: The skills, perspectives, and values needed for effective political involvement.

Politics: Influencing the allocation of scarce resources (Mason et al., 2016).

Population health: The aggregation of healthcare outcomes within specified groups of individuals and the distribution of outcomes among these groups.

Poverty: When an individual or group of individuals lacks human needs because they simply cannot afford to meet these needs.

Poverty thresholds: Income amounts set by the government that account for household size and earnings. A family whose income falls below this threshold is considered to be living in poverty.

Preceptor: An experienced nurse who facilitates and evaluates student learning in the clinical area over a specified time period of time (Billings & Halstead, 2013, p. 327).

Precision medicine: The focus is on identifying specific approaches that will be effective for patients based on individualized genetic, environmental, and lifestyle factors.

Primary prevention: Actions taken to modify health behaviors such as diet, sedentary behavior, or smoking toward preventing or managing a chronic condition such as heart disease or cancer. An example is reducing one's dietary fat intake to help lower cholesterol levels and prevent one from exceeding recommended cholesterol guidelines.

Principalism: A methodology used to resolve dilemmas arising in health care by appealing to abstract moral principles.

Professional malpractice: A type of negligence that results when a professional person fails to perform his or her professional duties in a reasonable manner.

Professional nursing organization: A collective entity of nurse members that has as its purpose enhancement of some element of patient care or the nursing profession.

Proficient: Someone with the experience to see a given situation in wholes rather than individual parts, who can analyze the situation and determine whether the typical picture is not materializing, and who can determine what needs to be revised within the plan of care in response (Benner, 1984).

Protected health information (PHI): As stipulated by U.S. law, any health information about an individual's status, his/her provision of health care, or payment for health care that is created or collected by a "covered entity." Covered entities include but are not limited to providers (including nurses), insurance companies, governmental entities, and auxiliary care staff including social workers.

Public health nursing: The field of nursing that specializes in improving the health care of the community or individuals in the community setting.

Public policy: Policy formed by governmental bodies (i.e., local, state, and federal legislation) and the regulations written from that policy.

Pull factors: Those factors that make migration to another country more attractive for education or practice than staying in the nurse's native country.

Push factors: Those factors that make it difficult to receive a basic or advanced education in nursing or to practice in the nurse's native country.

Qualitative studies: Descriptive research in which variables are not quantified numerically to describe a phenomenon of interest. Qualitative research is used to examine subjective human experience by using non-statistical methods of analysis (Borbasi & Jackson, 2012). It is associated with naturalistic inquiry, which explores the complex experience of human beings.

Quality management: A method for ensuring that all the activities necessary to design, develop, and implement a product or service are effective and efficient with respect to the system and its performance.

Race: A social classification that denotes a biologic or genetically transmitted set of distinguishable physical characteristics.

Radiation: A ubiquitous form of energy that can come from either human-made sources such as medical devices or natural sources such as the sun.

Randomized controlled trial (RCT): Experimental research that is the strongest design to support a cause and effect relationship. Subjects are randomly assigned to a treatment group or a control group.

Reporting system: A system for blame-free reporting of a system or process failure or the results of proactive risk assessments (TJC, 2016).

Respondeat superior: A legal doctrine, which holds that the employer is responsible for the actions of its employees that occur within the scope of the employment relationship.

Role transition: A process within the transition experience related to formation of a new identity as an independent provider of care. Assimilation to the new role requires both personal and institutional support.

Rural: Any area outside of the urban classification and having less than 2,500 people.

Safety culture: The product of individual and group beliefs, values, attitudes, perceptions, competencies, and patterns of behavior that determine the organization's commitment to quality and patient safety (TJC, 2016).

Satisfaction: A measure of the quality of a service or organization based on consumer or employee perceptions. Satisfaction ratings provide outcome measurement, contributing to consumerism and improvement processes to increase productivity and retention.

Secondary prevention: Interventions focused on early detection and screening of disease, such as tuberculosis skin testing.

Self-determination: The right of every individual to control his or her own person free from interference from others.

Sensemaking: The ability to reconstruct and interpret incoming information anew in ambiguous, complex, and evolving situations (Klein, Moon, & Hoffman, 2006).

Sharp end: Frontline personnel at the operations point of the organization; for example, at the point of patient care in a healthcare organization (Reason, 1997).

Slips and lapses: Execution failures or "errors which result from some failure in the execution and/or storage of an action sequence, regardless of whether or not the plan which guided them was adequate to achieve its objective" (Reason, 1990, p. 9).

Social determinants of health: Factors that can contribute to an individual's overall health status. These factors may include social-economic aspects, physical environment, and individual behaviors or characteristics.

Social media: Forms of electronic communication (such as websites for social networking and microblogging) through which users create online communities to share information, multimedia, ideas, personal messages, and other content.

Social policy: Policy decisions that are made to promote the welfare of the public.

St. Thomas' Hospital: A hospital in London where Florence Nightingale established the Nightingale School of Nursing.

Stacking: A cognitive decision-making strategy for dealing with multiple care delivery requirements, including a mental list of to-be-done tasks and a strategy for preventing error and/or minimizing bad outcomes (Sitterding & Ebright, 2015).

Standard of care: The degree of care, expertise, and judgment exercised by a reasonable person under the same or similar circumstances.

Standards of practice: The criteria against which professional practice is measured.

Stereotyping: Consigning cultural attributes to a group of people based on assumptions, opinions, or attitudes.

Swing beds: Excess hospital beds that are designated for patients needing long-term skilled nursing care.

Systematic reviews: Summaries of evidence obtained by researchers on a specific topic or clinical problem. They use a rigorous step-by-step process to identify, synthesize, and evaluate research studies to answer a specific clinical question and to make conclusions about best evidence.

Telehealth: Healthcare services delivered, managed, and coordinated by nurses and other healthcare providers using electronic information and telecommunications technologies.

Telemedicine: A component of telehealth focusing on medicine's approach to deliver, manage, and coordinate care via telecommunications technologies.

Tertiary prevention: Strategies that will slow disease progression, limit disability from a disease, and restore individuals to their optimal level of functioning.

Test plan: A blueprint for the licensing examination that outlines the examination's content areas and the percentage of questions devoted to each content area.

Tetanus: A potential health threat for persons who sustain wound injuries and is virtually 100 percent preventable with vaccination (CDC, 2014).

The Joint Commission: The nation's predominant standards-setting and accrediting body in health care. Its comprehensive accreditation process evaluates an organization's compliance with quality and safety standards and other accreditation requirements.

Tort law: Law that establishes rules for socially reasonable conduct.

Trade-offs: Decision resolutions that involve conflicting choices between highly unlikely but highly undesirable events and highly likely but less catastrophic ones (Woods et al., 2010).

Triage: A French word meaning *to sort*. During a disaster, it is the process of deciding who is to be treated first, who can wait, and whose life cannot be saved (Beach, 2010).

Universal healthcare access: Has three components: physical accessibility in terms of being able to reach services, financial affordability in terms of not causing financial hardship, and acceptability to those seeking services (WHO, 2014).

Urban area (UA): An area that encompasses 50,000 or more people.

Urban cluster (UC): An area that encompasses at least 2,500 people but less than 50,000 people.

Vector: A living organism that transmits an infective agent (such as a bacteria or virus) to a host, such as a human.

Vulnerable populations: Groups of individuals who are likely to have compromised access to health care and, therefore, are more likely to have poorer health outcomes, including higher mortality rates, compared to less vulnerable groups.

Years of life lost (YLL): Estimate of the number of years a person has lost because of premature death.

References

American Association of Critical-Care Nurses. (2016). *Standards for acute and critical care nursing practice.* Retrieved from http://www.aacn.org/wd/practice/content/standards.for.acute.and.ccnursing.practice.pcms?menu=

American Nurses Association. (n.d.). Healthy Nurse, Healthy Nation™. Retrieved from http://www.nursingworld.org/healthynurse

American Nurses Association. (1979). *The study of credentialing in nursing: A new approach.* Kansas City, MO: Author. Retrieved from http://www.nursecredentialing.org/CredentialingDefinitions

American Nurses Association. (2015). *Nursing: Scope and standards of practice* (3rd ed.). Silver Spring, MD: Author.

Beach, M. (2010). *Disaster preparedness and management.* Philadelphia, PA: F.A. Davis.

Benner, P. (1984). *From novice to expert: Excellence and power in clinical nursing practice.* Menlo Park, CA: Addison-Wesley.

Billings, D. M., & Halstead, J. A. (2013). *Teaching in nursing: A guide for faculty.* Amsterdam, The Netherlands: Elsevier Health Sciences.

Borbasi, S., & Jackson, D. (2012). *Navigating the maze of research.* Chatswood, Sydney, Australia: Mosby Elsevier.

Centers for Disease Control and Prevention. (2014). *Emergency wound management for healthcare professionals.* Retrieved from http://www.cdc.gov/disasters/emergwoundhcp.html

Centers for Disease Control and Prevention. (2015). *Chronic disease overview.* Retrieved from http://www.cdc.gov/chronicdisease/overview/index.htm

Global Citizen Initiative. (n.d.). *Definition of the global citizen.* Retrieved from http://www.theglobalcitizensinitiative.org

Health Resources and Services Administration. (n.d.). *Shortage designation: Health professional shortage areas & medically underserved areas/populations.* Retrieved from http://www.hrsa.gov/shortage/

Human Factors and Ergonomics Society. (2016). About HFES. Retrieved from www.hfes.org/web/AboutHFES/about.html

Huybrecht, S., Loeckx, W., Quaeyhaegens, Y., De Tobel, D., & Mistiaen, W. (2011). Mentoring in nursing education: Perceived characteristics of mentors and the consequences of mentorship. *Nurse Education Today, 31*(3), 274–278.

Institute of Medicine. (2000). *To err is human: Building a safer health system.* Washington, DC: National Academy Press.

Klein, G., Moon, B., & Hoffman, R. F. (2006). Making sense of sensemaking I: Alternative perspectives. *IEEE Intelligent Systems, 21*(4), 70–73.

Langer, E. J. (1989). *Mindfulness.* Reading, MA: Addison-Wesley.

Mason, D. J., Gardner, D. B., Outlaw, F. H., & O'Grady, E. T. (2016). *Policy and politics in nursing and health care* (7th ed.). St. Louis, MO: Elsevier.

Melnyk, B. M., & Fineout-Overholt, E. (2015). *Evidence-based practice in nursing and healthcare: A guide to best practice* (3rd ed.). Philadelphia, PA: Lippincott.

National Council of State Boards of Nursing. (1995). Delegation: Concepts and decision-making process. National Council Position Paper. Retrieved from https://nursing.iowa.gov/sites/default/files/media/delegation1.pdf

National Council of State Boards of Nursing. (2011). *What you need to know about nursing licensure and boards of nursing.* Chicago, IL: Author.

National Council of State Boards of Nursing (2016). National guidelines for nursing delegation. *Journal of Nursing Regulation, 7*(1), 5–14.

Reason, J. (1990). *Human error.* Cambridge, MA: Cambridge University Press.

Reason, J. (1997). *Managing the risks of organizational accidents.* Burlington, VT: Ashgate.

Sitterding, M. C., & Ebright, P. (2015). Information overload: A framework for explaining the issues and creating solutions. In M. C. Sitterding & M. Broome (Eds.), *Information overload* (pp. 11–33). Silver Spring, MD: American Nurses Association.

The Joint Commission. (2016). *Patient safety systems (PS).* Retrieved from https://www.jointcommission.org/assets/1/18/PSC_for_Web.pdf

U.S. Department of Health and Human Services, Office of Disease Prevention and Health Promotion. (n.d.). *Healthy People 2020: Disparities.* Retrieved from http://www.healthypeople.gov/2020/about/foundation-health-measures/Disparities

Vance, S. (2012). *The influence game: 50 insider tactics from the Washington, D.C. lobbying world that will get you to yes.* Hoboken, NJ: John Wiley & Sons.

Watson, J. (1979). *Nursing: The philosophy and science of nursing.* Boston, MA: Little Brown.

Woods, D. D., Dekker, S., Cook, R., Johannesen, L., & Sarter, N. (2010). *Behind human error* (2nd ed.). Burlington, VT: Ashgate.

World Health Organization. (1978). *Declaration of Alma-Ata.* Retrieved from http://www.who.int/publications/almaata_declaration_en.pdf

World Health Organization. (2010). *Framework for action on interprofessional education & collaborative practice.* Geneva, Switzerland: Author. Retrieved from http://apps.who.int/iris/bitstream/10665/70185/1/WHO_HRH_HPN_10.3_eng.pdf?ua=1

World Health Organization. (2014). *What is universal health coverage?* Retrieved from http://www.who.int/features/qa/universal_health_coverage/en/

Index

Italicized page locators indicate a figure; boxes and tables are noted with *b* and *t* respectively.